AN ATLAS OF
VETERINARY DENTAL RADIOLOGY

EDITED BY

Donald H. DeForge, VMD

Fellow of the Academy of Veterinary Dentistry
Fellow of the World Academy of Radiosurgery

Ben H. Colmery III, DVM

Diplomate, American Veterinary Dental College

IOWA STATE UNIVERSITY PRESS / AMES

An Atlas of **Veterinary Dental Radiology**

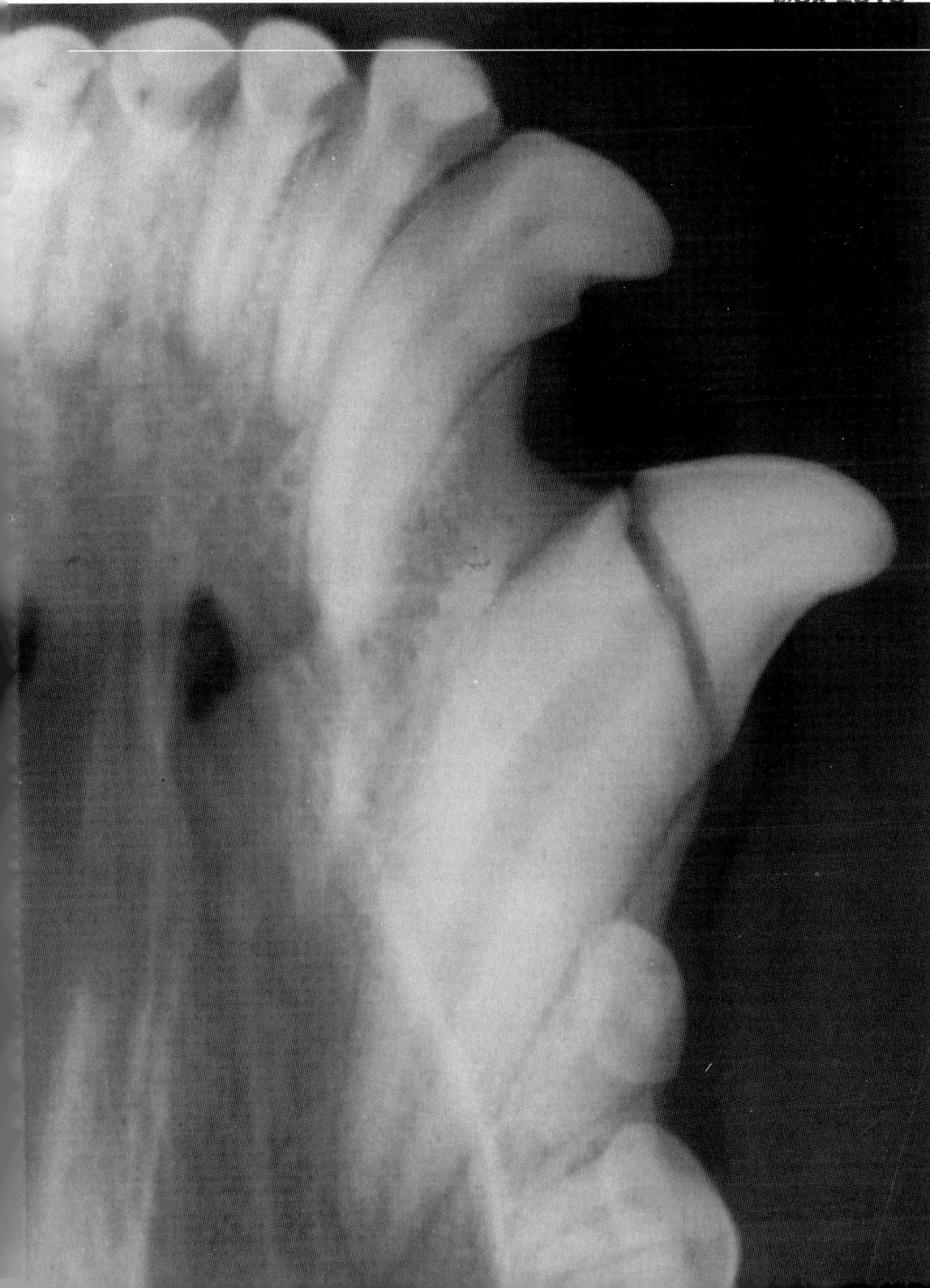

Ben H. Colmery III is a diplomate of the American Veterinary Dental College. He graduated from Michigan State University in 1968. After graduation, he entered private practice and over several years developed the practice into an American Animal Hospital Association Certified Hospital. He has practiced as chief of dentistry at the Animal Medical Center in New York City and is currently the staff dentist and oral surgeon at Michigan Veterinary Specialists.

Donald H. DeForge is a fellow of the Academy of Veterinary Dentistry and a fellow of the World Academy of Radiosurgery. He graduated from the University of Pennsylvania in 1971 and is the owner/director of the Milford Veterinary Hospital and the Animal Dental Center in Milford, Connecticut. He also operates the Connecticut Dental Referral Service, a referral practice in veterinary dentistry and oral surgery that services the New England states and New York, New Jersey, and Pennsylvania and offers postgraduate education in both dental radiology and dental radiographic interpretation, on site or by mail.

Figures A2.1 and A2.2 are reprinted with permission of DentaLabels, 19 Norwood Ave., Kensington, CA 94707.

Iowa State University Press
2121 South State Avenue, Ames, Iowa 50014

Orders: 1-800-862-6657
Office: 1-515-292-0140
Fax: 1-515-292-3348
Web site: www.isupress.edu

♾ Printed on acid-free paper in the United States of America

First edition, 2000

Library of Congress Cataloging-in-Publication Data

An atlas of veterinary dental radiology / edited by Donald H. DeForge, Ben H. Colmery III.—1st ed.
    p. cm.
  Includes bibliographical references.
  ISBN 0-8138-2997-6 (alk. paper)
    1. Veterinary dentistry. 2. Veterinary radiology—Atlases. I. DeForge, Donald H.
  II. Colmery, Ben H. III.

SF867.A85 2000
636.189′7607572—dc21   99-049133

Last digit is the print number: 9 8 7 6 5 4 3 2 1

CONTENTS

PART TWO   FELINE   115

FOREWORD

To watch the evolution of veterinary dentistry over two decades has been an inspiring event. Veterinary dentistry has largely evolved through the foresight and hard work of an ever-increasing number of dedicated individuals. To those pioneer men and women our whole profession and the pet-owning public owe a great deal. In a relatively short time veterinary dentistry has progressed from ignorance and neglect to a discipline of science and understanding.

The last 10 years have seen the development of increasingly detailed and comprehensive textbooks dedicated to this field. A large amount of our knowledge was originally extrapolated from human dental research. This has been greatly enhanced with research and clinical experience undertaken on domestic pets.

An area of veterinary dentistry that has been incompletely covered up to now is that of dental radiology. Many of the early textbooks may have covered how to take radiographs, but a void in interpretation of dental radiographs has been apparent for some time.

An Atlas of Veterinary Dental Radiology is one of those books that will immediately become a compulsory acquisition to anyone performing veterinary dentistry, whether the undergraduate or the specialist. The editors' passion for radiology is immediately evident in this text. The contributors and review committee read like a who's who of veterinary dentistry. This atlas introduces normals and shows abnormals that are faced daily in all intradisciplines of veterinary dentistry and oral surgery.

The editors are to be congratulated on bringing together such a talented group of people to produce an atlas that will become the benchmark of veterinary dental radiology. I believe everybody will enjoy this atlas, and I commend it to you.

Stephen Coles, BVSc, MACVSc (Veterinary Dentistry)
Diplomate, American Veterinary Dental College
Melbourne, Australia

PREFACE

Veterinary dentistry has been crawling out of the dark ages for over 30 years. The American Veterinary Dental Society has celebrated the twenty-third year of its founding in 1966. Eleven years after the establishment of the AVDS, the Academy of Veterinary Dentistry was born. In 1988, the American Veterinary Dental College was recognized by the AVMA. In its evolution, veterinary dental textbooks have emerged that have set this field apart from the other disciplines in veterinary medicine and surgery. *Concepts in Veterinary Dentistry* by Tholen, which devoted a chapter to dental radiology, was the first textbook to be published in this new era. Many excellent texts in veterinary dentistry have followed.

Since this beginning, veterinary dental radiology has evolved into an essential component of veterinary dentistry. High-detail intraoral film is mandatory and currently the film of choice when evaluating oral pathology. Without the information provided by dental radiology, treatment planning, therapy, and follow-up become impossible. In this textbook, we have attempted to cover all disciplines of dentistry. This is not a "how to fix it" book of therapy, but an actual uncovering of a new world of oral x-ray images to allow the novice as well as the specialist an opportunity to view what has not been seen or has been overlooked. The saying, you won't find it if you do not look for it, is the hallmark of the veterinary dental radiologist. This textbook will offer those who unfold its pages an opportunity to sort out the normal from the abnormal in radiologic diagnosis. It will unveil what has been ignored and will expand the clinical database. Most importantly, it will encourage the use of dental radiology in veterinary practices. As more and more intraoral films are used, new conditions will be uncovered. This will lead to better treatment plans and less pain and suffering for the pet, zoo, and domestic animal population. This textbook is a starting point for a journey to new frontiers. It is the first step. We hope you will enjoy taking this black and white passage from normal to abnormal; from canine to feline; and from multiple zoo species to lagomorph/rodent pets in oral radiology.

It is important for the reader to realize that this textbook has been a labor of love for all of its authors (see Contributors). This is not the work of two editors, but a combined effort of the leaders in veterinary dentistry internationally. We call it "our" atlas because it belongs to veterinary dentistry as a group and not to any one of us separately. Each author was chosen for his or her expertise in the area of presentation. Their comments and evaluations are based on firsthand experience with each case and are not abstract thoughts. While we all recognize that there may be several ways to manage a problem, recognition of the problem is the first step. We present the textbook as a primary diagnostic tool. It is our sincere hope that this contribution will become a cornerstone of veterinary dental radiology and the foundation of a valid resource library for many years to come.

Dr. Donald H. DeForge
Dr. Ben H. Colmery III

CONTRIBUTORS

[The numbers in brackets indicate chapters where contributions were made.]

Mary Suzanne Aller [9]
DVM, MS
Diplomate, American Veterinary Dental College

Dr. Aller has been a diplomate of the American Veterinary Dental College since 1991. She graduated from Virginia Polytechnic Institute and State University in 1975 with a BS in biology. She then attended the Ohio State University College of Veterinary Medicine, receiving the DVM degree in 1979, and the MS degree in veterinary pathobiology in 1980. She developed her interest in veterinary dentistry while in private small animal practice in Northern Virginia and joined the American Veterinary Dental Society. She became a charter member of the Academy of Veterinary Dentistry in 1987. In 1994, she opened an exclusive dental referral service for small animals with Dr. Charles A. Williams in Vienna, Virginia. She continues to write and lecture at numerous continuing education meetings throughout the United States to spread the word of veterinary dentistry.

Dr. Aller would like to gratefully acknowledge Karen Towe, certified AHT, for her assistance with the Normal Feline chapter.

Jamie G. Anderson [7]
DVM, MS, RDH
Diplomate, American College of Veterinary Internal Medicine
Diplomate, American Veterinary Dental College

Dr. Anderson received a BS degree in dental hygiene from the University of Southern California Dental School and is a registered dental hygienist with expertise in periodontics. She received her BS degree in animal science, MS degree in comparative pathology, and DVM degree from the University of California–Davis. Her specialty training was performed at the University of Pennsylvania. Dr. Anderson is in private specialty practice in Sacramento, California.

James M.G. Anthony [3, 11, 14, 16]
BSc (Agr), DVM, MRCVS, Dipl. EVDC
Fellow of the Academy of Veterinary Dentistry
Diplomate, American Veterinary Dental College

Dr. Anthony is a graduate of the Western College of Veterinary Medicine in Saskatchewan, Canada. He was the first Canadian to become a charter fellow of the Academy of Veterinary Dentistry in 1987 and a diplomate of the American Veterinary Dental College in 1989. He has lectured and taught veterinary dentistry internationally and has published many papers and articles. Dr. Anthony has also taught veterinary dentistry at the Atlantic Veterinary College (University of Prince Edward Island), La Medecine Veterinaire (University of Montreal), and the Ontario Veterinary College (University of Guelph). He is a consultant for veterinary dentistry for the Metro Toronto Zoo, the Vancouver Aquarium, and many practices across Canada. He coordinates and teaches the Pacific Dental Service Study Club and mentorship group. He resides in Vancouver, British Columbia, where he has a private veterinary dental referral practice and conducts clinical research.

Gary B. Beard [6]
DVM
Diplomate, American Veterinary Dental College

Dr. Beard, a graduate of Auburn University, practiced veterinary medicine at the AAHA Certified Goodwood Animal Hospital in Baton Rouge for over 25 years. During this time he was a co-founder and president of the American Veterinary Dental Society; co-founder, charter fellow, and first president of the Academy of Veterinary Dentistry; and a member of the organizing committee and charter diplomate of the American Veterinary Dental College.

In 1982, along with Drs. Tom Mulligan, Chuck Williams, Peter Emily, and Mr. Gerry Selin, the C.E. Seminars group was formed. Under the sponsorship of the American Animal Hospital Association and Henry Schein, over 16,000 veterinarians and veterinary technicians were given courses in various levels of veterinary dentistry including periodontics, endodontics, orthodontics, restoratives, crowns, and radiology. These courses, which included didactic lectures and step-by-step, hands-on lab sessions, were models for programs still in use in the teaching of veterinary dentistry.

In 1991, Dr. Beard received the AAHA Veterinarian of the Year, Fido Award for his pioneering efforts in the field of veterinary dentistry and in 1995 was awarded the Peter Emily Service Award from the College of Veterinary Dentistry.

Dr. Beard left private practice in 1992 to return to Auburn University where he presently serves as Assistant Dean of Outreach at the College of Veterinary Medicine and teaches dentistry.

Jan Bellows [4]

DVM, DACVP

Diplomate, American Veterinary Dental College
Diplomate, American Board of Veterinary Practitioners

Dr. Bellows received his undergraduate degree from the University of Florida (1968–1971). His graduate degree was obtained from the Auburn School of Veterinary Medicine in 1975, and he completed his postgraduate work in 1975–1976 at the Animal Medical Center in New York City by participating in a medical and surgical internship. He is now the owner and operator of the Pet Health Care Center located in Pembroke Pines, Florida.

Dr. Bellows has received many postgraduate awards including the AAHA Excel-Award for postgraduate examination in 1985, the Florida VMA Gold Star Award in 1986 and 1987, and the Broward County VMA–Clarence Dee Award in 1986. He was also awarded the status of diplomate of the American Board of Veterinary Practitioners in 1986, which was rectified in 1994. He is a fellow of the Academy of Veterinary Dentistry (1987) and a diplomate of the American Veterinary Dental College (1990).

He has contributed many publications to the field of animal dentistry and has presented multiple educational programs throughout the United States. Currently, he is involved in many different dental research projects.

Laura D. Braswell [16]

DDS

Laura D. Braswell is a periodontist in private practice in Atlanta, Georgia. After teaching at the Emory University School of Dentistry, she joined the research facility. Dr. Braswell is currently involved in nonhuman primate studies at Yerkes Regional Primate Research Center at Emory University. As the staff dentist at Zoo Atlanta, she has worked with many exotic species, from the great apes to large cats and elephants. Dr. Braswell is an honorary fellow of the Academy of Veterinary Dentistry (1994) and consults with veterinarians on animal dental care.

Linda L. Brooks [16]

DVM

Linda Brooks practices veterinary dentistry and small animal medicine at Northeast Veterinary Hospital in the mountains of North Georgia. She received her Doctorate of Veterinary Medicine from the University of Georgia in 1980. Dr. Brooks is past president of the American Veterinary Dental Society and currently is a veterinary dental consultant at Zoo Atlanta.

Ben H. Colmery III [8]

DVM

Diplomate, American Veterinary Dental College

Dr. Colmery graduated from Michigan State University with a BS degree and a DVM degree in 1968. Following graduation, he entered a small animal private practice in Ann Arbor, Michigan. Two years later he purchased the practice and developed it into an American Animal Hospital Association Certified Hospital. In 1993 he left Ann Arbor and joined the staff of the Animal Medical Center in New York City as Chief of Dentistry. In 1995, Dr. Colmery joined Michigan Veterinary Specialists, again as the staff dentist/oral surgeon.

Dr. Colmery's interest in dentistry started shortly after graduation when he realized the oral cavity had been largely ignored in veterinary school. Too many pets were presented with oral cavity problems that were not covered in lectures or textbooks. This was the beginning of a 25-year effort to better understand and treat the oral cavity problems of companion animals. During this period, Dr. Colmery was also on the adjunct faculty at Michigan State University treating animals and lecturing to students. He has coauthored a textbook on veterinary dentistry and published numerous articles for various journals and textbooks. He conducts funded research and is a consultant to the pharmaceutical industry. In addition, he has lectured worldwide on dentistry to students, colleagues, and the public. He is a cofounder of the American Veterinary Dental Society, a charter fellow of the Academy of Veterinary Dentistry, and a charter diplomate of the American Veterinary Dental College. He is a past president of the Michigan Veterinary Medical Association, the Academy of Veterinary Dentistry, and the Wastenaw Academy of Veterinary Medicine. He is a member of the Phi Zeta Veterinary Honor Society and a past recipient of the American Veterinary Dental College Peter Emily Award. Outside of veterinary medicine, he is a past president of the Ann Arbor Western Kiwanis and has volunteered his time for the National Ski Patrol System and Boy Scouts.

David A. Crossley [17]

BVetMed, MRCVS, Dipl. EVDC

Fellow of the Academy of Veterinary Dentistry

Dr. David Crossley attended the Royal Veterinary College in London, where he obtained his Bachelor of Veterinary Medicine degree in 1978. Following qualification, he returned to the northwest of England and spent 9 years working as an assistant in a small animal practice before setting up his own practice. He recently sold his practice in order to concentrate on his special interests in oncology, dentistry, and surgery. Dr. Crossley has now joined the surgical team at the Animal Medical Center, Manchester, where he operates his veterinary dental referral service. He is a fellow of the Academy of Veterinary Dentistry (1993).

Linda J. DeBowes [1]

DVM, MS

Diplomate, American College of Veterinary Internal Medicine
Diplomate, American Veterinary Dental College

Dr. DeBowes is an associate professor and Head of Small Animal Medicine at Kansas State University. She graduated from the College of Veterinary Medicine at Washington State University in 1981 and received her MS degree from Kansas State University in 1985. Dr. DeBowes is a diplomate of the American College of Veterinary Internal Medicine (Internal Medicine) and of the American Veterinary Dental College.

Donald H. DeForge [1, 13]

VMD

Fellow of the Academy of Veterinary Dentistry

Fellow of the World Academy of Radiosurgery

Dr. DeForge is a 1971 graduate of the University of Pennsylvania. He is the hospital director of the Milford Veterinary Hospital and operates the Connecticut Dental Referral Service, a referral practice in veterinary dentistry and oral surgery that services primarily the New England states and New York, New Jersey, and Pennsylvania. The referral service also offers postgraduate education in dental radiology. Dental radiographic interpretation is also available on site or by mail.

Dr. DeForge lectures on small animal dentistry and oral surgery, emphasizing practical applications for the general practitioner. He has been the dentistry and oral surgery contributor to *DVM Newsmagazine* since 1993. He has also published clinical reports in the *Journal of Veterinary Dentistry*. He is editor and publisher of *Veterinary Dentistry Report*, an encapsulated summary of the most up-to-date applications of veterinary dentistry in small animal practice.

As a fellow of the Academy of Veterinary Dentistry and a clinical researcher, he studies products and equipment that may improve or enhance veterinary dentistry. Fixed crown prosthodontics, guided tissue regeneration with bioceramic bone grafts, dental radiology, and implantology advancements are his major interests in veterinary dentistry. Dr. DeForge received the 1996 Northeast Practitioner of the Year Award from the American Animal Hospital Association. Also in 1996, he was the recipient of the American Veterinary Dental College's Peter Emily Resident Award. This annual award is sponsored by Pharmacia and UpJohn Animal Health and goes to an individual exhibiting high ideals and a commitment to furthering the field of veterinary dentistry.

Edward R. Eisner [15]

DVM

Diplomate, American Veterinary Dental College

Dr. Eisner is a Cornell graduate; he received his bachelor degree in 1960 and his veterinary degree in 1964. Dr. Eisner has practiced small animal dentistry in the Denver metro area since 1964 and has operated a veterinary dental referral practice serving the Rocky Mountain region since 1983. As a diplomate of the American Veterinary Dental College, he is recognized as a board certified specialist in veterinary dentistry.

Dr. Eisner is on the advisory boards of the *Journal of Veterinary Dentistry* and *Veterinary Forum*. He has published more than three dozen scientific papers, has written several textbook chapters, and is the author of two books on the subject of dentistry. A popular speaker, he has delivered frequent presentations on animal dentistry both nationally and internationally since 1980.

Dr. Eisner would like to acknowledge the contributions made by Linda Klippert, CVT, University of Illinois, College of Veterinary Medicine, Department of Clinical Medicine, Urbana, Illinois, and by Katherine A. Jennings, CVT, Denver Veterinary Dental Service, Denver, Colorado.

Peter Emily [16]

DDS

A graduate of the Creighton University School of Dentistry, Dr. Emily received postgraduate training in oral pathology, periodontics, and endodontics at Denver General Hospital and the University of Pennsylvania. His active interest in veterinary dentistry started in 1962, and he continues to be a consultant to veterinarians throughout the United States and in several foreign countries. Dr. Emily has been an American Kennel Club confirmation judge for many years and is a consultant in dentistry to the American Kennel Club and the Senior Dog Judges Association. He conducts intramural and continuing education courses at universities and in many parts of the world. He has authored three veterinary dentistry texts and numerous articles. Dr. Emily is an honorary fellow of the Academy of Veterinary Dentistry and an honorary diplomate of the American Veterinary Dental College. Annual awards presented by the American Veterinary Dental College are named in his honor. In 1992, Dr. Emily became the only professional outside the veterinary profession to receive the American Animal Hospital Association Award of Merit for outstanding contributions to veterinary medicine.

Michael R. Floyd [Appendix 2]

DVM

Fellow of the Academy of Veterinary Dentistry

Dr. Floyd graduated from the University of California–Davis in 1961 and became a fellow in the Academy of Veterinary Dentistry in 1988. He designed a state-of-the-art veterinary dental clinic and operatory, the Orinda Veterinary Dental Service, in Orinda, California, in 1995. Dr. Floyd received, in 1991, the Alumni Achievement Award from the University of California–Davis for contributions in veterinary medicine and pioneering in veterinary dentistry. In 1993 he was honored with the Excellence in Continuing Education Award by the California Academy of Veterinary Medicine.

The "Modified Triadan System: Nomenclature for Veterinary Dentistry" was written by Dr. Floyd and was published in the *Journal of Veterinary Dentistry* in 1991. Its common usage in veterinary dentistry has enabled more accurate communication to occur in both written and spoken applications.

Cecilia Gorrel [13]

BSc, MA, Vet MB, DDS, MRCVS, Dipl EVDC

Honorary Fellow of the Academy of Veterinary Dentistry

Dr. Cecilia Gorrel is qualified as a Doctor of Dental Surgery, an oral pathologist, and a veterinary surgeon. Dr. Gorrel is actively involved, as an independent consultant, in research into oral diseases in the dog and cat. She also runs veterinary dentistry and oral surgery referral clinics. She is president of the British Veterinary Dental Association and of the European Veterinary Dental Society. Dr. Gorrel is also an honorary fellow of the Academy of Veterinary Dentistry. Dr. Gorrel lectures and tutors courses in veterinary dentistry and oral surgery both in the United Kingdom and abroad. She has written numerous articles on veterinary dentistry and coauthored the *Handbook of Small Animal Oral Emergen-*

cies by Gorrel, Penman, and Emily, published by Pergamon Press in 1993, as well as the *Manual of Small Animal Dentistry*, published by the British Small Animal Veterinary Association in 1995.

B. Jean Hawkins [1]
MS, DVM
Fellow of the Academy of Veterinary Dentistry
Diplomate, American Veterinary Dental College

Dr. Hawkins received her Doctor of Veterinary Medicine degree from Louisiana State University and served her internship in small animal medicine at Auburn University. She is a fellow of the Academy of Veterinary Dentistry and a diplomate of the American Veterinary Dental College.

Dr. Hawkins, who also acts as a veterinary dental consultant, wrote *Veterinary Dentistry in Your Clinic©*, a sixteen-hour course she teaches in private clinics and for veterinary associations. She has also produced instructional videotapes on three topics in veterinary dentistry: orthodontics, canine toothbrushing, and the veterinarian-based dental unit. In addition, she produced *Applied Dentistry for Veterinary Practice*, a videotape presented at the 1992 Waltham Symposium. Dr. Hawkins organized and taught the veterinary dentistry curricula at Auburn University, Oregon State University, and Washington State University. She has held several offices, including president, in the American Veterinary Dental Society and for five years was editor of the society's *Journal of Veterinary Dentistry*. She serves on the Board of Directors and the Credentials Committee of the Academy of Veterinary Dentistry, as well as the Credentials and Appeals Committees of the American Veterinary Dental College. Dr. Hawkins founded, and codirected from 1981 to 1984, a companion animal–human bond project known as PALS: People and Animals, Loving and Sharing.

In addition to her enthusiastic participation in continuing education programs regionally and nationally, in 1993 Dr. Hawkins was a featured speaker at the World Small Animal Veterinary Congress in Berlin and for the Japanese Animal Hospital Association in Japan. Dr. Hawkins is the recipient of the American Animal Hospital Association Region VI Service Award and the Alan J. White Memorial Lecture Award of the British Small Animal Veterinary Association.

Dr. Hawkins' areas of interest include therapy and prevention of periodontal disease in small animal practice; client understanding of pets' dental needs; and veterinary technician training in dentistry.

Philippe R. Hennet [4]
Diplomate, European Veterinary Dental College
Diplomate, American Veterinary Dental College

Philippe Hennet graduated from the Ecole Veterinaire de Toulouse, France, in 1988, and he subsequently completed a junior internship there in small animal surgery. He worked on a research project on endodontics in dogs with the Toulouse Dental School from 1987 to 1989 and presented the results of this work in his veterinary degree thesis in 1990. After one and one-half years in small animal practice, he moved to the United States, where he completed a research fellowship and clinical residency program in veterinary dentistry at the Veterinary School of the University of

Pennsylvania, Philadelphia. He is a diplomate of the American Veterinary Dental College. He returned to France where he is currently running a referral specialty practice based in Neuilly-sur-Seine. He consults at the Alfort Veterinary School (Paris) and Lyon Veterinary School and is also an independent scientific consultant for companies and research projects. He is the current president of the French Veterinary Dental Association (GEROS/CNVSPA) and the current president-elect of the European Veterinary Dental Society (EVDS). He is the author of many publications in French and English and lectures worldwide on veterinary dentistry.

Steven E. Holmstrom [5]
DVM
Diplomate, American Veterinary Dental College
Fellow of the Academy of Veterinary Dentistry

Dr. Holmstrom received his degree from the University of Missouri in 1972. He is a director at the Companion Animal Hospital in Belmont, California, which has referral specialists in dentistry, surgery, oncology, and internal medicine. He is also an instructor of veterinary dentistry for animal health technicians at Foothill College. Dr. Holmstrom is a diplomate of the American Veterinary Dental College, a fellow of the Academy of Veterinary Dentistry, past president of the Academy of Veterinary Dentistry, and past president of the American Veterinary Dental College. He is also a coauthor of *Veterinary Dental Techniques*, published by W. B. Saunders. The text has been published in English, Japanese, and Spanish.

Thomas H. Kavanagh [6]
DVM
Diplomate, American Veterinary Dental College
Fellow of the Academy of Veterinary Dentistry

Dr. Kavanagh is a private practitioner and the owner of the Village Animal Clinic, P.C., 34415 Grand River, Farmington, Michigan, an oral medicine and oral surgery referral practice. He is also an assistant adjunct professor for the Department of Small Animal Clinical Sciences at Michigan State University. Dr. Kavanagh has practiced referral dentistry for 15 years, has lectured veterinarians and veterinary students, and has mentored alternate pathway candidates for entry to the American Veterinary Dental College.

M. Lynne Kesel [1]
DVM, MA

Dr. Kesel is an associate professor at Colorado State University in Fort Collins, Colorado. As a member of the Department of Clinical Sciences, she teaches and supervises veterinary students in small animal elective surgery and dentistry. She also performs advance dental procedures in the Veterinary Teaching Hospital.

Dr. Kesel received her DVM from Colorado State University in 1981 and practiced laboratory animal medicine for 8 years. In 1989, she assumed her present position as a clinical veterinary dentist and lecturer. She also holds an MA in fine arts and in biomedical illustration.

Heidi B. Lobprise [10]

DVM

Diplomate, American Veterinary Dental College

Dr. Lobprise graduated from Texas A&M Univeristy in 1983. She is currently an associate at the Dallas Dental Service Animal Clinic in Dallas, Texas. She is a diplomate of the American Veterinary Dental College. She heads the AVDC Exam Chair, was the Training Program chair for 1996–1997, and was the president of the American Veterinary Dental Society for the 1996–1997 year. Dr. Lobprise is also a coauthor of *Veterinary Dentistry: Principles and Practice*.

Kenneth F. Lyon [14]

DVM

Diplomate, American Veterinary Dental College

Dr. Lyon is a diplomate of the American Veterinary Dental College and a charter fellow of the Academy of Veterinary Dentistry. He is the current president of the Academy and serves on the Board of Directors of the American Veterinary Dental College and the American Veterinary Dental Society. He is chairman of the Journal of Veterinary Dentistry–Journal Management Committee and served as editor-in-chief of the *Journal of Veterinary Dentistry* from 1991–1995. Dr. Lyon is a 1980 graduate of the University of Minnesota College of Veterinary Medicine (DVM) and a graduate of the University of Arizona (BS). In 1993, he received the American Veterinary Medical Association Practitioner Research Award, given in recognition of outstanding accomplishments in veterinary medical research by a practicing veterinarian for his study of feline subgingival resorptive lesions. Dr. Lyon has veterinary dental specialty practices at Mesa Veterinary Hospital, Ltd. in Mesa, Arizona, and the Southwest Veterinary Specialty Center in Tucson, Arizona.

Sandra Manfra Marretta [3, 11]

DVM

Diplomate, American Veterinary Dental College

Diplomate, American College of Veterinary Surgeons

Dr. Manfra Marretta received her DVM degree from Cornell University in 1977. Following graduation she completed an internship and surgical residency at the Animal Medical Center in New York City. Following her training at the Animal Medical Center she joined a small animal practice in Staten Island, New York, for 2 years. In 1984, she returned to the Animal Medical Center for a dental residency with Mark Tholen, DDS. In 1985, she became a diplomate of the American College of Veterinary Surgeons, and in 1988 she became a charter diplomate of the American Veterinary Dental College. She remained at the Animal Medical Center as a senior staff surgeon and director of oral medicine and surgery until 1990. In 1990, she relocated to Urbana, Illinois, and is an associate professor in Small Animal Surgery and Dentistry at the University of Illinois.

Dr. Manfra Marretta is the author of over one hundred publications. She is the winner of numerous awards including the Animal Medical Center's Veterinarian of the Year Award, the Norden Distinguished Teacher Award, and the University of Illinois College of Veterinary Medicine's All-Round Excellence Award for Excellence in Teaching, Research, and Service.

Ashley Oakes [Introduction]

DVM

Diplomate, American Veterinary Dental College

Dr. Oakes received her DVM degree from the University of Florida, College of Veterinary Medicine in 1989. She completed her veterinary dental residency training in Baton Rouge, Louisiana, in 1993. During this time, she held a position as a clinical instructor of dentistry at the Louisiana State University, School of Veterinary Medicine. Dr. Oakes is a diplomate of the American Veterinary Dental College.

After completing her residency program, Dr. Oakes moved to Colorado, where she served as the veterinary dentist for a multi-doctor small animal and emergency care hospital. She now operates her own veterinary dental referral practice at Tampa Bay Veterinary Referral, Inc., in Largo, Florida.

Ayako Okuda [10, 11, 14]

BVSc, PhD, DSc

Dr. Okuda, from Japan, is known internationally for her contributions in basic and clinical research in animal dentistry. She has authored numerous journal articles and publications. She is a member of the International Association for Dental Research, the American Society of Bone and Mineral Research, the American Veterinary Dental Society, the Japanese Association for Oral Biology, the Japanese Society of Veterinary Science, Japan Veterinary Medical Association, the Japanese Small Animal Dental Society, Ladies Association of Veterinarians, and the Japanese Animal Hospital Association.

Anna Fong Revenaugh [7, 12, Appendix 1]

DVM

Diplomate, American College of Veterinary Radiology

Dr. Revenaugh is a 1989 graduate of the University of California, School of Veterinary Medicine. As a student she was awarded the Thomas Millman Fellowship in Veterinary Radiology. Dr. Revenaugh entered the radiology residency program at the University of Pennsylvania after several years in private practice. The residency was completed in 1995. Currently Dr. Revenaugh has a radiology consultation and mobile ultrasound service (Animal Imaging Specialties) in Sacramento, California.

Eva M. Sarkiala-Kessel [12]

DVM, PhD

Diplomate, American Veterinary Dental College

Dr. Kessel graduated from the College of Veterinary Medicine, Helsinki, Finland, in 1984. She continued her studies toward her PhD degree at the same university from 1989 to 1994. In 1992 she began her dental residency under the instruction of Dr. Colin Harvey at the University of Pennsylvania. She completed this residency in 1994. She is now practicing at Allpets Clinic in Boulder, Colorado.

Chris J. Visser [14]
BVSc, DVM MRCVS
Diplomate, American Veterinary Dental College

Dr. Visser is a diplomate of the American Veterinary Dental College, a charter fellow of the International Academy of Veterinary Dentistry, and a member of the American Veterinary Dental Society. As an AVMA recognized board-certified veterinary specialist, he performs endodontics, periodontics, orthodontics, operative dentistry, restorations, oral pathology and radiology, dental orthopedics, oral surgery, and treatment of oral diseases and neoplasia.

Dr. Visser has been a veterinarian since 1964. He qualified in South Africa and, after completing the American Veterinary Practice Examination in 1980, established a practice in Scottsdale, Arizona. He practices veterinary dentistry at the Aid Animal Dental Clinic associated with the Aid Animal Clinic in Scottsdale. He is an associate editor of endodontics for the *Journal of Veterinary Dentistry*. He is the author of numerous articles and a featured lecturer at many veterinary seminars.

Robert B. Wiggs [2]
DVM
Diplomate, American Veterinary Dental College
Charter Fellow of the Academy of Veterinary Dentistry

Dr. Wiggs graduated in 1973 from Texas A&M University. He is currently the owner/director of the Dallas Dental Service Animal Clinic in Dallas, Texas. He is also an adjunct assistant professor for the Department of Biomedical Science at Baylor College of Dentistry, a part of the Texas A&M University system. He is a charter fellow of the Academy of Veterinary Dentistry, and a diplomate of the American Veterinary Dental College. He was president elect of that same organization for 1996–1998. Dr. Wiggs is also the immediate past president of the American Veterinary Dental Society. Dr. Wiggs has received many awards including the Peter Emily Award from the American Veterinary Dental College in 1994, the Texas A&M Outstanding Alumnus—Companion Animal in 1995, and the TVMA Companion Animal Practitioner of the Year award in 1996. Dr. Wiggs is also the coauthor of *Veterinary Dentistry: Principles and Practice*.

Photography Acknowledgment

Mr. Douglas Thayer
Media Department
University of Pennsylvania
School of Veterinary Medicine

Special Acknowledgment from Dr. Colmery

This textbook of veterinary dental radiology represents a heroic effort by its principal author, Dr. Donald DeForge. The area of veterinary dental radiology is basically uncharted territory with few textbooks available to the veterinary profession. This text is an attempt to present a complete dental atlas that is still considered portable. As technology evolves and digital imaging becomes mainstream, the text will continue to serve as a reference. As oral radiology is used in more species, new reference chapters will be added to future editions. In time, textbooks dedicated to individual species and subdisciplines will appear. This is needed information.

Only those who have written and published a text can appreciate the dedication required to complete the project. Countless hours were spent gathering and reviewing the individual chapters. This text and atlas has been peer reviewed to assure completeness and accuracy. Countless phone calls, faxes, and e-mails were made to the contributors, photographer, and publisher. Countless hours were lost from work and family life. But all the effort was worth the sacrifice. The result speaks for itself.

With the utmost respect and sincerity, thank you, Dr. DeForge.

Ben H. Colmery III, DVM
Diplomate, American Veterinary Dental College

Special Acknowledgment from Dr. DeForge

This text could never have been completed without the effort of many more people than the contributing authors mentioned here. The people behind the camera in an epic movie receive minor credit on the movie screen. The people behind the creation of a book many times are never acknowledged. To those who have not been mentioned, a special thank you from the editors.

On my own home front, there are four people who must not be forgotten. First my brother, Jerry DeForge, who was always present for encouragement and advice, must be acknowledged. He has spent hours organizing the chapters, helping with computer entry, and assisting me in author communications over a 5-year period. Similarly, Denise DeForge, my daughter, was always available as needed. She consulted on chapter layout and computer entry and became the on-staff text troubleshooter. Sandy Sanders, former chief dental technician at the CT Dental Referral Service must be acknowledged for her assistance in x-ray editing, processing, and chapter ordering. Lastly, to Jane Chiodo, the main typist for the text, a special thank you. Jane never complained when hour after hour of rewrites were placed in front of her.

To each of you, a thank-you from the bottom of my heart. Without you, we would never have been able to accomplish our dream. Because of this, I offer a part of this dream to each of you. This text belongs to you as well as to all of the authors who have worked so hard to bring it to reality.

Donald H. DeForge, VMD
Fellow of the Academy of Veterinary Dentistry
Fellow of the World Academy of Radiosurgery

Review Consultants

Diplomates of the American Veterinary Dental College:

Dr. James Anthony
Dr. James Auvil
Dr. Gary Beard
Dr. Paul Cleland
Dr. Peter Emily
Dr. Loic Legendre
Dr. Heidi Lobprise
Dr. Ken Lyon
Dr. Robert Wiggs

Diplomate of the American College of Veterinary Radiology:

Dr. Anna Fong Revenaugh

Diplomates of the European Veterinary Dental College:

Dr. Loic Legendre
Dr. James Anthony

INTRODUCTION Radiology Techniques

Dr. Ashley Oakes

An understanding of radiology imaging principles is necessary to generate diagnostic oral films. Intraoral radiology provides better isolation of teeth than the extraoral radiographic technique. Eliminating superimpositioning and image distortion and achieving sharpness and detail on oral radiographs require that specific positioning techniques be employed. Once these techniques have been learned and mastered, accurate dental films can be produced to help ensure the proper diagnosis and treatment of a case.

Projection Geometry and Positioning Techniques

Sharpness and resolution are important criteria for the production of a quality dental radiograph. *Sharpness* is defined as the measure of how well a boundary between two areas of contrasting radiodensity is delineated. *Resolution* is the visualization of relatively small objects which are close together. Both of these parameters are influenced by the same geometric principles and the following factors will increase sharpness and resolution: 1) a small focal spot (preset in dental x-ray machines), 2) elimination of motion (object or dental x-ray machine), and 3) the appropriate type of x-ray film. As film grain size decreases, sharpness and resolution increase. Intensifying screens and double emulsion films decrease sharpness and resolution.

Penumbra is a broad fuzzy zone at the edges of the image caused by photons originating from different sites on the tungsten target focal spot. Penumbra can be minimized by increasing the distance between the focal spot and the object using a long, open-ended cylinder. This allows utilization of only those x-ray photons whose paths are almost parallel to the primary x-ray beam. Decreasing the distance between the object and the film and using the smallest focal spot possible will also help decrease penumbra.

Image size distortion is a function of focal spot-to-film and object-to-film distance. As the focal spot-to-film distance increases and the object-to-film distance decreases, size distortion is minimized. Image shape distortion results in unequal magnification of different parts of the object, which occurs when not all parts of the object are at the same focal spot-to-object distance. This can be minimized by placing the film parallel to the object and aiming the x-ray beam perpendicular to the object and the film.

Bisecting Angle and Paralleling Techniques

The bisecting angle technique was developed to minimize image distortion caused by the inability to place the dental film parallel to the central axis of the tooth. Placing the film parallel to the teeth in the maxillary arcade and anterior mandible is particularly difficult because of the flat palate and impeding soft-tissue structures of the mandibular symphysis. To utilize the bisecting angle technique, the film is placed as close to the tooth as possible and the primary x-ray beam is aimed perpendicular to the plane which bisects the angle created by the plane of the central axis of the tooth and the plane of the dental film. The bisecting angle is the imaginary plane which divides the angle created between the tooth and the film into two equal parts. Distortion of the tooth is minimized but is still present because the film is closer to the crown of the tooth than it is to the root apex. Therefore, image magnification occurs in an apical direction, but the length will be altered. If the tube head angle is too obtuse to the bisecting angle, the tooth will be foreshortened. If the tube head angle is too acute, then the tooth will be elongated.

The paralleling technique was developed to help eliminate the distortion created by the differences in the object-film distance that occur when using the bisecting angle technique. When the paralleling technique is used, the film is placed parallel to the object. In order to achieve parallelism, the film must be moved medially into the oral cavity and, therefore, farther away from the object (tooth). This will create some image magnification and loss of detail as the object-to-film distance is increased. To minimize the loss of detail, long cones are used. Placing the film away from the tooth and maintaining the parallel position can be difficult. In some cases it is impossible to achieve parallelism between the tooth and the dental film. If the film is angled no more than 20 degrees from true parallelism, however, distortion will be minimal.

Object Location and the Buccal Object Rule

More than one view may be necessary to localize an object such as an impacted tooth. Two views taken at 90 degrees to one another will give a three-dimensional picture of the object's position. An occlusal view (dorsoventral or ventrodorsal) and a periapical view (buccal-lingual) of the mandible and anterior maxilla are very useful for object localization. Occlusal views of the distal portion of the maxilla are more difficult to interpret because of the superimposition of the anterior portion of the skull.

The buccal object rule (tube shift technique or Clark's rule) is useful for object localization as well as for isolating structures for better visualization. Objects which are *lingual* to a reference point (for example a specific tooth or tooth root) will move in the *same* direction as the change in position of the tube head (either rostrally or distally); objects *buccal* to the reference point move *opposite* the direction of the tube head. An acronym to help remember this rule is SLOB, which stands for same-lingual, opposite-buccal. This technique is used frequently in veterinary dentistry to isolate the palatal (lingual) and buccal roots of the maxillary fourth premolars and molars. For example, if the tube head is moved rostrally, the palatal (lingual) root of the upper fourth premolar will be the most rostral root on the radiograph and the mesiobuccal root will be distal to the palatal root. To change the position of the tube head, the perpendicular angle to the bisecting angle is maintained, and the tube head is simply angled obliquely at the object in either a slightly more anterior or a slightly more posterior oblique view.

Intraoral Radiography in the Dog and Cat

Dog skulls can vary significantly between breeds, from the brachycephalic pug to the dolicocephalic greyhound. The brachycephalic breeds are the most difficult to master the intraoral technique on because of the tooth crowding and rotation that are present. These animals usually require additional oblique views to help isolate tooth roots. The dolicocephalic breeds are easier to achieve a good intraoral study on because the teeth are well separated; however, they usually require the use of more dental film because of the extra length of the jaws.

Intraoral radiographs of the mandibular premolars and molars are obtained by using the standard radiographic technique. The film is placed on the lingual side of the teeth and parallel to the central axis of the teeth. The dental x-ray beam is then aimed perpendicular to the film. This is the only area in the oral cavity of the dog and cat where the standard technique can be used. In some dogs and cats it may be difficult to use this technique on the most rostral premolars because of interference of the mandibular symphysis, which will not allow ventral placement of the film to get the apical extent of the tooth roots. The bisecting angle technique will be needed for views of such premolars, and for views of the rest of the dentition.

The mandibular incisors can usually be radiographed on one dental film. The animal is placed in dorsal or lateral recumbency with the dental film as close to the incisors as possible on the lingual side. The cone is then centered over the first incisors pointing in a caudal direction with the x-ray beam aimed perpendicular to the bisecting angle. The apices of both mandibular canines can be obtained in this view if the dental film extends far enough cau-

dally. The frenulum of the tongue may prevent proper placement of the intraoral film in some pets, particularly cats. If this becomes a problem, the tongue can be placed between the teeth and the film. This will result in increased soft-tissue density, and the radiographic technique (kVp, mA) may have to be adjusted, but this is not usually necessary. The crowns of the canine teeth will be distorted in this rostrocaudal view. If a radiograph of the mandibular canine crowns is desired, the x-ray tube can be shifted lateral to the tooth and aimed at the bisecting angle.

To obtain a radiograph of the mandibular first, second, and third premolars in a dog and the third premolars in the cat where the symphysis prevents proper parallel placement of the film, place the animal in dorsal recumbency. Position the film on the lingual side of the teeth as close to the teeth and ventral border of the mandible as possible. Direct the cone at the teeth from a lateral position and aim the x-ray beam at the bisecting angle.

The maxillary incisors are radiographed with the same technique as is used for the mandibular incisors except that the animal is placed in sternal or lateral recumbency. The apices of the maxillary canines are usually superimposed over the first and second premolars in this view. The maxillary canines should be radiographed from a lateral or rostrocaudal oblique view using the bisecting angle technique. In large breed dogs the root apex and crown of the maxillary canine may not fit on one film on the lateral view, and two views may be necessary to assess the whole tooth. The oblique rostrocaudal view usually allows visualization of the entire tooth on one film.

Radiographs of the maxillary premolars and molars are commonly taken with the bisecting angle or, less frequently, the paralleling technique, because the flat palate makes it difficult to place the film parallel and in close apposition to the tooth roots. To radiograph these teeth the animal is placed in sternal or lateral recumbency. For the bisecting angle technique, the film is placed as close to the tooth as possible on the lingual side of the dentition.

If the paralleling technique is used, the film is moved medially toward the center of the palate while keeping it parallel to the tooth. The object-to-film distance must be increased so that the entire image will be recorded on the film. If the film is placed too close to the tooth, the root apices will not be projected on the dental film.

Maxillary premolars one through three can be viewed with the tube head placed lateral to the teeth. If the animal has crowding and/or rotation of these teeth, additional views in a rostrocaudal oblique position may be required to improve visualization of tooth roots.

Rostrocaudal and/or caudorostral oblique views are needed to isolate the different tooth roots of the maxillary fourth premolar and the first and second molar teeth. A rostrocaudal view of premolar four provides an isolated view of the anterior tooth roots, but the distal root will be superimposed over the first molar. An additional view of the tooth from the caudorostral oblique projection will isolate the distal root well, and the anterior roots will be superimposed over the third premolar. The tooth roots of the molar teeth will be superimposed by their crowns, so the technique may need to be adjusted to penetrate the additional structures.

In cats and in brachycephalic dogs, the zygomatic arch may be superimposed over the maxillary premolar tooth roots. If the cone is placed in a rostrocaudal oblique position, the zygomatic arch can be shifted off the area of interest.

When one is learning the positioning techniques for intraoral dental radiographs, it is easiest to place the dog or cat in sternal recumbency for views of the maxillary dentition, in dorsal recumbency for views of the anterior mandible, and in lateral recumbency for views of the mandibular premolars and molars. As one masters the technique, the animal can be left in lateral recumbency (as many veterinarians perform dental procedures with the animal in this position) and the views taken following the same principles. To radiograph the anterior teeth in lateral recumbency the animal's head is propped on a towel to prevent interference of the treatment table with the tube head. Film holders are often needed for many of these views to keep the film from moving once it is placed in proper position. Gauze squares and foam forms are useful for this purpose. Table I.1 is a technique chart to serve as a reference for taking intraoral radiographs with a dental x-ray machine and intraoral film.

Table I.1. Reference chart for taking intraoral radiographs with a dental x-ray machine and intraoral film.

Exposure Time for D Speed Intraoral Dental Film
Cats   0.1–0.3 seconds
Dogs   0.2–0.5 seconds

Dental Machine
70 kVp
1-15 mA
12" FFD

Intraoral Dental Film

Intraoral dental film is composed of an emulsion and a base. The emulsion records the radiographic image. It contains silver halide crystals and is held to the base by a gelatin matrix. Intraoral dental film is a double emulsion film, which means both sides of the film base are coated with emulsion. An advantage of double emulsion film is that less radiation is required to make the diagnostic image.

The film base is a piece of clear plastic that is tinted blue to enhance image quality. The base contains an embossed dot for film orientation so the animal's left and right sides can be identified. The side of the film with the raised (convex) dot is the side, which faced the radiation.

An intraoral dental film packet has four main components. The film itself is wrapped in black paper to protect it from light exposure. The back of the film contains lead foil to shield the film from back scatter radiation, which could cause film fog. These components are then wrapped in a paper or plastic outer wrap, which is moisture resistant. A color-coded tab on the back of the packet identifies the speed of the film and the number of films in the packet.

Film speed is a qualitative description of how fast the film reacts to radiation to record an image. The speed of x-ray film ranges from A (slowest) to F (fastest). Intraoral dental film is available in D and E speeds. The exposure time of E speed film is 50 percent less than D speed, but there is less sharpness and more film fogging with E speed film. Either film is acceptable for use, but in human dentistry there is a desire to convert dentists to the use of E speed film only because the decrease in image quality is not significant enough to warrant the increased radiation exposure to the patient.

The speed of the film is an inherent quality and is based on the size of the silver halide crystals. The larger crystals are more sensitive to radiation and require shorter exposure times. However, these larger crystals are the cause of the decreased image sharpness. Film speed can be increased slightly by increasing the temperature at which the film is processed, but this results in increased film fog and graininess.

Intraoral dental film comes in three common sizes: periapical, bitewing, and occlusal. The composition of the film does not vary in the different film sizes. In veterinary medicine the periapical and occlusal sizes are used primarily. Periapical films are used to evaluate the crown, root, and periapical region and come in three sizes: size 0 ($7/8" \times 1 3/8"$), size 1 ($15/16" \times 1 9/16"$), and size 2 ($1 1/4" \times 1 5/8"$). Size 0 is used commonly in cats and small breed dogs. Size 2 is used for medium and large breed dogs and for single tooth studies such as an endodontic case. Size 1 film is narrow and is used for anterior projections in humans, but it is not commonly used in veterinary dentistry.

Occlusal film is size 4 film and is used to evaluate a larger area of the mandible or maxilla than would be seen on a single periapical film. It is commonly used for full-mouth dental radiograph studies in medium to large breed dogs to get more teeth per film with each radiation exposure. The dimensions of size 4 film are $2 1/4" \times 3"$.

X-ray Film Image Formation and Processing

X-ray photons strike the silver halide crystals in the film emulsion to produce the "latent image" of the structure(s) being radiographed. The silver halide crystals contain bromide, iodide, and silver ions, some free interstitial silver ions, and latent image sites. The x-ray photons react primarily with the bromide ions within the crystals to cause the release of an electron from the ion. The electron moves through the emulsion and activates other bromide ions to release more electrons. These migrating electrons eventually become trapped in the latent image sites in the halide crystal. The latent image sites then become negatively charged by the electrons. The positive charge of the free interstitial silver ions causes them to move to the negatively charged latent image site where the silver ion gains an electron to become an atom of metallic silver.

When the x-ray film is exposed to the developer solution, these silver atoms initiate the conversion of the other silver ions in the silver halide crystal to a grain of metallic silver. The greater the number of silver atoms per halide crystal, the more sensitive it is to the developer solution. The developer converts the metallic silver to black metallic silver, which can be visualized. The fixer solution rinses away the silver halide crystals that were not irradiated to clear the film and allow visualization of the image.

The developer solution is a reducing agent (supplies or donates electrons) which is catalyzed by the metallic silver in the latent image sites. This ensures that the silver ions in the irradiated crystals are reduced and converted to black metallic silver first. If the film is left in the developer too long, the developer will eventually reduce the unexposed silver halide crystals, and the film will be too dark (overdeveloped). Overdevelopment of the film results in chemical film fog. The initial development of a film is slow, then it hits a rapid density increase phase, and then it slows down dramatically. This final slow phase is reached after the exposed crystals have been reduced and delineates the time when the film should be removed from the developer to prevent overdeveloping.

The *density* of the x-ray film is the overall degree of darkening. The variation in the film density results from the uneven distribution of developed (exposed) and undeveloped (unexposed) crystals.

Processing Solutions and Techniques

To manually process x-ray films, the film is placed in the developer for 4½ to 5 minutes at 68 degrees Fahrenheit. Once properly developed, it is rinsed in clean circulating water for 15 to 20 seconds. The water rinse serves to slow the development process and remove the alkaline activator, which would neutralize the acidic fixer solution.

The fixing solution contains a clearing agent, acidifier, preservative, and hardener. The clearing agent works rapidly on the unreacted silver halide crystals to increase their solubility and rinse them away. If the film is left in the fixer too long, the clearing agent will start to remove the grains of metallic silver and decrease the density of the film. The acidifier serves to neutralize any developer solution which may remain in the film emulsion after rinsing. The hardener hardens the gelatin to prevent damage to the film with handling, and it aids film drying. The film should be in the fixing solution for at least 10 minutes.

The final washing of the film is very important to remove all processing chemicals. Improper washing will leave chemicals which will discolor and stain the film. Films should be washed in clean running water for no less than 20 minutes. The emulsion can be washed off completely if the film is left in the water too long (i.e., overnight). After the film is washed the excess water is shaken off, and the film is placed on a drying stand to dry. Ideally, moderately warm circulating air is used to dry the films, but the films should not be blown dry with direct air from a fan.

Rapid processing chemicals are often used to shorten procedural time, particularly in veterinary dentistry, because the animals are under general anesthesia. It is very convenient to use a Chairside Darkroom™ (Rinn) and rapid processing solutions so the films can be developed and viewed directly in the dental operatory. Rapid processing solutions are similar in composition to the conventional processing solutions, but they are more concentrated. Processing films in these solutions usually requires 10 to 20 seconds in the developer and 1 to 2 minutes in the fixer solution.

Films processed with the rapid processing chemicals do not gain the same degree of contrast as films processed by conventional solutions, and they may discolor over time. To help prevent these problems, the film can be read immediately after it has been in the fixer for 1 minute, but then it should be placed back in the fixer solution for 10 to 15 minutes, followed by the wash for 20 minutes before drying.

It is necessary to change the developer and fixer solutions when they become exhausted. Exhaustion of the developer solution results in films that have reduced density and contrast. When solutions become turbid, they should be changed. The fixer should be changed when the developer is changed. A "reference film" can be used to monitor film processing when the chemicals are first changed. This film is kept on hand (placed on view box) to serve as a comparison to subsequent films. As the chemicals become exhausted, the films will lose density and contrast. This will signal the time to replace the developer and fixer.

Automatic film processors can be used for dental film. The main advantage of this system is the decrease in film processing time. Most machines are able to develop, fix, wash, and dry the film in 4 to 6 minutes. Automatic processors made specifically for dental films work best because the rollers are the appropriate size for the small dental films.

The automatic processors designed for larger films can be used if the dental film is taped to a film which is the appropriate size for that processor. There are some disadvantages with this technique, however. First, the area on the dental film covered with tape will not be developed. Second, the dental film often becomes dislodged from the tape in the processor. This can cause other films to jam, or the dislodged film may stick to another film and ruin it. Because of these problems, this method is not recommended.

The density and contrast of automatically processed films tend to be consistent; however, the quality is not as high as with manually processed films. This results from the higher temperature and concentration of the developer solution in the automatic processor. Other disadvantages of this system are the increased purchase and maintenance costs. A darkroom should be maintained in case the automatic processor malfunctions.

Dental Film Mounts

Once the films have dried they should be mounted in plastic or cardboard dental film mounts. The mounts protect the films and allow them to be placed in a systematic fashion for viewing. Film mounts come in a wide variety of styles to hold a single film or multiple films. If the films are placed in the mounts with the embossed dot positioned so the raised side is toward the viewer, the animal's left side should be mounted on the right and the animal's right side on the left. When the films are mounted in this way, the animal's mouth will have the same relationship as the films in the mount to the viewer.

An alternative method is to mount the animal's left side on the left and its right side on the right so that the teeth are oriented to the viewer as if the viewer were inside the mouth looking out at the teeth.

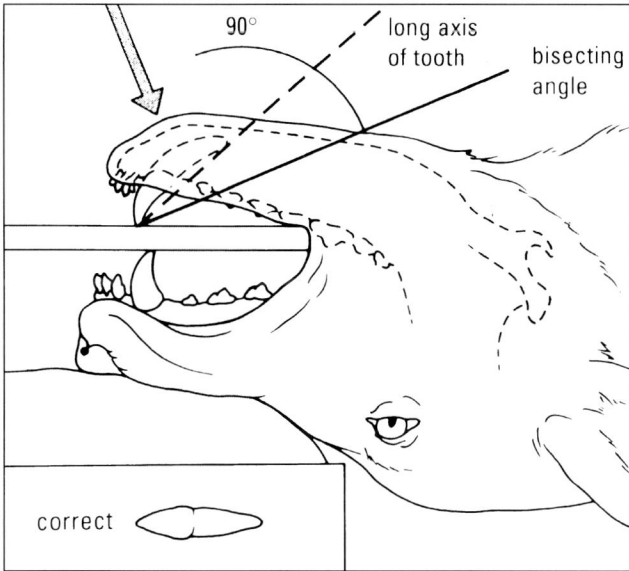

FIGURE 1.1

Bisecting angle technique, producing an accurate image of the tooth.

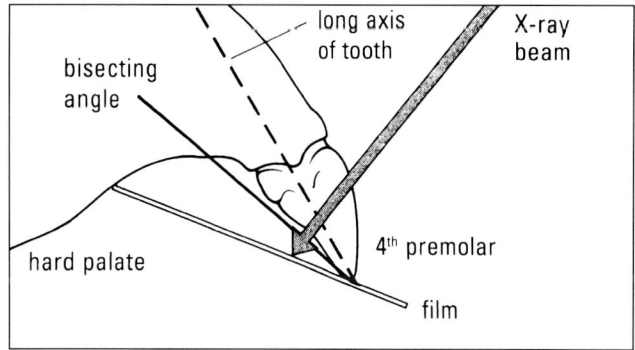

FIGURE 1.2

Parallel technique for intraoral radiography.

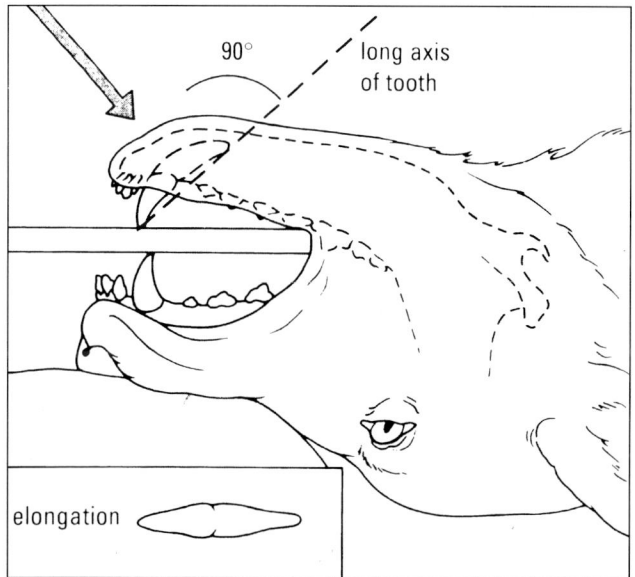

FIGURE 1.3

Dental x-ray film angled toward the long axis of the upper fourth premolar, without bending the film or missing the apex.

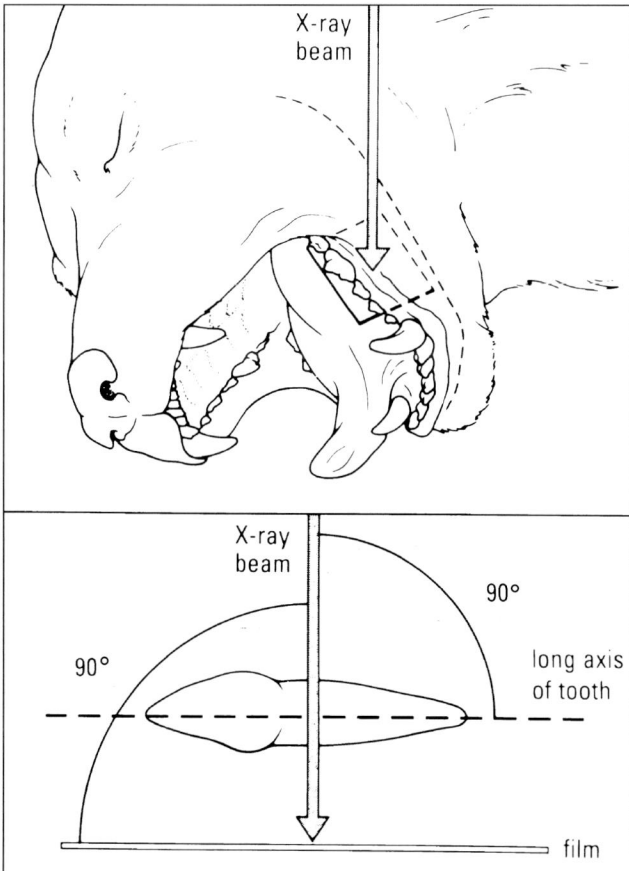

FIGURE 1.4

Directing the x-ray beam at right angles to the long axis of the tooth, elongating the tooth's image.

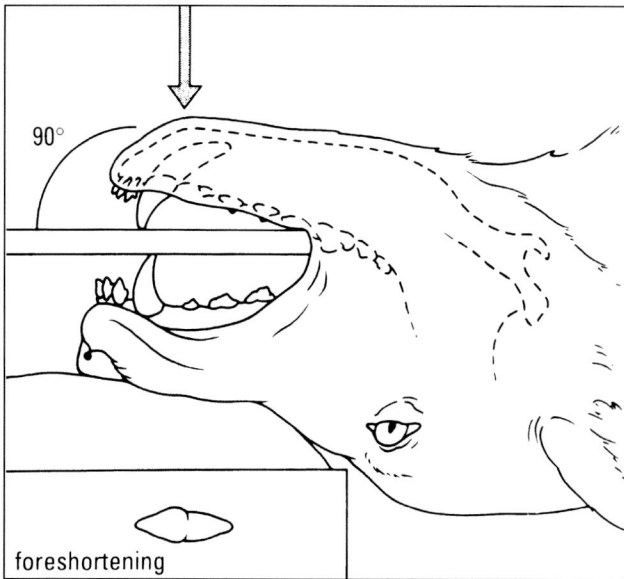

FIGURE 1.5

Directing the x-ray beam at right angles to the film, shortening the tooth's image.

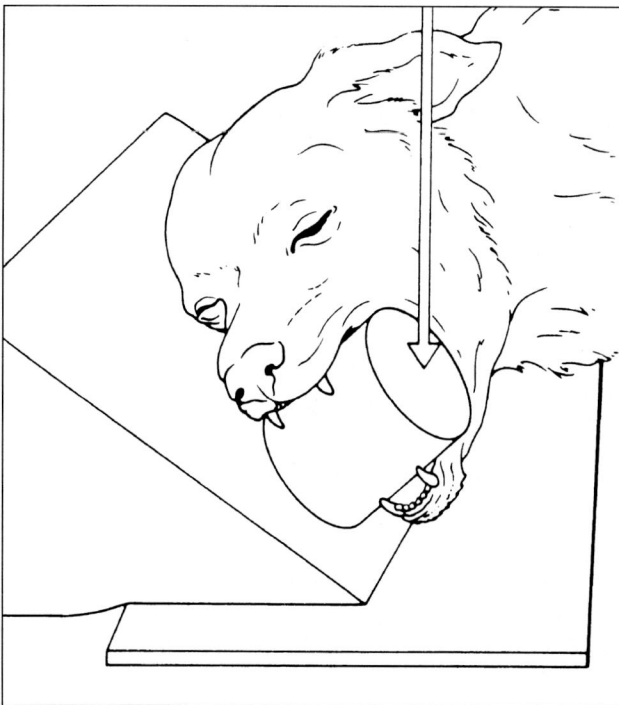

FIGURE 1.6

Oblique lateral technique for radiography of the right mandibular premolars.

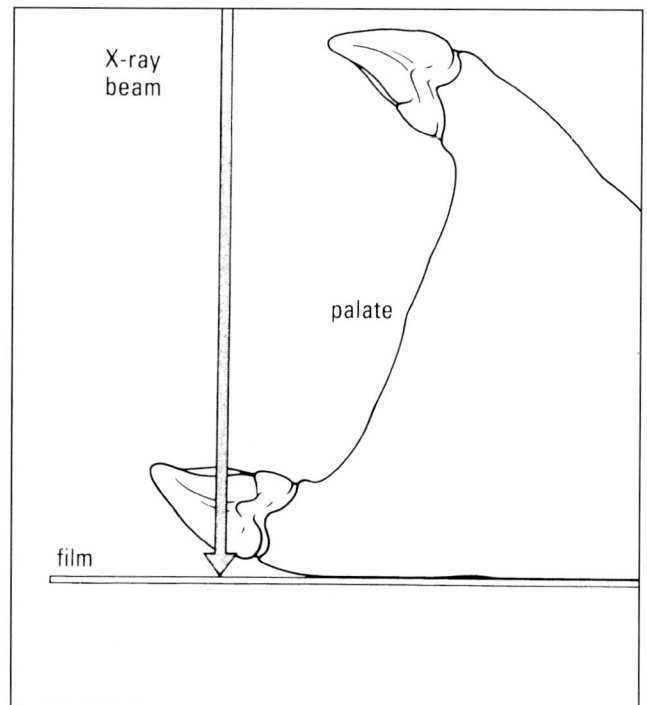

FIGURE 1.7

Extraoral parallel technique for radiography of the upper premolars.

PART ONE   Canine

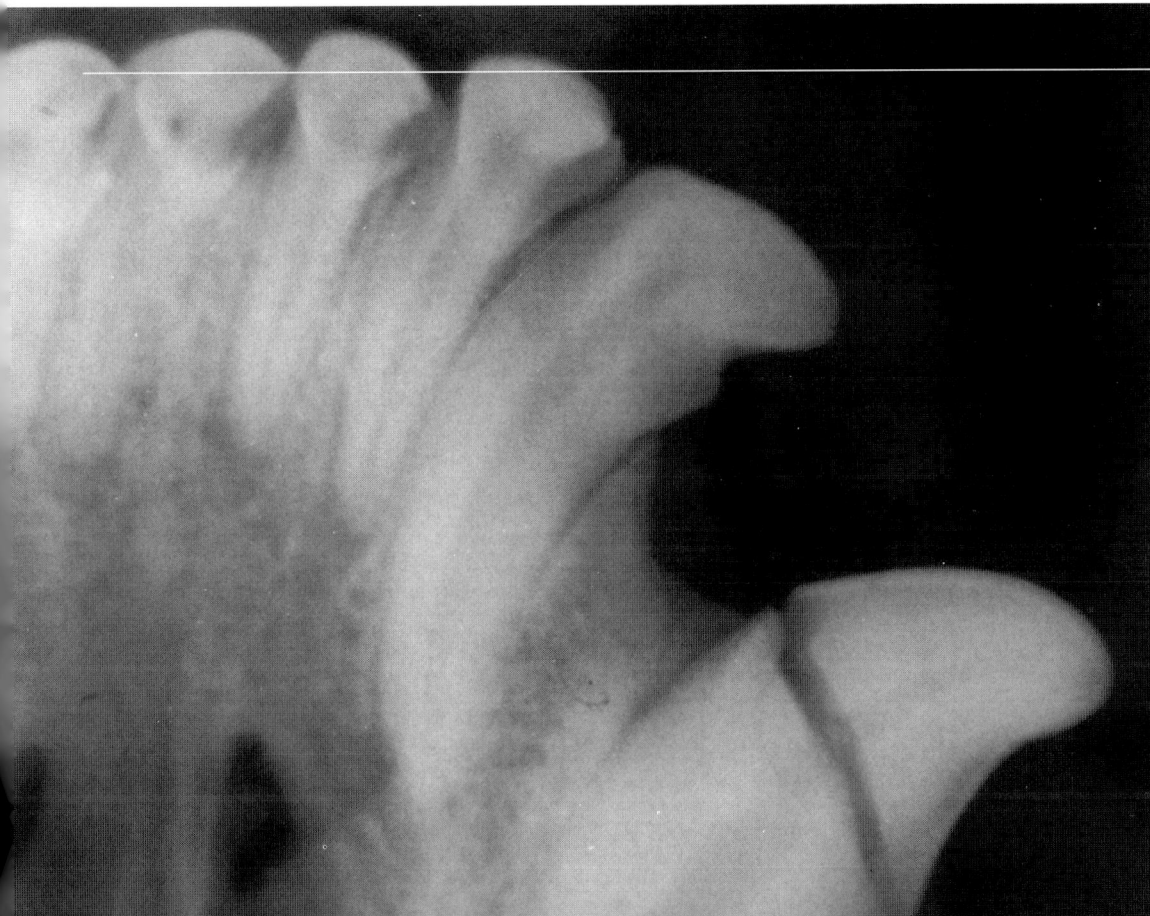

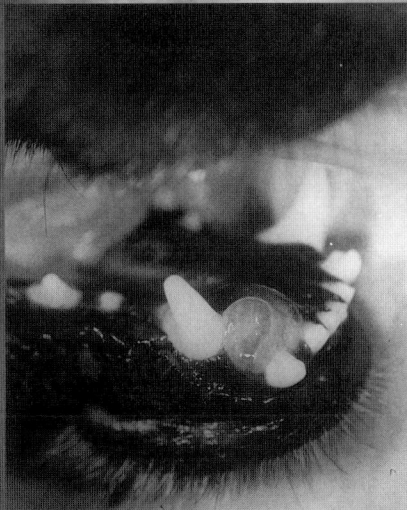

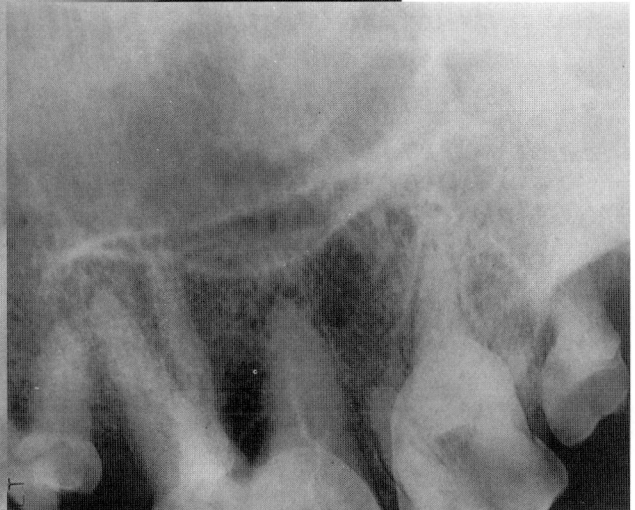

1 Normal Canine Intraoral Radiographic Anatomy

Dr. Linda J. DeBowes
Dr. Donald H. DeForge

Dr. M. Lynne Kesel
Dr. B. Jean Hawkins

FUNCTIONAL ANATOMY OF TEETH AND RELATED STRUCTURES

Dr. M. Lynne Kesel

The permanent dentition for adult dogs, which is composed of forty-two teeth, is:

2 (Incisors 3/3, Canines 1/1, Premolars 4/4, Molars 2/3) = 42.

The teeth of dogs and cats are functionally adapted to their dietary needs. The cat, as a strict carnivore, has only sharp, pointy teeth designed for capturing prey and rendering it into digestible portions. The dog, however, with its more omnivorous tastes, also has molar surfaces in the caudal mouth which have flat, grinding surfaces.

All teeth have the same basic anatomy. The tooth crown, which is covered with enamel, is that portion of a tooth which is visible above the gingival margin (originating at the CEJ, the cemento-enamel junction) during any stage of eruption. The enamel is similar to bone in that it is made up of the same calcium phosphates of the apatite type, but greatly exceeds bone, cementum, and dentin in the inorganic component of the crystallites. These crystallites are laid down in slightly flattened hexagonal rods, which are generally perpendicular to the surface of the tooth. Enamel thickness varies greatly but is generally thickest at the apex of the crown. Enamel can be chipped loose from the underlying dentin; in such cases it always has an abrupt, sharp edge perpendicular to the dentin. Such an edge can be ground down for smoothness, but undermined enamel will always chip off if the supporting dentin is not present.

The body of the tooth is formed of dentin, a modified, dense bone (the ivory of elephants). The dentin surrounds the tooth pulp, the live portion of the tooth; odontoblasts, which line the pulp, constantly deposit dentin throughout the life of the pulp. Primary dentin is pre-eruption dentin; secondary dentin is that which is normally laid down during maturation; and tertiary dentin is that which is laid down in response to stimulus, such as attrition. Each odontoblast leaves behind a nonmineralized process as it builds dentin inward. As the diameter of the pulp decreases, the odontoblastic processes get closer together. Although tiny (0.5-3 μm), the interdentinal tubules, which contain cytoplasm of the odontoblastic processes as well as axons from the nerve plexus of the tooth pulp, make the dentin porous. This is abundantly clear when trauma to a tooth causes hemorrhage to color the dentin with hemoglobin, or when a nonvital tooth turns gray. The presence of living odontoblastic processes undoubtedly accounts for the resilience of a live tooth, as opposed to the brittleness of a dead one. The axons of the pulpal nerves account for sensitivity when dentin is exposed.

The tooth pulp has abundant blood and lymph vessels and an abundant nerve supply. The vast majority of its cellular elements are fibroblasts, although undifferentiated cells also exist. In most dogs and cats, the apex of the tooth root forms a delta for the entrance of the nerves and vessels, and the apex is tightly constricted. In contrast to humans, the apex terminates in an open canal. There can be accessory canals for blood supply along the length of the root. The presence of a blood supply allows the tooth pulp to support inflammation. Pulpitis, whether caused by mechanical, thermal, infectious or other insult, results from the same biological changes as in any other tissue. The sensory result is pain. Pulpitis most always results in pulpal necrosis.

Embryologically, the tooth crown derived its shape from the developing tooth bud (dental papilla) and enamel epithelium. Odontoblasts are induced by this structure to produce dentin, after which ameloblasts produce enamel adjacent to predentin, covering it. Thus the tooth begins as a bell-shaped structure which lengthens to form the complete crown and then the root. The first enamel and dentin are formed at the apex of the crown, then make concentric and longer layers on the outside (enamel) and inside (dentin) of the tooth. The final layers of enamel, at the base of the crown, form a ring around the crown rather than covering the entire crown continuously.

When the enamel organ has reached its final size, Hertwig's epithelial root sheath takes over the growth of the root. If the tooth is single rooted, the sheath merely forms into a circle, but if two or three roots are to be formed, it duly forms into more than one circle at the base of the crown. Hertwig's sheath is a layer of undifferentiated cells which induce odontoblasts for the root formation. The sheath typically stays in place and apparently is largely responsible for the eruption of the tooth. Typically only half of the root is formed when a tooth begins to erupt. Constriction of the diaphragm of the sheath is responsible for the tapering of the root tip. Cementum is formed late in root formation. Cellular elements evolve among the fibrils of the protodentin at the outer surface of the root. It takes various times for the root tips to close after full eruption, as much as 18 months for canine (cuspid) teeth. This has implications for endodontic therapy, as a wide open tooth root cannot tolerate a standard root canal. However, fortunately, Hertwig's epithelial root sheath can still proliferate and close the root apex in the face of a devitalized pulp if infection is controlled (apexification). The odontocytes continue to lay down dentin throughout the life of the tooth, until the pulp chamber is virtually eliminated.

Enamel defects and errors in coronal morphology may be due to hereditary or environmental influences. Any febrile illness that affects epithelial cells will cause a disruption of the enamel organ; in the past, many dogs who had distemper in puppyhood exhibited enamel dysplasia of several teeth that were in the same stage of development when the tooth was infected. Physical trauma is usually the cause when only one or two teeth have enamel deficits. Extraction of deciduous teeth has damaged permanent crowns, as has merely bumping into objects.

The periodontium bears the same relationship to teeth as the earth does to fence posts or trees. No matter what the strength of the objects embedded within them, the supporting substances must function correctly or the objects are lost. Because the primary cause of loss of teeth of small animals is periodontal disease, examination of the form and function of the periodontium must be our first step in our struggle to understand periodontitis.

Simply put, the periodontium consists of the periodontal ligament, which anchors the tooth in the bony socket (the alveolus, a portion of or extension of the bone of the jaw), which, in turn, is covered by oral epithelium. The most important thing to remember about these tissues—connective tissue, bone and epithelium—is that they are dynamic and responsive. They enjoy a rich supply of blood and lymph vessels and nervous tissue, which, for ease of illustration, is usually omitted from drawings and is therefore often ignored.

To begin a close examination of the periodontium, from the tooth outward, we must begin with a tooth structure. Cementum covers the tooth root from the cementoenamel junction to the apex, becoming thicker toward the tip of the root. Cementum is analogous to periosteum, in that it is a live tissue covering the modified bone, dentin. It contains cellular elements, connective tissue, and a mineralized matrix to anchor fibers of the periosteal ligament extruded from it. These fibers intermesh with fibers from alveolar bone (Sharpey's fibers) to form the periodontal ligament.

The periodontal ligament fibers, which are nonmineralized and therefore radiolucent between the tooth root and the dense alveolar bone of the socket, are aligned to suspend the tooth evenly in the socket. The ligament acts as a shock absorber during mastication or trauma. Solidly anchored teeth would be much more likely to shatter or to cause supporting bone to break. This ligament, like others in the body, is responsive to stress. Disuse will cause it to weaken, and pressure (to a point) will strengthen it. If torn, as in trauma, the ligament can repair itself rapidly. Excessive pressure, as in improper orthodonture, can kill cellular elements and cause loss of the periodontal ligament, which leads us

to another function of the ligament—physical separation of tooth root and bone. Although dentin is considered a dense, modified bone, it is unlike bone in that it does not continuously remodel after it is once set down. However, if osteoclasts from the surrounding bone are allowed into dentin, they will resorb the mineral matrix. If they are deep within the bone of the jaw, osteoblasts follow the osteoclasts and lay down normal bone. (In shallow osteoclastic resorption, such as that found at the cementoenamel junction in feline resorptive lesions, the osteoclasts are not followed by osteoblasts). Tooth roots not protected by periodontal ligament, are therefore resorbed and replaced by normal bone, which is less dense and weaker than dentin. The result of bone replacement is loss of the anchoring quality of the tooth and, therefore, loss of the crown.

The bony socket of the tooth, the alveolus, is lined by dense cortical bone, from which Sharpey's fibers originate for the periodontal ligament. The density of this bone is demonstrated in radiographs as a white line, or "lamina dura," just outside of the periodontal ligament. The surrounding bone is cancellous, except where alveolar bone joins the cortical bone of the jaw at the open end of the tooth socket. The alveolar processes of the mandible are part of a dental ridge, a continuity of the jaw that is particularly evident in the mandible. When teeth have never been present, the dental ridge is absent, and if enough time has elapsed after an extraction, the dental ridge atrophies due to lack of stress by tooth roots, and a depression occurs.

The oral epithelium lies over the bone. In healthy, young periodontium, the tissue of the gingiva forms a fibrous connection to the neck of the tooth just apical to the CEJ. Then the gingiva reflects over the enamel to form the flap of the free (or marginal) gingiva. This flap of tissue defines the gingival sulcus, that gingiva which clings to the base of the tooth like a rubber sheet to a wet bathtub when healthy. A healthy free gingiva tapers to a thin edge coronally. Next to the enamel, which is too slick a surface to allow attachment, lies a special tissue, sulcular epithelium. This nonkeratinized epithelium has minimal intracellular connections and is only a few cells thick, allowing it to be the remnant of the epithelial tissue that formed the enamel organ and which was left in place as the tooth erupted through it.

From the extremity of the marginal epithelium, for varying widths away from the crown of the tooth, the gingiva covering the tooth and bone is attached. This tissue is parakeratinized epithelium with an obvious basement membrane over a connective tissue matrix. This tissue is closely adhered to the bone via rete pegs, which are visible as pinpoint shallow depressions in its surface, giving the tissue a stippled appearance. The attached gingiva has the ability to form and reform attachments to the tooth or bone. When healthy, it maintains a pink color, except where it is pigmented. It is permeated by an extensive blood supply, which allows for rapid repair after damage due to mastication and other trauma. The attached gingiva, with its fibrous attachments to tooth and bone, protects the periodontal ligament and alveolar bone from invasion by microbes.

The palatal epithelium, or masticatory mucosa, is similar to attached gingiva. It, too, is closely adhered to bone and is well vascularized, with its blood supply coming from the rostral and caudal palatine arteries, which run parallel to the dental arcade on each side. It is thrown up into rugal folds (rugae), which probably aid in swallowing.

The oral mucosa is continuous with the attached gingiva at the mucogingival junction (MGJ). The oral mucosa is thin and loosely attached to underlying bone. Its blood supply is less extensive than that of the attached gingiva, and generally runs at a right angle to the line of the attached gingiva, an important consideration when considering surgery. The mucosa is elastic to allow free movement of the jaws and lips. It is not, strictly speaking, periodontal tissue, as it never will be directly adjacent to a tooth in a healthy periodontium.

Periodontal tissues have the capability to heal themselves in a dynamic equilibrium between insult and repair. Oral gingival trauma, whether mechanical, thermal, or other, is quickly repaired unless damage covers a broad area and cellular elements cannot repair or replicate. Loss of attached gingiva leads to loss of the tooth, due to anaerobic microbial attack at the periodontal ligament. The usual cause of loss of teeth, however, is periodontitis. When plaque is not cleaned off the teeth in a regular fashion, whether by mastication of elastic fibers or by brushing, the number of aerobic bacteria in the plaque increases, and their metabolites cause inflammation in adjacent marginal gingiva. The first sign of inflammation is reddening and swelling of the leading edge of the gingiva due to increased circulation and capillary permeability. The sulcular epithelium secrets antibodies as inflammatory and phagocytic cells are mobilized to the areas of the sulcus. The rounding of the leading edge of the marginal gingiva allows plaque to enter the sulcus, after which the population of bacteria changes to anaerobic. Gingivitis in some animals is largely an inflammatory response to oral flora in the gingival sulcus. This may result in a massive influx of inflammatory cells, leading to gingival

and mucosal friability (lymphocytic/plasmacytic stomatitis in cats) or to fibrous hypertrophy (nonacanthomatous epulis or "reactive gingiva"), which is seen mainly in dogs. The presence of bacteria in the gingival sulcus often leads to attack of the periodontal ligament and bone by lytic substances produced by bacteria and phagocytic cells. Once an active infection occurs, pus is readily seen from pockets produced by loss of bone and periodontal ligament. In most pets, these pockets may become quite deep, becoming more and more efficient at protecting bacterial troublemakers from cleansing action. Gingival hypertrophy, in which a false periodontal pocket is formed, should be treated by gingivoplasty, in which the extraneous tissue is surgically excised to reestablish a healthy sulcus.

In most animals, once alveolar bone has been destroyed, the marginal gingiva recedes due to lack of support and the roots of the teeth are exposed. In humans, the recession of gingiva is commonly a millimeter a decade, but compensatory apical widening of attached gingiva also occurs so that octogenarians may still have adequate attached gingiva but appear very "long in the tooth" because of the gingival recession. Although this gingival widening probably occurs in dogs and cats as well, the progress of loss often exceeds compensatory mechanisms, and necrosis and loss of periodontal ligament and bone allows infection to travel apically. If a pocket of infection can be adequately cleaned of necrotic cementum and soft tissue, gingiva may reestablish a light attachment to the dentin. Gingiva will not attach to necrotic surfaces. If attached gingiva has been lost over a limited portion of the tooth root, sliding gingival flap surgery may be utilized to provide protective attached gingiva after totally cleaning the exposed tooth root. The important thing to remember is that alveolar bone will not reestablish a coronal border unassisted, and reestablishment of a healthy gingiva is only a salvage operation.

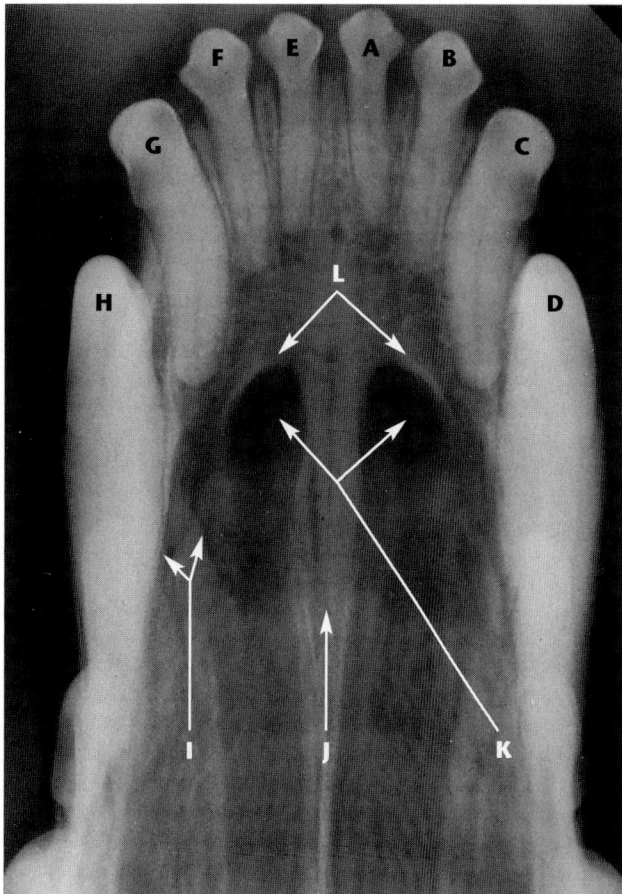

FIGURE 1.1

Contributing Author:
Donald H. DeForge

Description: Normal anatomy.

Points Identified:

A. 101	E. 201
B. 102	F. 202
C. 103	G. 203
D. 104	H. 204

I. Lateral border of nasal bone
J. Palatine suture
K. Palatine fissures
L. Palatine process of incisive bone

Common Errors: Without tube angulation, the apices of 104, 204 are not visible.

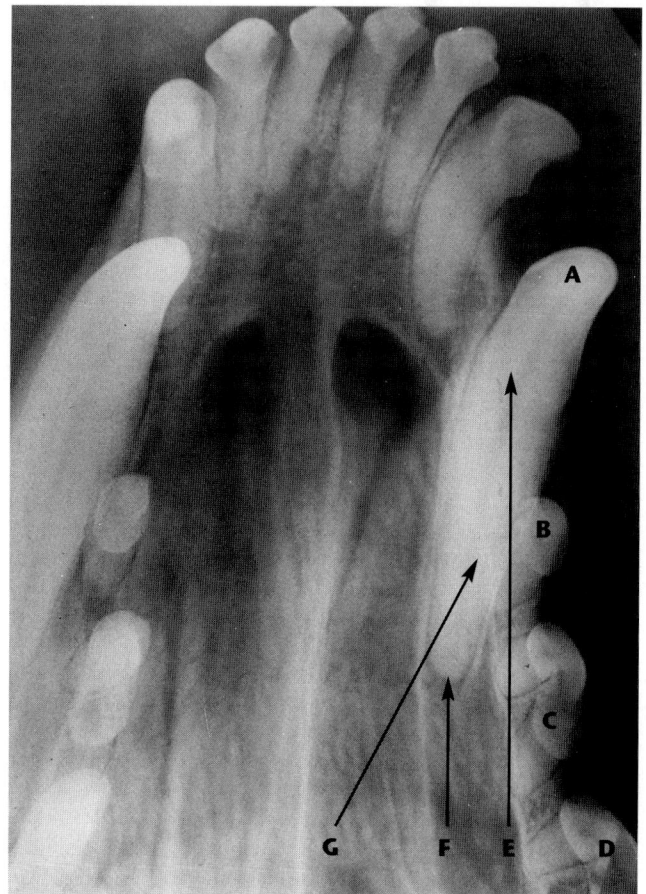

FIGURE 1.2

Contributing Author:
Donald H. DeForge

Description: Normal anatomy.

Points Identified:

A. 204
B. 205
C. 206
D. 207
E. Pulp canal 204
F. Apex 204
G. Root canal 204

Diagnostic Keys: G. With angulation of the x-ray head using the rostral bisecting angle, the apex is now clearly visible. With rotation of the tube to the right using the rostral bisecting angle technique, the apex of 104 would be visible.

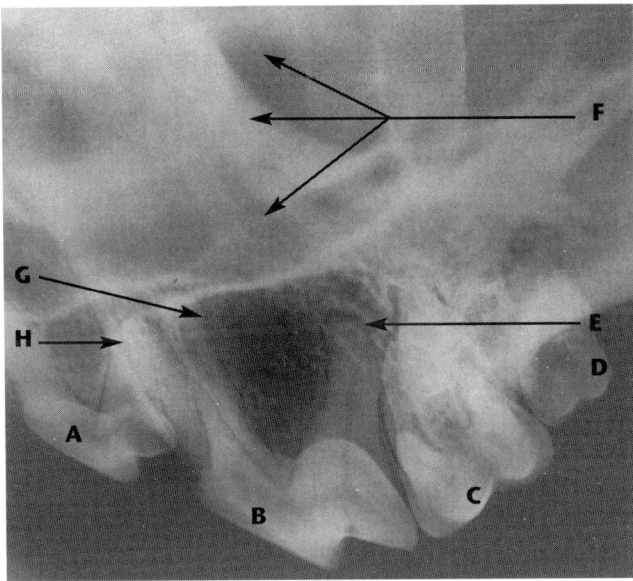

FIGURE 1.3

Contributing Author:
Donald H. DeForge

Description: Normal anatomy.

Points Identified:

  A. 207
  B. 208
  C. 209
  D. 210
  E. Distal root 208
  F. Maxillary sinus
  G. Palatal root 208
  H. Mesial buccal root 208

Common Errors: G. The mesiobuccal root of 208 is superimposed on the distal root of 207. (To separate the roots of 208, the tube was positioned in a caudal rostral position with correct bisecting angle. This places the palatal root in the center. The angle was too acute, superimposing the mesiobuccal root of 208 on the distal root of 207.)

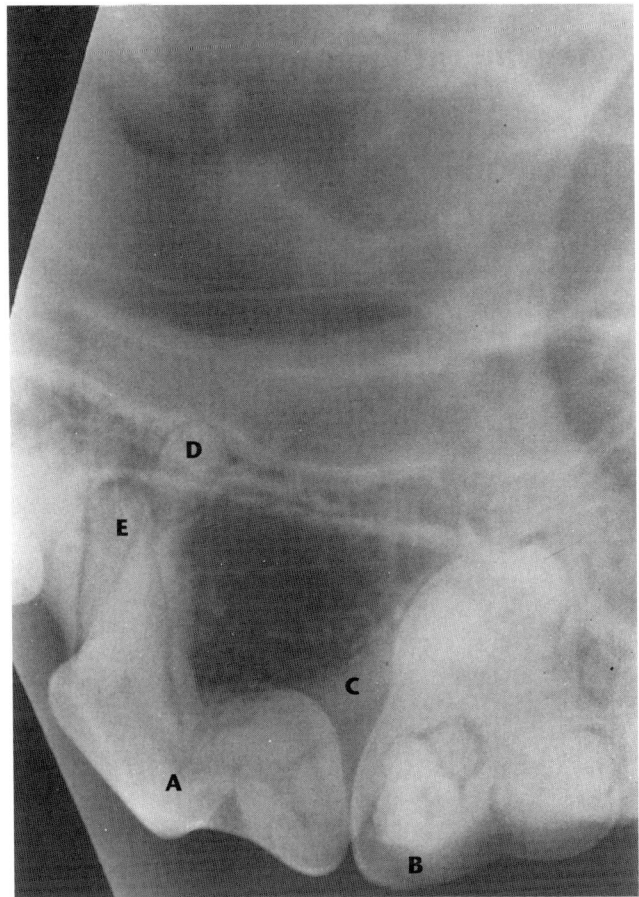

FIGURE 1.4

Contributing Author:
Donald H. DeForge

Description: Normal anatomy.

Points Identified:
  A. 108
  B. 109
  C. Distal root 108
  D. Mesiobuccal root 108
  E. Palatal root 108

Common Errors: This projection was taken in the cranial rostral bisecting angle position with the tube head too far forward. The mesiobuccal and palatal roots have been separated, but now the distal root is buried in 109.

FIGURE 1.5

Contributing Author:
Donald H. DeForge

Description: Normal anatomy.

Points Identified: 208

- A. Mesiobuccal root
- B. Palatal root
- C. Distal root

Diagnostic Keys: In this view, 208 has been taken with bisecting angle in the caudal rostral position. The mesiobuccal root is the most forward, the palatal root is in the center, and the distal root stands alone.

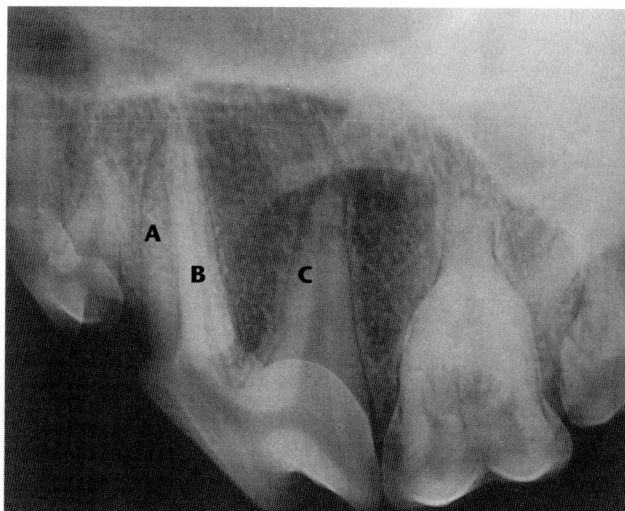

FIGURE 1.6

Contributing Author:
Donald H. DeForge

Description: Normal anatomy.

Points Identified: 208

- A. Distal root
- B. Palatal root
- C. Mesiobuccal root

Diagnostic Keys: Perfect separation of all three roots of 208. Taken with the bisecting angle, caudal rostral projection. This placed the palatal root in the center, the mesiobuccal root and the distal root standing alone.

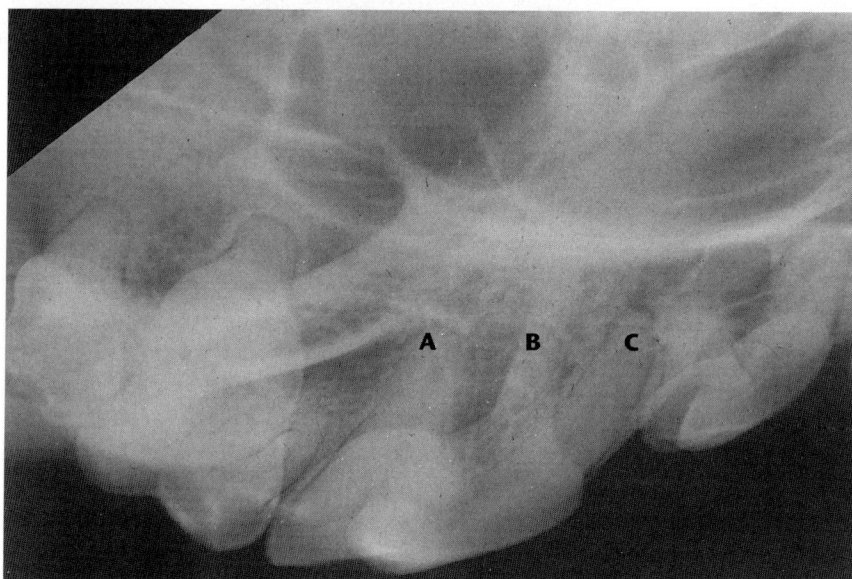

FIGURE 1.7

Contributing Author:
Donald H. DeForge

Description: Normal anatomy—mature tooth (8 years old).

Points Identified: 108

- A. Mesiobuccal root
- B. Palatal root
- C. Distal root
- D. Pulp horn

Diagnostic Keys: Note the perfect separation of the three roots of 108 and the narrow pulp canals with osteolytic changes occurring around distal root apex. It is important when planning endodontic treatment to have perfect visualization of endodontic anatomy.

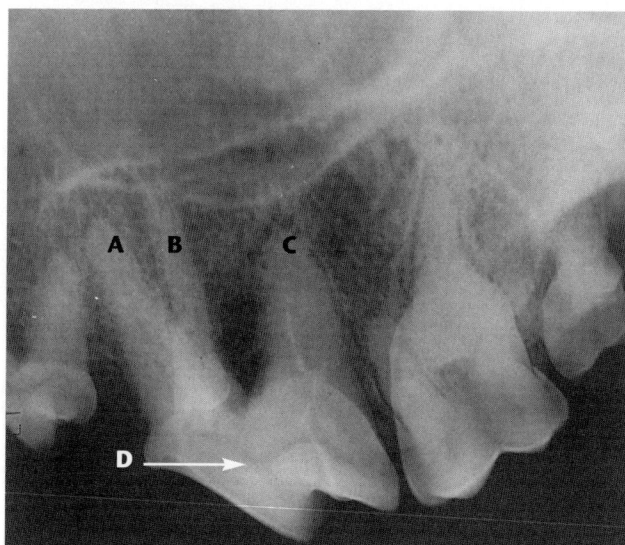

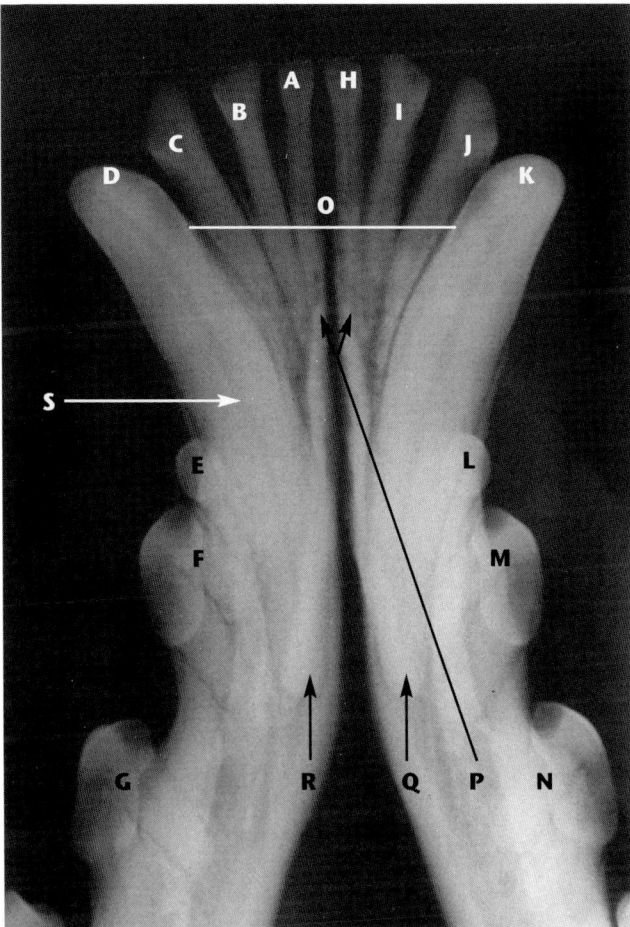

FIGURE 1.8

Contributing Author:
Donald H. DeForge

Description: Normal anatomy.

Points Identified:

A. 301	H. 401
B. 302	I. 402
C. 303	J. 403
D. 304	K. 404
E. 305	L. 405
F. 306	M. 406
G. 307	N. 407

O. Crestal bone—incisors
P. Mandibular symphysis
Q. Apex 404
R. Apex 304
S. Root canal 304

Diagnostic Keys: O. The bone level is abnormally low in this patient (i.e., horizontal bone loss).

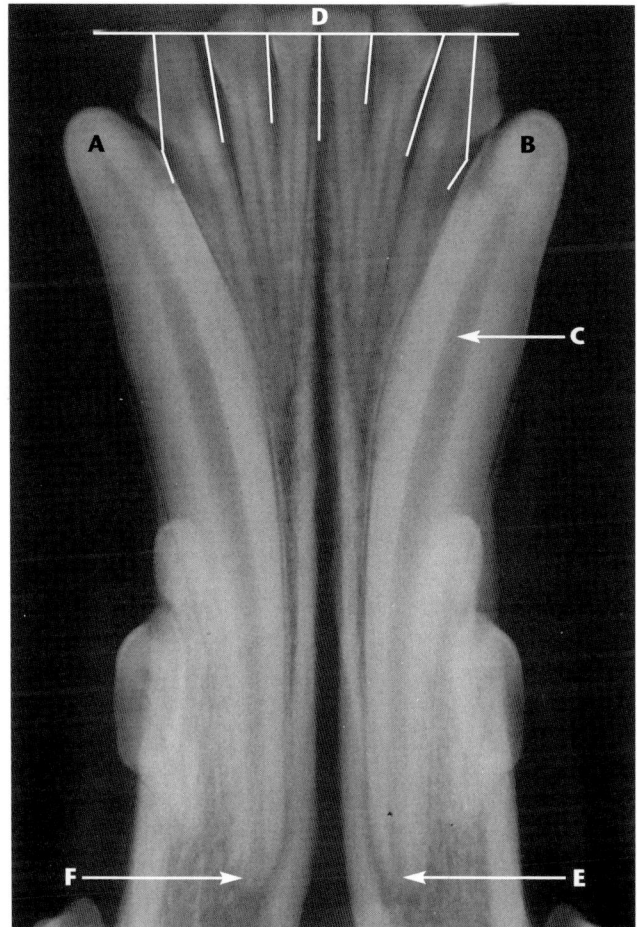

FIGURE 1.9

Contributing Author: Linda J. DeBowes

Description: Normal anatomy.

Points Identified:

A. 304
B. 404
C. Large pulp canal—immature animal (6 months old)
D. Crestal bone—incisors
E. Apex 404
F. Apex 304

Diagnostic Keys: D. In a normal patient, bone level in the incisor area is slightly below the CEJ. E,F. Questionable if apices are now closed.

Common Errors: A,B. Notice the elongation of the canine teeth due to improper bisecting angle. (See introduction for correct technique.)

FIGURE 1.10

Contributing Author: Linda J. DeBowes

Description: Normal anatomy.

Points Identified:

A. Pulp canals
B. Apices

Diagnostic Keys: Same as Figure 1.9 except patient is 4 months old. Notice the wide pulp canals. Notice that the apex is open as compared to Figure 1.9.

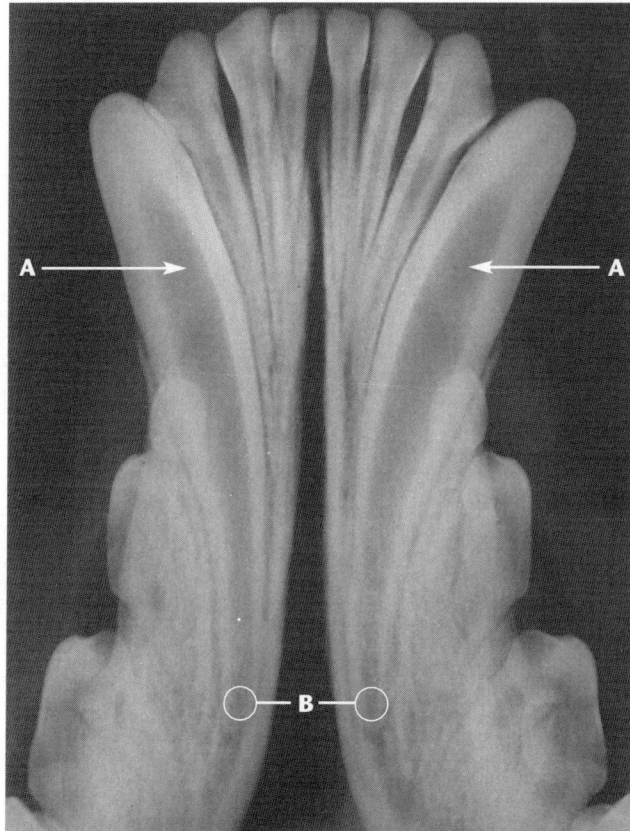

FIGURE 1.11

Contributing Author:
Donald H. DeForge

Description: Normal anatomy.

Points Identified:

A. 306   D. 309
B. 307   E. 310
C. 308   F. 311

G. Mandibular canal
H. Ventral cortex of mandible
I. Root canal

Diagnostic Keys: Note the narrowness of the root canal (I) as compared to the root canal (I) in Figure 1.14. (Figure 1.11: 4-year-old patient; Figure 1.14: 6-month-old patient)

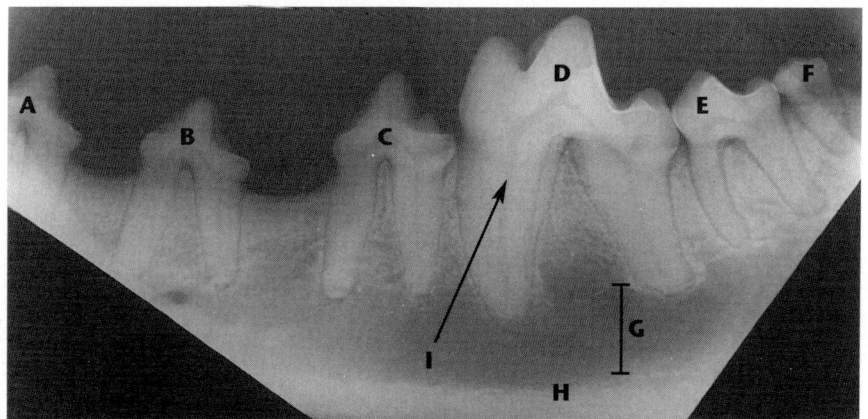

FIGURE 1.12

Contributing Author: Linda J. DeBowes

Description: Normal anatomy.

Points Identified:

A. 406
B. 407
C. 408
D. 409

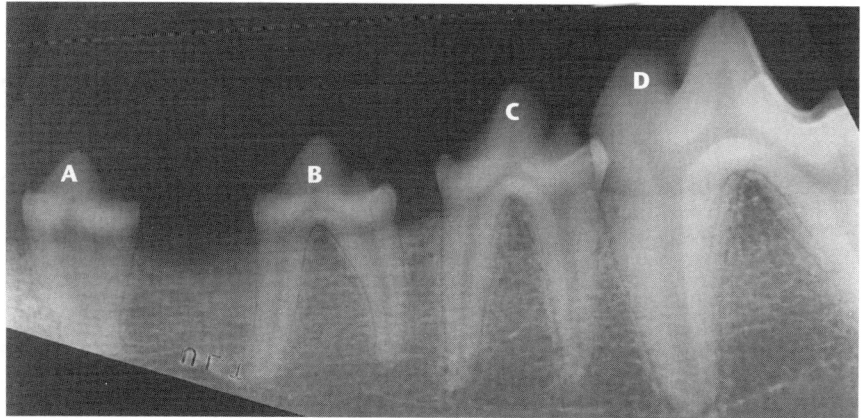

FIGURE 1.13

Contributing Author:
Donald H. DeForge

Description: Normal anatomy.

Points Identified:

A. Mental foramen
B. Furcation crestal bone
C. Enamel 410
D. Dentin 409
E. Invagination line of intraradicular groove

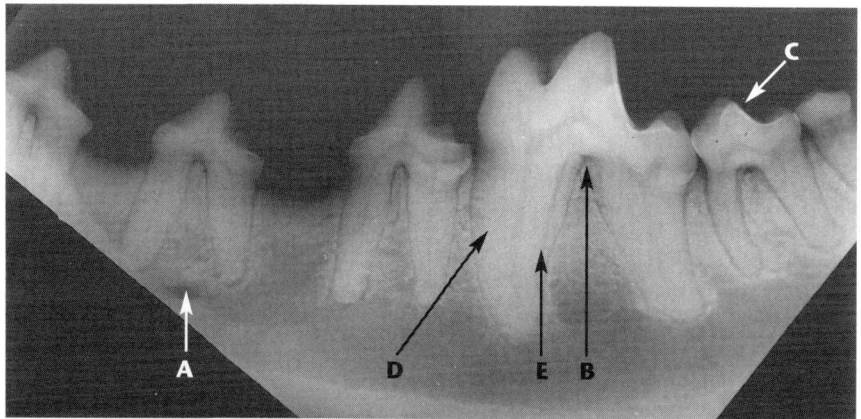

FIGURE 1.14

Contributing Author: Linda J. DeBowes

Description: Normal anatomy.

Points Identified:

A. 408   C. 410
B. 409   D. 411

E. Pulp chamber
F. Pulp horn
G. Periodontal ligament space (radiolucent)
H. Lamina dura (radiopaque)
I. Mandibular canal
J. Root canal

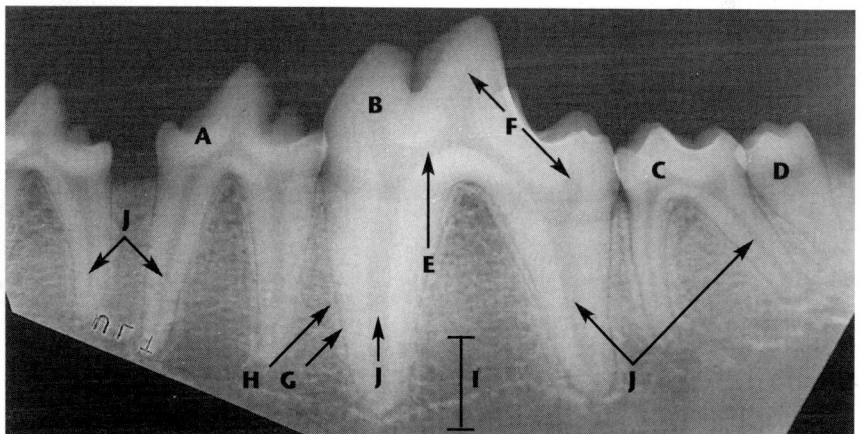

FIGURE 1.15

Contributing Author: Linda J. DeBowes

Description: Normal anatomy.

Diagnostic Keys: Same teeth shown as in Figure 1.12 at 10 months of age.

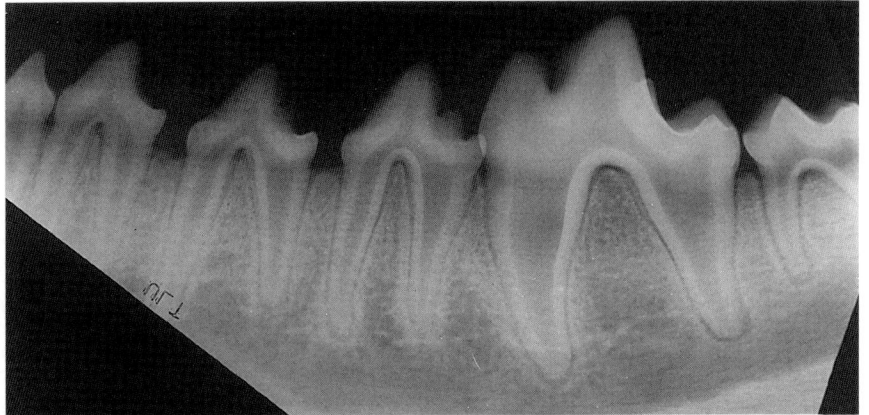

FIGURE 1.16

Contributing Author: Linda J. DeBowes

Description: Normal anatomy.

Points Identified:

A. Mandibular condyle
B. Mandibular fossa of the temporal bone

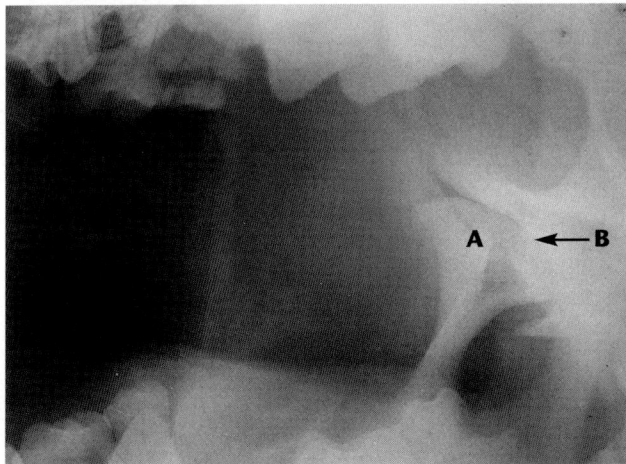

FIGURE 1.17

Contributing Author: Linda J. DeBowes

Description: Normal anatomy.

Points Identified:

A. Mandibular condyle
B. Mandibular fossa of the temporal bone
C. Retroglenoid process of the temporal bone

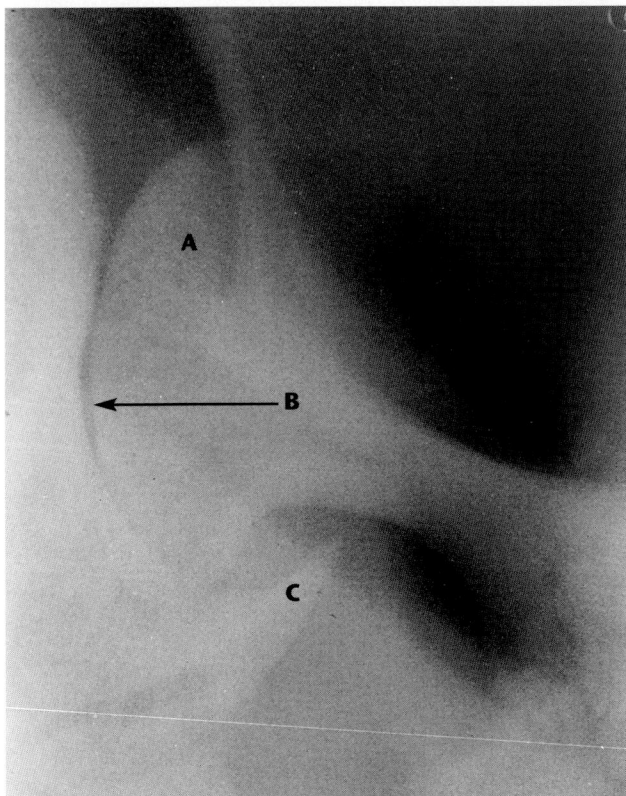

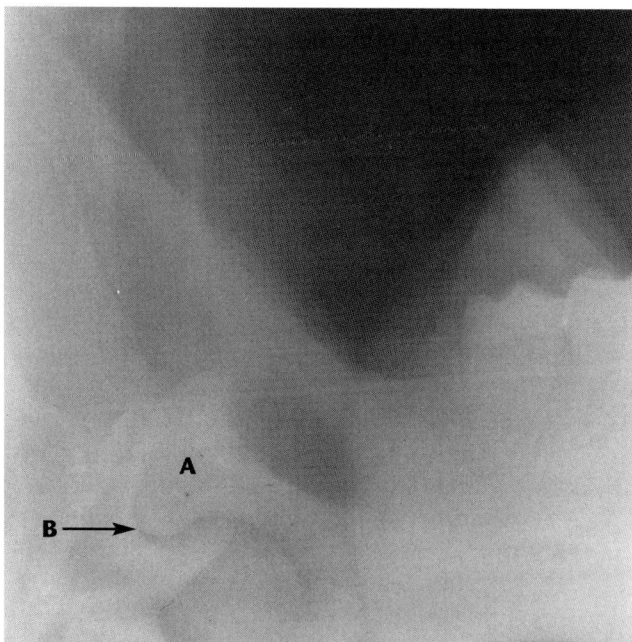

FIGURE 1.18

Contributing Author: Linda J. DeBowes

Description: Normal anatomy.

Points Identified:

A. Mandibular condyle
B. Mandibular fossa of the temporal
   bone

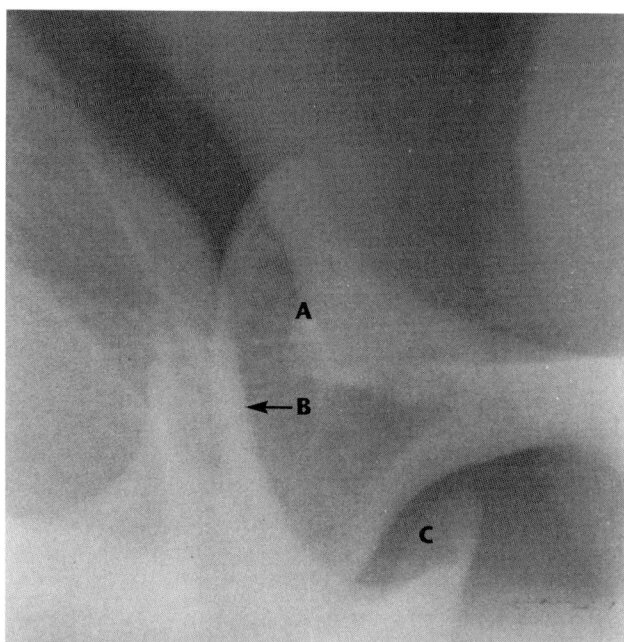

FIGURE 1.19

Contributing Author: Linda J. DeBowes

Description: Normal anatomy.

Points Identified:

A. Mandibular condyle
B. Mandibular fossa of the temporal
   bone
C. Retroglenoid process of the temporal
   bone

2 Canine Pedodontics

Dr. Robert B. Wiggs

INTRODUCTION

The following situations are shown on the radiographs in this chapter.

Normal Anatomy
- Pre-eruption of deciduous tooth buds in a newborn
- Pre-eruption of permanent tooth buds
- Deciduous teeth undergoing resorption for exfoliation
- Mixed dentition (4 months)
- Permanent immature (open apex)
- Intraradicular grooves

Developmental Abnormalities of Deciduous Teeth
- Missing deciduous teeth
- Supernumerary deciduous teeth pre-eruption
- Supernumerary deciduous teeth erupted
- Fusion tooth deciduous
- Gemination deciduous tooth
- Retained deciduous premolars

Acquired Abnormalities of Deciduous Teeth
- Fractured

Developmental Abnormalities of Permanent Teeth
- Missing permanent teeth
- Supernumerary permanent teeth erupted
- Supernumerary permanent tooth in anomalous site
- Peg tooth

- Fusion tooth permanent
- Gemination permanent tooth
- Dilacerated crown
- Microdontia
- Enamel hypocalcification (unerupted teeth)
- Retained deciduous with permanent impacted teeth
- Hard tissue impaction (mandibular cuspid)
- Impacted deformed tooth
- Dilacerated root
- Supernumerary roots
- Fused roots and ribbon canals
- Lateral canals

Acquired Abnormalities of Permanent Teeth (Crown Fractures)
- Apexigenesis—pulp capping procedure
- Apexigenesis bridge formation
- Apexification—procedure
- Apexification root closure

Oral Cleft Palates
- Wry mouth
- Primary cleft palate
- Secondary cleft palate
- Odontoma
- Dens in dente

Other Developmental Abnormalities
- Craniomandibular osteopathy

Normal Anatomy

FIGURE 2.1

Contributing Author: Robert B. Wiggs

Description: Pre-eruption permanent tooth bud identification, in the maxilla and incisal area of a 7-week-old female Doberman.

Points Identified: Permanent maxillary root incisor tooth buds (101, 102, and 103) and permanent right canine tooth bud (104).

A. 101	E. 501
B. 102	F. 502
C. 103	G. 503
D. 104	H. 504

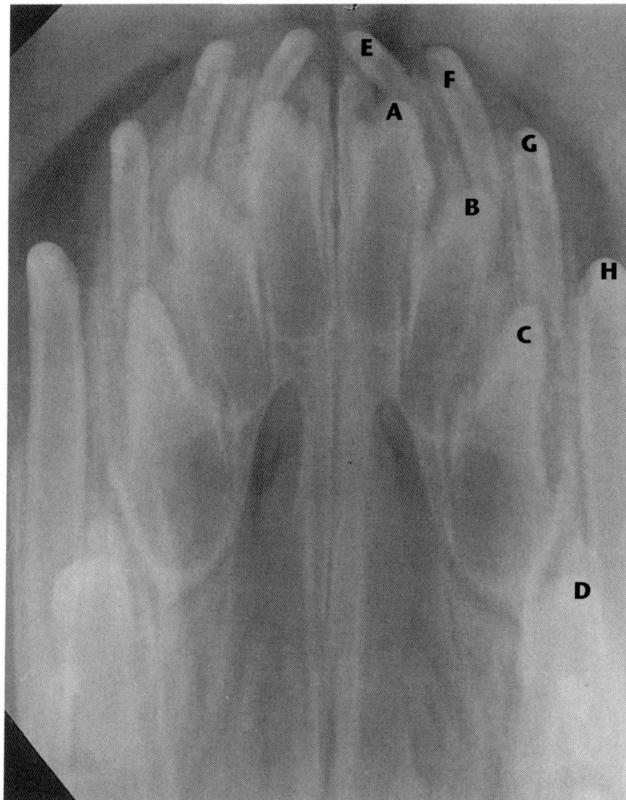

FIGURE 2.2

Contributing Author: Robert B. Wiggs

Description: Pre-eruption permanent tooth bud identification, in the maxilla of a 7-week-old female Doberman.

Points Identified: Permanent maxillary right premolar tooth buds (105, 106, 107, and 108). Note how permanent tooth bud for 107 sits mesial to (forward of) its deciduous counterpart (507).

A. 105	E. 506
B. 106	F. 507
C. 107	G. 508
D 108	

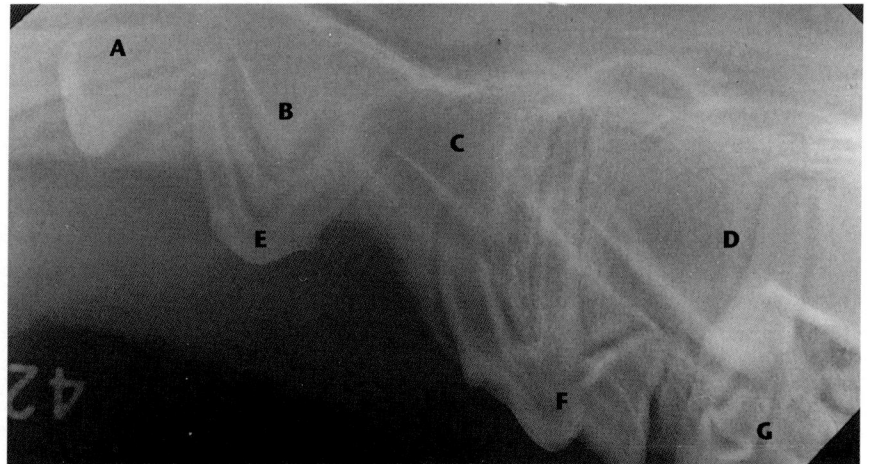

FIGURE 2.3

Contributing Author: Robert B. Wiggs

Description: Pre-eruption permanent tooth bud identification in the maxilla of a 7-week-old female Doberman.

Points Identified: Permanent maxillary right molar tooth buds. Note that maxillary molars 109 and 110 have no deciduous counterparts.

A. 109
B. 110

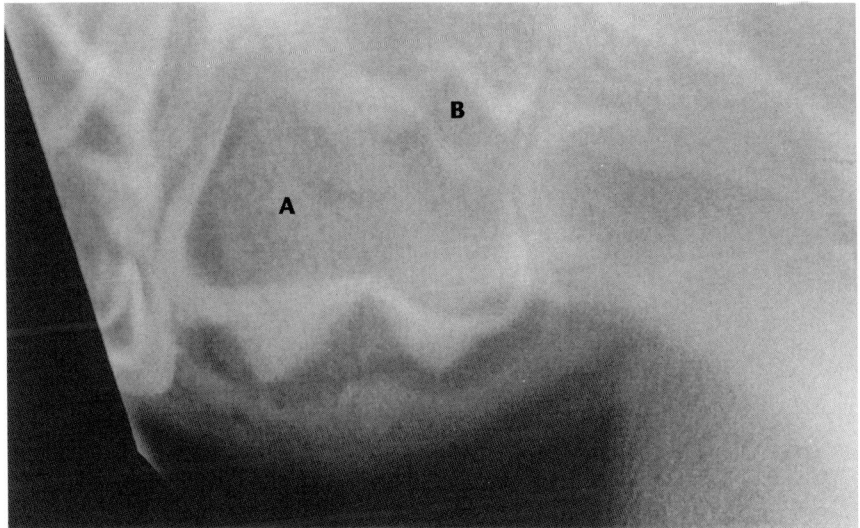

FIGURE 2.4

Contributing Author: Robert B. Wiggs

Description: Pre-eruption permanent tooth bud identification, in the mandible of a 7-week-old female Doberman.

Points Identified: Permanent mandibular right incisor tooth buds (401, 402, and 403) and permanent right canine tooth bud (404).

A. 401   E. 801
B. 402   F. 802
C. 403   G. 803
D. 404   H. 804

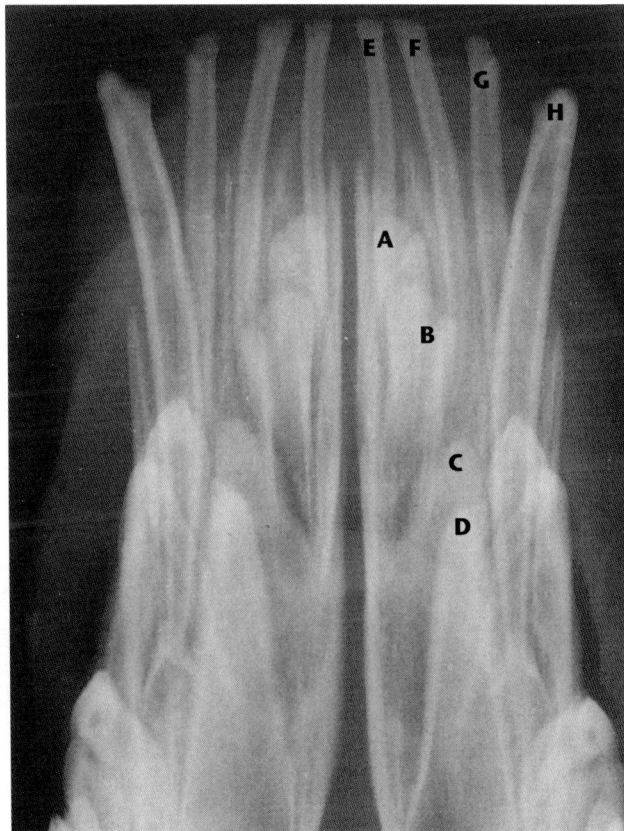

FIGURE 2.5

Contributing Author: Robert B. Wiggs

Description: Pre-eruption permanent tooth bud identification, in a composite film of the mandible of a 7-week-old female Doberman.

Points Identified: Permanent mandibular right premolar tooth buds (405, 406, 407, and 408) and permanent right molar tooth buds (409, 410, and 411).

- A. 405
- B. 406
- C. 407
- D. 408
- E. 409
- F. 410
- G. 411
- H. Deciduous cheek teeth

Diagnostic Keys: Notice that the tooth buds 401 to 410 are in the horizontal ramus, while 411 (mandibular third molar) is in the vertical ramus. Tooth buds 311 and 411

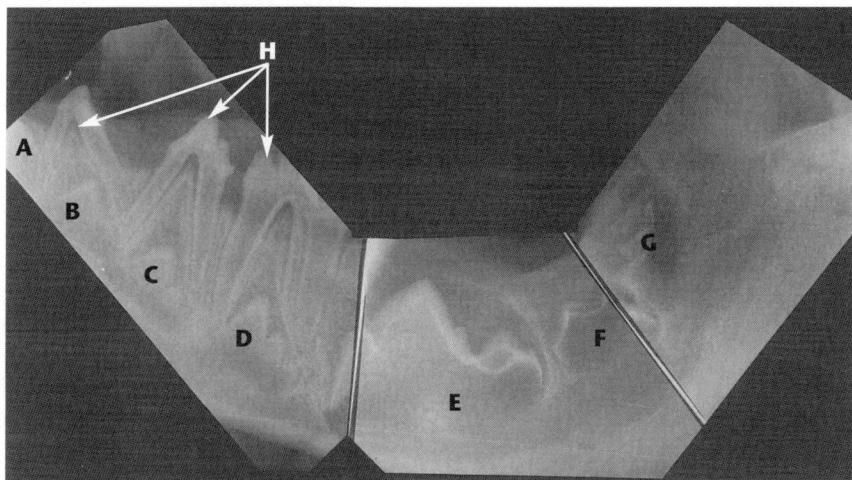

(mandibular third molars), being in the vertical ramus at an early age, are the most difficult tooth buds to isolate to identify. The mouth should be propped open and the film placed intraorally, parallel to the vertical ramus. The PID (position indicating device) should be placed at approximately a 45 degree dorsal angle to the film. This is the reverse of the 45 degree vertical angle to film typically used for the other mandibular teeth.

Please note the permanent second lower molar tooth buds (310 and 410) may also be found in the vertical ramus at an early age.

FIGURE 2.6

Contributing Author: Robert B. Wiggs

Description: Deciduous root resorption without permanent tooth buds present.

Points Identified: Mandibular deciduous cheek teeth 707 and 708. This is an example of the importance of pedodontic radiology in purebreds. A primary normal dentition does not guarantee that a permanent tooth is present.

- A. 707
- B. 708

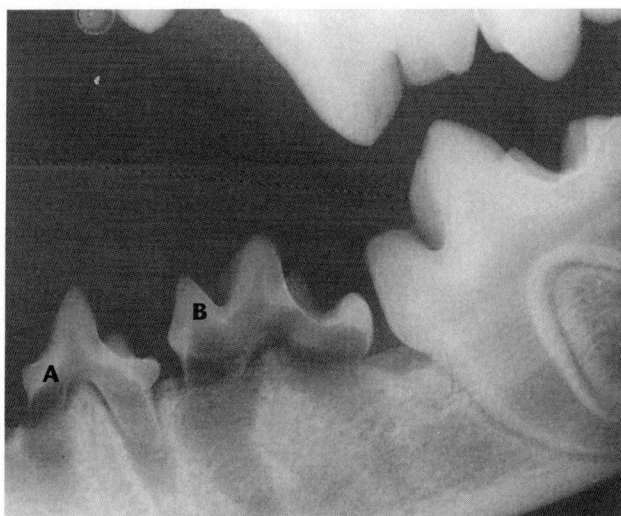

FIGURE 2.7

Contributing Author: Robert B. Wiggs

Description: Maxilla of a 6-month-old male German shepherd puppy. Mixed dentition (combination of deciduous and permanent teeth *erupted* in the mouth at the same time).

Points Identified: Permanent tooth buds. Deciduous teeth 603/604 and 503/504, still present. Note also open root apices of the erupted permanent maxillary incisors.

A. 101	H. 203
B. 102	I. 204
C. 103	J. 205
D. 104	K. 503
E. 105	L. 504
F. 201	M. 603
G. 202	N. 604

Diagnostic Keys: Note the large open root apices of the immature permanent developing teeth. This is a normal finding for this age. The apices close to form an apical delta as the teeth mature.

Common Errors: Primary and deciduous tooth buds are often confused.

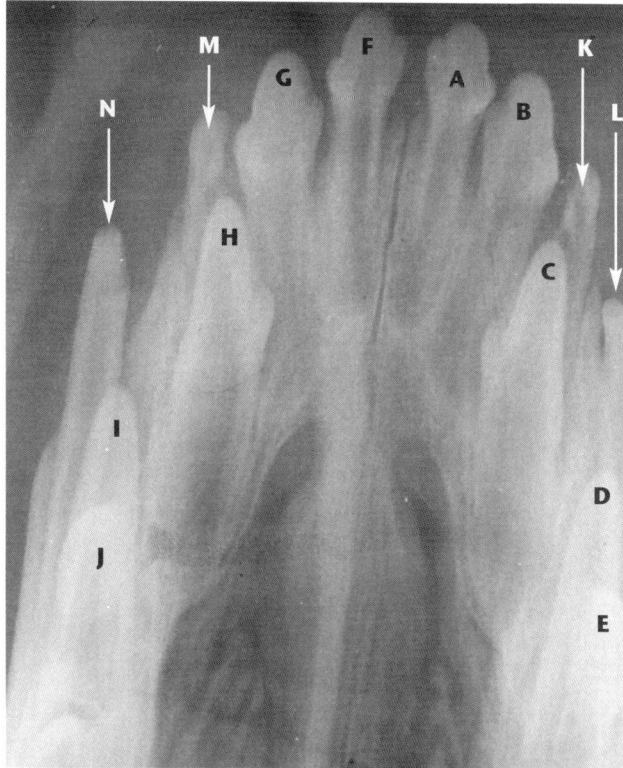

FIGURE 2.8

Contributing Author: Robert B. Wiggs

Description: Permanent immature teeth with open apices.

Points Identified: It is very important to determine if open apices are present if endodontic treatment becomes necessary.

A. Open apices of mandibular canines

Diagnostic Keys: Loss of density in deciduous root structure.

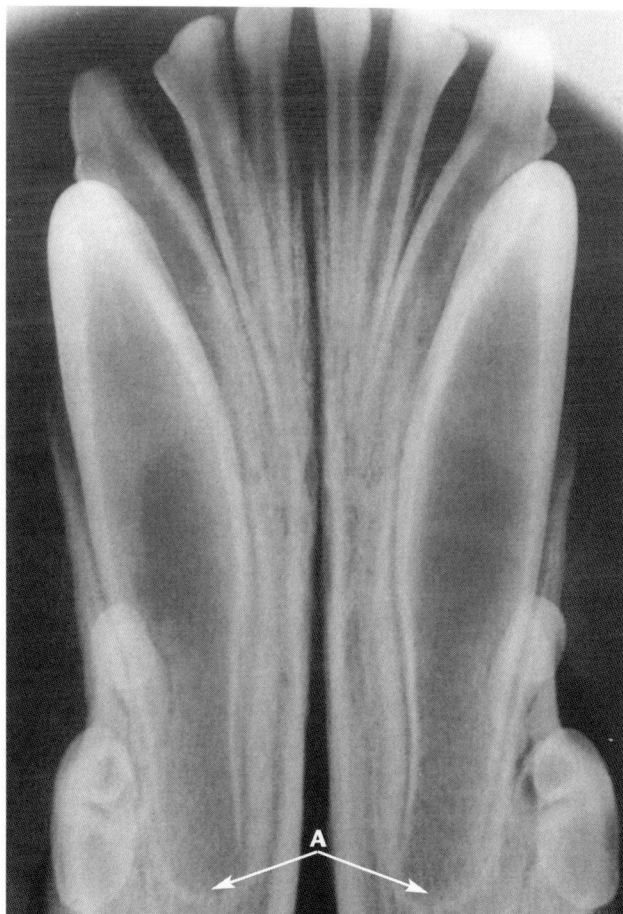

FIGURE 2.9

Contributing Author: Robert B. Wiggs

Description: Right mandibular cheek teeth in a 7-month-old male Labrador retriever.

Points Identified: Normal medial root intraradicular groove of the right mandibular first molar (409), which is found in many cheek teeth's intraradicular root structure.

A. 409
B. Normal medial root intraradicular groove

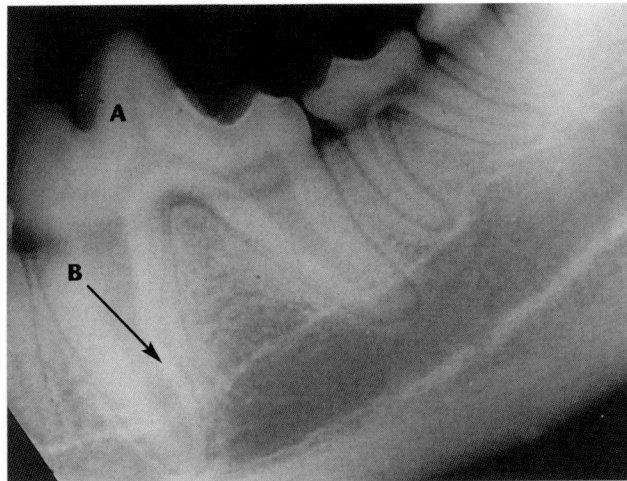

Developmental Abnormalities of Deciduous Teeth

FIGURE 2.10

Contributing Author: Robert B. Wiggs

Description: Missing deciduous teeth and their successional replacements in the mandible of an 11-week-old female Doberman.

Points Identified: Deciduous teeth and permanent tooth buds.

A. 302	J. 406
B. 303	K. 702
C. 304	L. 703
D. 305	M. 704
E. 306	N. 706
F. 402	O. 802
G. 403	P. 803
H. 404	Q. 804
I. 405	R. 806

Diagnostic Keys: Lack of deciduous teeth (701 and 801) and permanent successional tooth buds (301 and 401). The lack of successional tooth buds, when deciduous precursors are missing, is a common genetic defect.

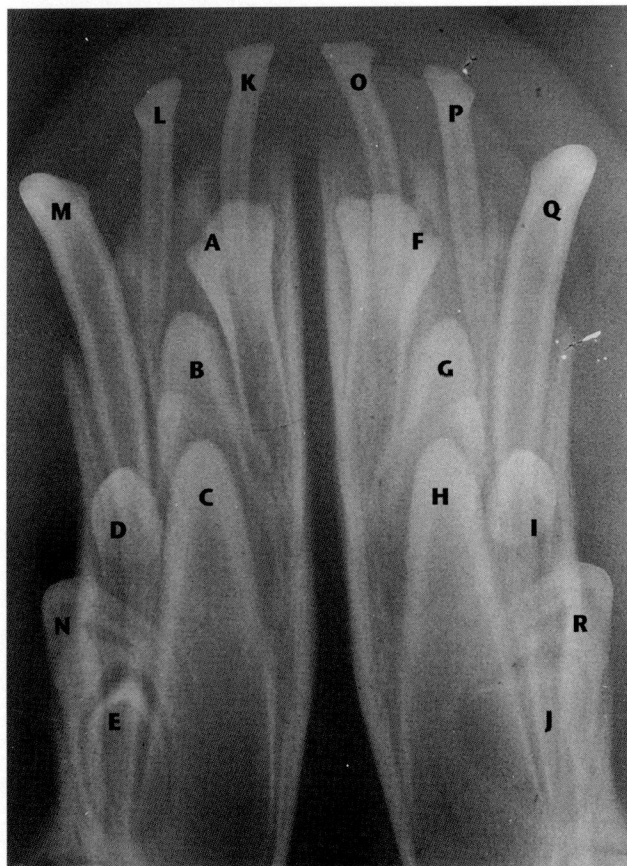

FIGURE 2.11

Contributing Author: Robert B. Wiggs

Description: Supernumerary deciduous teeth and successional tooth buds in the maxilla of a 9-week-old female Boxer puppy.

Points Identified: Supernumerary deciduous teeth and permanent tooth buds. Secondary anatomy would indicate the supernumeraries to probably be central incisors (S501 and S101).

A. S101	J. S501
B. 101	K. 501
C. 102	L. 502
D. 103	M. 503
E. 104	N. 504
F. 201	O. 601
G. 202	P. 602
H. 203	Q. 603
I. 204	R. 604

Diagnostic Keys: Supernumerary deciduous tooth (S501), and permanent successional

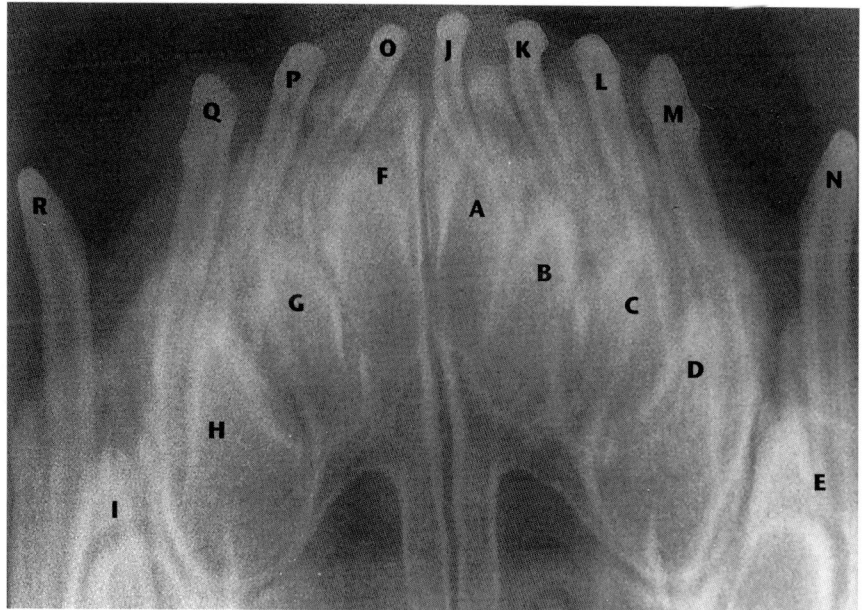

tooth bud (S101). Supernumerary permanent successional tooth buds are common in the genetic condition of supernumerary teeth when supernumerary deciduous precursors are present.

FIGURE 2.12

Contributing Author: Robert B. Wiggs

Description: Fusion deciduous maxillary incisor teeth in 8-week-old male boxer puppy.

Points Identified: Fused deciduous maxillary right central (501) and intermediate (502) incisor teeth.

A. 101	E. Fused 501/502
B. 102	F. 503
C. 103	G. 504
D. 104	

Diagnostic Keys: Note there are the normal number of permanent successional tooth buds in the right quadrant giving additional credence of the double-crowned deciduous tooth being a fusion tooth.

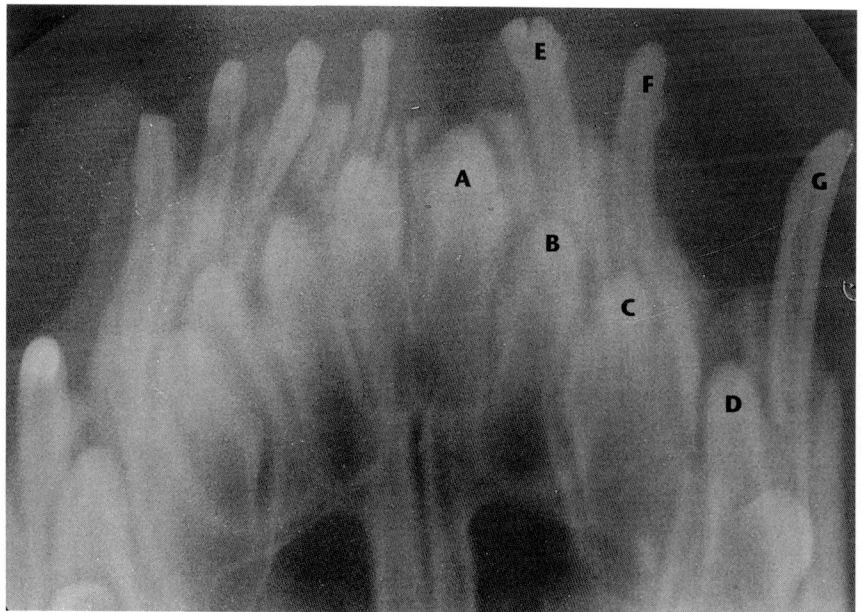

FIGURE 2.13

Contributing Author: Robert B. Wiggs

Description: Gemination deciduous maxillary right cuspid (504).

Points Identified: Note the double crown.

Diagnostic Keys: True fusion canine teeth are not possible since in the dog there is only one canine tooth per quadrant. *Therefore, double-crown or -bodied canine teeth must be some form of gemination rather than fusion.*

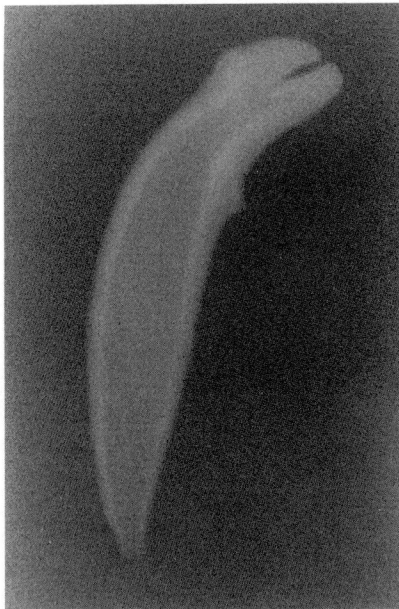

Acquired Abnormalities of Deciduous Teeth

FIGURE 2.14

Contributing Author: Robert B. Wiggs

Description: Fractured deciduous maxillary right canine (504) in a 10-week-old male Doberman.

Points Identified: Fractured cusp tip of maxillary right canine (504) with pulp chamber exposure.

    A. 504, fractured tip

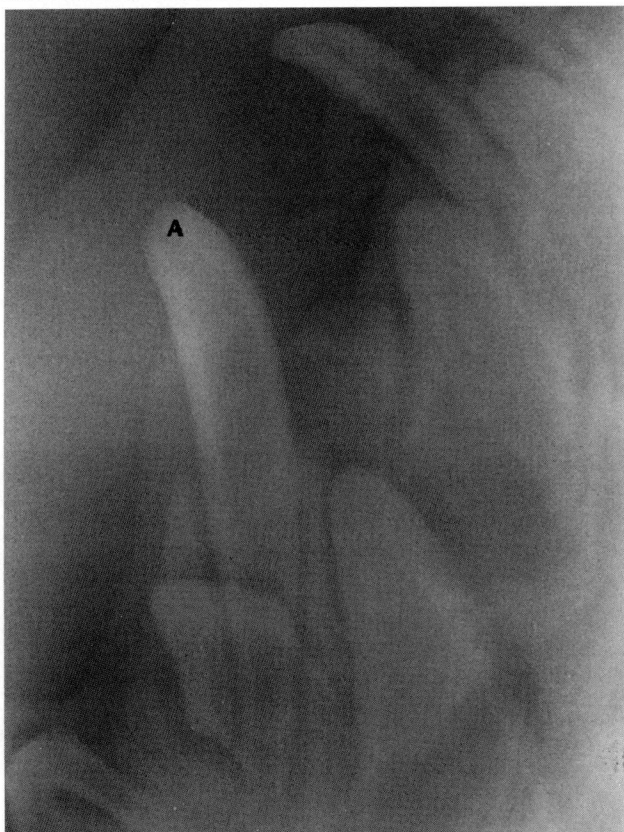

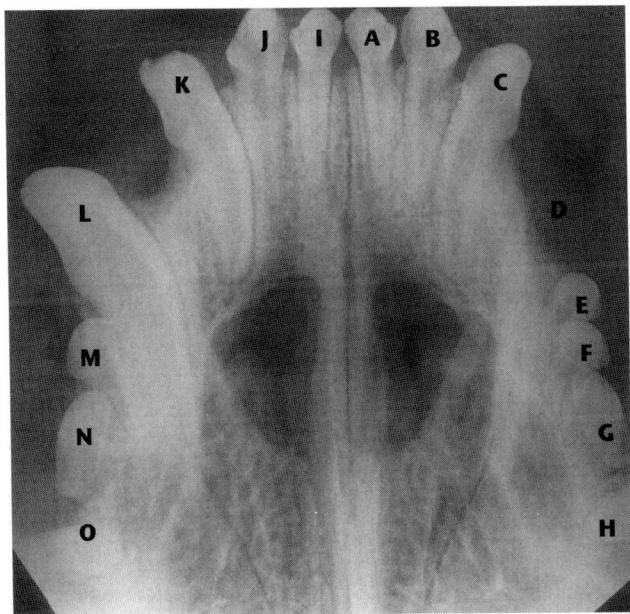

FIGURE 2.15

Contributing Author: Robert B. Wiggs

Description: Missing permanent tooth in the maxilla of a 7-month-old female boxer.

Points Identified: Missing permanent maxillary right canine (104), supernumerary right first premolar (S105), and rotation of both third premolars (107 and 207).

A. 101	I. 201
B. 102	J. 202
C. 103	K. 203
D. 104 (missing)	L. 204
E. S105	M. 205
F. 105	N. 206
G. 106	O. 207
H. 107	

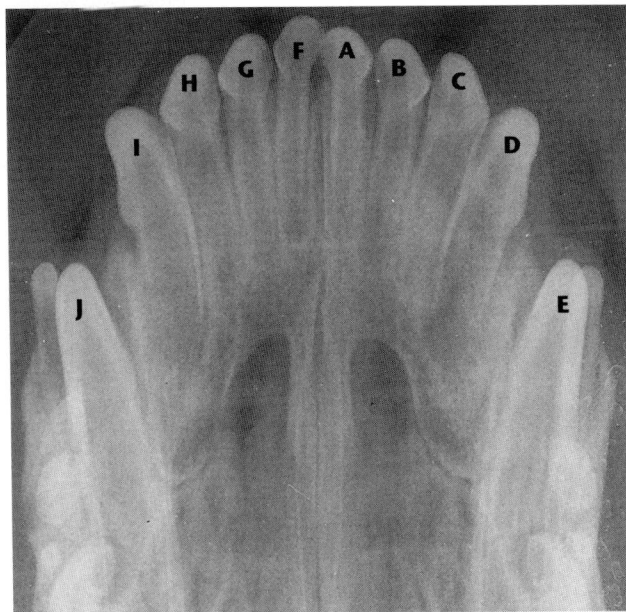

FIGURE 2.16

Contributing Author: Robert B. Wiggs

Description: Supernumerary permanent maxillary incisors in a 6-month-old female boxer.

Points Identified: Eight permanent incisors. Supernumerary maxillary first or central incisors (S101 and S201).

A. S101	F. S201
B. 101	G. 201
C. 102	H. 202
D. 103	I. 203
E. 104	J. 204

FIGURE 2.17

Contributing Author: Robert B. Wiggs

Description: Supernumerary permanent maxillary incisor erupted in an anomalous site (palatally).

Points Identified: Supernumerary maxillary left incisor (S202). From the secondary anatomy, it would appear to be a supernumerary second or intermediate incisor.

A. 101	E. 202
B. 102	F. S202
C. 103	G. 203
D. 201	

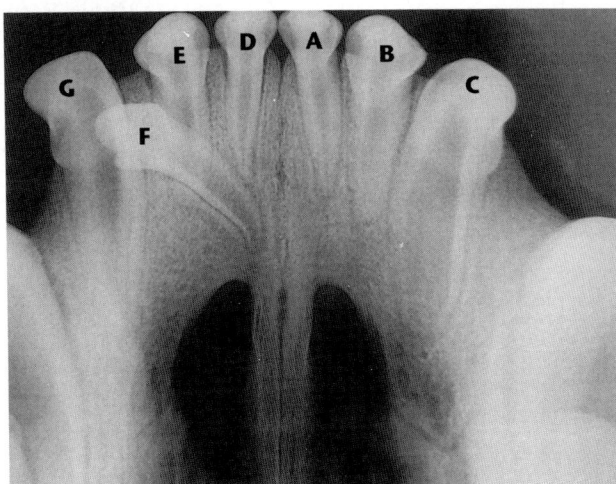

FIGURE 2.18

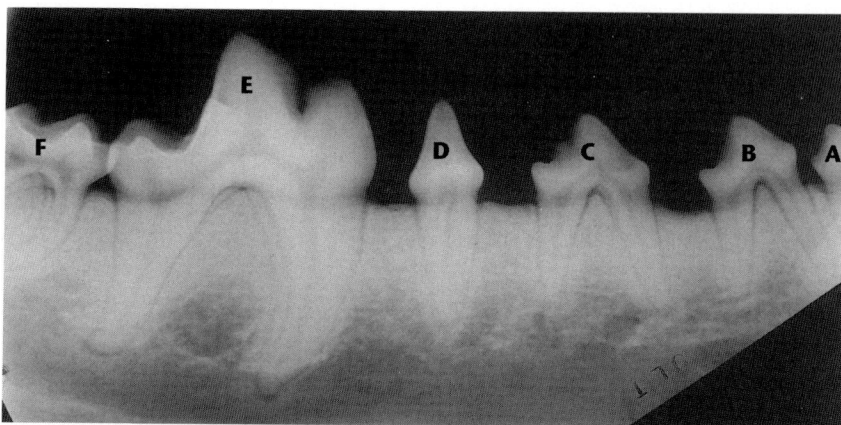

Contributing Author: Robert B. Wiggs

Description: Left side of the mandible in a 10-month-old male beagle.

Points Identified: The permanent mandibular left fourth premolar has a single root with a simple cusp crown and is a peg tooth (308).

A. 305	D. 308
B. 306	E. 309
C. 307	F. 310

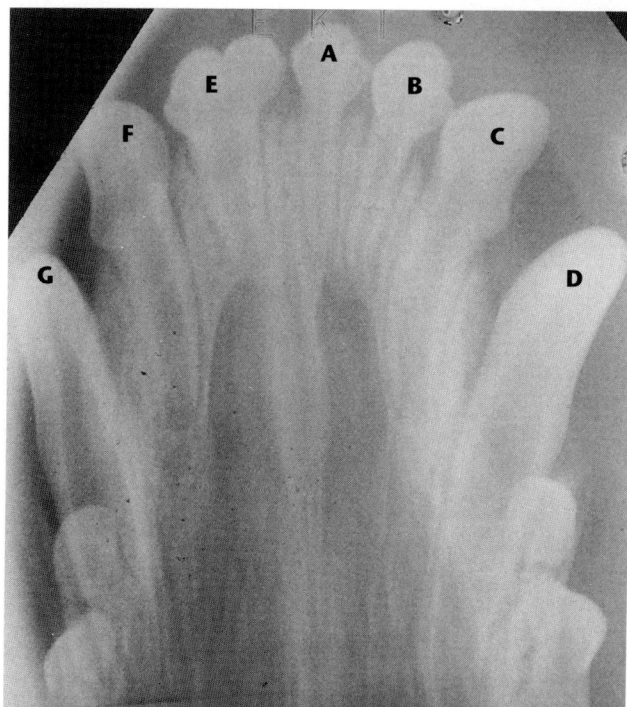

FIGURE 2.19

Contributing Author: Robert B. Wiggs

Description: Maxilla in a 6-month-old male cairn terrier.

Points Identified: The permanent maxillary left first (201) and second (202) incisors have fused into a single tooth.

A. 101	E. Fused 201/202
B. 102	F. 203
C. 103	G. 204
D. 104	

Diagnostic Keys: Notice there is only two left incisors and that the first has a double-headed crown. This distinguishes fusion from gemination.

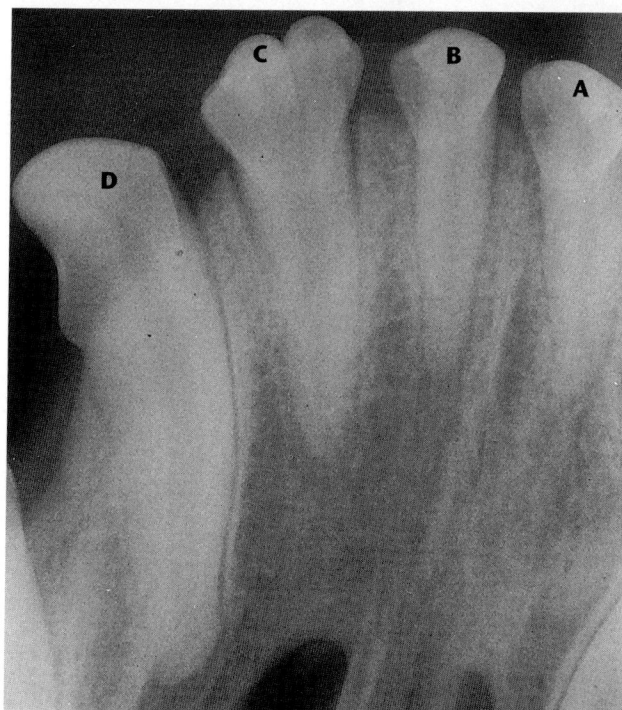

FIGURE 2.20

Contributing Author: Robert B. Wiggs

Description: Maxilla of a 9-month-old male German shepherd.

Points Identified: Permanent maxillary left gemination second incisor (G202).

A. 101
B. 201
C. G202
D. 203

Diagnostic Keys: Note the three left maxillary incisors. The second has a double crown, indicating that it is a gemination tooth (G202). Because all incisors are present, this is *gemination* rather than fusion.

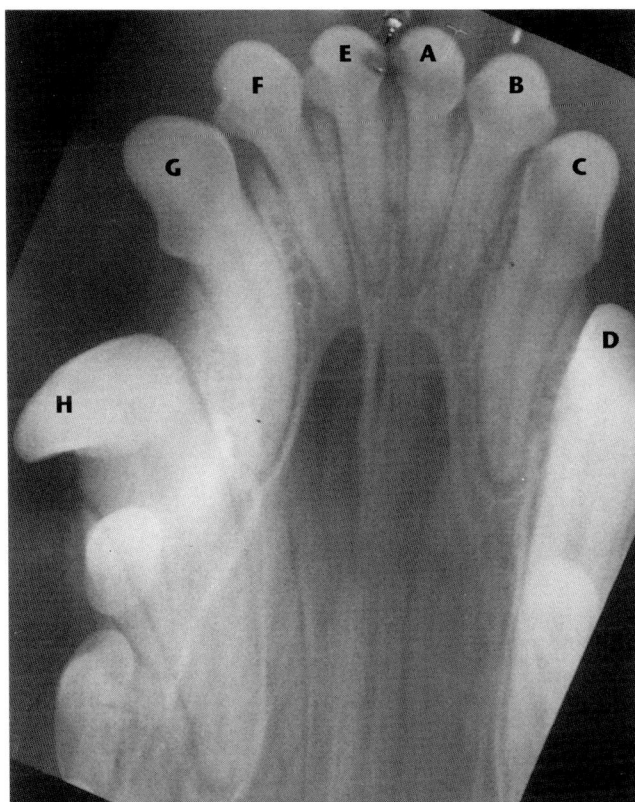

FIGURE 2.21

Contributing Author: Robert B. Wiggs

Description: Dilacerated crown of a permanent maxillary left canine in a male Shetland sheepdog.

Points Identified: The permanent maxillary left canine tooth (204) has an acute angulation or dilaceration of the crown. Dilaceration can be identified in crown and root systems of teeth.

A. 101	E. 201
B. 102	F. 202
C. 103	G. 203
D. 104	H. 204, dilacerated crown

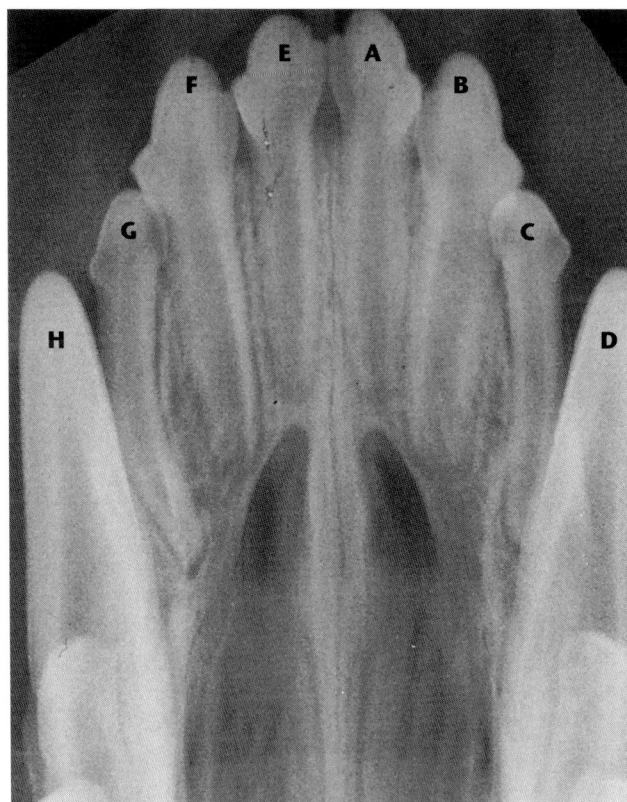

FIGURE 2.22

Contributing Author: Robert B. Wiggs

Description: Maxilla of a 6-month-old Australian shepherd.

Points Identified: Both permanent maxillary third, or corner, incisors are microdontia teeth (103 and 203).

A. 101	E. 201
B. 102	F. 202
C. 103	G. 203
D. 104	H. 204

Diagnostic Keys: Note the reduced crown size of the corner incisors (103 and 203). The reduced diameter of the crown will typically result in a root structure that is reduced in diameter correspondingly.

FIGURE 2.23

Contributing Author: Robert B. Wiggs

Description: Enamel hypocalcification or hypoplasia of permanent teeth in the mandible of a 6½-month-old male Labrador retriever.

Points Identified: The permanent mandibular left third incisor (303) shows irregular crown shape and poor root development indicating probable enamel hypocalcification. Additionally, the left canine tooth (304) also shows an irregular crown surface. Note the absence of 302 with possible root remnants present.

A. 301	E. 401
B. 302	F. 402
C. 303	G. 403
D. 304	H. 404

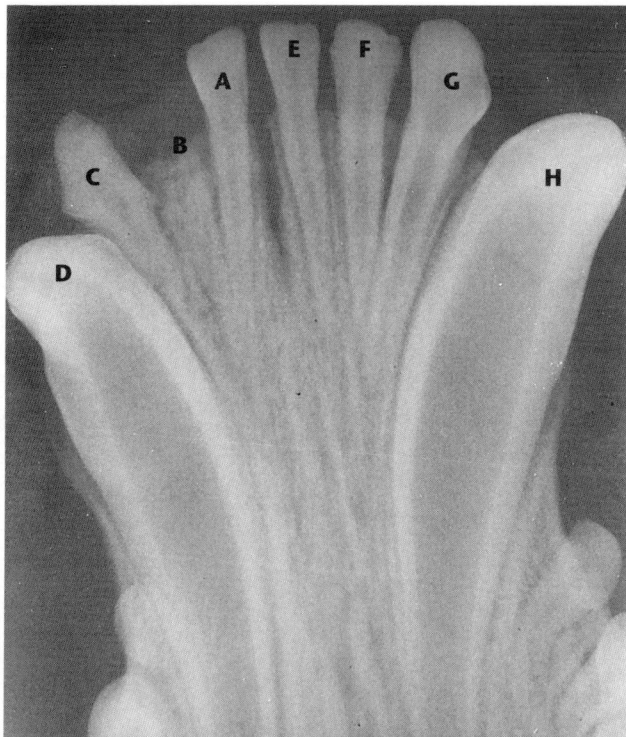

FIGURE 2.24

Contributing Author: Robert B. Wiggs

Description: Retained deciduous teeth, in an 11-month-old female Maltese.

Points Identified: The deciduous mandibular cheek teeth (806, 807, and 808), even with their root structures almost completely resorbed, have been retained over their permanent successors (406, 407, and 408). Note the crowding between 408 and 409 with a perfect area for periodontal disease to form in the interproximal space.

A. 806
B. 807
C. 808
D. 406
E. 407
F. 408
G. 409
H. Interproximal space

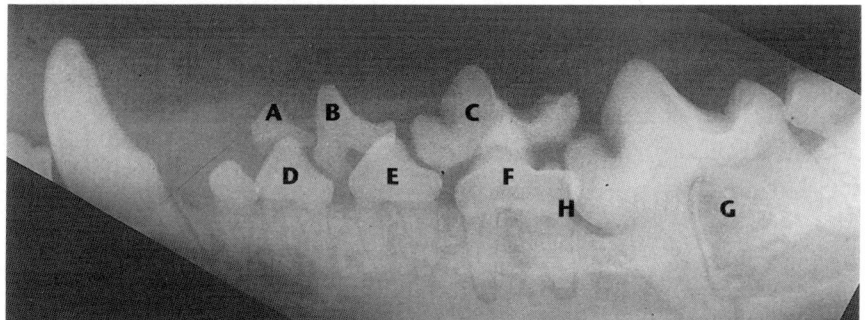

FIGURE 2.25

Contributing Author: Robert B. Wiggs

Description: Hard tissue tooth impaction in the mandible of a male German shepherd.

Points Identified: The permanent mandibular left canine tooth (304) impacted within the bone or hard tissue of the mandible.

    A. 304
    B. 404

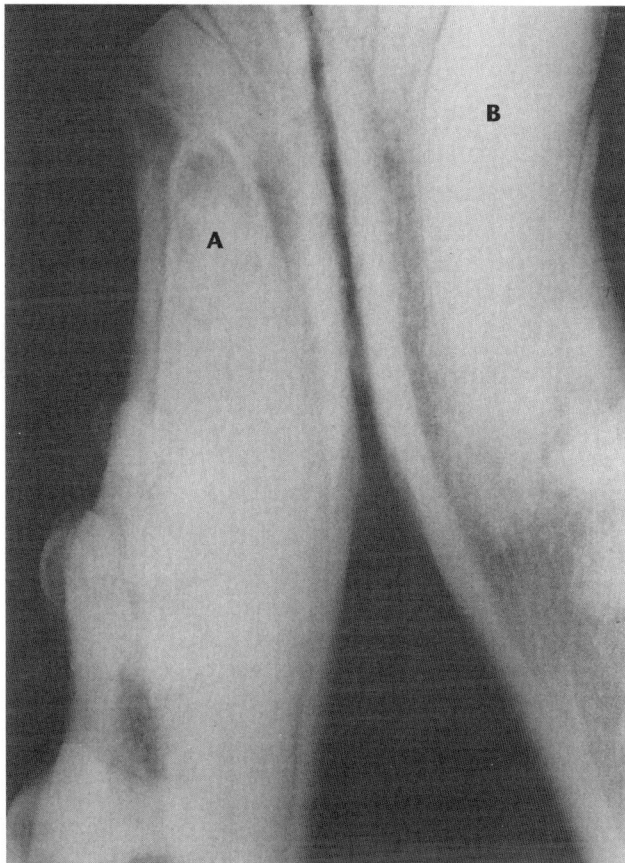

FIGURE 2.26

Contributing Author: Robert B. Wiggs

Description: Tooth impacted in the maxilla due to its malformation.

Points Identified: The permanent maxillary right canine (104) is microdontic, has a crown malformation, and is impacted in the bone or hard tissue.

    A. 104

Diagnostic Keys: When the crown is small in diameter, the root structure will typically also be reduced accordingly.

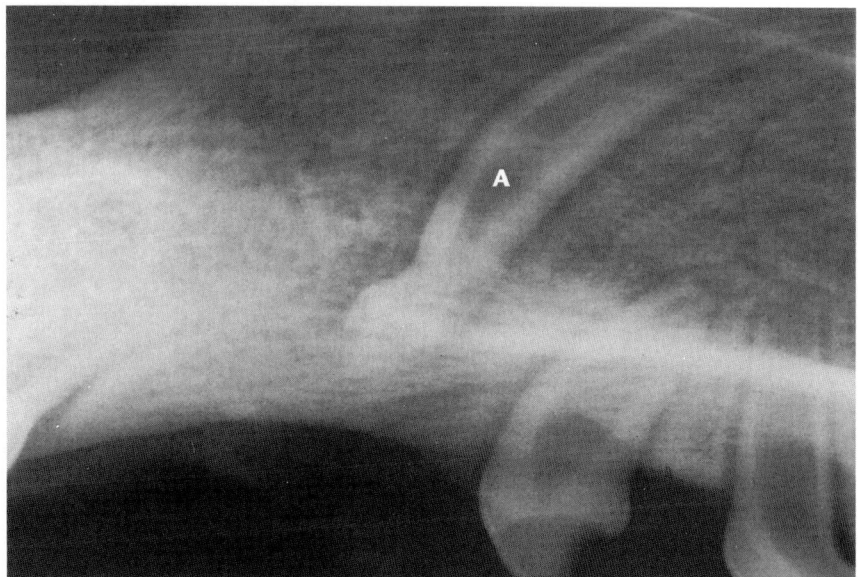

FIGURE 2.27

Contributing Author: Robert B. Wiggs

Description: Dilacerated root in the maxilla of a 7-month-old Shetland sheepdog.

Points Identified: The deciduous maxillary right third incisor (503) has been retained, deflecting the permanent successor's (103) development. This may have resulted in a dilacerated or crooked root.

A. 101
B. 102
C. 103
D. 104
E. 201
F. 202
G. 203
H. 204
I. 503

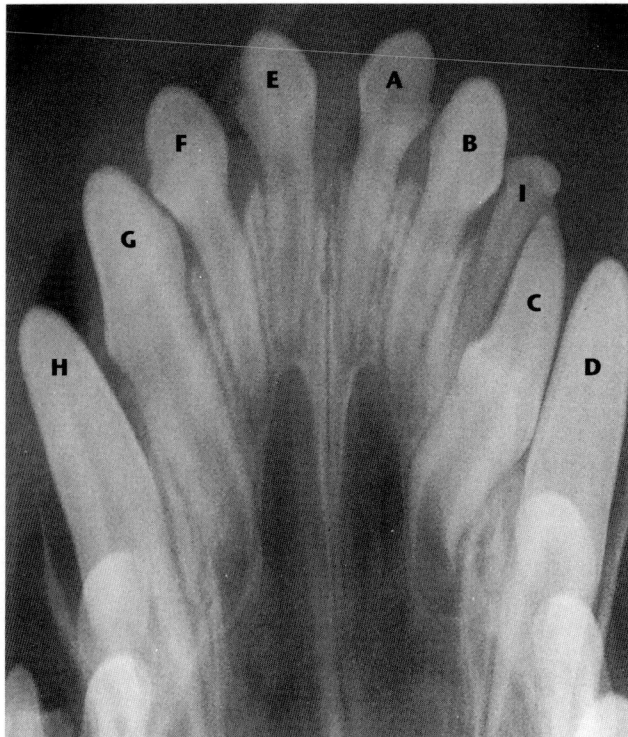

FIGURE 2.28

Contributing Author: Robert B. Wiggs

Description: Supernumerary rooted tooth in the maxilla of an 11-month-old Akita.

Points Identified: The permanent maxillary right third premolar (107) has a supernumerary third root. The upper fourth premolar (108) had been extracted at 6 months of age, due to trauma from being kicked by a horse.

A. 106
B. 107
C. 108 (missing)
D. Three roots on 107

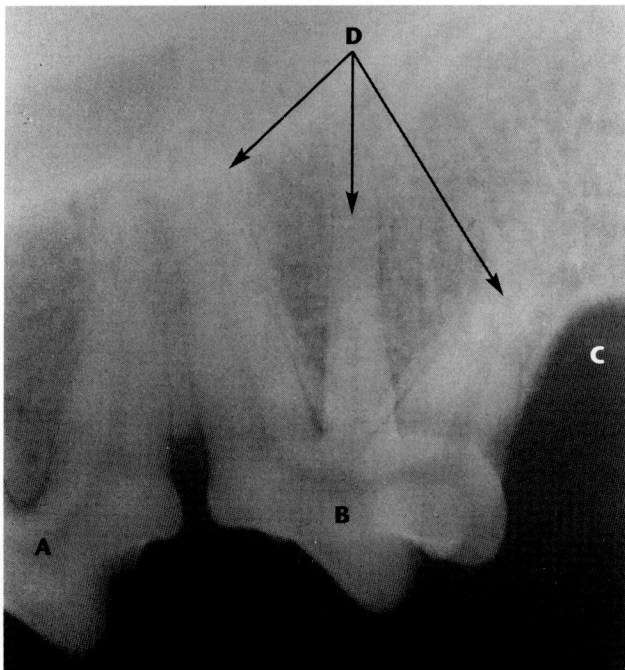

FIGURE 2.29

Contributing Author: Robert B. Wiggs

Description: Fused roots and ribbon endodontic canal in a permanent molar.

Points Identified: The permanent maxillary right first molar (109) has fused distal and palatal roots. Note the large continuous or ribbon canal connecting the two roots. Not all fused roots have ribbon canals. Dorsoventral view (left figure) and distomesial view (right figure).

    A. Ribbon canal
    B. Fused roots

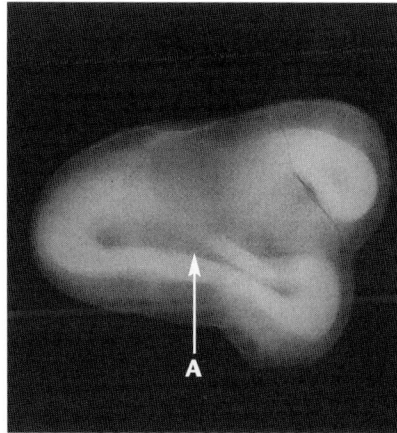

A

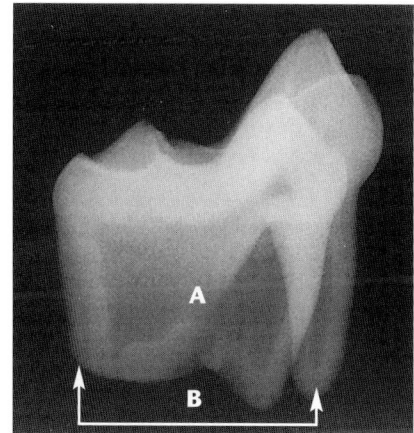

B

FIGURE 2.30

Contributing Author: Robert B. Wiggs

Description: Lateral or accessory canal in the endodontic root canal system of the distal root of a permanent maxillary premolar in a 4-year-old female Australian shepherd.

Points Identified: The endodontically treated permanent maxillary left fourth premolar (208). Notice the radiopaque obturation material has entered a lateral or accessory canal leading off the main endodontic root canal system of the intraradicular surface of the distal root. Notice the slight overfill of the lateral canal into the associated radiolucent area.

    A. Lateral or accessory canal
    B. Slight overfill of the lateral canal
    C. Radiolucent area

Diagnostic Keys: Most lateral canals are suspected from radiolucencies lateral to the root structure of endodontically compromised teeth. Typically, they are actually diagnosed either radiographically, during root canal procedures when radiopaque material is compacted into them, or by visual assessment upon extraction. This tooth must be followed carefully with postendodontic radiology to confirm that extensive pathology is not coexistent with the lateral canal (which would lead to endodontic failure).

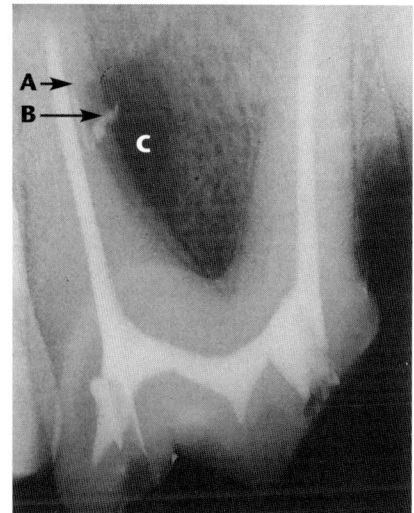

Acquired Abnormalities of Permanent Teeth (Crown Fractures)

FIGURE 2.31

Contributing Author: Robert B. Wiggs

Description: A direct pulping procedure (i.e., vital pulpotomy) of the permanent mandibular left canine (304) with pulp exposure in a still vital tooth. The pulp capping was performed in hopes of maintaining the tooth's vitality and stimulating continued root maturation and apical closure (apexogenesis) of the tooth in an 8-month-old female rottweiler.

Points Identified: Notice the open apex of the permanent mandibular left canine (304) and the radiopaque therapeutic material containing a calcium hydroxide base in the coronal segment of 304.

    A. Vital pulp capping agent
    B. 304
    C. Thin root walls
    D. Open apex

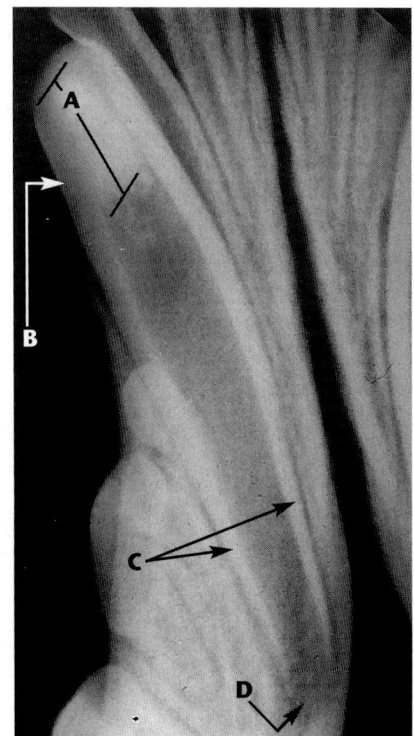

FIGURE 2.32

Contributing Author: Robert B. Wiggs

Description: Apexogenesis or the probable success of a direct pulping procedure of the permanent mandibular left cuspid (304). This is a follow-up radiograph of the previous radiograph shown in Figure 2.31, approximately 5½ years later.

Points Identified: Notice the dentinal bridge in the coronal segment of 304, the narrowing of the pulp cavity, thickening of the dentinal walls of the root canal, and the closure of the root apex, all indicating continued maturation and vitality of the tooth following the pulp capping procedure.

    A. Dentinal bridge
    B. 304
    C. Thickening of root walls
    D. Closed apex

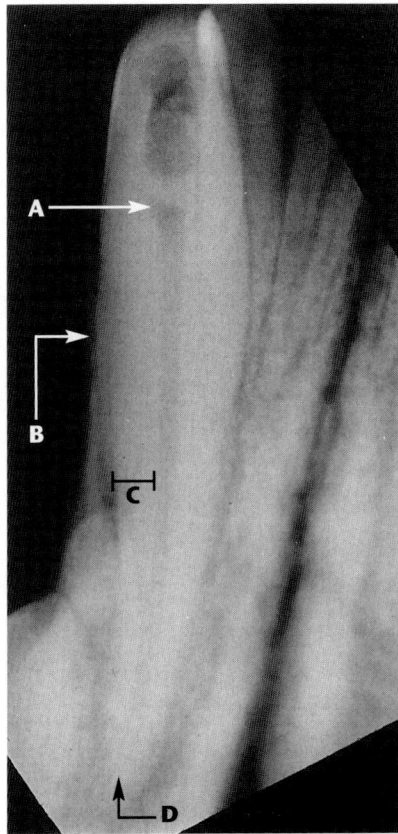

FIGURE 2.33

Contributing Author: Robert B. Wiggs

Description: An apexification procedure of a nonvital permanent mandibular left canine (304), in hopes of stimulating root closure (apexification) of the tooth in a 7½-month-old male Standard Poodle. Apexification therapy is performed in teeth with open apices, stimulating root closure so that a standard root canal therapy can be performed on the tooth to maintain function.

Points Identified: Open apex of permanent mandibular left canine (304). Radiopaque therapeutic material containing a calcium hydroxide base in the root canal.

    A. 304
    B. Therapeutic root canal filling material
    C. Open apex

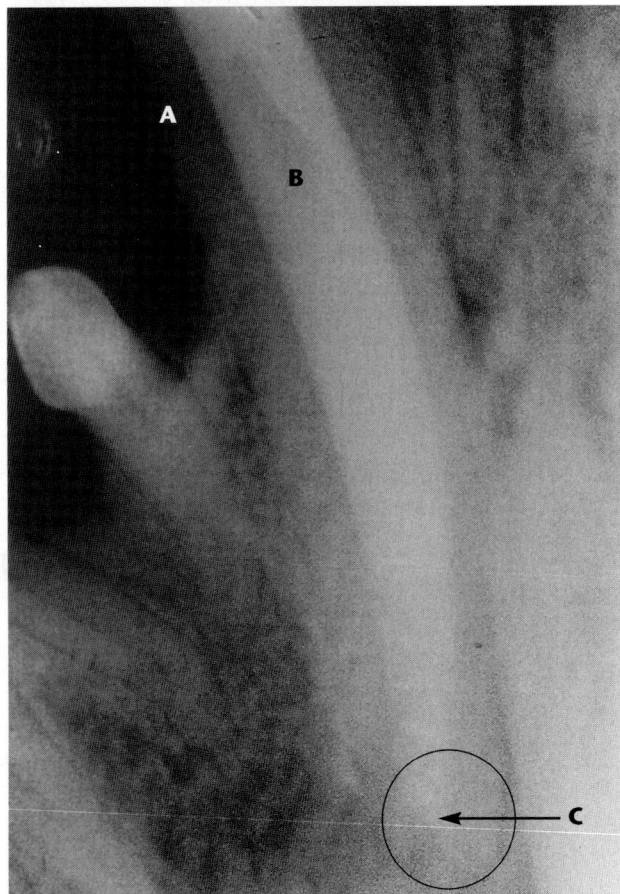

Oral Cleft Palates

FIGURE 2.34

Contributing Author: Robert B. Wiggs

Description: Maxillary wry mouth in a 4-month-old male German shepherd.

Points Identified: Note the reduced development of the left side incisal bone area, resulting in a curvature or wry effect of the maxilla to the left.

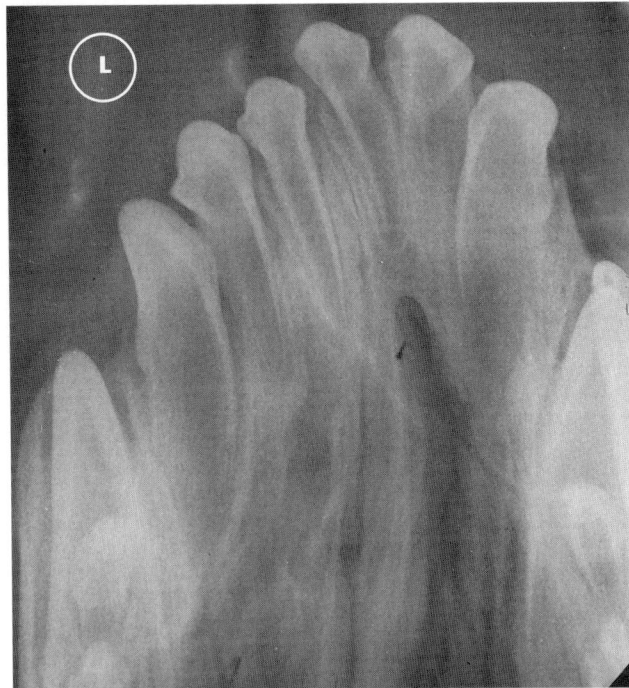

FIGURE 2.35

Contributing Author: Robert B. Wiggs

Description: Bilateral primary cleft palate in a 4-month-old female dachshund.

Points Identified: Note primary clefts; these typically express themselves physically as cleft lips. The incisal bone and the maxilla have failed to completely link together; this is a result of both maxillary processes failing to fully develop and properly migrate. Also note that 201 and 202 have fused, and that the deciduous and permanent third incisors (103, 203, 503, 603) are distal to the cleft.

- A. 103
- B. Fused 201/202
- C. 203
- D. 503
- E. 603
- F. Primary clefts

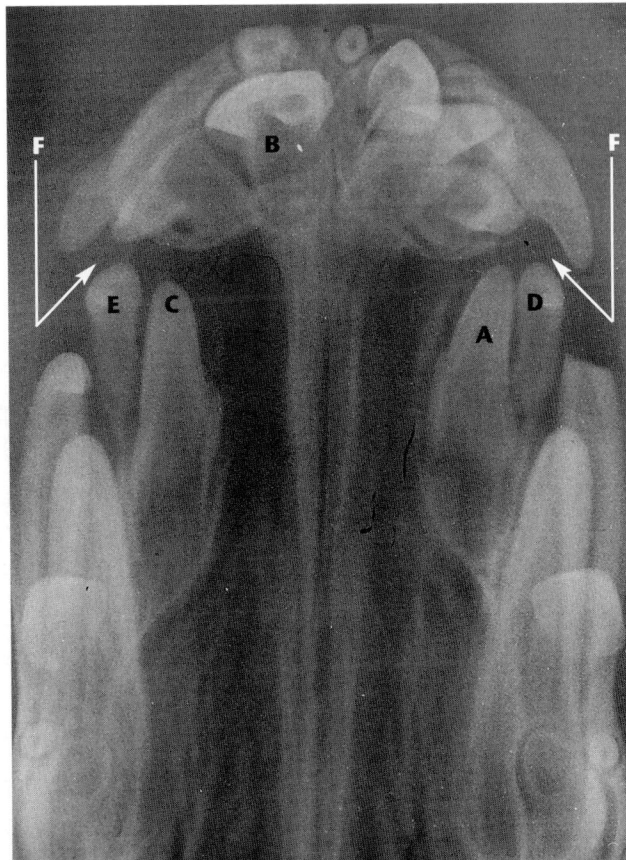

FIGURE 2.36

Contributing Author: Robert B. Wiggs

Description: A bilateral secondary cleft resulting in a cleft palate in a 7-month-old female basenji.

Points Identified: Note the large radiolucent areas behind the incisal teeth extending well back into the hard palate. This condition typically occurs due to the palatal plates of the maxillary process failing to develop and fuse with the opposite palate and the nasal septum.

A. Bilateral secondary cleft palate

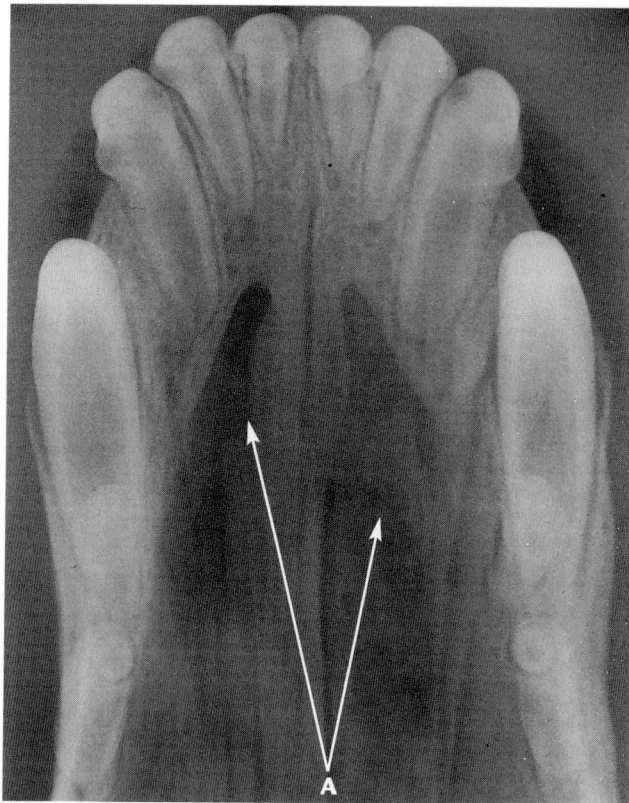

FIGURE 2.37

Contributing Author: Robert B. Wiggs

Description: Odontoma in a 3-month-old male basset hound.

Points Identified: Notice the severe displacement of the deciduous teeth and permanent tooth buds.

A. 101	K. 501
B. 102	L. 502
C. 103	M. 503
D. Odontoma	N. 504
E. 104	O. 506
F. 105	P. 601
G. 201	Q. 602
H. 202	R. 603
I. 203	S. 604
J. 204	

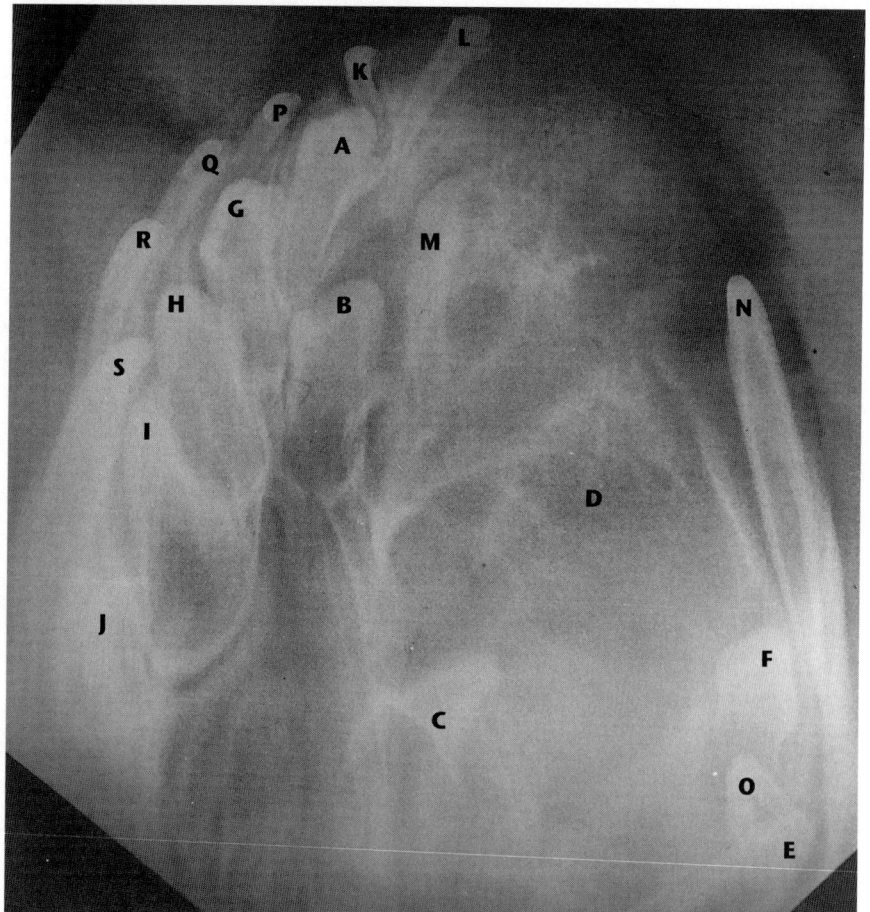

FIGURE 2.38

Contributing Author: Robert B. Wiggs

Description: Dens in dente 209 palatal root.

Points Identified:

A. Typical "tooth within a tooth" structure

Diagnostic Keys: A developmental tooth anomaly in which there is a deep invagination of lingual or palatal surface lined wholly or partially with enamel.

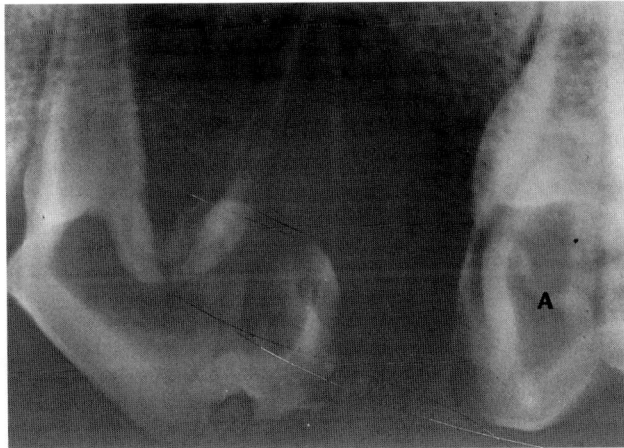

Other Developmental Abnormalities

FIGURE 2.39

Contributing Author: Robert B. Wiggs

Source: Film contributed by Bruce J. Kerns, DVM.

Description: Craniomandibular osteopathy in a 6-month-old Labrador.

Points Identified: Excessive periosteal new bone shown in mid- to caudal mandible. This patient is exhibiting no temporomandibular joint (TMJ) problems at this point. This condition usually ceases when the dog is skeletally mature.

A. Excessive periosteal proliferation

Diagnostic Keys: Mostly seen in small breeds (i.e., West Highland white terriers, etc.). Can also be seen in large breeds.

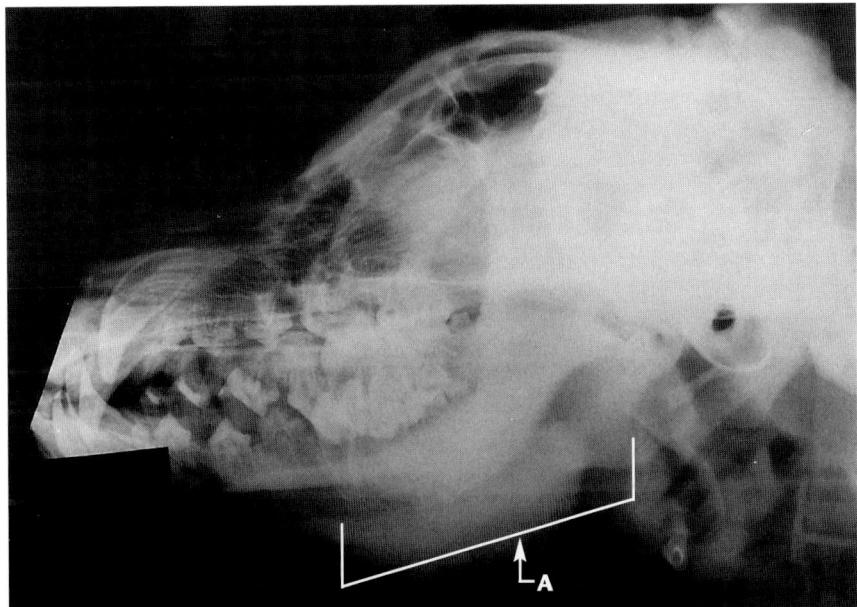

3 Canine Endodontics

Dr. Sandra Manfra Marretta
Dr. James M.G. Anthony

INTRODUCTION

Dental radiography is essential in the accurate diagnosis and treatment of endodontic disease in dogs. Numerous radiographic findings may aid in the diagnosis and confirmation of endodontic disease. Following the diagnosis of endodontic disease, dental radiography is required in the administration and postoperative evaluation of endodontic therapy.

Radiographic Diagnosis of Endodontic Disease

Endodontic disease in dogs is most frequently associated with acute dental trauma resulting in pulpal exposure. Other less common causes of endodontic disease in dogs include: rapid attrition, advanced periodontal disease, deep dental caries, and thermal or electrical injuries. Dental radiographs are imperative when attempting to assess the extent of endodontic pathology. Dental radiographs can depict the following radiographic changes commonly associated with endodontic disease: radiographic loss of tooth structure to the pulp canal, changes in the lamina dura, periapical lysis, apical lysis, large endodontic systems, destruction of periodontal structures, an sclerosis or lysis associated with osteomyelitis.

Radiographic Loss of Tooth Structure to the Pulp Canal

Dental radiographs may aid in the confirmation of tooth structure loss to the pulp canal. Usually this can be determined on gross examination of the tooth with a dental explorer; however, dental radiographs confirm the clinical examination (Figures 3.1–3.3).

Changes in the Lamina Dura

An important landmark in radiographic diagnosis of endodontic disease is the lamina dura or compact layer of bone lining the alveolus that appears as a thin white line next to the periodontal ligament. As the contents of an infected pulp exude through the apex, they cause changes in the shape and continuity of the lamina dura and in the width and shape of the periodontal ligament[1] (Figures 3.4 and 3.5).

Periapical Lysis

Periapical lysis refers to lysis of the bone around the apex of an affected tooth root and is commonly associated with chronic endodontic disease. This lesion appears as a dark halo around the apex of the root. When a multirooted tooth is affected with endodontic disease, one, two, or three roots may develop periapical lysis (Figures 3.6, 3.7, and 3.8).

Apical Lysis

Apical lysis refers to lysis of the apex of the root. This lesion appears as a destructive lesion of the apex of the root with only the coronal portion of the root remaining intact (Figure 3.9).

Large Endodontic Systems

Teeth with endodontic systems proportionally larger than their contralateral counterparts may be seen in teeth with endodontic disease. The larger endodontic system may be caused by a failure of the normal deposition of dentin because of pulpal injury at an early age. Larger endodontic systems my alternatively be secondary to endodontic resorption (Figures 3.10 and 3.11).

Destruction of Periodontal Structures

Endodontic disease and periodontal disease may occur concurrently in the same tooth. The classification and prognostic factors of endodontic-periodontic lesions in the dog has been previously described.[2] The three categories of endodontic-periodontic lesions include: Class I, endodontic-periodontic lesions; Class II, periodontic-endodontic lesions; and Class III, true combined endodontic and periodontic lesions.

A Class I lesion is usually caused by a fractured tooth, and grossly there is a narrow and difficult-to-probe "drainage canal" which exits near the gingival margin. Radiographically, Class I lesions have a typical J-shaped lesion around the apex with a narrower periodontal pocket at the alveolar crest (Figures 3.12, 3.13, and 3.14).

A Class II lesion is usually caused by a deep periodontal pocket extending to the apex of the tooth. Periodontal probing reveals a wide, deep periodontal pocket. Radiographically there is a wide, deep periodontal space extending to the apex (Figure 3.15).

Class III, true combined endodontic and periodontic lesions, occurs infrequently. Class III lesions have a wide, deep periodontal pocket and a fractured crown with pulpal exposure. Radiographically, a Class III lesion would typically have pronounced periapical lysis secondary to the fractured tooth with a deep, wide periodontal pocket.

Sclerosis or Lysis Associated with Osteomyelitis

Chronic endodontic disease may result in severe secondary osteomyelitis. Radiographic changes associated with osteomyelitis secondary to chronic endodontic disease include proliferation and lysis of the surrounding bone (Figures 3.16 and 3.17A-D).

Dental Radiography in the Treatment of Endodontic Disease

Dental radiography is essential in the successful perioperative management of endodontic disease. The different aspects of radiographic evaluation of endodontic therapy include preoperative, intraoperative, immediate postoperative, and long-term postoperative assessment.

Prior to the administration of endodontic therapy the tooth should be assessed radiographically. Preoperative radiographs will demonstrate the size of the endodontic system, the degree of apical formation, and the presence of root fractures, occluded canals, and abnormal root structure.

Size of the Endodontic System

Young dogs and cats have wide endodontic systems. As the animal ages, the endodontic system becomes more narrow (Figures 3.18 and 3.19).

Apical Formation

When an immature tooth is fractured it is important to radiograph the tooth because the type of endodontic therapy recommended will vary based on the presence or absence of an apex. Formation of an apex will permit administration of conventional endodontic therapy. The absence of an apex will necessitate alternative therapeutic modalities including a pulpotomy or apexogenesis in a vital immature tooth or an apexification procedure or extraction in a nonvital tooth (Figures 3.20 and 3.21).

Root Fractures

Prior to the administration of endodontic therapy a tooth should be radiographed to evaluate for the presence of root fractures. Failure to diagnose root fractures prior to the administration of therapy may result in failure of the endodontic procedure (Figure 3.22).

Occluded Canals

Older calicified root canals may appear radiographically as a very thin radiolucent line. These older restricted canals may not be amenable to complete debridement because of difficulty instrumenting the canal to the apex (Figure 3.23).

Abnormal Root Structure

Prior to the administration of endodontic therapy, it is important to reveal any abnormalities in the root structure. Abnormalities in root structure that may alter the endodontic therapeutic plan include additional roots and severely curved canals (Figure 3.24).

Intraoperative Radiography (Conventional Endodontic Therapy)

Dental radiography can be an important factor in the successful completion of an endodontic procedure. Immediately prior to the creation of a coronal endodontic access, a radiograph should be taken to help determine the ideal coronal access point. Teaching models, previously described, can also aid in the creation of the ideal coronal access point.[3-5] In the creation of one teaching model, barium markers were placed over the "ideal" endodontic access sites which were then used as guides for creation of the access sites (Figures 3.25, 3.26, and 3.27). An ideal coronal access point ensures a straight-line access to the apex and helps prevent iatrogenic perforation of the pulpal floor or pulp canal and metal fatigue, which may result in the breaking of endodontic files during conventional endodontic therapy (Figures 3.28, 3.29, and 3.30).

Intraoperative radiographs should be taken once the operator feels that the file has reached the apex. A radiograph at this time will confirm that the file has indeed reached the apex (Figure 3.31).

During the endodontic procedure, if bleeding persists either the pulp has not been completely removed or the apex of the tooth has been perforated. A radiograph can delineate between these two causes of persistent intraoperative hemorrhage (Figure 3.32).

After filling the root canal with the endodontic filling material but prior to placement of the restorative material in the access site, a radiograph should be taken to ensure complete filling of the canal (Figures 3.33, 3.34, and 3.36). Once a complete fill has been achieved the access site can be restored and a final postoperative radiograph is taken (Figures 3.35 and 3.37).

Intraoperative Radiography (Surgical Endodontic Therapy)

The initial radiographic assessment for surgical endodontic therapy is the same as conventional endodontic therapy since surgical endodontic therapy is preceded by conventional endodontic therapy. Immediately prior to the creation of a surgical endodontic access, a radiograph should be taken to help determine the ideal surgical access point. Teaching models previously described can aid in the creation of the ideal surgical access point[6] (Figure 3.38). A postoperative radiograph is taken following placement of the retrograde amalgam filling (Figure 3.39).

Long-Term Postoperative Radiography (Pulpotomies and Conventional and Surgical Endodontic Therapy)

Long-term postoperative radiography is imperative in the evaluation of endodontic procedures. The purpose of long-term postoperative radiography following pulpotomies and conventional and surgical endodontic therapy is to evaluate the success or failure of the procedure. Long-term postoperative radiographs following a successful pulpotomy will demonstrate a dentinal bridge 6 months postoperatively (Figure 3.40). An unsuccessful pulpotomy procedure may appear 6 months postoperatively with a failure to deposit secondary dentin, a failure of apical formation, and/or periapical lysis. Long-term postoperative radiographs of successful conventional and surgical endodontic procedures will demonstrate no further evidence of periapical lysis, while unsuccessful conventional and surgical endodontic procedures will demonstrate periapical or apical lysis (Figure 3.41).

Failure to adequately utilize dental radiography in the management of endodontic disease in dogs can have devastating results. Conversely, proper utilization of dental radiography can serve to improve the veterinarian's diagnostic skills and management of endodontic disease in the dog.

References

1. Harvey CE, Emily PP. Endodontics (clinical and radiographic examination). In *Small Animal Dentistry*. Philadelphia:WB Saunders, 1993, 162–65.

2. Manfra Maretta S, Schloss AJ, Klippert LS. Classification and prognostic factors of endodontic-periodontic lesions in the dog. *Jour Vet Dent* 9(2):27–30 (1992).

3. Manfra Marretta S, Golab G, Anthony JMG, Cloran J, Klippert LS. Development of a teaching model for coronal access to the canine dentition. *Jour Vet Dent* 9(4):11–17 (1992).

4. Manfra Marretta S, Golab G, Anthony JMG, Cloran J, Klippert LS. Ideal coronal endodontic access points for the canine dentition. *Jour Vet Dent* 10(4):12–15 (1993).

5. Visser CJ. Coronal access of the canine dentition. *Jour Vet Dent* 8(4):12–16 (1991).

6. Manfra Marretta S, Eurell J, Klippert LS. Development of a teaching model for surgical endodontic access sites in the canine. *Jour Vet Dent* (accepted July 1994).

X-RAY PLATES

FIGURE 3.1

Contributing Author:
Sandra Manfra Marretta

Description: Radiograph of a 4-year-old Labrador retriever following a fall. Note the fractured maxillary canine crown with extension of the fracture line through the pulp canal.

Points Identified: Fracture in 204. There is no radiographic evidence of endodontic pathology (root apex) at this time.

A. Short oblique fracture through pulp canal, 204

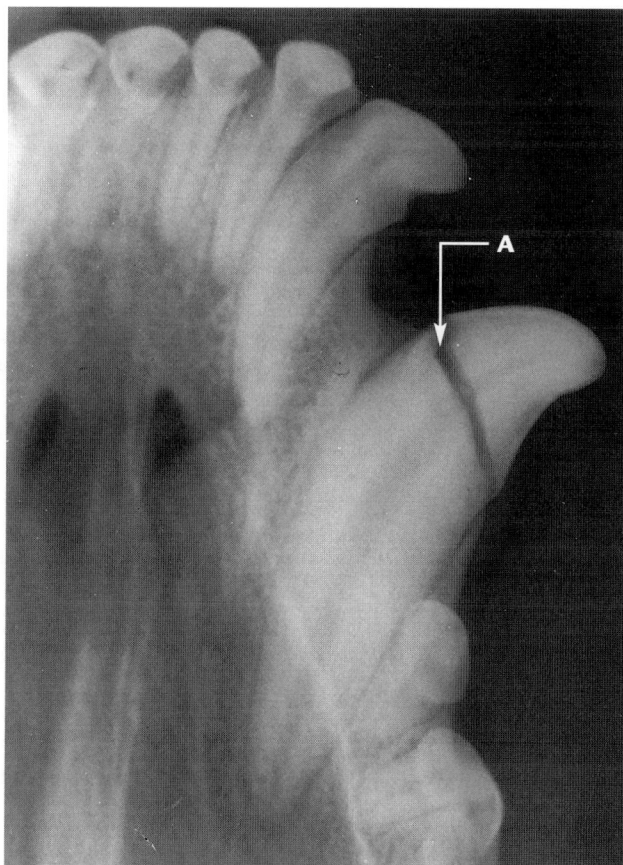

FIGURE 3.2

Contributing Author:
Sandra Manfra Marretta

Description: Radiograph of the rostral mandible of a 7-year-old Doberman pinscher with a history of difficulty eating and hypersalivation. Note the several worn crowns of the incisors and canine teeth. Radiographically the pulp of these teeth appears to be exposed. Pulpal exposure was confirmed with a dental explorer.

Points Identified:

A. Attrition of canines and incisors with pulp exposure
B. Apical osteolysis
C. Root resorption

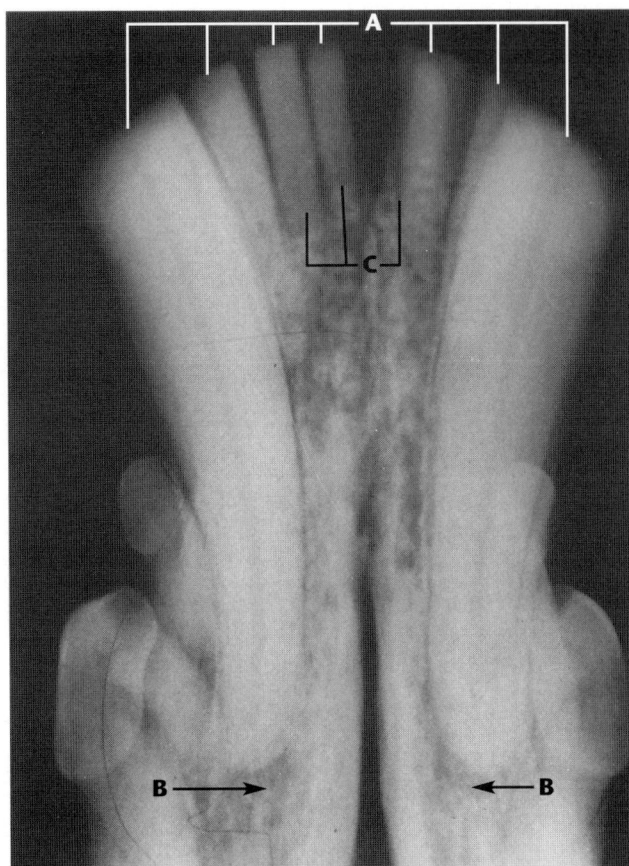

FIGURE 3.3

Contributing Author:
Sandra Manfra Marretta

Description: Radiograph of a 7-year-old basset hound with severe dental caries of the right second mandibular molar (410). Note the periapical lysis of both the mesial and distal roots because of endodontic disease secondary to the loss of crown structure.

Points Identified: 410, crown already amputated and roots hemisected.

A. Periapical pathology due to endodontic disease, 410
B. Hemisected roots, 410

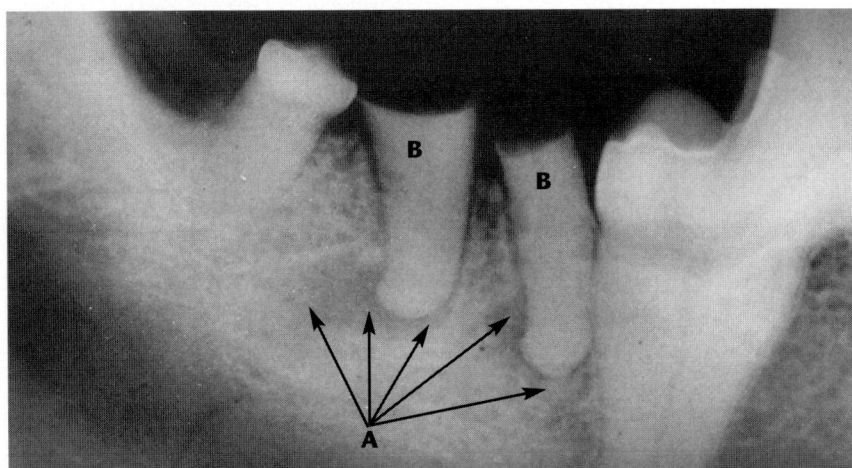

FIGURE 3.4

Contributing Author:
Sandra Manfra Marretta

Description: The fractured maxillary right second incisor in this 1-year-old golden retriever demonstrates a loss of detail of the lamina dura around the apex when compared to the lamina dura of the intact maxillary left second incisor.

Points Identified: Root apex showing inconsistent apical detail that is consistent with early endodontic pathology.

    A. 102, root apex
    B. 202, root apex

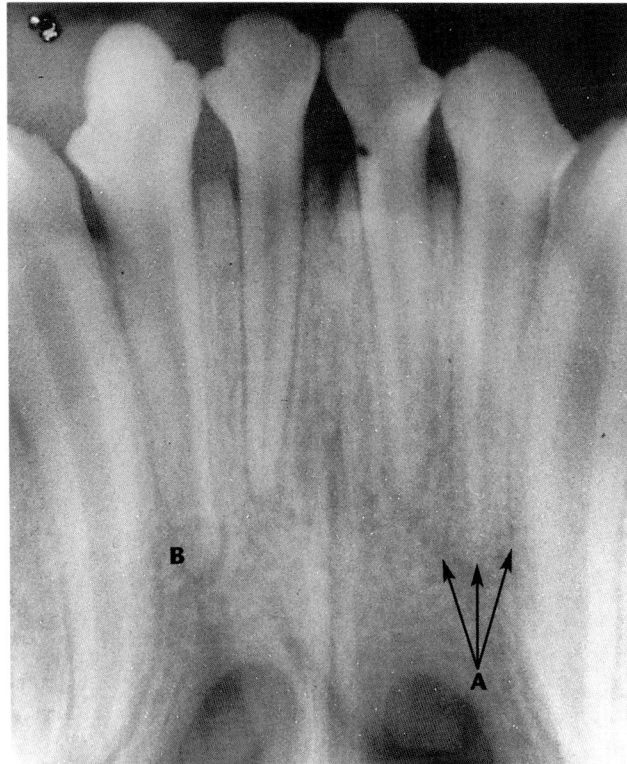

FIGURE 3.5

Contributing Author:
Sandra Manfra Marretta

Description: Left maxillary fourth premolar (208) with a slab fracture and secondary pulpal exposure. Note the loss in shape and continuity of the lamina dura in the apical region of the distal root.

Points Identified:

    A. 208
    B. Apical pathology of distal root

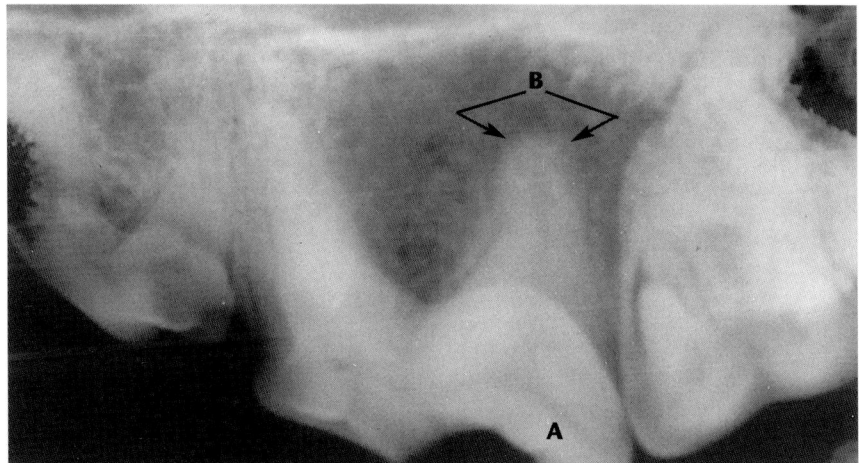

FIGURE 3.6

Contributing Author:
Sandra Manfra Marretta

Description: Intraoperative radiograph of a 2-year-old mixed breed dog who was presented with a fractured right mandibular canine tooth (404). Note the lysis around the apex of the canine tooth.

Points Identified:

A. 404
B. Periapical lytic area

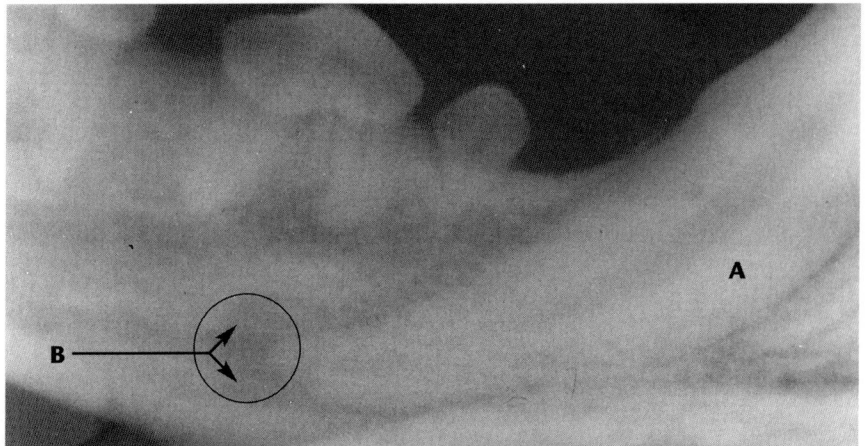

FIGURE 3.7

Contributing Author:
Sandra Manfra Marretta

Description: Radiograph of the mandibular first molar (309) of a 4-year-old Shetland sheepdog. Note the periapical lysis around the mesial and distal roots.

Points Identified:

A. 309
B. Periapical lysis involving both roots

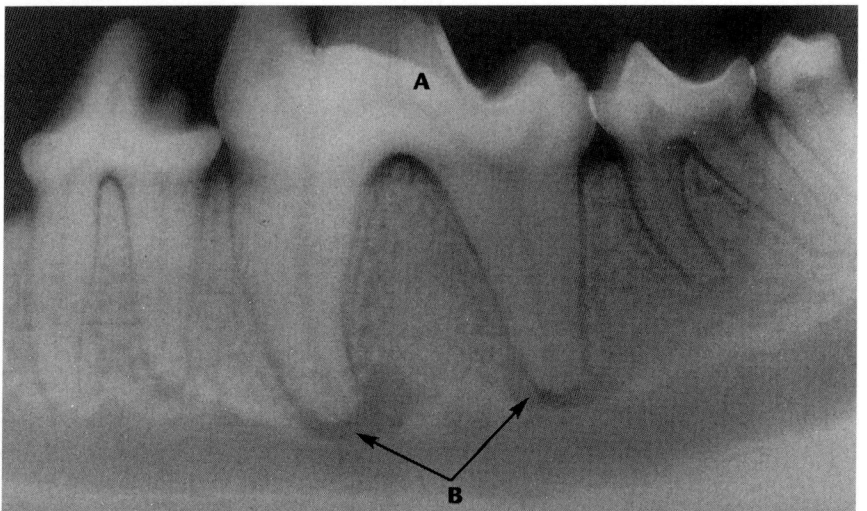

FIGURE 3.8

Contributing Author:
Sandra Manfra Marretta

Description: Radiograph (using the caudal oblique bisecting angle technique) of a 10-year-old mixed breed dog presented because of left-sided facial swelling in the region of the maxillary fourth premolar (208). The maxillary fourth premolar was fractured and the pulp was chronically exposed. Note the large area of radiolucency around the apex of the distal root and the smaller areas of radiolucency around the apices of the mesiobuccal and palatal roots.

Points Identified: 208. Palatal root appears central on x-ray between the mesiobuccal (rostral) and distal roots. All three roots show periapical lytic areas.

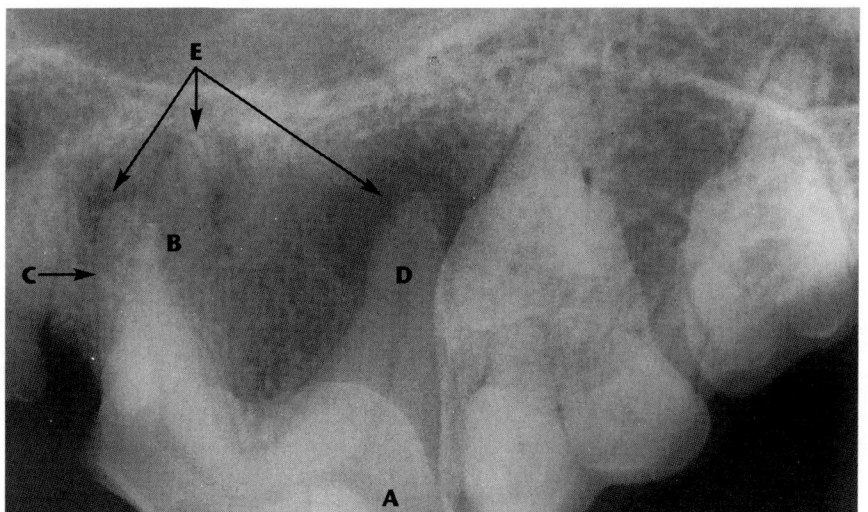

A. 208
B. Palatal root
C. Mesiobuccal root (rostral)
D. Distal root
E. Periapical lytic areas

FIGURE 3.9

Contributing Author:
Sandra Manfra Marretta

Description: Fractured maxillary fourth premolar (108) in a 10-year-old Shetland sheepdog; demonstrates partial apical lysis of the distal aspect of the distal root.

Points Identified: Partial apical lysis of the distal aspect of the distal root of 108.

    A. 108
    B. Apical lysis of distal root

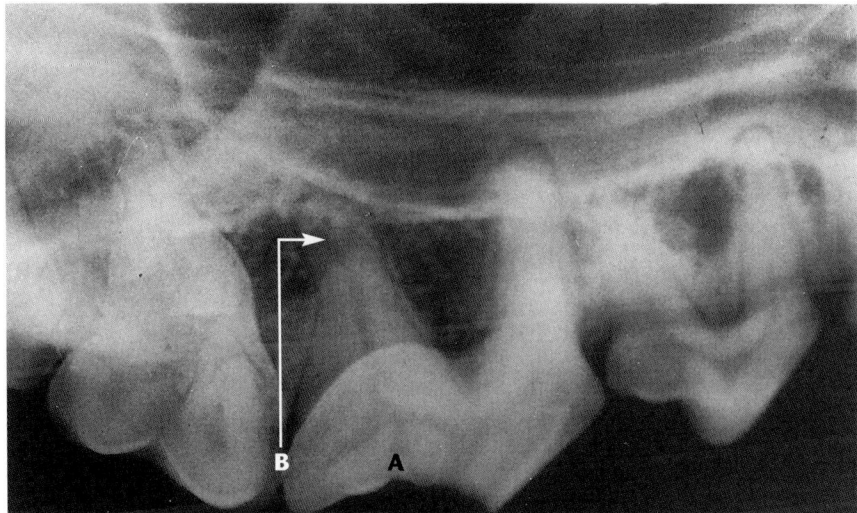

FIGURE 3.10

Contributing Author:
Sandra Manfra Marretta

Description: Rostral maxillary radiograph of a 9-year-old Labrador retriever presented because of a gray discolored maxillary left first incisor (201) which was fractured but without pulpal exposure. Note the asymmetry of the root canals of the two central incisors: the left incisor tooth (201) has a larger root canal than the right incisor (101).

Points Identified: Central incisors (101, 201) and increased root canal space in 201.

    A. 101
    B. 201
    C. Increased root canal space
    D. Apical lucency

Diagnostic Keys: Increased pulp/root canal space is indication that with pulpal pathology dentinogenesis has ceased. This patient needs endodontic care.

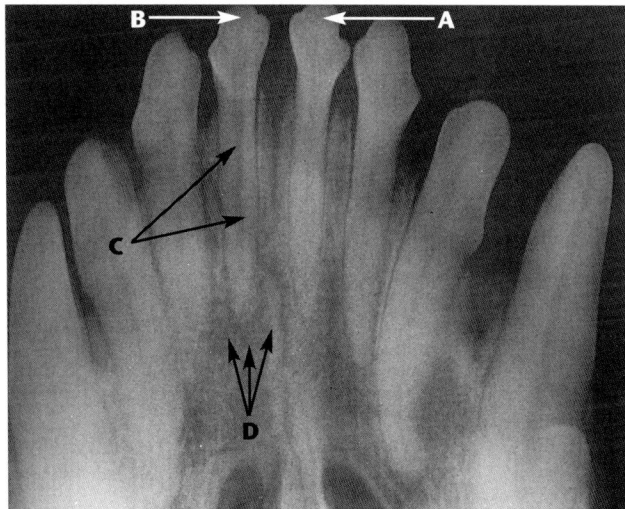

FIGURE 3.11

Contributing Author:
Sandra Manfra Marretta

Description: Rostral mandibular radiograph of a 9-year-old German shepherd presented because of a severely worn left mandibular canine tooth (304) with chronic pulpal exposure. Note the asymmetry of the root canal of the two mandibular canine teeth (304, 404). Also note the rough, irregular apical portion of the root of the left canine tooth.

Points Identified:

A. 304
B. 404
C. Apical lytic area
D. Increased pulp/root chamber

Diagnostic Keys: Apical lytic areas plus increased pulp/root chamber indicate pulp death and early cessation of dentinogenesis.

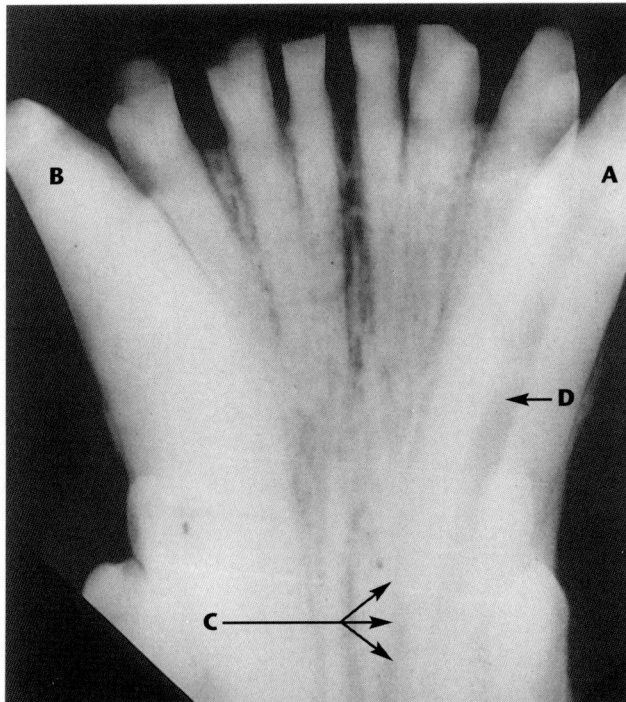

FIGURE 3.12

Contributing Author:
Sandra Manfra Marretta

Source: Manfra Marretta et al. Classification and prognostic factors of endodontic-periodontic lesions in the dog. *Jour Vet Dent* 9(2):27–30. 1992. With permission.

Description: Radiograph of a lower first molar (309) depicting the typical radiographic appearance of a Class I endo-perio lesion. Note the J-shaped lesion associated with the mesial root and the narrower periodontal pocket at the alveolar crest.

Points Identified:

A. 309
B. J-shaped lesion, mesial root
C. Apical lytic area, distal root

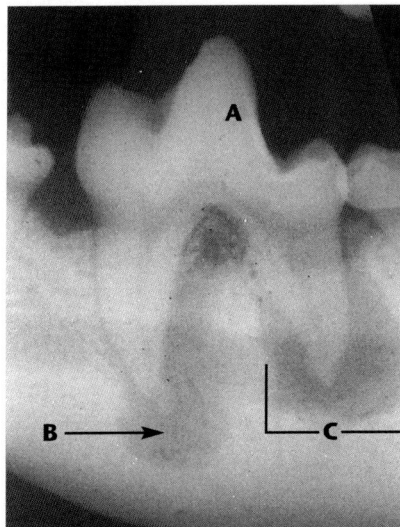

FIGURE 3.13

Contributing Author:
Sandra Manfra Marretta

Description: Radiograph of the maxillary canine tooth of a 3-year-old Doberman pinscher. This tooth was fractured, exposing the pulp, when the dog was less than 1 year old. The dog presented with ipsilateral nasal discharge and a draining tract at the mucogingival line. Note the severe destruction of the periodontium secondary to the endodontic lesion.

Points Identified: Aftereffects of long-term endodontic disease postpulpal death.

   A. 104
   B. Damaged apex and periodontium

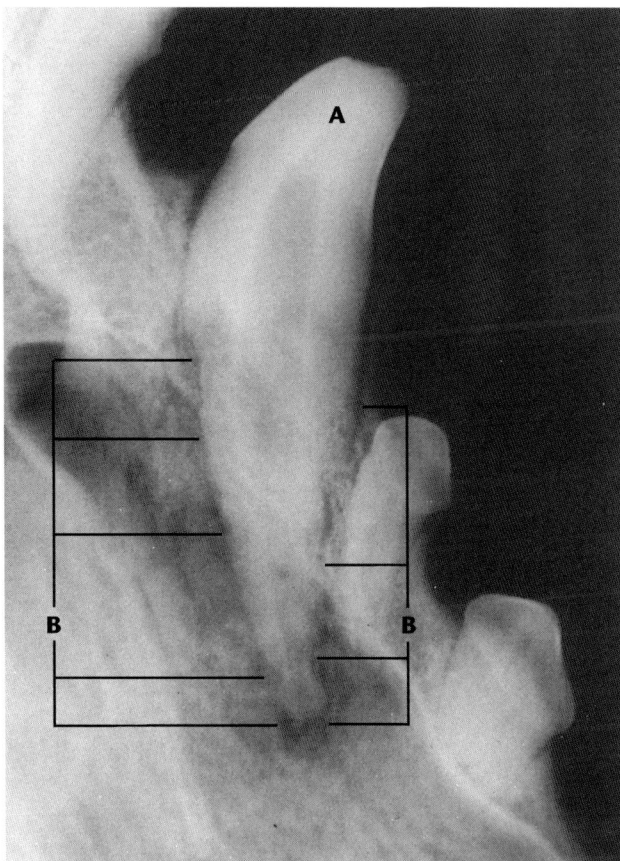

FIGURE 3.14

Contributing Author:
Sandra Manfra Marretta

Description: A 30-degree caudal oblique projection of the upper right fourth premolar (108) in a 3-year-old mixed breed dog presented because of a hyperplastic erythematous gingival mass on the buccal aspect of the gingiva margin of the fourth premolar. No fractures evident. There was a narrow periodontal pocket on the buccal aspect of the distal root. Note the J-shaped lesions associated with the distal and palatal roots.

Points Identified: Caudal oblique projection places palatal root between mesiobuccal (rostral) and distal roots. Severe periapical pathology present.

   A. 108
   B. Mesiobuccal (rostral) root
   C. Palatal root
   D. Distal root
   E. J-shaped lesions

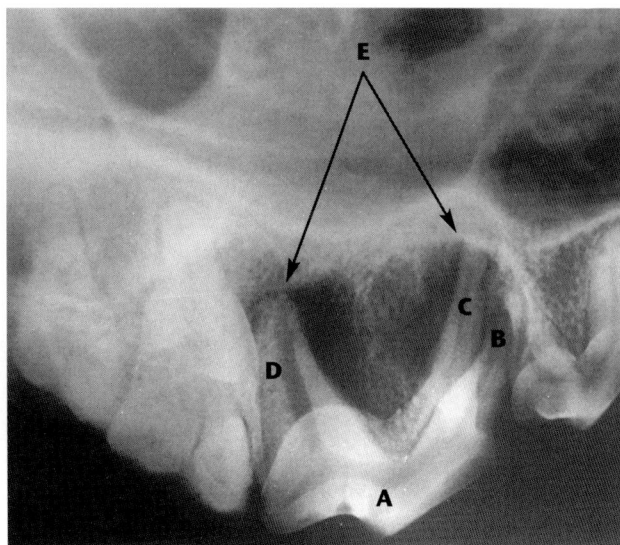

FIGURE 3.15

Contributing Author:
Sandra Manfra Marretta

Source: Manfra Marretta et al. Classification and prognostic factors of endodontic-periodontic lesions in the dog. *Jour Vet Dent* 9(2): 27-30. 1992. With permission.

Description: Radiograph of a lower first molar (409) which depicts the typical radiographic appearance of a Class II perio-endo lesion. Note the wide periodontal space extending to the apex of the distal root. The mesial root has periapical lysis secondary to migration of bacteria from the distal root through the endodontic system with extrusion of infected pulp contents to and beyond the apex of the mesial root.

Points Identified:

A. 409
B. Wide periodontal space around apex of distal root
C. Periapical lysis, mesial root

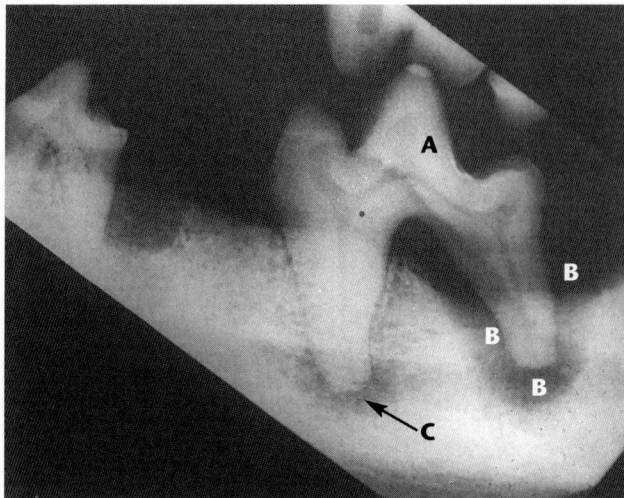

FIGURE 3.16

Contributing Author:
Sandra Manfra Marretta

Description: Radiograph of the right mandibular first molar (409) in a 7-year-old Chihuahua presented because of swelling of the right mandible in the region of the right first molar. A purulent cutaneous draining tract was present ventral to the tooth. An inflammatory reaction was confirmed on cytologic examination. Note the significant horizontal bone loss present indicating longstanding periodontal disease. In addition, note the lysis of the mandible secondary to the chronic osteomyelitis as a result of severe periodontal disease.

Points Identified: Osteomyelitis of mandible.

A. 409
B. Lysis of mandible
C. Osteomyelitis of mandible; apical lysis
D. Combined perio-endo lesion from advanced periodontitis

Diagnostic Keys: Dental radiology is imperative prior to extraction to prevent iatrogenic trauma to the mandible. Client should be shown this x-ray before proceeding with extraction. Osseoconductive bone material and postextraction antibiotics are imperative with acrylic splinting.

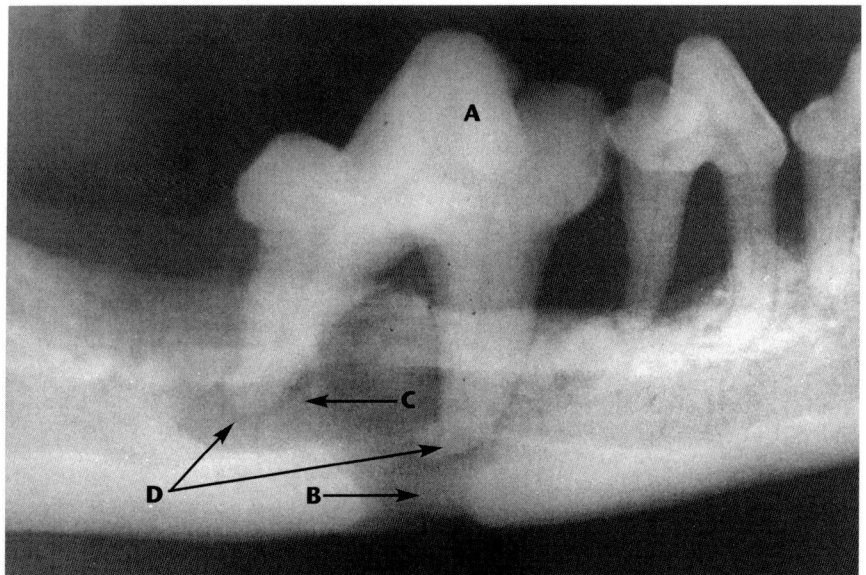

FIGURE 3.17A–H

Contributing Author:
Sandra Manfra Marretta

Source: Provided courtesy of John Losonsky, Dipl. ACVR, Veterinary Clinical Medicine, University of Illinois.

Description: CAT scan performed on a 7-year-old shar pei who was presented because of severe bony swelling of the left hemimandible. A tentative diagnosis of a mandibular tumor was made, and a CAT scan was performed to help delineate the tumor margins. Note the proliferation and lysis of bone around the left hemimandible in the region of the fractured left canine tooth (see arrows). A histopathologic examination of the bone confirmed the diagnosis of osteomyelitis. The bony mandibular swelling resolved following extraction of the left canine tooth.

Points Identified: Lysis and proliferation of bone around left hemimandible (see arrows on Figures 3.17 C–H).

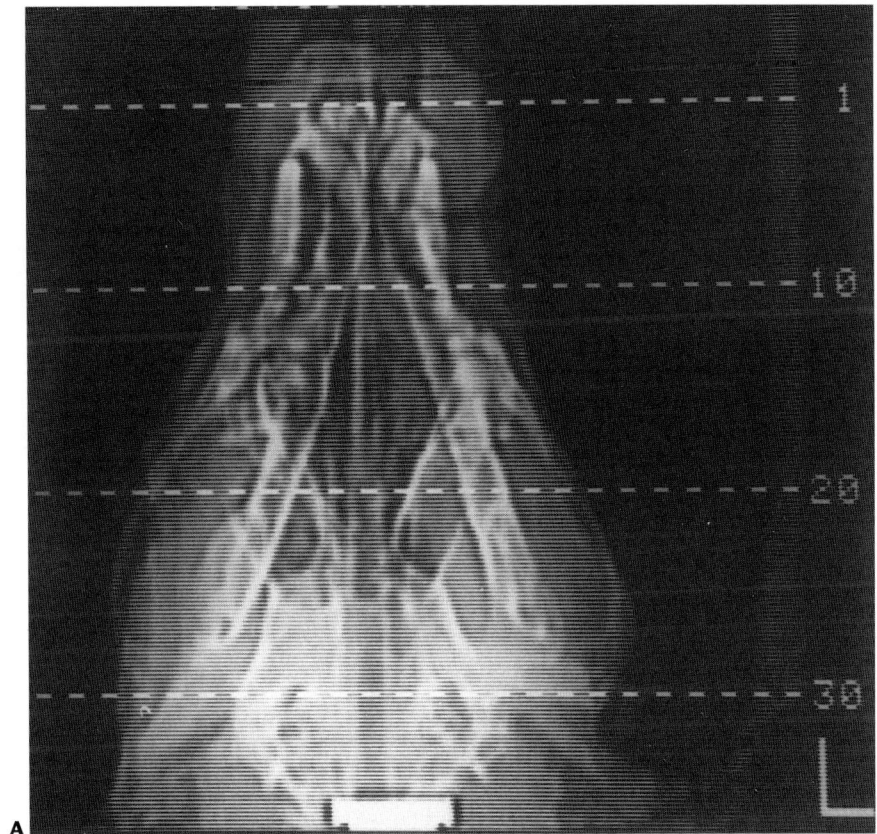

A

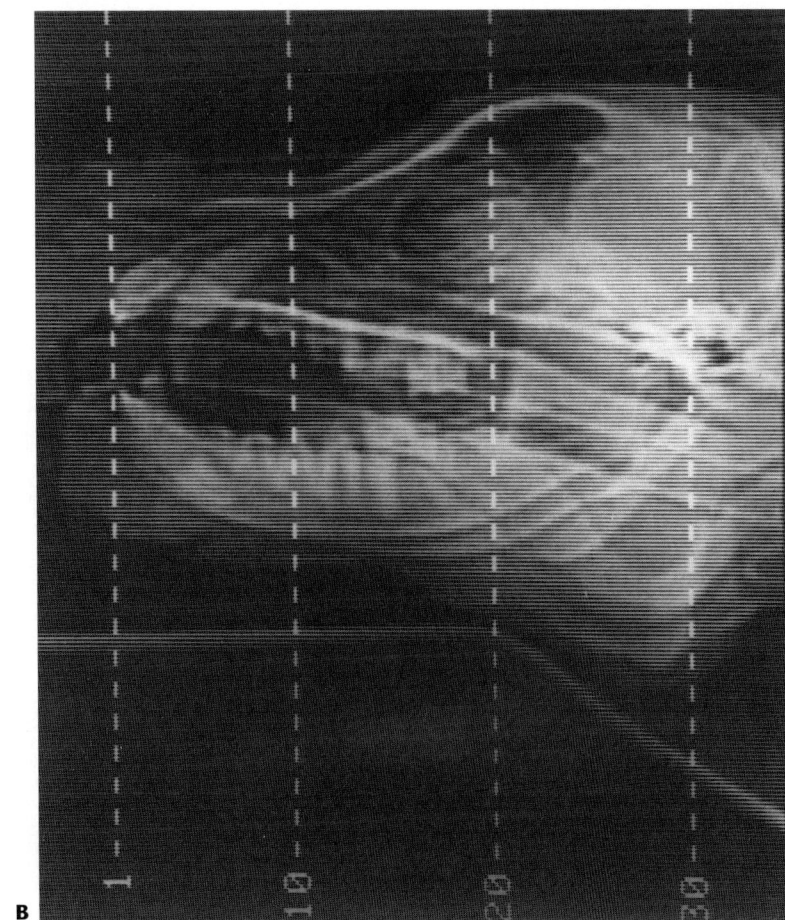

B

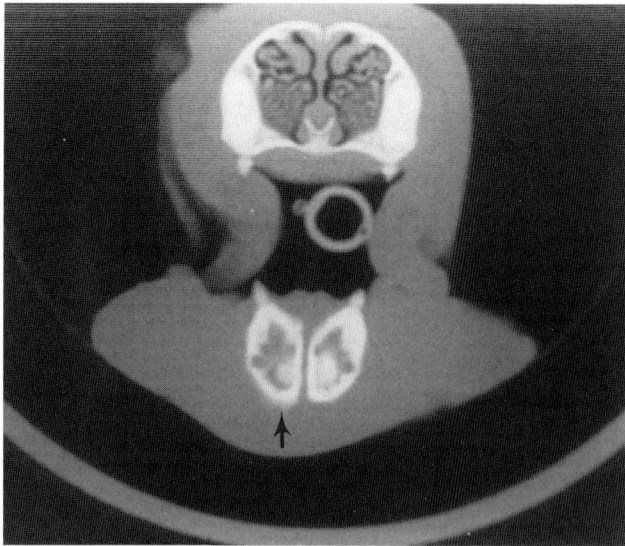

C

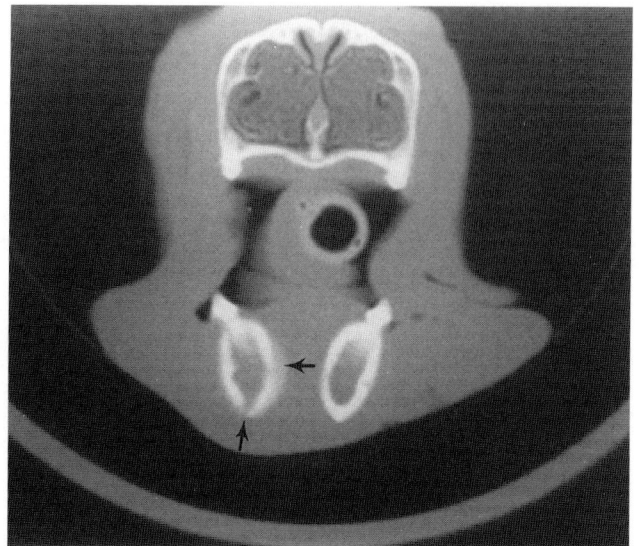

F

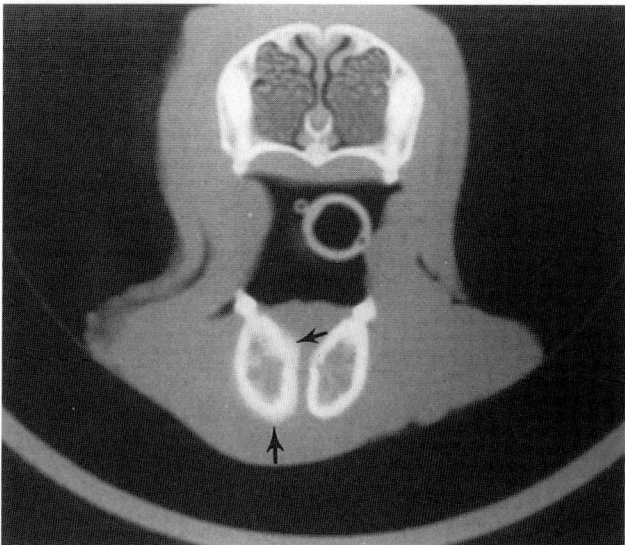

D

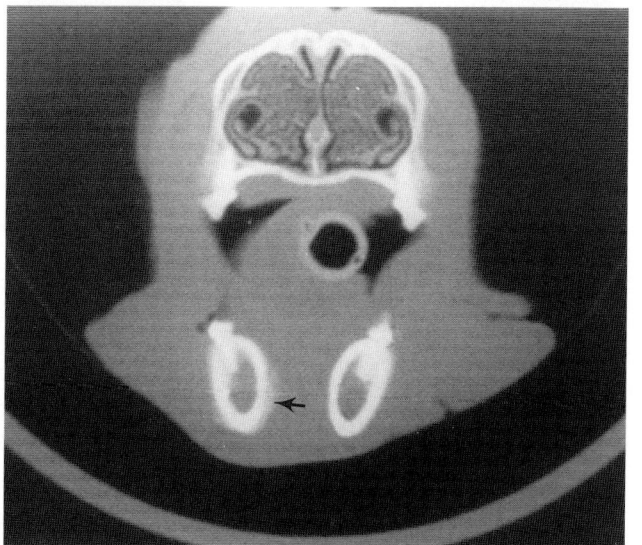

G

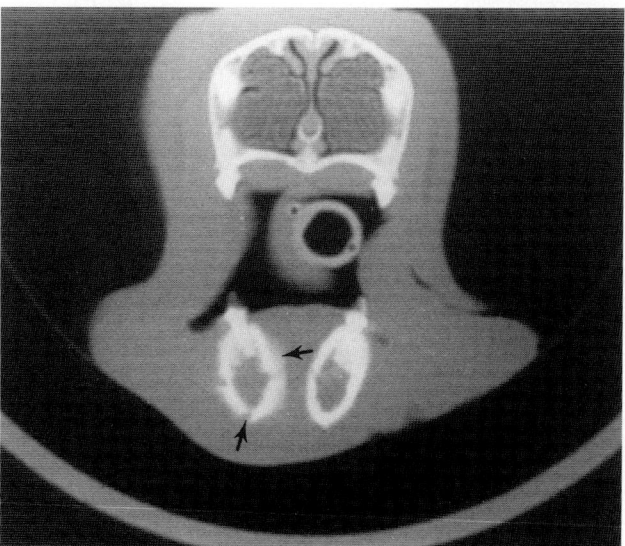

E

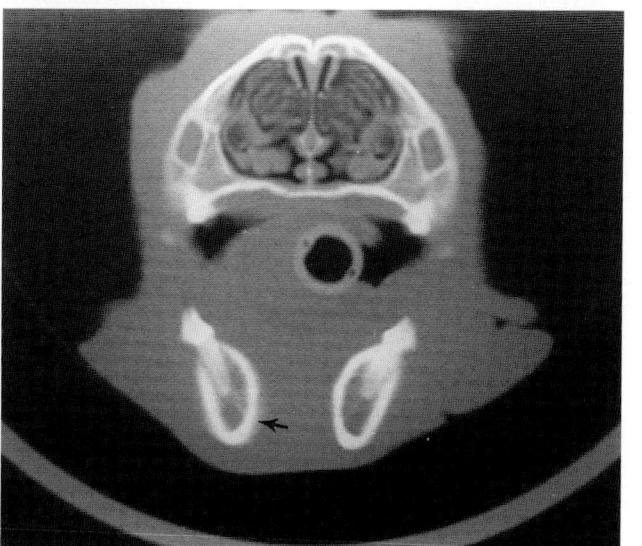

H

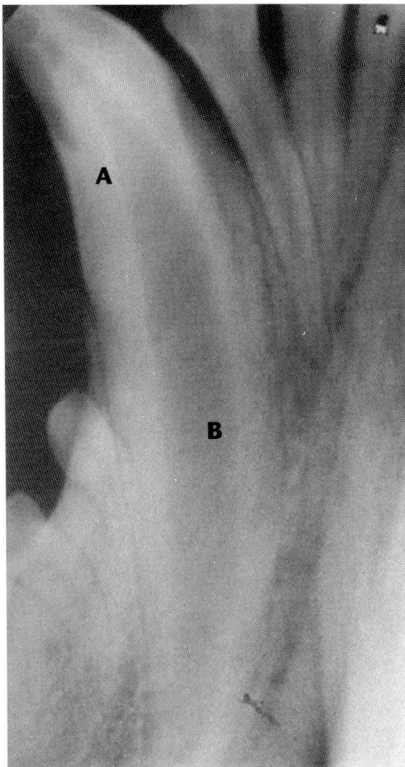

FIGURE 3.18

Contributing Author:
Sandra Manfra Marretta

Description: Radiograph of the mandibular canine tooth of a 1-year-old Labrador retriever demonstrating the wide endodontic system present in young dogs.

Points Identified:

A. 304
B. Pulp/root canal, immature canine (304)

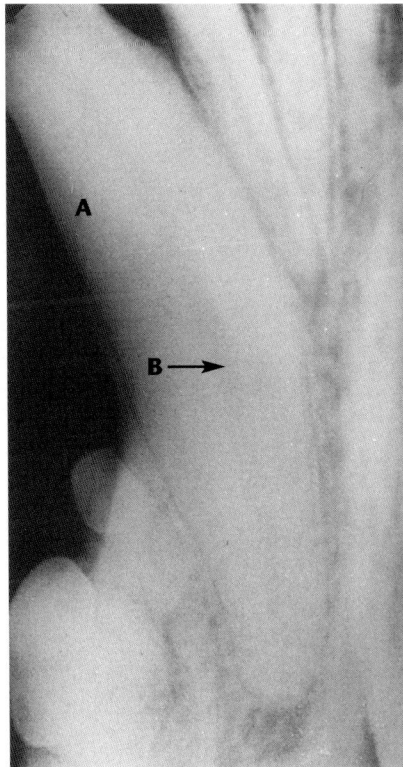

FIGURE 3.19

Contributing Author:
Sandra Manfra Marretta

Description: Radiograph of the mandibular canine tooth of a 6-year-old German shepherd dog demonstrating the narrower endodontic system present in older dogs.

Points Identified:

A. 304
B. Pulp/root canal, older canine (304)

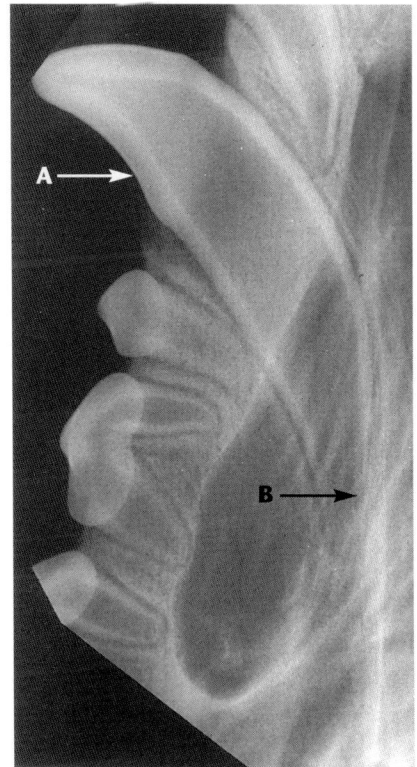

FIGURE 3.20

Contributing Author:
Sandra Manfra Marretta

Description: Radiograph of the maxillary canine tooth of a 6-month-old dog demonstrating incomplete apical formation.

Points Identified:

A. 104
B. Open apex, immature tooth

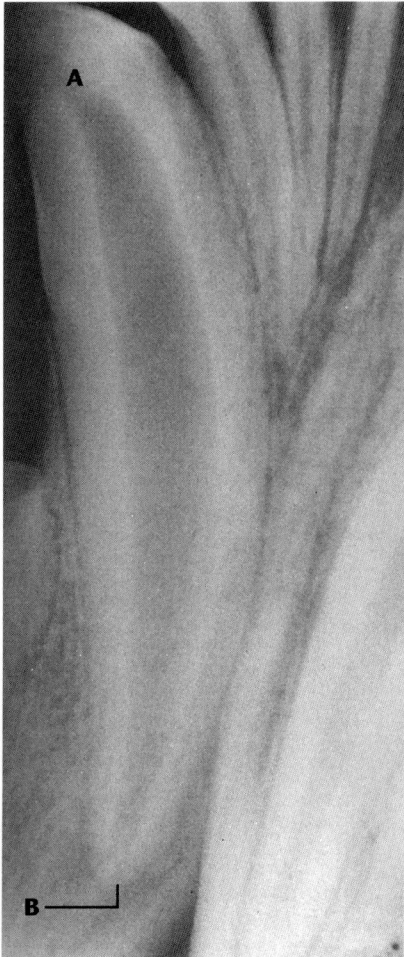

FIGURE 3.21

Contributing Author:
Sandra Manfra Marretta

Description: Radiograph of a mandibular canine tooth (404) with complete apical formation.

Points Identified:

A. 404
B. Closed apex

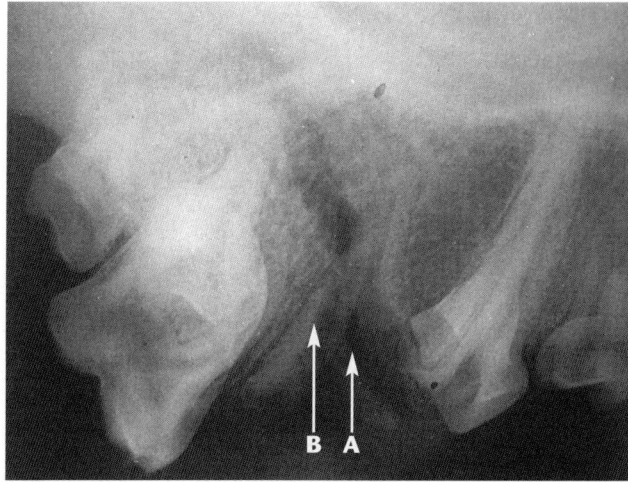

FIGURE 3.22

Contributing Author:
Sandra Manfra Marretta

Description: Radiograph of a root fracture in maxillary fourth premolar 208. This fracture was presented as part of an oral trauma examination caused by an auto accident.

Points Identified:

A. Short oblique fracture, mesiobuccal root, 208
B. Complex fracture distal root, 208

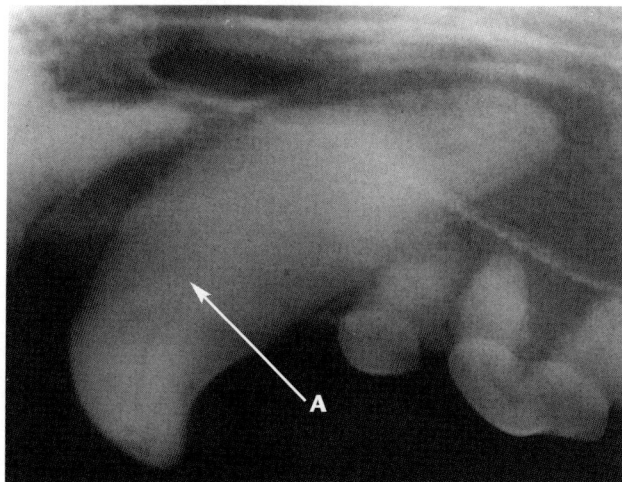

FIGURE 3.23

Contributing Author:
Sandra Manfra Marretta

Description: Radiograph of a gray, discolored, maxillary canine tooth (104) of a 9-year-old golden retriever, demonstrating an occluded or restricted canal.

Points Identified:

A. Restricted or narrowed canal, 104

Diagnostic Keys: Note that the canal is seen as a very thin radiolucent line. With the aging animal there is a closing down of pulp/root canal size as secondary dentin is laid down by odontoblasts.

FIGURE 3.24

Contributing Author:
Sandra Manfra Marretta

Description: Radiograph demonstrating the severe curvature normally present in the maxillary third incisor (103) in a dog.

Points Identified:

A. 103 (normal curvature)

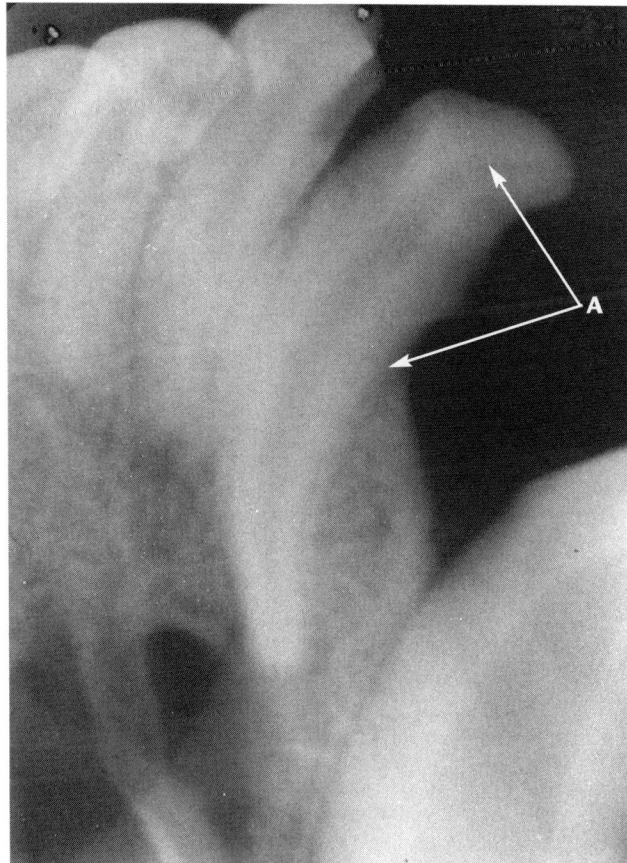

FIGURE 3.25

Contributing Author:
Sandra Manfra Marretta

Source: Manfra Marretta et al. Development of a teaching model for coronal access to the canine dentition. *Jour Vet Dent* 9(4): 11–17. 1992. With permission.

Description: Radiographs of the maxillary canine tooth from a teaching model for coronal access to the canine dentition.

Points Identified: Labiopalatal (top series) and mesiodistal (bottom series) radiographs of maxillary canine.

A. Initial radiographs
B. Barium markers on ideal access point (see bright spot on radiographs)
C. K-files in root canals

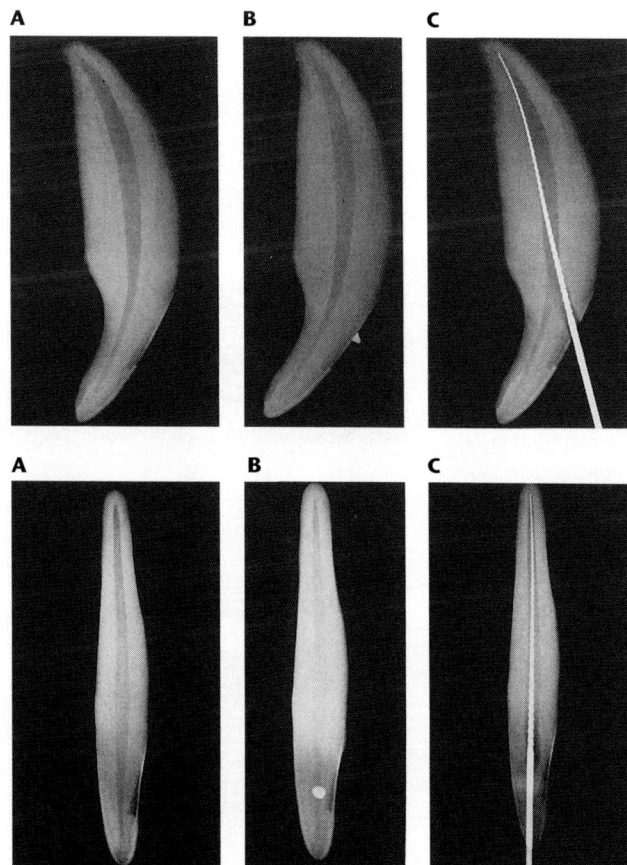

FIGURE 3.26

Contributing Author:
Sandra Manfra Marretta

Source: Manfra Marretta et al. Development of a teaching model for coronal access to the canine dentition. *Jour Vet Dent* 9(4): 11-17. 1992. With permission.

Description: Radiographs of the mandibular fourth premolar from a teaching model for coronal access to the canine dentition.

Points Identified: Buccolingual (top series) and mesiodistal (bottom series) radiographs of mandibular fourth premolar.

   A. Initial radiographs
   B. Barium markers on ideal access points (see bright spots on radiographs)
   C. K-files in root canals

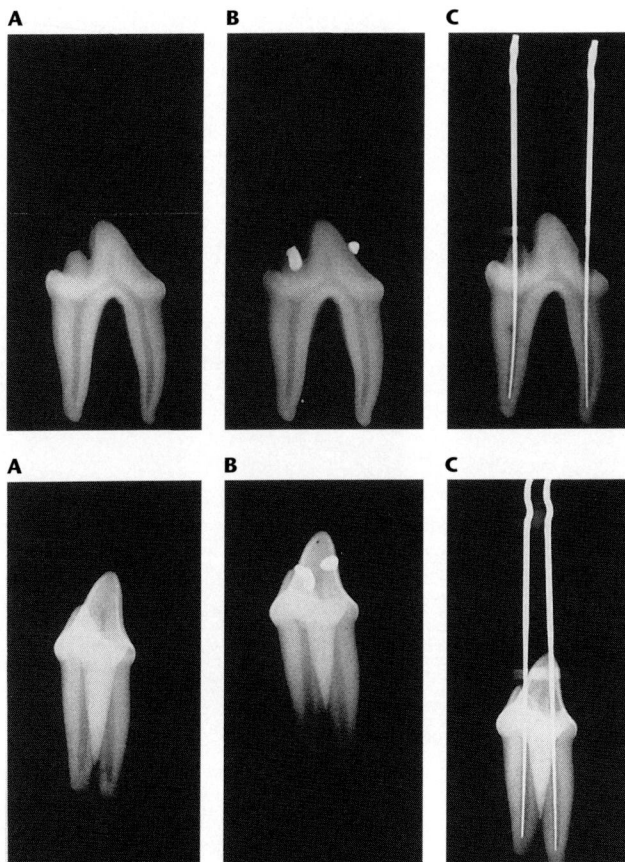

FIGURE 3.27

Contributing Author:
Sandra Manfra Marretta

Source: Manfra Marretta et al. Development of a teaching model for coronal access to the canine dentition. *Jour Vet Dent* 9(4): 11-17. 1992. With permission.

Description: Radiographs of the maxillary fourth premolar from a teaching model for coronal access to the canine dentition.

Points Identified: Buccopalatal (top series) and distomesial (bottom series) radiographs of maxillary fourth premolar.

   A. Initial radiographs
   B. Barium markers on ideal access points (see bright spots on radiographs)
   C. K-files in root canals

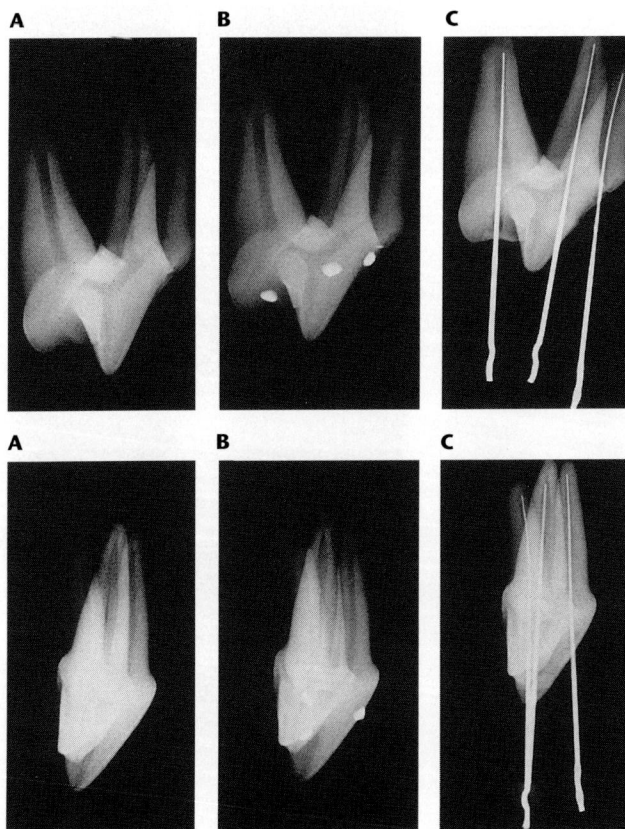

FIGURE 3.28

Contributing Author:
Sandra Manfra Marretta

Description: Radiograph of a maxillary canine tooth in a 10-year-old dog, demonstrating an inadequate coronal access. Note the abrupt bend in the file where the shaft meets the cutting edge of the file. Also note the failure of the file to reach the apical portion of the root canal.

Points Identified:

A. 104
B. Improper access to pulp canal

Common Errors: This inappropriate coronal access may result in breaking the file within the pulp canal.

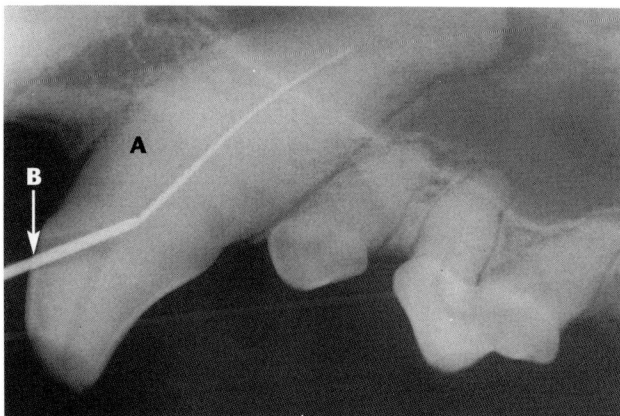

FIGURE 3.29

Contributing Author:
Sandra Manfra Marretta

Description: Rostral mandibular radiograph of a 3-year-old German shepherd dog with bilateral mandibular canine pulpal exposure secondary to rapid dental attrition. Note the broken file in the left mandibular canine root canal.

Points Identified:

A. 304
B. Broken file in pulp canal (instrument disarticulation)

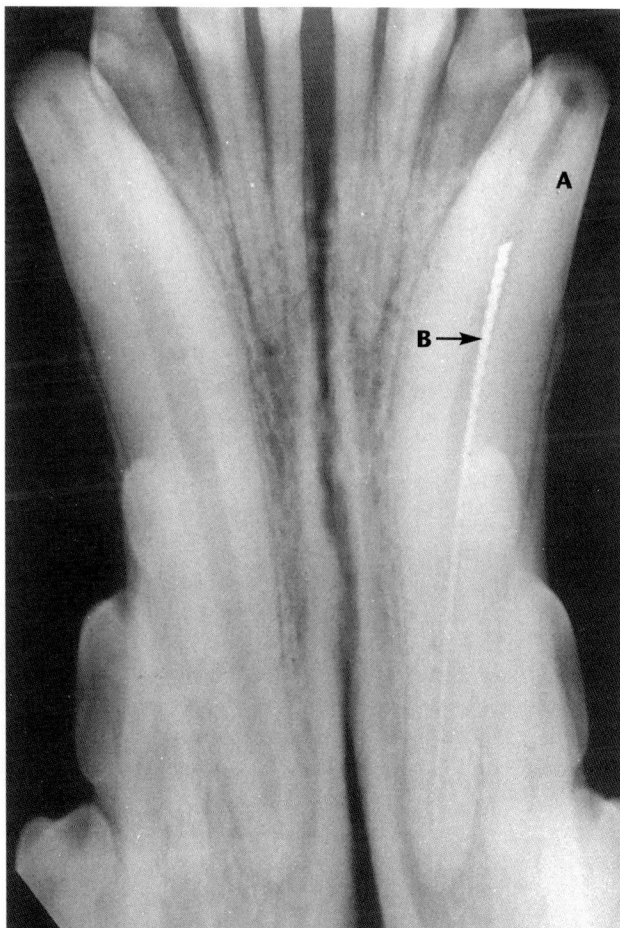

FIGURE 3.30

Contributing Author:
Sandra Manfra Marretta

Description: Postoperative radiograph of the dog in Figure 3.29. Note that an adequate apical fill has been achieved even though the broken file was not able to be retrieved. The restorative base utilized in this endodontic procedure was Ketac-fil, which is radiolucent.

Points Identified:

A. 404
B. Adequate fill in canal with trapped file

Diagnostic Keys: If adequate apical fill could not be accomplished and the file were nonretrievable, surgical endodontics would be necessary.

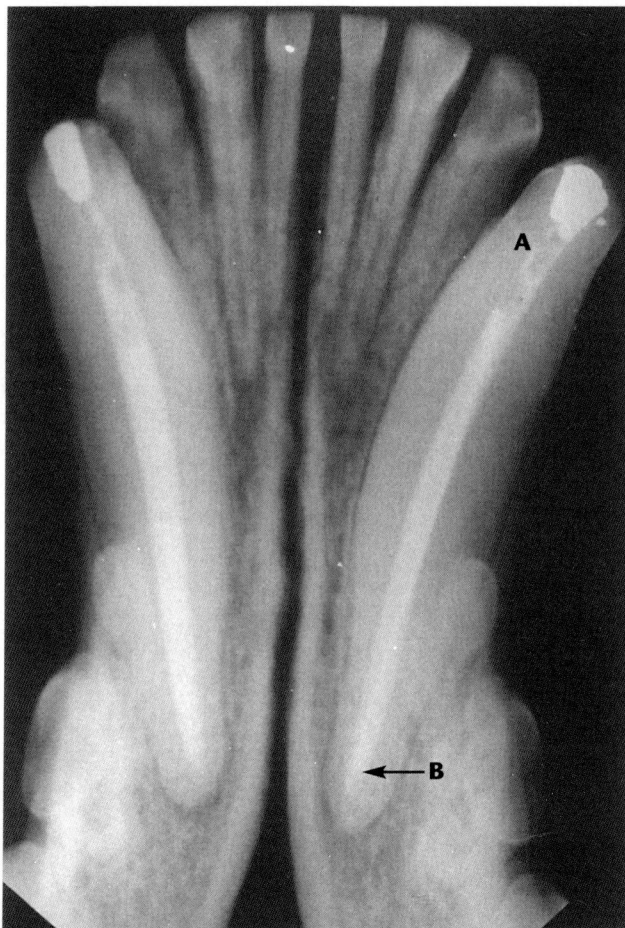

FIGURE 3.31

Contributing Author:
Sandra Manfra Marretta

Description: Radiograph of a mandibular canine tooth, confirming that the file has reached the apex.

Points Identified:

A. File
B. File reaches most apical extent of root canal

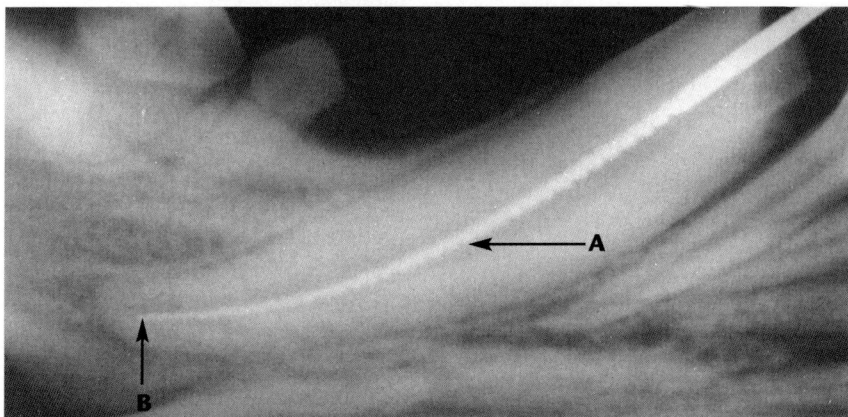

FIGURE 3.32

Contributing Author:
Donald. H. DeForge

Description: Radiograph of a maxillary canine (104) with perforated apex. The file has perforated the apex of this tooth and was the cause of persistent intraoperative hemorrhage. The file was withdrawn to the apex, hemorrhage subsided, and an apexification procedure was completed.

Points Identified:

A. 104
B. File perforating the apex

Diagnostic Keys: A nonvital immature tooth with an open apex is treated with apexification, an endodontic treatment, that involves closure of the root apex by cementum formation (osteocementum), stimulated by the presence of Ca(OH)$_2$.

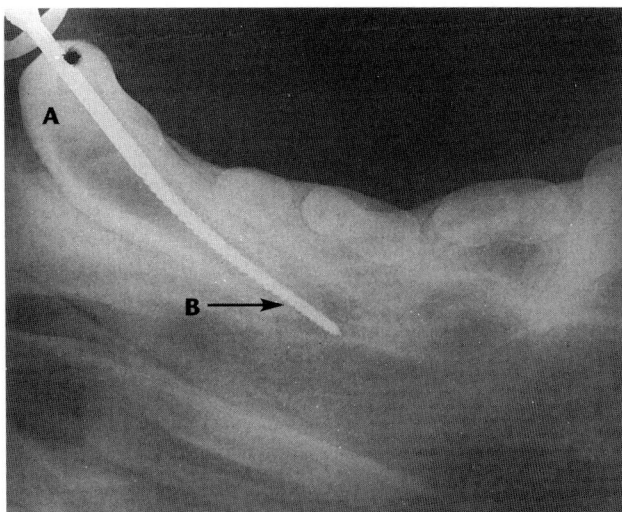

FIGURE 3.33

Contributing Author:
Sandra Manfra Marretta

Description: Radiograph of a maxillary canine tooth (104) with inadequate apical fill.

Points Identified:

A. 104
B. Blackened, radiolucent area, showing incomplete fill

Diagnostic Keys: This endodontic procedure will fail. Obturating material must be removed and debridement repeated until apical one-third of root canal system is completely sealed.

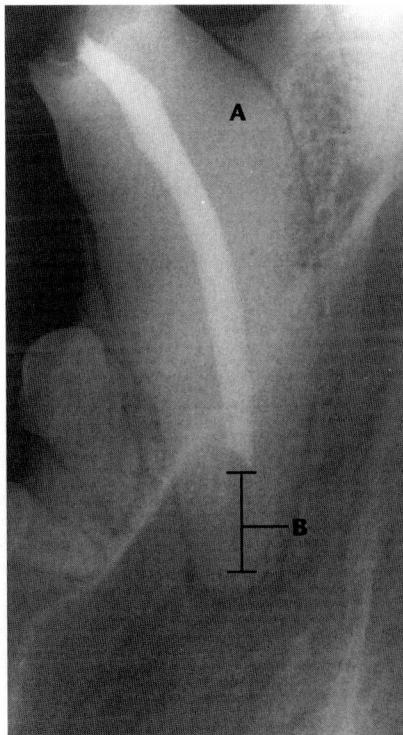

FIGURE 3.34

Contributing Author:
Sandra Manfra Marretta

Description: Radiograph demonstrating adequate fill of a fractured maxillary right second incisor (102).

Points Identified:

    A. 102
    B. Adequate fill

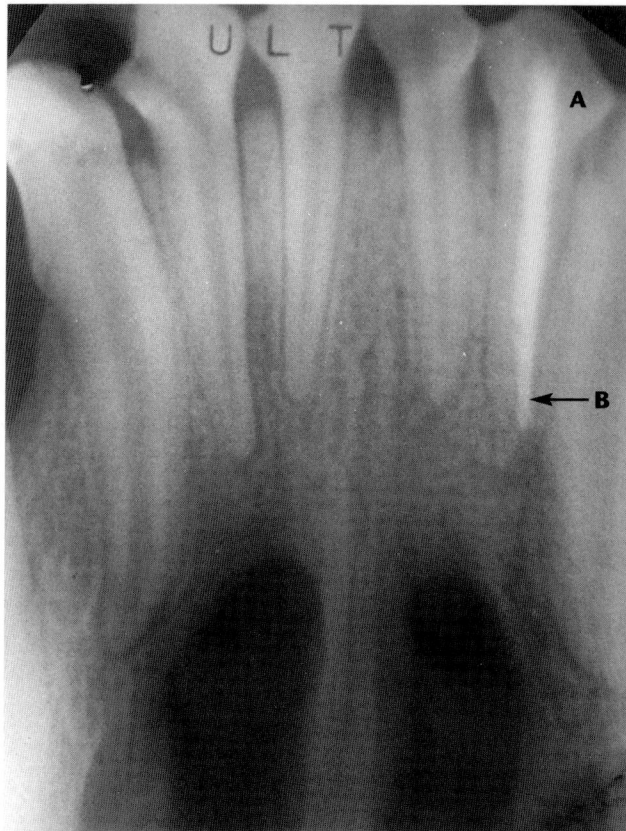

FIGURE 3.35

Contributing Author:
Sandra Manfra Marretta

Description: Radiograph demonstrating appropriate placement of an amalgam restoration in the incisor tooth pictured in Figure 3.34.

Points Identified: Proper undercut for mechanical lock in amalgam restoration.

    A. 102
    B. Proper undercut for mechanical lock

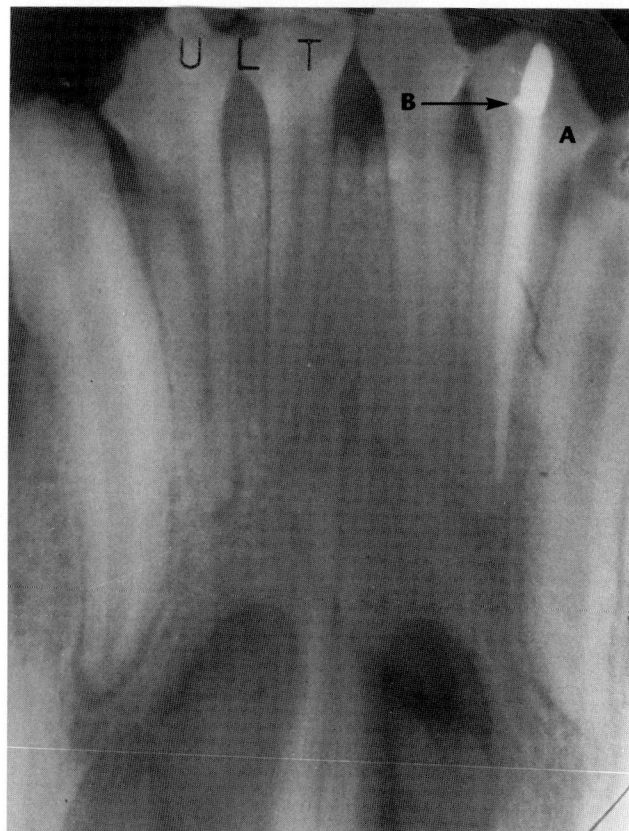

FIGURE 3.36

Contributing Author:
Sandra Manfra Marretta

Description: Radiograph demonstrating questionable fill in a fractured mandibular canine tooth (404).

Points Identified:

  A. 404
  B. Radiolucent zone below obturating termination

Diagnostic Keys: The fuzzy radiolucent zone below the obturating termination may be a continuation of the apical root canal that is unfilled. This patient will probably have a successful endodontic conclusion, but should be followed closely radiographically in 3, 6, and 12 months. New three-dimensional filling techniques with heated gutta percha allow thermoplasticized sealants to flow into the terminal apex for complete filling.

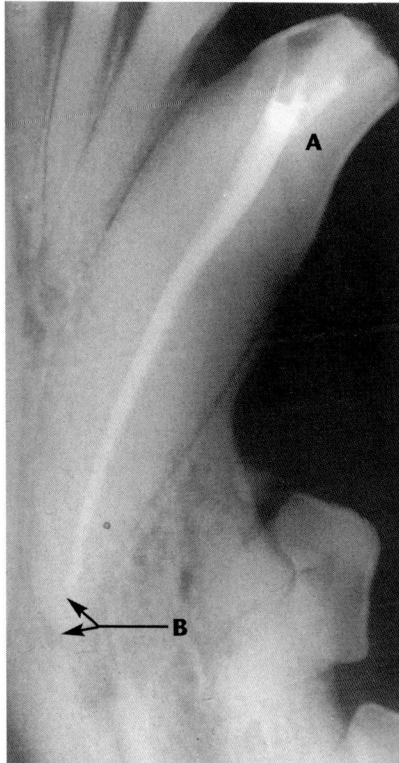

FIGURE 3.37

Contributing Author:
Sandra Manfra Marretta

Description: Radiograph demonstrating appropriate placement of amalgam restorations in the access sites of the canine tooth pictured in Figure 3.36.

Points Identified: 404. Amalgam restorations at multiple access sites.

  A. 404
  B. Amalgam restorations

Common Errors: When possible, avoid multiple access sites. Multiple access sites lead to weakening of coronal structure and increase directly the potential for crown fracture. This patient would benefit from full jacket crown restorative care.

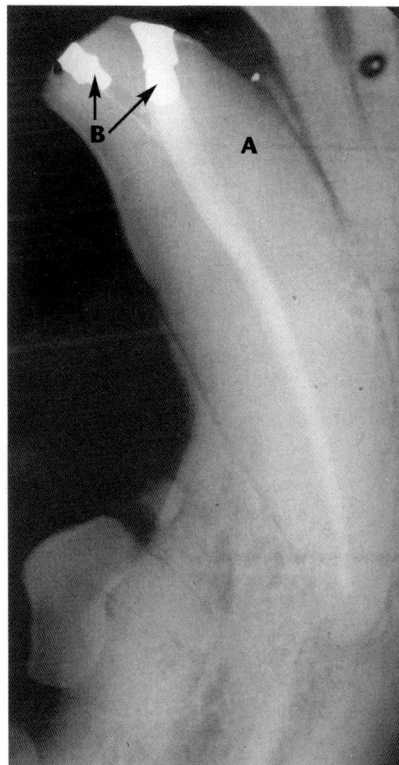

FIGURE 3.38

Contributing Author:
Sandra Manfra Marretta

Source: Manfra Marretta et al. Development of a teaching model for surgical endodontic access sites in the canine. *Jour Vet Dent*, accepted July 1994. With permission.

Description: Radiographs of the first mandibular molar from a teaching model created for ideal surgical access sites. Note that an apicoectomy has been successfully performed through the small but adequate surgical site.

Points Identified:

A. Endodontic file in mesial root canal
B. Barium marker placed over ideal surgical access site
C. Surgical access site

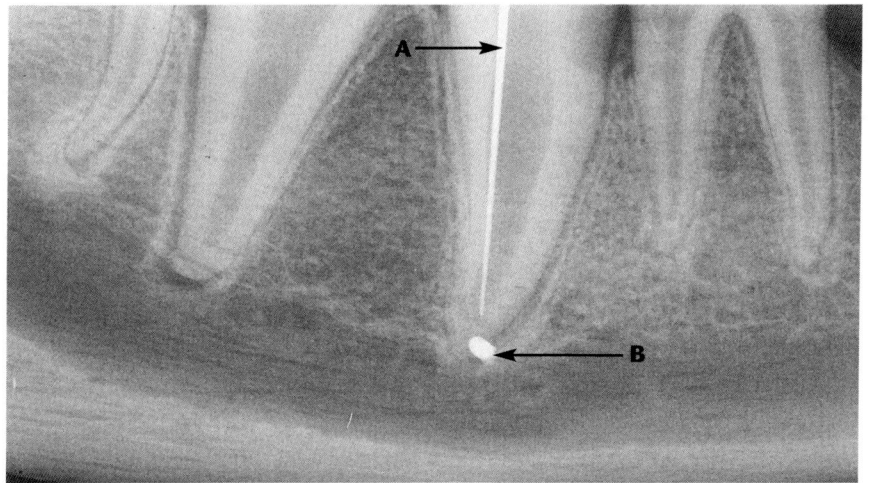

A

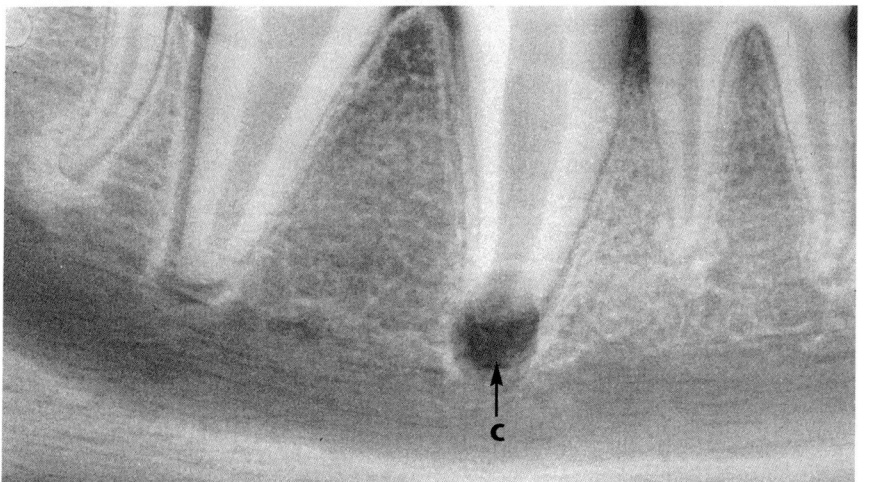

B

FIGURE 3.39

Contributing Author:
Sandra Manfra Marretta

Description: Postoperative radiograph of
the maxillary canine tooth in a 9-month-old
weimaraner that had a fractured canine tooth
with pulpal exposure and severe facial swelling
over the apex of the affected tooth. Note the
retrograde amalgam restoration of the apicoectomy site.

Points Identified: Retrograde fill in a surgical endodontic treatment.

    A. 104
    B. Retrograde fill

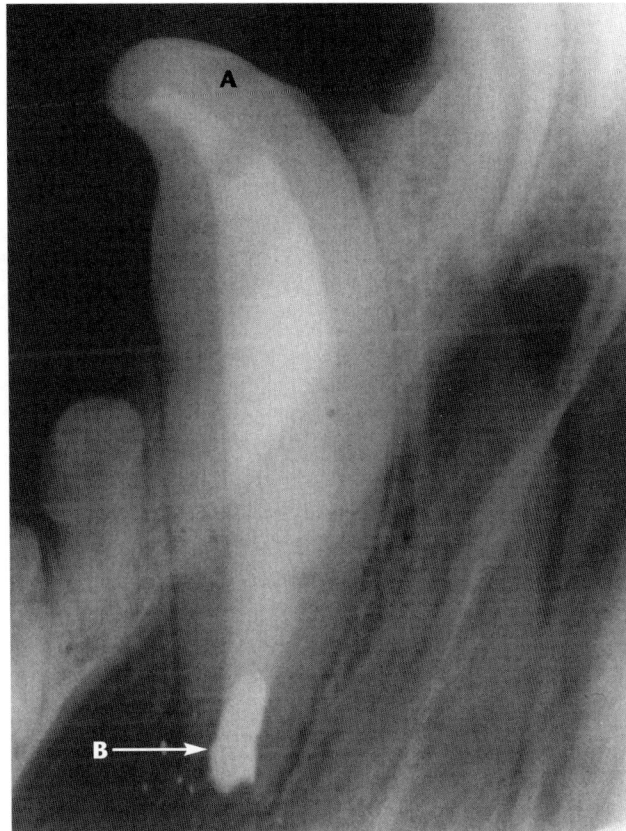

FIGURE 3.40

Contributing Author:
Sandra Manfra Marretta

Description: Radiograph of a 3-month
postoperative successful pulpotomy case with a
dentinal bridge (104). Note that the dot at the
radicular termination at the apex is a film artifact.

Points Identified:

    A. 104
    B. Dentinal bridge
    C. Film artifact

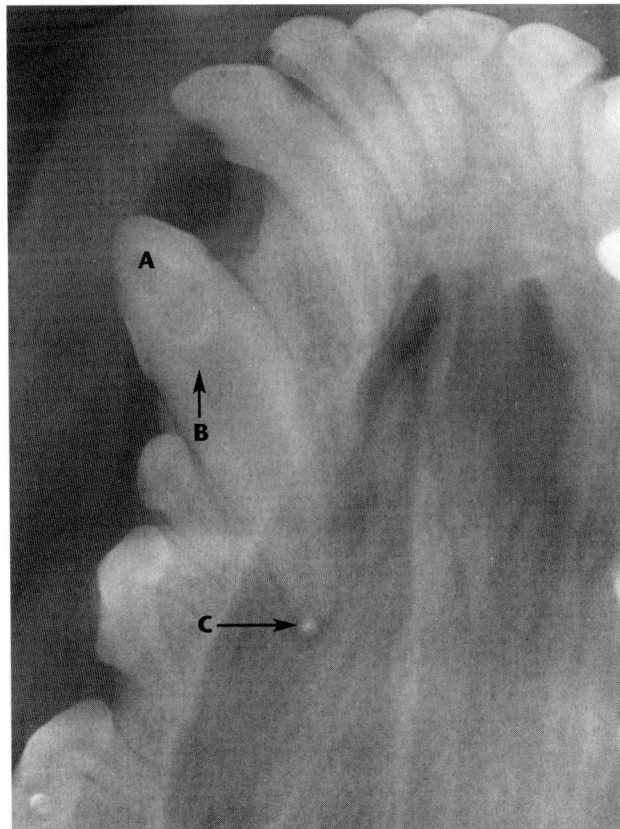

FIGURE 3.41

Contributing Author:
Sandra Manfra Marretta

Description: Radiograph of the maxillary canine tooth in a 13-year-old beagle who had inadequate conventional endodontic therapy 6 years prior to this radiograph. There was a draining tract present at the mucogingival line near the distal aspect of the canine tooth. Note the resorption of the endodontic filling and lysis of the distal aspect of the apex in this endodontic failure.

Points Identified: Endodontic failure denoted by root resorption and periradicular lysis.

A. 204
B. Root resorption and periradicular lysis

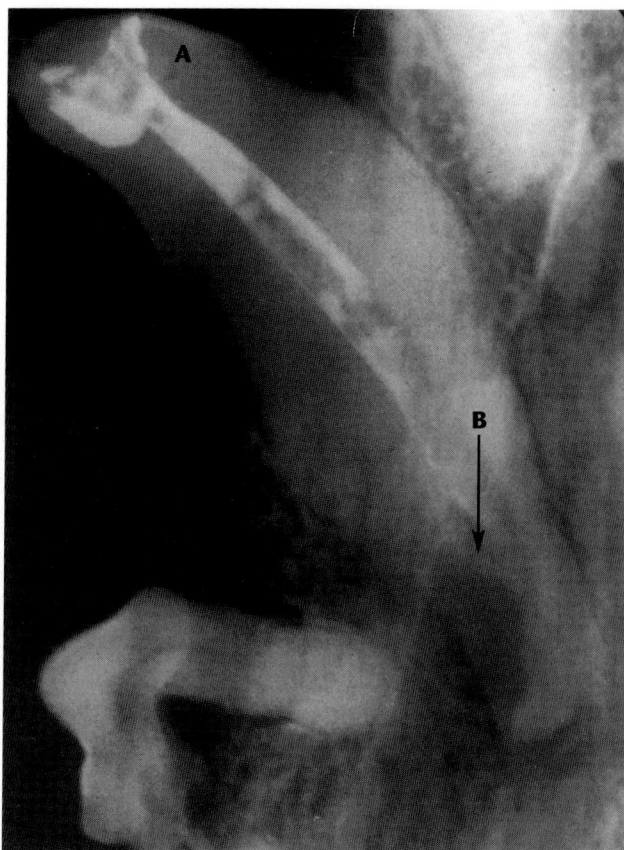

4 Canine Periodontics

Dr. Philippe R. Hennet
Dr. Jan Bellows

INTRODUCTION: RADIOGRAPHIC DIAGNOSIS

Advanced periodontitis with soft tissue, bony, and tooth surface changes is commonly seen in companion animals. Treatment may include subgingival root planing, periodontal surgery, partial tooth resection with endodontic treatment of the remaining root(s), or total extraction. Radiography plays an essential role in determining the extent of periodontal disease and therapy. Radiographs are evaluated for alveolar bone changes, interdental bone height fluctuation, presence of the lamina dura, trabecular patterns, periodontal ligament space, and other osseous and tooth surface changes.

Radiographs show two-dimensional representations of three-dimensional structures. At times, radiographs may not adequately show the severity of disease. Early destructive bone lesions sometimes are not radiographically observable. Buccal and lingual alveolar bone are particularly difficult to evaluate because of superimposition and summation. In addition to the radiographic findings, the clinician should rely on clinical examination, including sulcular depths, tooth mobility, and appearance of the attached gingiva, in order to decide on the best treatment plan.

Normal Radiographic Anatomy

Normal, healthy alveolar bone has a characteristic appearance on radiographs. The alveolar crests are situated approximately 2 to 3 mm apical to the cementoenamel junction of the teeth. The shape of the alveolar crests may vary from rounded to flat. Between anterior teeth, the alveolar crest will usually appear pointed. Between posterior teeth the alveolar crest will be parallel to a line between the adjacent cementoenamel junctions, where the enamel thins and disappears. The alveolar crests will be continuous with the lamina dura of the adjacent teeth, and only the interproximal portions of the lamina dura and the periodontal ligament are visible. The buccal and lingual areas are not seen in the radiograph. Widening of the periodontal ligament space and loss of lamina dura can be interpreted as resorption of the alveolar bone.

The overall height of the alveolar crest bone in relationship to the cementoenamel junction gives evidence of whether loss of bone has occurred. The distribution of bone loss is classified as either localized or generalized depending on the number of areas affected. Localized bone loss occurs in isolated areas; generalized bone loss involves the majority of the crestal bone. Initially, peri-

odontitis usually develops as a localized erosion of the alveolar crest. Bony changes cannot be radiographically detected until they are relatively advanced. As the severity of the periodontitis increases, more alveolar bone is destroyed and the process becomes generalized.

Established Periodontitis

In the advanced stages of periodontitis, pocket formation can extend from 6 to 12 mm (normal sulcal depth being 3 mm in the canine species). Radiographically, these pockets can present as vertical or horizontal bony defects affecting the alveolar bony plates. The alveolar bone forms four walls around the tooth: (1) buccal, (2) lingual-palatal, (3) mesial, and (4) distal. Horizontal bone loss is used to describe the radiographic appearance of the loss of bone height in the region of several adjacent teeth. In horizontal bone loss the buccal, lingual, and interdental bone have been resorbed. This we describe as a suprabony pocket where the entire thickness of crestal bone is lost. A suprabony pocket has its base coronal to the alveolar crest. The true gingival pocket involves attachment loss, apical migration of the junctional epithelium, and transformation of the junctional epithelium into pocket epithelium. It is important to understand these changes because although they may not be evident radiographically in the early stages, they will warrant further x-ray rechecks for monitoring the progression or cessation of periodontal pathology. In advanced periodontitis it is not uncommon, in the anterior teeth, to radiographically visualize up to 50 percent loss of interdental septal bone. This destructive process radiating from excessive plaque formation will cause a widening of the interdental septa as bone loss progresses.

The second form of bony loss is the infrabony pocket, also described as infra-alveolar vertical bone loss. The infrabony pocket has its base apical to the alveolar crest. These vertical or infrabony pockets have been classified in humans in relationship to pocket morphology. The same classification is used in animals:

1. One-wall bony pocket: One osseous wall is remaining and bone is missing on three walls of the defect.
2. Two-wall bony pocket: The defect is bordered by two remaining walls.
3. Three-wall bony pocket: Three walls are remaining in this de-

fect, with bone missing on only one face.

4. Four-wall bony pocket: This is also called a "cup" or "moat" bony defect. Four bony walls remain around the tooth as the defect surrounds the tooth (i.e., tooth in a "cup" or tooth "surrounded by a moat").

The morphology of the bone loss, radiographically as well as on probing exam, is important to the patient for planning further treatment. The amount of bone present will directly relate to the potential for osseous regeneration or the need for extensive periodontal surgery with bone replacement. The inconsistent bony margin makes the morphology of the pocket even harder to describe at times. In addition, the bony lesion can be superimposed on the root of the affected tooth, leading to even further difficulty in interpretation. The root surface and interdental spaces can be covered with soft tissue to the cementoenamel junction (CEJ), making the lesion clinically nonprobable yet reasonably well evidenced by x-ray.

Furcation exposures come from bone loss at the bifurcation of multirooted teeth. It is sometimes difficult to determine radiographically whether the interradicular space is involved unless there is a radiolucent area in the region of the furcation. Only advanced furcations where both cortical plates are gone will be easily recognized on radiographs. Class I (incipient) furcation exposure exists when the tip of a probe can just (<1 mm) enter the furcation area. Bone still fills most of the area where the roots meet. Class II (definite) furcation exposure exists when the probe tip extends more than 1 mm horizontally into the area where the roots converge. Class III (through and through) lesions exist secondary to advanced periodontal disease. The alveolar bone has eroded to a point that the explorer probe passes through the defect unobstructed. Alveolar dehiscence exists when the alveolar cortical bone is resorbed along the entire length of the root. Radiographically, there will be a radiopaque line surrounding the affected root.

All of the above radiographic changes are progressive as periodontal disease worsens. Because of this, radiology becomes a very important tool in periodontal treatment change and ultimate patient prognosis.

X-RAY PLATES

FIGURE 4.1

Contributing Authors:
Jan Bellows and Philippe R. Hennet

Description: Combined periodontic-endodontic lesion of retained mandibular deciduous last premolar. (The endodontic-periodontic relationship—Class II, perio-endo lesion, primarily periodontal with secondary endodontic involvement.)

Points Identified:

A. Root resorption, mesial and distal roots
B. Apical osteolytic zone, mesial root
C. Furcation resorption site (distal root)
D. Furcation exposure (Class III)

Diagnostic Keys: Apical granuloma, horizontal bone loss.

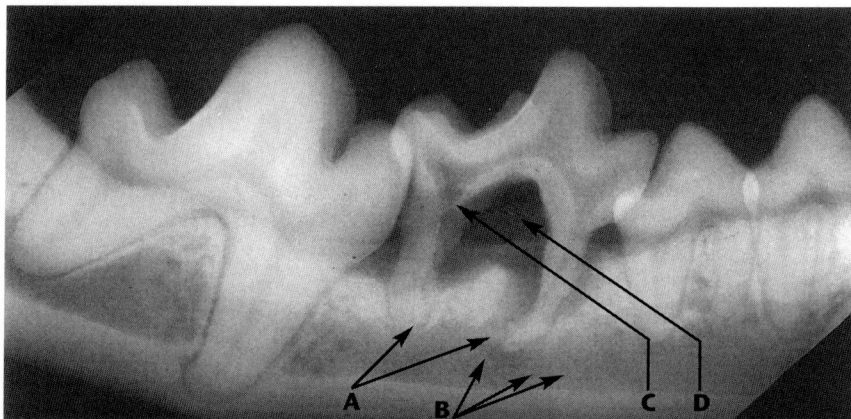

FIGURE 4.2

Contributing Authors:
Jan Bellows and Philippe R. Hennet

Description: Juvenile periodontitis affecting mandibular incisors.

Points Identified:

A. Vertical bone loss
B. Apical osteolytic pathology, incisors
C. Mandibular symphysis

Diagnostic Keys: Wide canal systems indicate immature teeth; central and middle incisors missing.

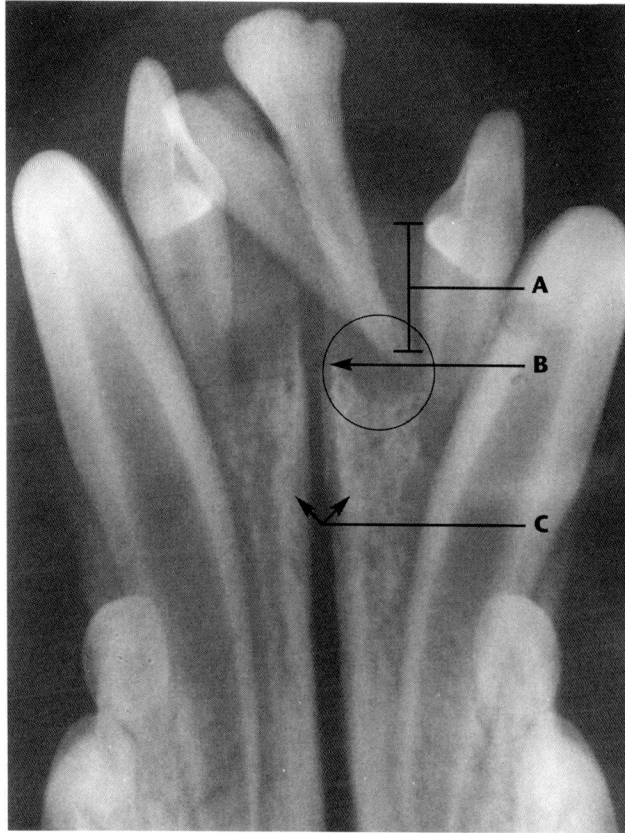

FIGURE 4.3

Contributing Authors:
Jan Bellows and Philippe R. Hennet

Description: Incipient periodontal disease.

Points Identified: Early bone loss.

A. Decreased density, interproximal and furcation bone

Diagnostic Keys: Decrease in bone density.

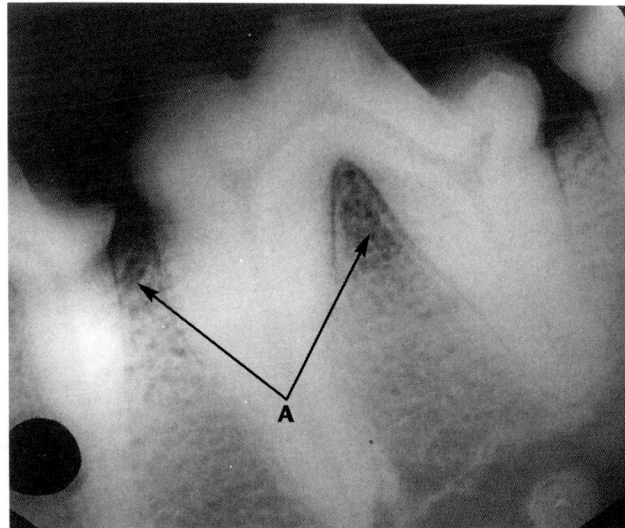

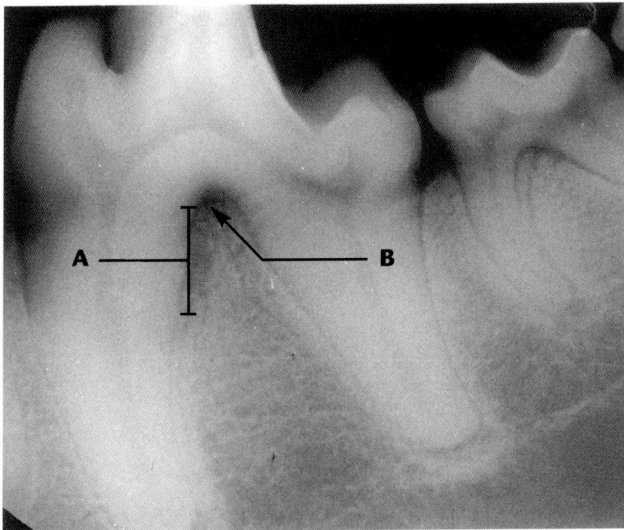

FIGURE 4.4

Contributing Authors:
Jan Bellows and Philippe R. Hennet

Description: Early periodontitis.

Points Identified: Vertical bone loss.

A. Vertical bone loss, distal surface of the mesial root of the mandibular first molar
B. Decreased bone density

Diagnostic Keys: Decrease of bone density.

Common Errors: Overlooking the extent of disease.

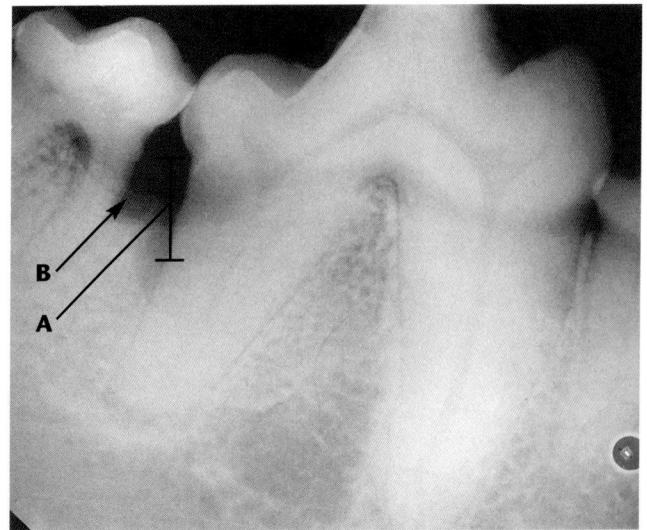

FIGURE 4.5

Contributing Authors:
Jan Bellows and Philippe R. Hennet

Description: Early periodontitis.

Points Identified: Vertical bone loss (mandibular).

A. Bone loss, distal surface of the distal root
B. Bone loss, mesial surface of the mesial root

Diagnostic Keys: Void on the distal surface.

Common Errors: Overlooking the extent of disease.

FIGURE 4.6

Contributing Authors:
Jan Bellows and Philippe R. Hennet

Description: Early to moderate periodontitis.

Points Identified: Bone loss and decreased bone density, mandibular first molar (309).

A. 309
B. Vertical bone loss, mesial surface, mesial root
C. Furcation bone loss, early stage
D. Vertical bone loss distal surface distal root 309

Diagnostic Keys: Loss of lamina dura density, mesial surface of the distal root of 309 and furcation. Vertical bone loss, mesial and distal surfaces, 309. Root remnant (distal root 308) and bony proliferation.

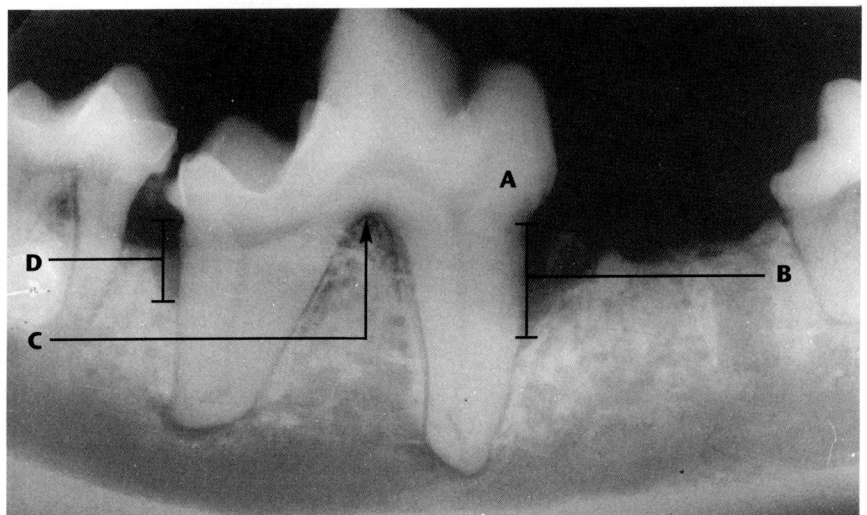

FIGURE 4.7

Contributing Authors:
Jan Bellows and Philippe R. Hennet

Description: Advanced periodontitis in the maxilla.

Points Identified:

A. Class III furcation exposure (208) between palatal and mesiobuccal roots and mesiobuccal and distal roots
B. Distal root
C. Palatal root
D. Mesiobuccal root

Diagnostic Keys: Loss of bony density and bone loss.

Common Errors: Overlooking combined perio-endo lesion in 206.

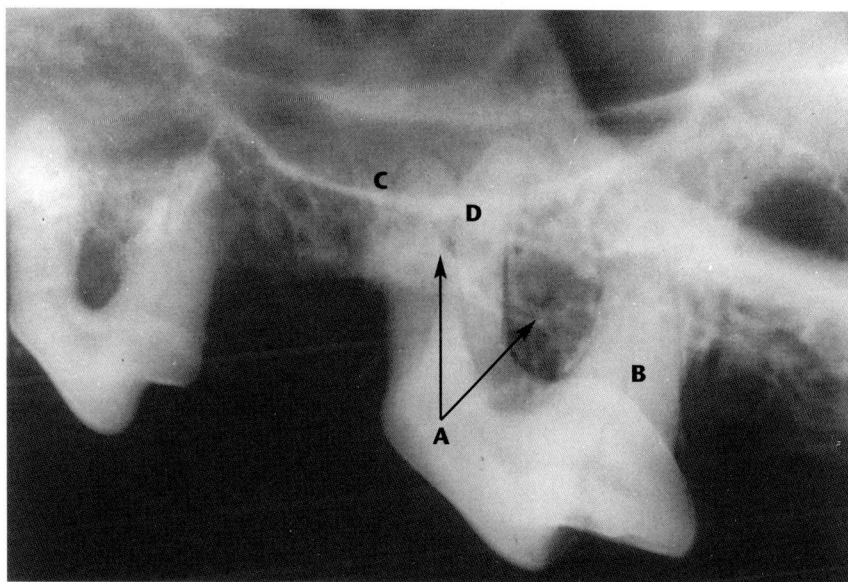

FIGURE 4.8

Contributing Authors:
Jan Bellows and Philippe R. Hennet

Description: Maxillary fourth premolar (108)—periodontitis.

Points Identified: Maxillary fourth premolar (108).

A. Vertical bone loss, interproximal 107/108
B. Vertical bone loss with furcation exposure 108

Common Errors: Overlooking the extent of disease.

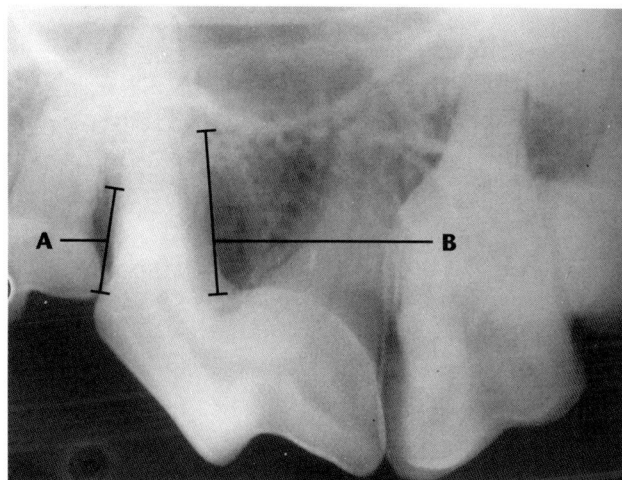

FIGURE 4.9

Contributing Authors:
Jan Bellows and Philippe R. Hennet

Description: Advanced periodontitis, incisors.

Points Identified: Maxillary incisors; horizontal bone loss with exposure of root surfaces (see bars on figure).

Diagnostic Keys: Bone loss.

Common Errors: Overlooking root resorption.

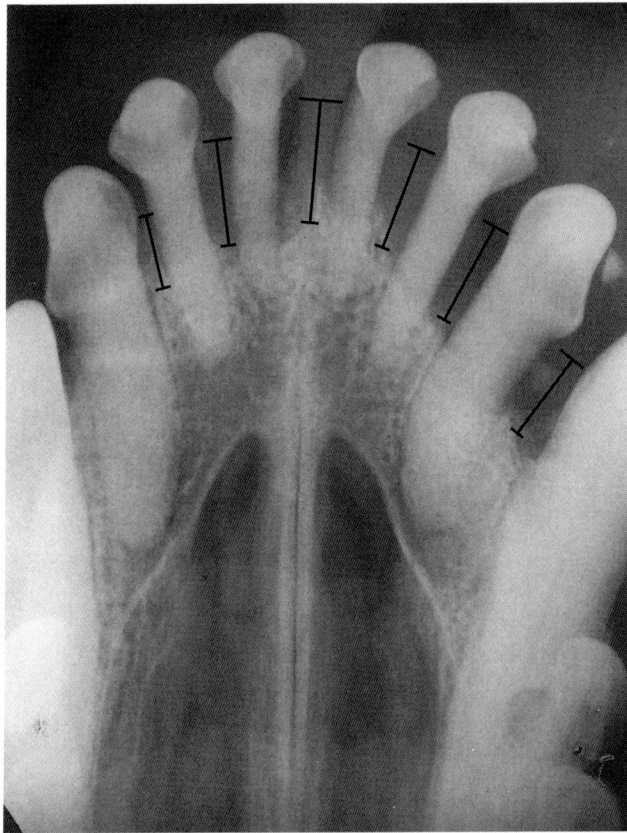

FIGURE 4.10

Contributing Authors:
Jan Bellows and Philippe R. Hennet

Description: End-stage periodontitis, mandibular incisors.

Points Identified:

A. Sclerosing osteomyelitis with advanced cortical bone resorption of the anterior mandibular area (see arrows).
B. Incisors with total loss of bony attachments.

Common Errors: Overlooking possible metabolic disease or neoplasia as a cause of bone loss.

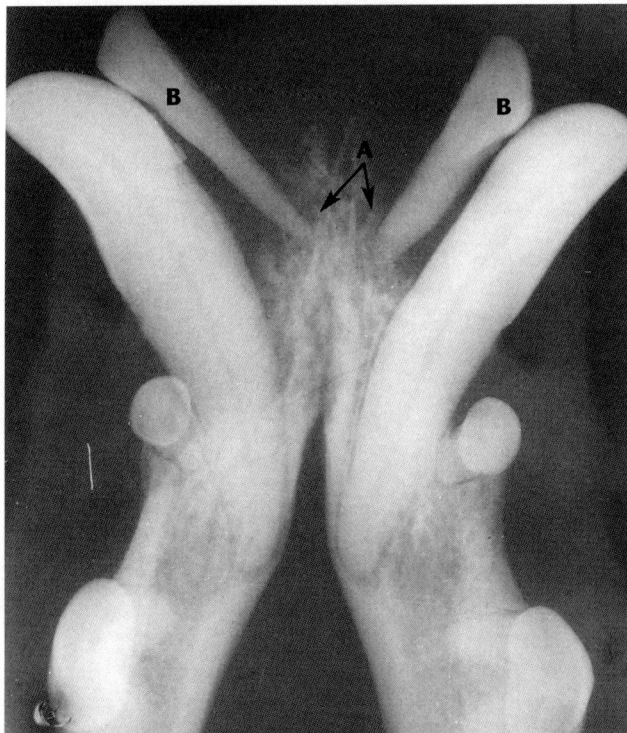

FIGURE 4.11

Contributing Authors:
Jan Bellows and Philippe R. Hennet

Description: Class II/perio-endo lesion.

Points Identified: 409

A. Primary periodontal lesion, distal root
B. Mesial root, periapical radiolucent halo, secondary endodontic lesion

Diagnostic Keys: Bone loss distal root; increased density, mesial root.

Common Errors: Overlooking the extent of disease.

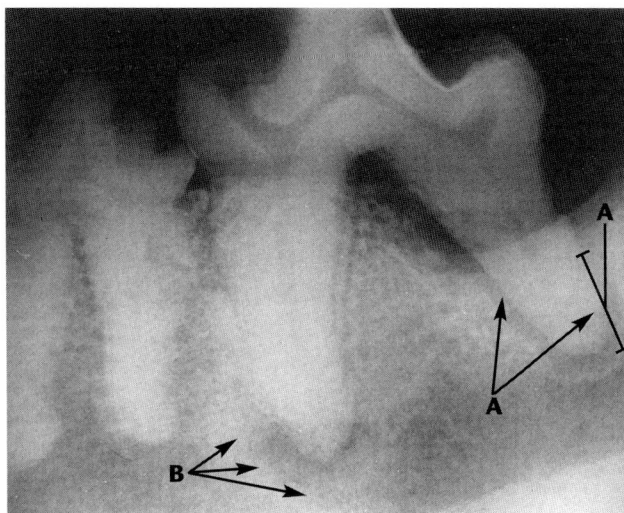

FIGURE 4.12

Contributing Authors:
Jan Bellows and Philippe R. Hennet

Description: End-stage periodontitis, maxillary fourth premolar (208).

Points Identified:

A. Distal root showing root length radiolucency, indicating pathology with severe bone loss
B. Mesiobuccal root with vertical bone loss (palatal root not shown in this projection)

Diagnostic Keys: Partial avulsion due to disease.

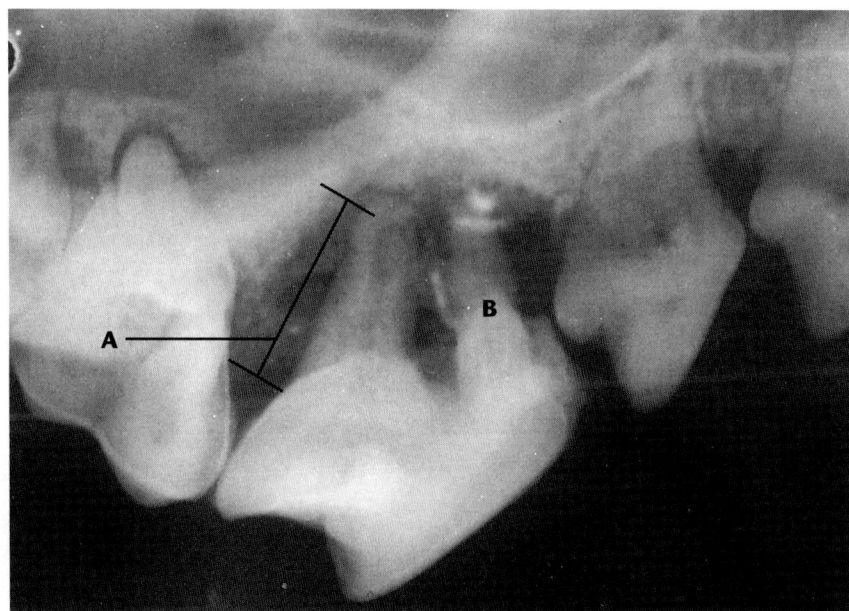

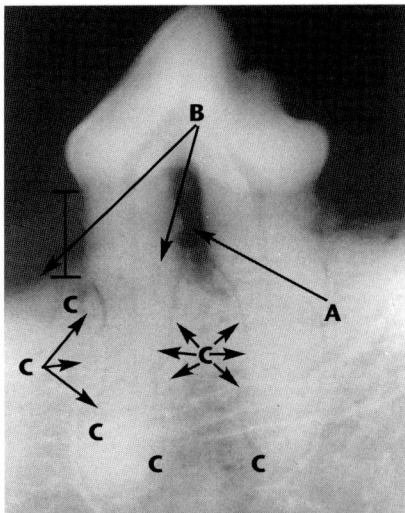

FIGURE 4.13

Contributing Authors:
Jan Bellows and Philippe R. Hennet

Description: Advanced periodontitis.

Points Identified:

A. Class III furcation exposure, 307
B. Horizontal bone loss
C. Root resorption and ankylosis

Diagnostic Keys: Bone loss; resorption.

Common Errors: Overlooking root resorption and ankylosis (Note: There is no condensing osteitis shown on this radiograph.)

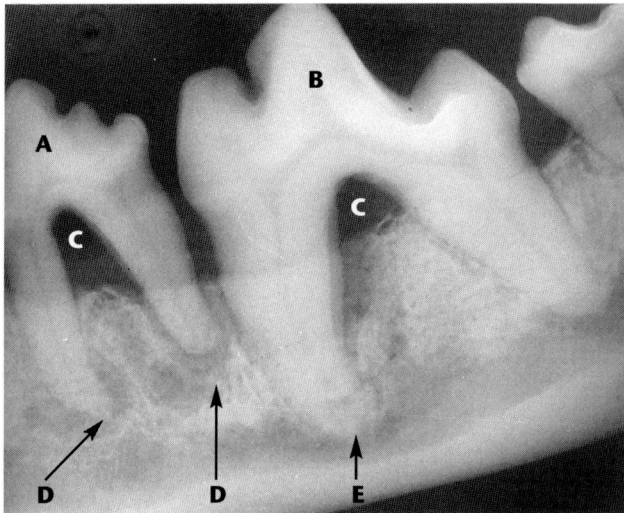

FIGURE 4.14

Contributing Authors:
Jan Bellows and Philippe R. Hennet

Description: Advanced periodontitis.

Points Identified:

A. 408
B. 409
C. Class III furcation exposure 408, 409
D. Resorption with periapical radiolucency, mesial root, 408
E. Infrabony periodontal disease in mesial root, 409, causing periapical lesions in mesial and distal roots

FIGURE 4.15

Contributing Authors:
Jan Bellows and Philippe R. Hennet

Description: Edentulous mandible.

Points Identified:

A. Residual sclerosing osteomyelitis, recently lost teeth

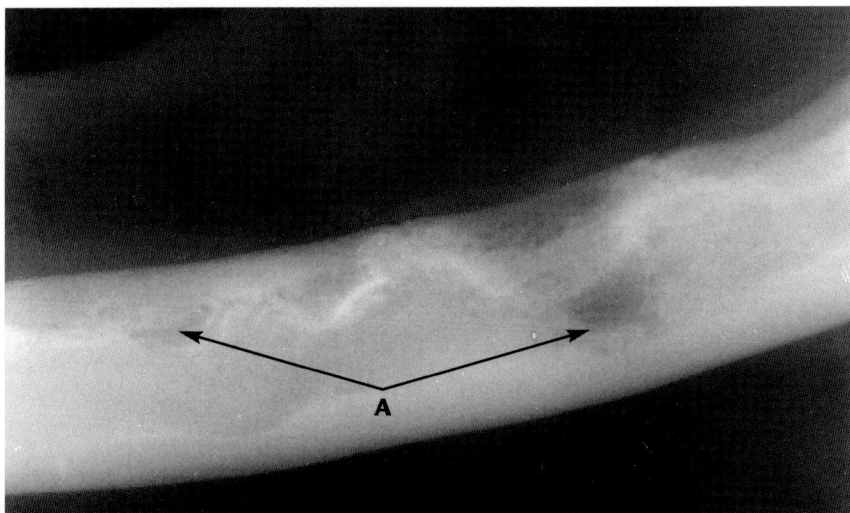

FIGURE 4.16

Contributing Authors:
Jan Bellows and Philippe R. Hennet

Description: Pathologic fracture, vomer/incisive bone.

Points Identified:

A. Bone loss, fracture lines

Common Errors: Overlooking the extent of the disease. Must biopsy site and review histopathology for definitive diagnosis.

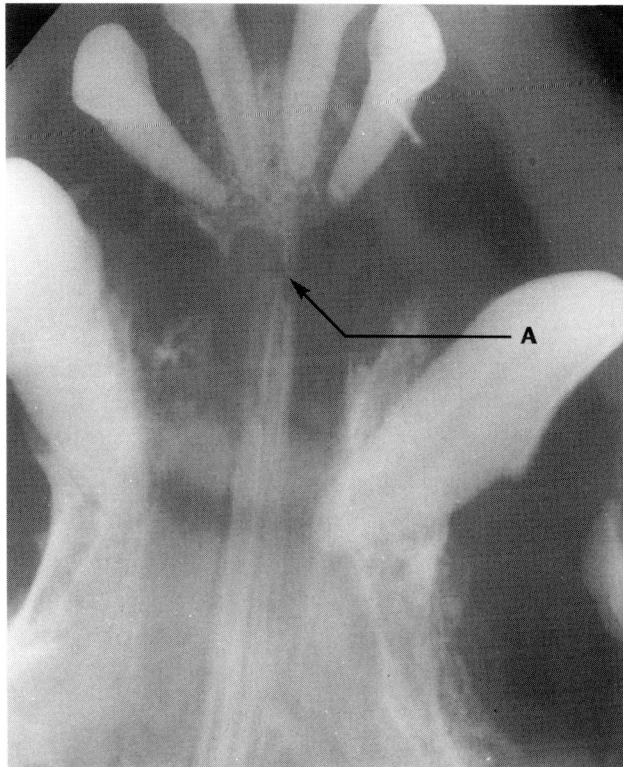

FIGURE 4.17

Contributing Authors:
Jan Bellows and Philippe R. Hennet

Description: Pathologic fracture in mandible.

Points Identified:

A. 407
B. 408
C. 409
D. Fracture line, mandibular vertical fracture at level of distal root
E. Teeth sectioned to be extracted

Diagnostic Keys: Bone loss.

Common Errors: Attempting extractions prior to radiography can lead to iatrogenic pathology. Note deep placement of 409's root in the mandibular canal in opposition with the ventral cortex of the mandible.

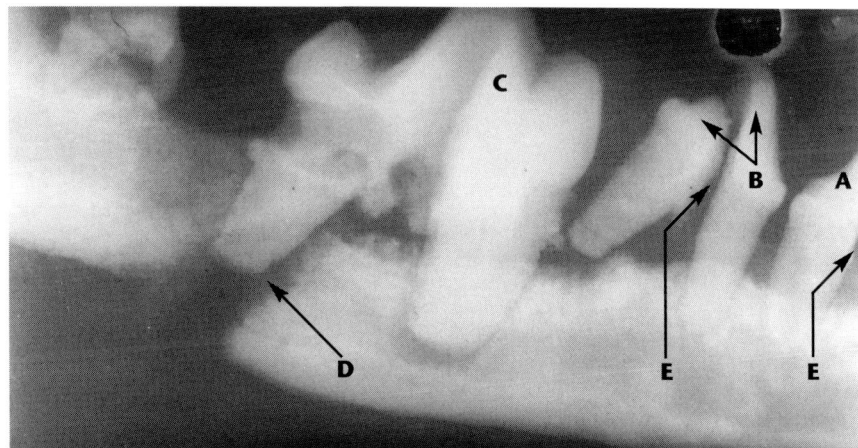

FIGURE 4.18

Contributing Author:
Donald H. DeForge

Description: Idiopathic dental root resorption.

Points Identified: 308, 310 (view A); 408, 410 (view B).

A. 308
B. 310
C. 408
D. 410
E. Mesial roots (310/410)—apical two-thirds of these roots are missing with patient showing no clinical signs related to these teeth.
F. Mesial roots (308/408)—early signs of resorption. Lesions of idiopathic root resorption originate in the apex and progress coronally.
G. Distal roots (308/408)—early signs of resorption. Lesions of idiopathic root resorption originate in the apex and progress coronally.

Diagnostic Keys: No clinical pathology is present. Radiographs show lack of root structure with trabecular bone replacing root.

Common Errors: Misdiagnosis of periodontal-endodontic lesions or primary endodontic lesions.

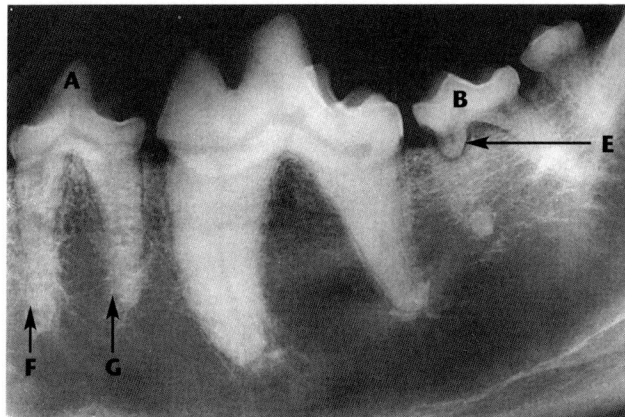

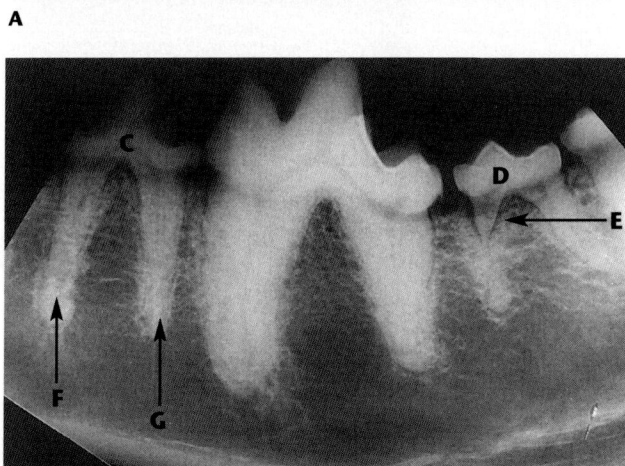

DIGITAL IMAGE ANALYSIS

Michael S. Reddy
Thomas W. Weatherford, III
C. Anne Smith
Brian D. West
Marjorie K. Jeffcoat
Thomas M. Jacks

Standard intraoral radiographs were made by fabricating custom occlusal registration appliances for each radiographic projection. An aluminum reference wedge was incorporated in each custom film holder to provide a density reference. In order to assure that the radiographs were assessed without knowledge of the identity of the dog or treatment group, a random number table was used to code each radiographic series.

A personal computer–based image processing work station was used to obtain quantitative measurements of bone loss. For each measurement, the radiograph (Figure 4.19) was placed under a video camera and digitized with 512 × 512 pixels of spatial resolution and 8 bits (256 gray levels) of contrast resolution. The first

radiograph was digitized and stored on an optical disk. The subsequent radiographic image was aligned to the initial image by manipulating it under a video camera. The images were corrected for variations in contrast and film tilt using computer algorithms. The second radiographic image was then subtracted from the first, with the resultant subtraction image showing areas of bone loss (dark areas) and bone gain (light areas) against a neutral gray background. Measurements of bone loss or gain were made along each root surface interactively using a mouse as the pointing device. The estimate of bone mass change was achieved by converting the subtraction image to a binary image of black and white using a variable operator-controlled threshold. The operator adjusted the threshold until the change appeared white against a background which was black. A morphologic filter was applied to the image to limit the remaining noise in the image. An erode operation was performed on the binary image to remove isolated pixel noise. A dilate operation was then performed to restore the areas of bony change to their approximate original size. Pseudocolor image enhancement was used to represent areas of bone gain as green and areas of bone loss as red. Regions of no change were displayed as the original shades of gray. The color-enhanced image was electronically added to the original radiograph so that the area of change could be visualized on the original radiograph image (Figure 4.20). A comparison of the mean change in gray level at the color enhancement region to the gray levels from the subtraction image of the reference wedge allowed calculation of the thickness of the lesion. The thickness and area measurements were used to calculate an index of bone mass change. Previous studies have indicated that the error in replicability of determination of areas was 4 percent and that calculated changes in bone mass correlated ($r^2 > 0.9$) with acutal changes in bone mass.

Source

This section was excerpted from: Alendronate treatment of naturally occurring periodontitis in beagle dogs by Michael S. Reddy, Thomas W. Weatherford, III, C. Anne Smith, Brian D. West, Marjorie K. Jeffcoat, and Thomas M. Jacks. *J Periodontol* 66(3). March 1995.

X-RAY PLATES

FIGURE 4.19

Contributing Authors:
Michael S. Reddy, Thomas W. Weatherford, III, C. Anne Smith, Brian D. West, Marjorie K. Jeffcoat, Thomas M. Jacks, The University of Alabama at Birmingham, School of Dentistry, Dept. of Periodontics

Description: Radiograph of mandibular premolar teeth in a beagle with horizontal bone loss due to periodontitis.

Points Identified: This film is base line film that will be utilized to determine progressive bone loss with the aid of digital subtraction radiography. See Figure 4.20.

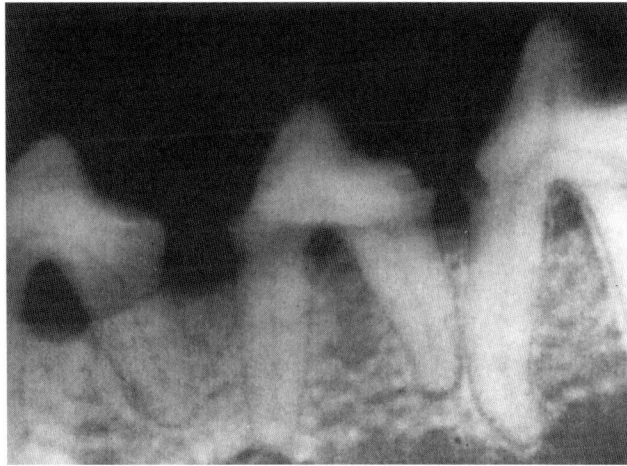

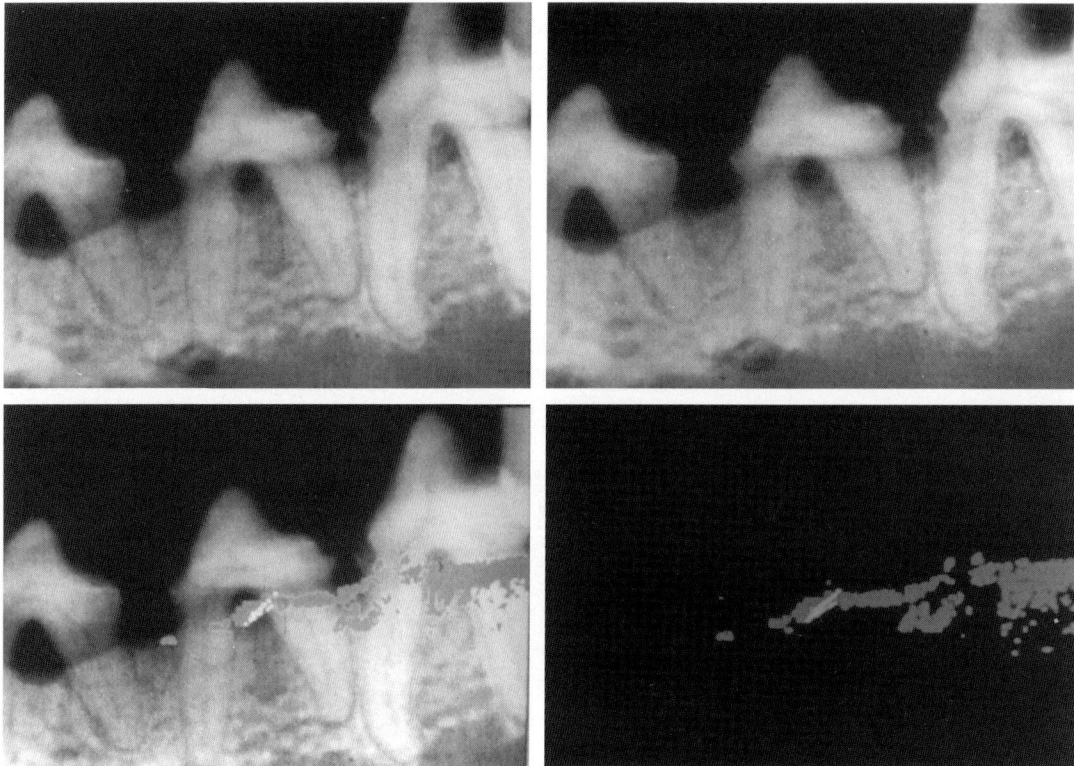

FIGURE 4.20

Contributing Authors:
Michael S. Reddy, Thomas W. Weatherford, III, C. Anne Smith, Brian D. West, Marjorie K. Jeffcoat, Thomas M. Jacks, The University of Alabama at Birmingham, School of Dentistry, Dept. of Periodontics

Description: Illustration of digital subtraction radiography. Upper right and left panels are radiographs taken 3 months apart. Lower right panel shows the area of progressive bone loss (in shades of red on the original plate). Lower left panel shows the area of progressive bone loss superimposed on the original radiograph.

Points Identified: Areas of progressive bone loss (flat gray areas in figures).

*(**See also** color plate.)*

5 Restorative Dentistry

Dr. Steven E. Holmstrom

INTRODUCTION: RESTORATIVE RADIOLOGY

While dental radiology is used relatively infrequently for restorative dentistry, it is used very commonly in procedures associated with restorative dentistry. For example, before, during, and after performing endodontic therapy, the practitioner must take dental radiographs. These radiographs are for the evaluation of the case prior to endodontics for diagnostics, intraoperatively to evaluate instrumentation and obturation of the canal, and finally postoperatively to evaluate the finished product. At 6 and 12 months after the procedure radiographs are taken to evaluate the results. Many restorative products will show up on dental radiographs, and the fill of the access site can be evaluated. However, more importantly, these radiographs are taken to evaluate whether or not there is good foundation on which to place the restoration. An excellent quality restoration over a poor quality root canal will give poor quality results. This chapter will radiographically compare some of the common filling materials: glass ionomers, composite resins, and amalgam. It will discuss the evaluation of teeth and the use of glass ionomers for the treatment of teeth with feline odontoclastic resorptive lesions (neck lesions). Teeth are commonly filled with composite resin restorative material, with amalgam, and by crown therapy. Appropriate and inappropriate filling techniques will be shown. Finally, the use of dental radiology for the evaluation of osseointegrated implants will be reviewed.

Comparison of Restorative Products

A small measuring spoon was used to cast portions of glass ionomer (Vitrebond™, 3M; Shofu II™, Shofu™), composite resin (Z-100™ and P-50™, 3M) and amalgam (Tytin™, Kerr). The amalgam, being made from metal, is the most radiodense, allowing no penetration of x-rays to the film. The glass ionomers and composites by themselves would be radiolucent. Radiodensity has been accomplished by adding minute radiodense particles.

Glass Ionomer Filling of Cervical Line Lesions

The first reason for the use of dental radiology in cervical line lesion restoration would be for the evaluation of the tooth for suitability of restoration. If there is resorption of the tooth root structure, restoration by itself has little hope for success.

Dental radiology can also be used to evaluate the fill of cervical line lesions. This evaluation should consist of observation for voids of restoration, overfills, or overhangs. Radiology can also be used as a follow-up months after the restoration to detect further tooth destruction.

Composite Resin Restoration

Dental radiology can be used to evaluate the appropriateness of a tooth to be restored. The radiographs can detect tooth fractures that may not be detected otherwise. The completeness of a fill with the restorative material can also be evaluated. Voids in the restoration may necessitate removal and replacement of the material. Radiographs can also detect overhangs or inappropriate fillings.

Dental radiology can be used as a follow-up to evaluate fractures, caries, and inflammatory root resorption after a restoration has been placed.

Amalgam Restoration

Amalgam is used as a restorative material, and may be evaluated in a fashion similar to that used for composite resins. However, due to its radiodensity, the restoration itself may obscure the view of some pathologies. For example, a fracture in a tooth may be covered by amalgam, making it nonvisible.

Crown Restoration

Radiology of the simple crown restoration has limited value, as most of the critical area to be evaluated is covered by the metal casting and is not visible. Some new ceramic extracoronal restorations are radiolucent. If root canal therapy has been performed, the radiograph should be evaluated for apical response (the absence or resolution of an apical abscess). The area of tooth around the crown should be evaluated for lucent areas that may represent decay formation due to poor marginal fit.

The placement of a deep post may be evaluated radiographically for appropriateness of fit of the restoration. The tooth should be evaluated on a periodic basis with multiple views for the presence of vertical root fractures that may be caused by the post (vertical fractures).

Implantology

There are many manufacturers of implants and many types of

implants that can be used. Dental radiology is used throughout the procedure for placing an implant. At first, dental radiographs are taken to evaluate the quantity and quality of the bone structure and as a guide for implant placement. After incising and reflecting the gingiva, a pilot hole is drilled. Radiographs are taken at this point to evaluate the direction and placement of the implant. One complication that radiographs may avoid is the misdirection of the implant. The final implant hole is then trephined with an ultra—low speed implant handpiece and drill guide. Trephining is stopped when the proper depth is reached as measured by preoperative radiographs and notches on the trephine drill.

After insertion of the implant, a radiograph is taken to evaluate the position of the implant. The patient is awakened and a three- to 6-month healing period begins. At this point, the patient is re-anesthetized and radiographs are taken to evaluate osseointegration. Osseointegration is noted by growth of bone into the implant and the absence of lytic areas around the implant. If osseointegra-

tion is successful, impressions are taken, and a crown is manufactured and placed.

This procedure is not without complications. Misdirection and penetration into adjacent teeth or poor alignment for the future crown can occur, even with dental radiology acting as a guide. Additionally, penetrating the nasal sinus and penetrating another tooth are complications that may be noted by dental radiology.

Summary

Dental radiology is an important tool in veterinary dentistry, and restorative/operative dentistry cannot be practiced without it. Its use in operative dentistry is primarily in the support of the other dental disciplines of endodontics and oral surgery. As new restorative materials become available to the veterinary dentist, radiology will continue to be paramount in their application and evaluation in operative dentistry.

X-RAY PLATES

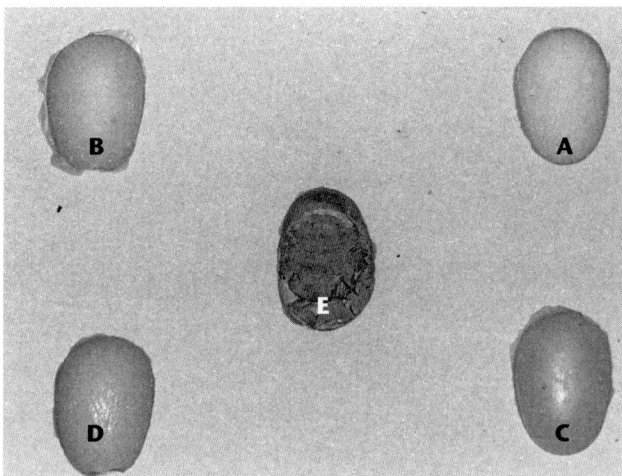

FIGURE 5.1

Contributing Author:
Steven E. Holmstrom

Description: Restorative material appearance; different densities of restorative materials.

Points Identified:

    A. Glass ionomer: Vitrebond™, 3M
    B. Glass ionomer: Shofu II™, Shofu™
    C. Composite: P-50™, 3M
    D. Composite: Z-100™, 3M
    E. Amalgam: Tytin™, Kerr

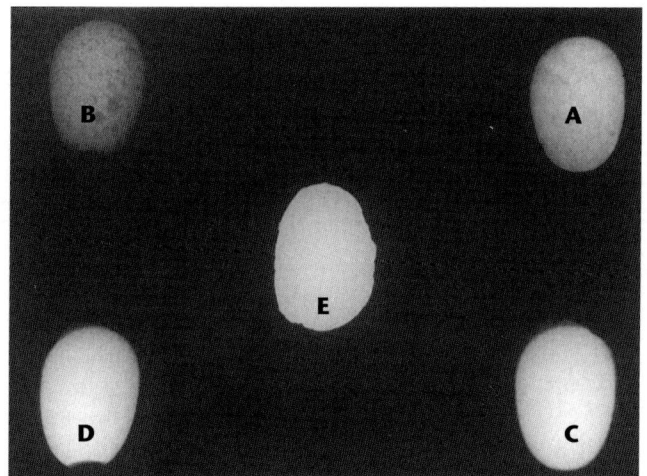

FIGURE 5.2

Contributing Author:
Steven E. Holmstrom

Description: Restorative x-ray density appearance. Radiographic densities vary because of product and fillers added to product.

Points Identified:

    A. Glass ionomers: Vitrebond™, 3M
    B. Glass ionomer: Shofu II™, Shofu™
    C. Composite: P-50™, 3M
    D. Composite: Z-100™, 3M
    E. Amalgam: Tytin™, Kerr

Diagnostic Keys: Amalgam, being made from metal, is most radiodense allowing no penetration of x-rays.

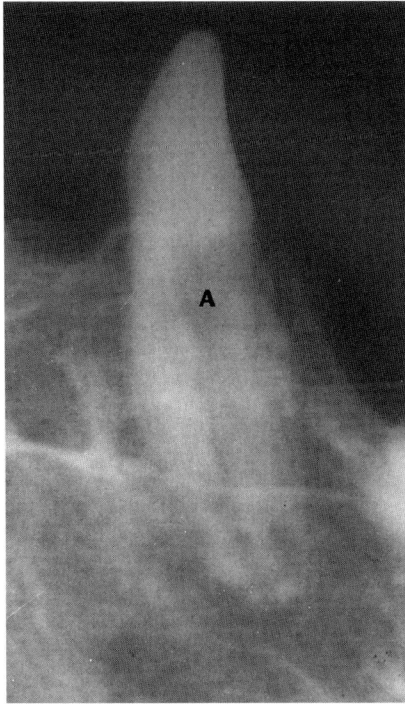

FIGURE 5.3

Contributing Author:
Steven E. Holmstrom

Description: Resorptive lesion, nonrestorable.

Points Identified:

A. Internal odontoclastic resorptive lesion, 204 feline

Diagnostic Keys: Internal moth-eaten structure of root system.

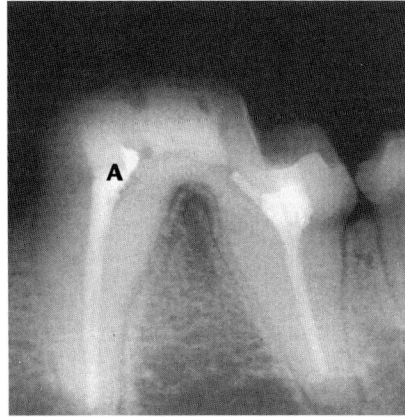

FIGURE 5.4

Contributing Author:
Steven E. Holmstrom

Description: Difficulties in restorative-operatory dentistry. In the mesial table of 409, a restorative material has been placed post–endodontic therapy.

Points Identified:

A. Void in restoration and improper fill

Diagnostic Keys: Note voids in walls of dentin where restorative has been placed. Microleakage will ensure failure in this case, with bacterial migration into dentin.

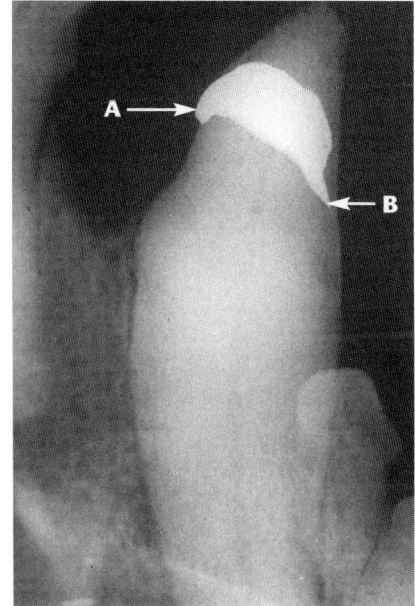

FIGURE 5.5

Contributing Author:
Steven E. Holmstrom

Description: Amalgam restoration 104.

Points Identified:

A. Overhang of amalgam
B. Irregular (pointed) fill

Diagnostic Keys: This application will lead to failure of restoration or microleakage. Apex of tooth must be evaluated for potential endodontic disease.

FIGURE 5.6

Contributing Author:
Steven E. Holmstrom

Description: Placement of post as pretreatment for extracoronal restoration (crown).

Points Identified:

A. Post

Diagnostic Keys: Posts which are too large or placed at an angle that exerts stress on pulp canal can result in vertical or oblique crown fractures.

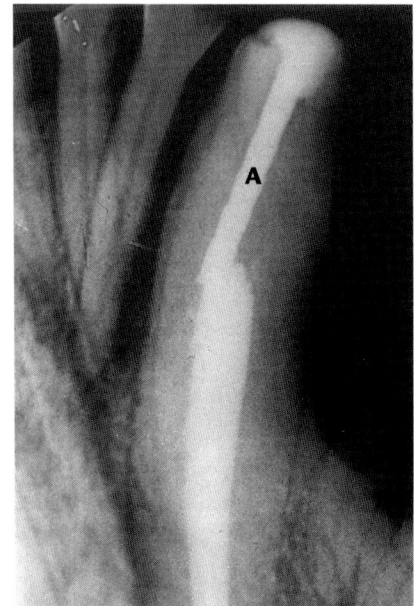

FIGURE 5.7

Contributing Author:
Steven E. Holmstrom

Description: Extracoronal treatment (titanium crown), 108. (Palatal root has been resected.)

Points Identified:

A. Opaque crown, 108

Diagnostic Keys: In opaque crowns marginal caries should be inspected on a routine yearly basis. At the same time, root apex endodontic x-rays should be taken. With new radiolucent ceramic crowns (not shown here) the tooth structure beneath the crown can also be evaluated.

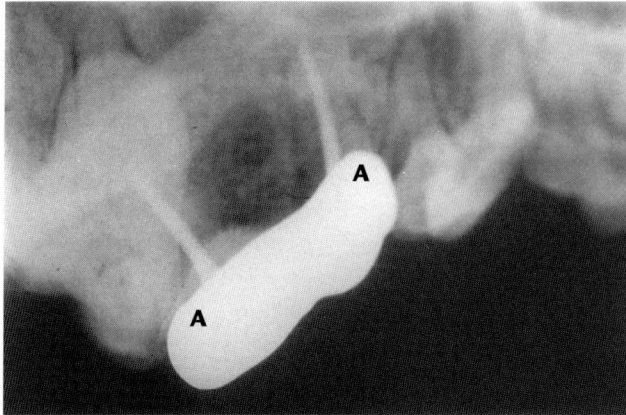

FIGURE 5.8

Contributing Author:
Steven E. Holmstrom

Description: Implantology—direction and placement of two implants.

Points Identified:

A. Implant (check for placement depth)
B. Implant (check for placement direction)

Diagnostic Keys: Radiographs are important to determine implant placement depth and avoid implant misdirection.

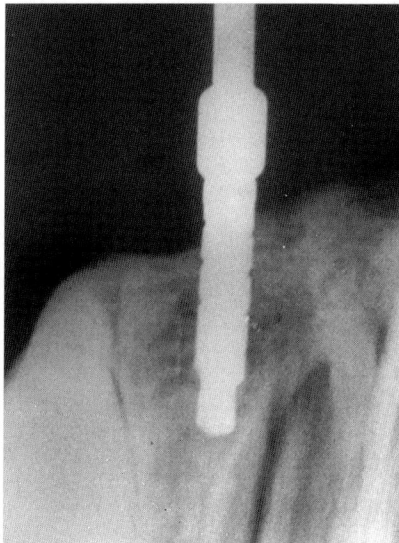

A

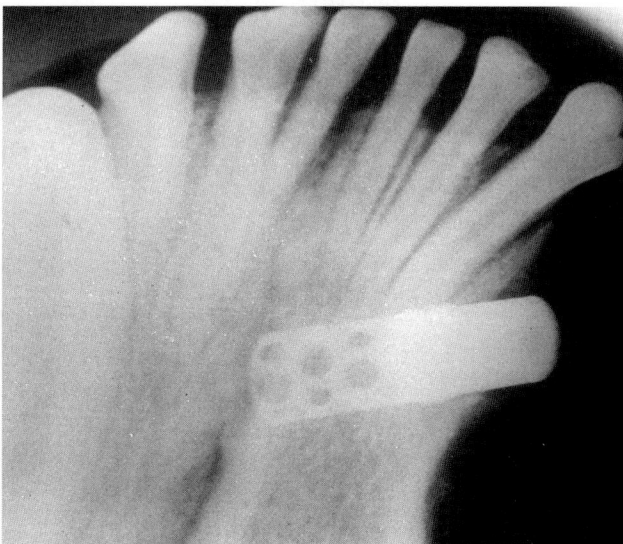

B

FIGURE 5.9

Contributing Author:
Steven E. Holmstrom

Description: Osseointegration

Points Identified:

A. Bone growth into implant

Diagnostic Keys: Osseointegration is noted by bone growth into the implant and the absence of lytic areas around the implant. The option of two implants being used to anchor pontics is a viable option in this patient.

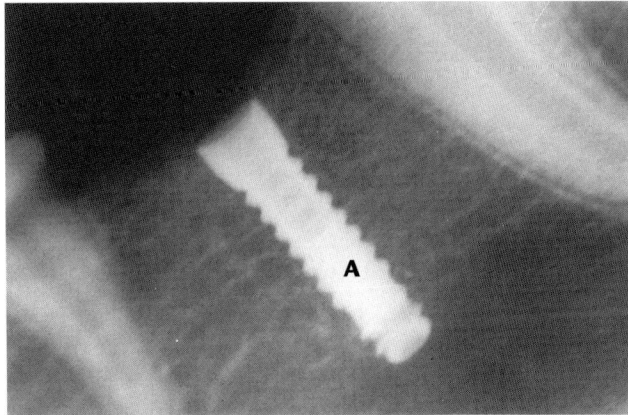

A

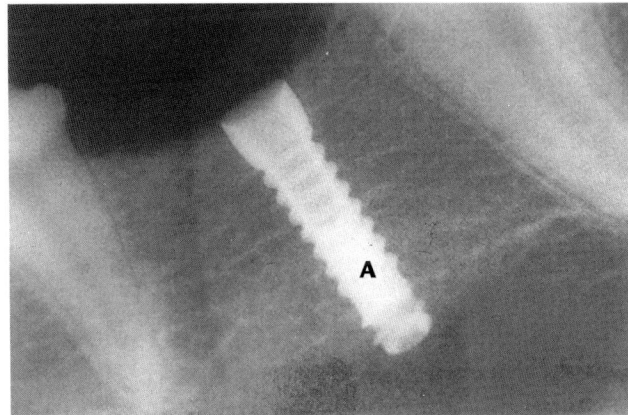

B

FIGURE 5.10

Contributing Author:
Steven E. Holmstrom

Description: Implantology.

Points Identified: Implant showing potential sinus perforation and incomplete osseointegraph. Note irregular border around the implant.

A. Implant—incomplete osseointegration

Diagnostic Keys: Potential for failure exists. Close and further radiographic follow-up is needed prior to pontic placement in this instance.

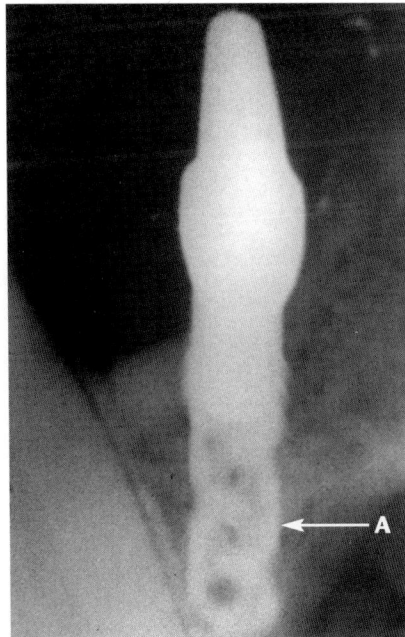

6 Orthodontics

Dr. Thomas H. Kavanagh
Dr. Gary B. Beard

INTRODUCTION

Orthodontic radiography is used before, during, and after operative procedures. Candidates for orthodontia may be screened for conditions that preclude treatment, allow a guarded prognosis, or indicate the probability of successful treatment. Interoperative radiographic evaluation will help avert complications by providing visualization of hard tissue changes before external evidence occurs.

Radiography is indicated in interceptive orthodontics in young animals, especially when exodontia of deciduous teeth is the treatment of choice. Documentation of adult dentition is essential. Absence of a permanent tooth bud will change the extraction options. Radiography is also indicated for planning treatment of impacted teeth.

In adult dentition, preoperative radiographic evaluation is made to detect hidden pathology that may interfere with movement of teeth, such as ankylosis, root resorption, dilacerated and/or bulbous roots, periapical disease, intraradicular lesions, immature periodontium, neoplasia, root agenesis, and the like. In addition, evaluation of anchor teeth will determine which teeth are suitable for use.

Radiography is used during treatment to monitor for complications such as extrusion, fracture, dehiscence, pulpal death, ankylosis, peridontitis, and root resorption. Postoperative films will reveal health and monitor periodontium regeneration. Lastly, dental radiographs are an integral part of the animal's records, which include signalment, orthodontic models, photographs, and charting.

X-RAY PLATES

FIGURE 6.1

Contributing Author:
Thomas H. Kavanagh

Description: A 3-month-old female Old English sheepdog with brachygnathia and lower deciduous cuspids fractured at the gum line. All permanent tooth buds are present. Arrows point to crypt cusps. Buds are semilucent.

Points Identified:

A. 301	F. 401
B. 302	G. 402
C. 303	H. 403
D. 304	I. 404
E. 305	J. 405

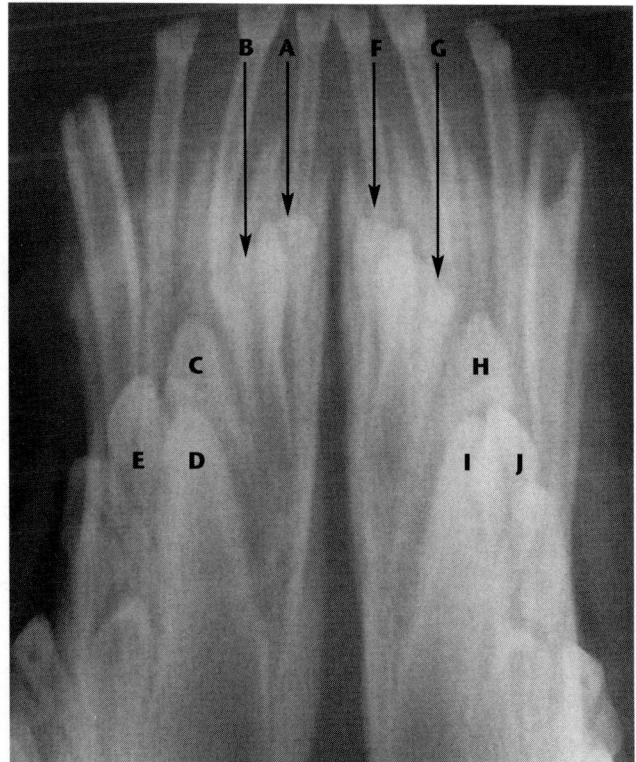

FIGURE 6.2

Contributing Author:
Thomas H. Kavanagh

Description: Tooth buds 104, 105, 204, 205.

Points Identified:

- A. 104
- B. 105
- C. 204
- D. 205

Common Errors: A common error is to confuse the locations of 105/104 and 205/204. To avoid this, follow the large buds of cuspids to their crowns.

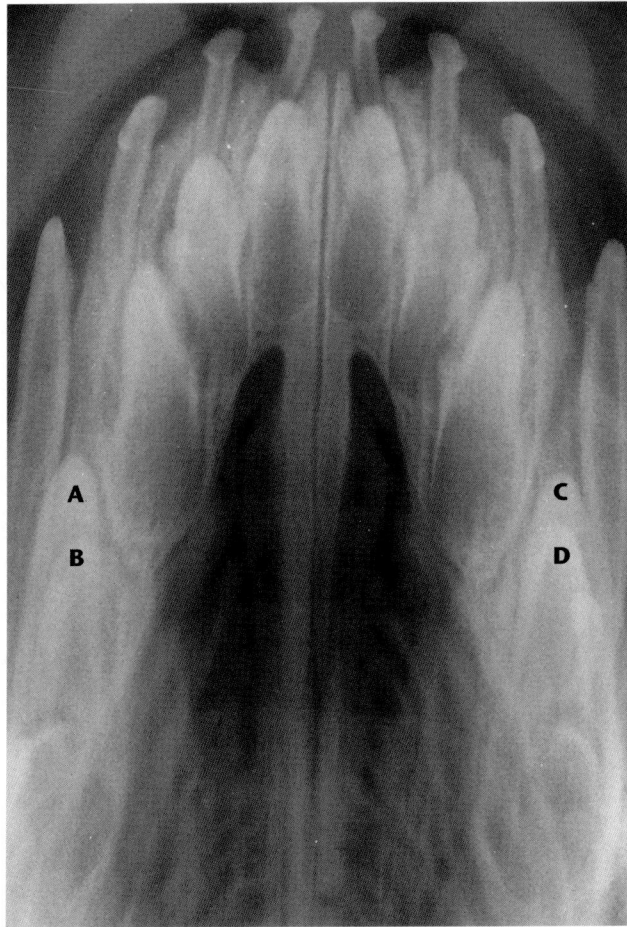

FIGURE 6.3

Contributing Author:
Thomas H. Kavanagh

Description: Linguoversion canines injuring the palate in an 8-week-old female standard poodle. Note that the lower canines erupt lingually to their predecessors.

Points Identified:

- A. 304
- B. 404

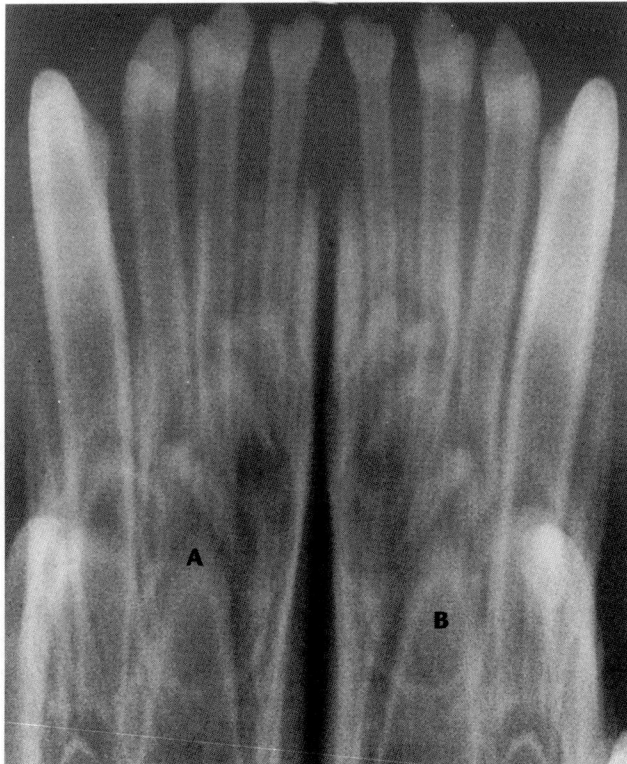

FIGURE 6.4

Contributing Author:
Thomas H. Kavanagh

Description: A 6-month-old female sheltie with linguoversion mandibular canines. Note open apices.

Points Identified:

A. 304
B. 404
C. Open apices

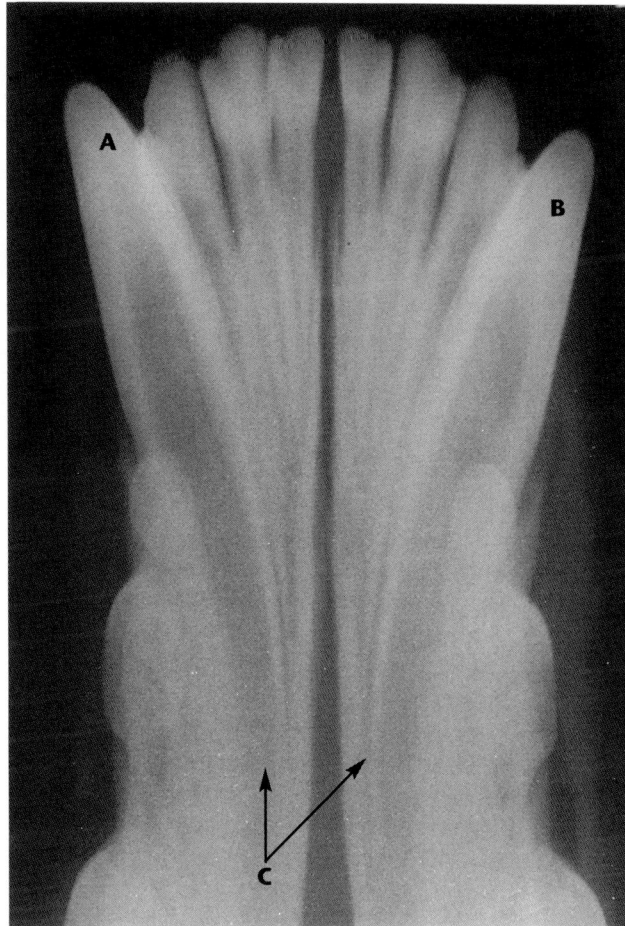

FIGURE 6.5

Contributing Author:
Thomas H. Kavanagh

Description: Occlusal view of a 9-week-old German shepherd female with a wry bite resulting in an anterior cross bite of 503/803, 502/802, 501/801, and deviation of the maxilla to the right. Note that all deciduous teeth have a corresponding tooth bud present.

Points Identified: Wry bite with deviation of maxilla to the right. Note the asymmetry of the incisive (premaxilla) bone.

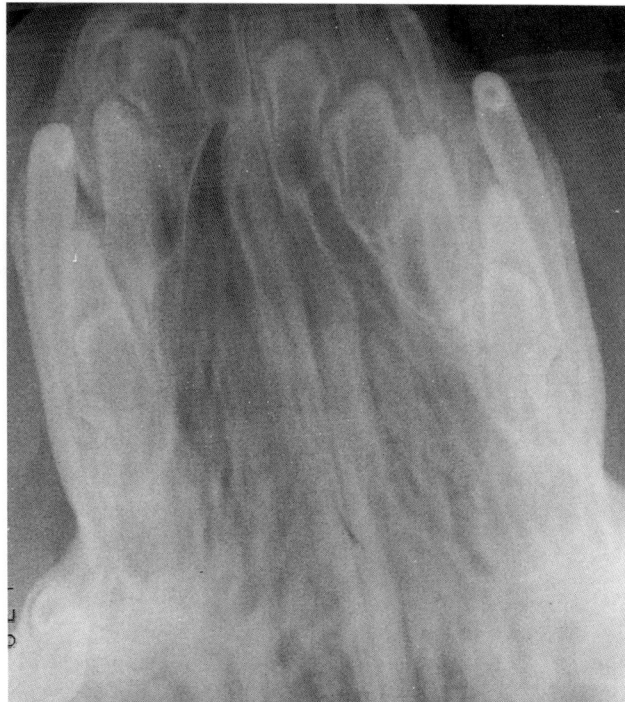

FIGURE 6.6

Contributing Author:
Thomas H. Kavanagh

Description: Enamel hypoplasia of 201. Note decreased size of root of 201. Note the asymmetry of the palatine fissure and incisive (premaxilla) bone.

Points Identified:

A. 201

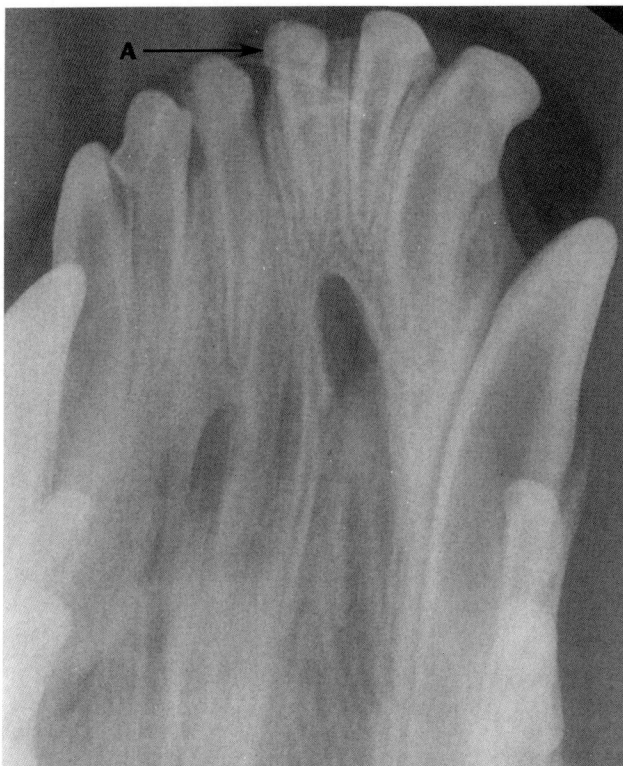

FIGURE 6.7

Contributing Author:
Thomas H. Kavanagh

Description: One year later at 18 months of age (see Figure 6.6). Even though the patient has a wry muzzle, all front teeth occlude in scissor occlusion. Of interest is trabecular radiolucency of 201. The canal width is similar to the contralateral counterpart, suggesting vital pulp.

Points Identified:

A. 201
B. A lamina dura is not distinguishable

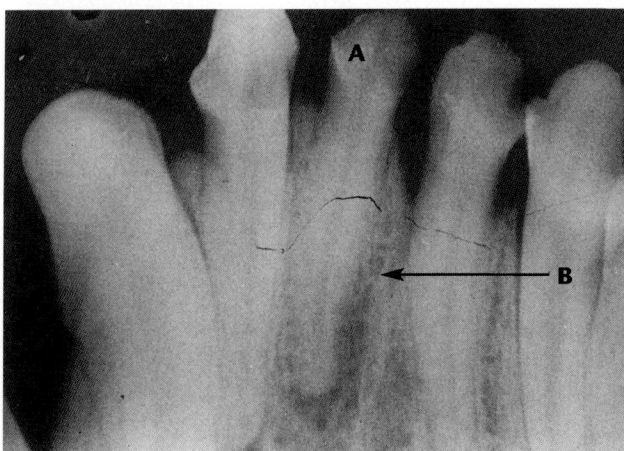

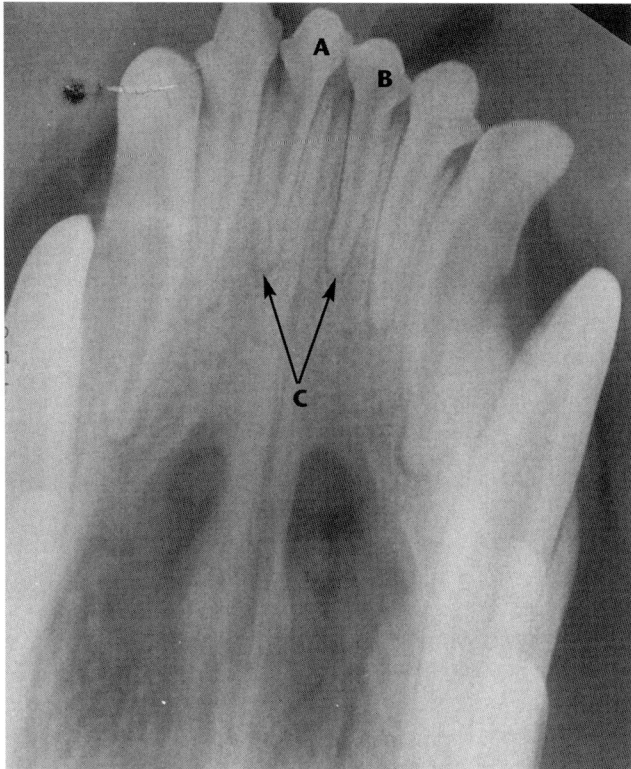

FIGURE 6.8

Contributing Author:
Thomas H. Kavanagh

Description: Anterior cross bite, 13-month-old female German shorthaired pointer; 102, 101, 201. This preoperative occlusal view shows short 102, 101, 201.

Points Identified: Note periapical radiolucencies in 101, 201 due to trauma from malocclusion. Radiographic monitoring will determine pulp vitality.

    A. 101
    B. 201
    C. Periapical radiolucency

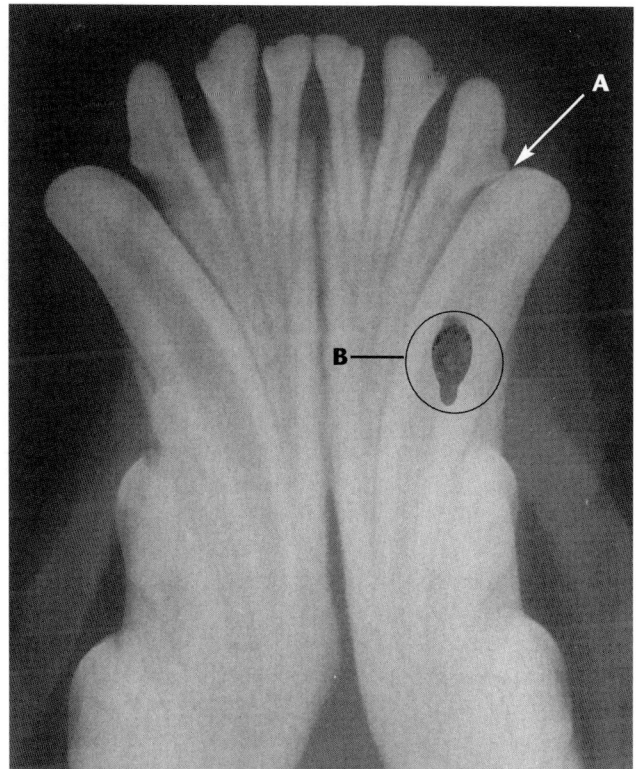

FIGURE 6.9

Contributing Author:
Thomas H. Kavanagh

Description: Same patient as in Figure 6.8, showing preoperative lower occlusal view. Note that 303 has contact with 304 interproximally. This is normal. All the other lower incisors are displaced facially and splayed due to the malocclusion. The apices are closed.

Points Identified: Note 303/304 interproximal contact. This may lead to periodontal pathology if not corrected with orthodontics. In any case it must be monitored.

    A. 303/304, interproximal contact
    B. Artifact

FIGURE 6.10

Contributing Author:
Thomas H. Kavanagh

Description: Same patient as in Figures 6.8 and 6.9; spring-loaded expansion device shown intraoperatively to treat anterior cross bite. There is much difficulty visualizing apices and the periodontium.

Points Identified:

A. Note expansion bar moving incisors
B. Device anchored to canines 104/204

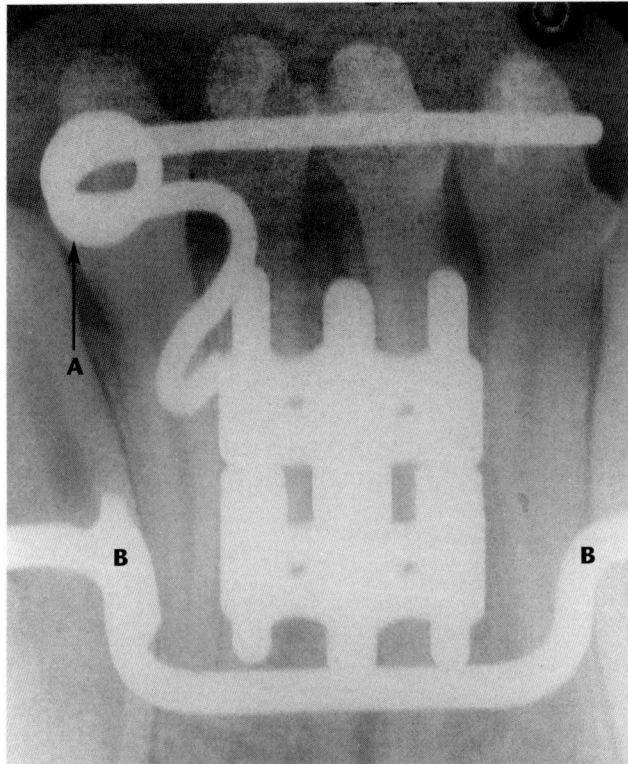

FIGURE 6.11

Contributing Author:
Thomas H. Kavanagh

Description: Same patient as in Figures 6.8–6.10. Postoperative film. Cannot verify that subject teeth have tipped into position, but there does appear to be decreased radiolucency of the root apices (101, 201).

Points Identified:

A. 101
B. 201
C. Area of decreased radiolucency (subjective)

Diagnostic Keys: This is subjective but decreased radiolucency could indicate that occlusive trauma has stopped. Another film should be taken in 6 months for comparison.

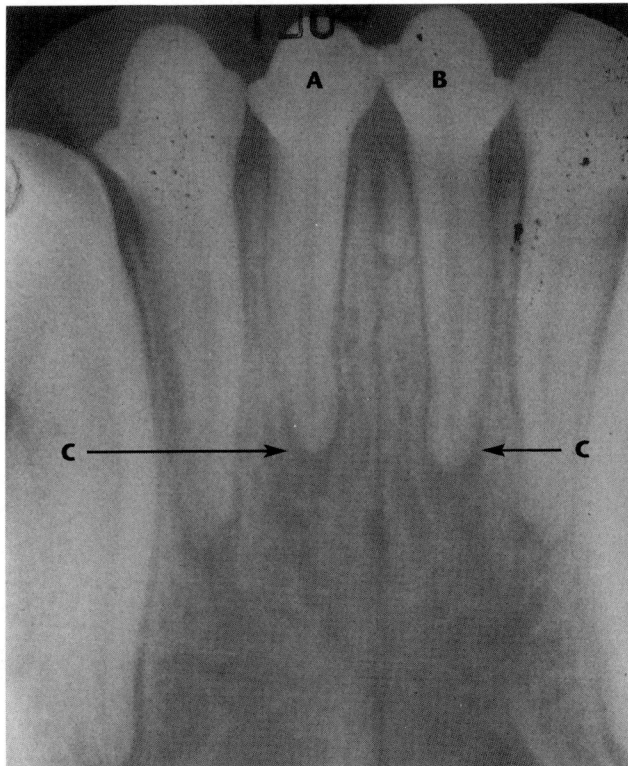

FIGURE 6.12

Contributing Author:
Thomas H. Kavanagh

Description: Radiograph of impacted incisor 201 in a 6-month-old female Gordon setter.

Points Identified:

A. 201, impacted incisor
B. Overlying bone

Diagnostic Keys: Note the overlying bone. Note the lack of a complete lamina dura, indicating ankylosis. The prognosis for eruption in this case is guarded due to the ankylosis and closed apex.

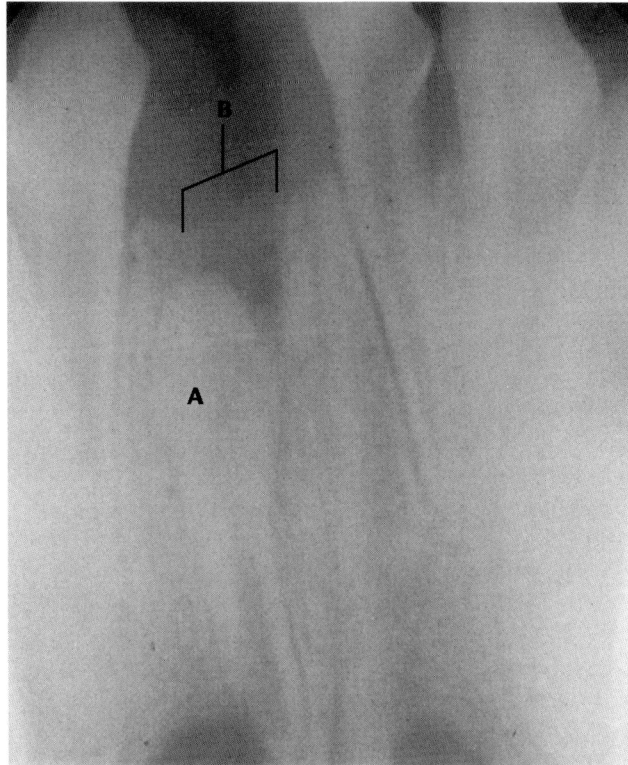

FIGURE 6.13

Contributing Author:
Thomas H. Kavanagh

Description: Occlusal view of a 9-month-old Shetland sheepdog with a mesioverted canine tooth (204). The maxillary canine tooth is displaced rostrally, hitting the upper third incisor tooth.

Points Identified: Note the vast difference between diastemas 103/104 and 203/204. Also, 204 has an apex much more distal than its 104 counterpart.

A. 103
B. 104
C. Large normal diastema 103/104
D. Decreased diastema 203/204

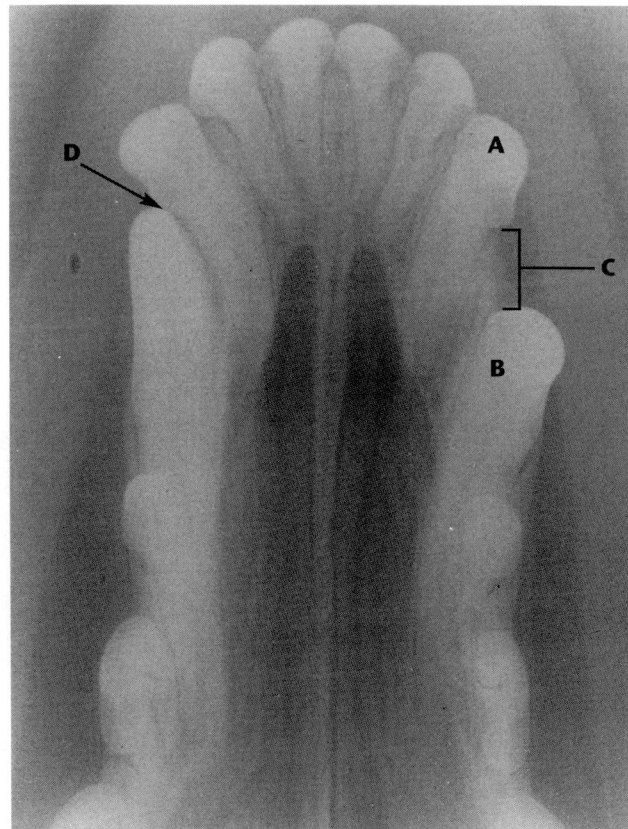

FIGURE 6.14

Contributing Author:
Thomas H. Kavanagh

Description: Same patient as in Figure 6.13. Orthodontic buttons placed on 204 and 208 to move tooth 204 with elastic chain. Interoperative iatrogenic pathology.

Points Identified:

A. Mesiobuccal root 208
B. Furcation/crestal bone widening
C. Tipping distal root 208 with extrusion
D. Increased interproximal space 208/209

Diagnostic Keys: Distal root apex pathology: wide furcative lamina dura and loss of interproximal contact between 208 and 209 indicate subluxation of 208. Vertical bone loss indicates iatrogenic periodontitis.

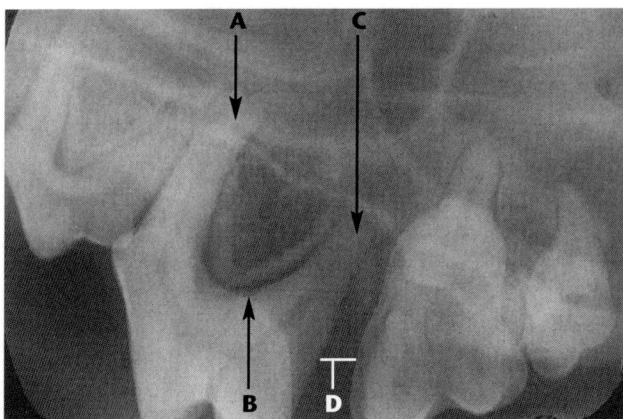

FIGURE 6.15

Contributing Author:
Thomas H. Kavanagh

Description: Same patient as in Figures 6.13 and 6.14. After 2 weeks of treatment for mesioversion tooth in a sheltie, the diastema space 203/204 is starting to increase.

Points Identified:

A. Diastema space 203/204
B. Orthodontic button to which elastic chain is attached (not shown, button on 208 to attach elastic chain distally)

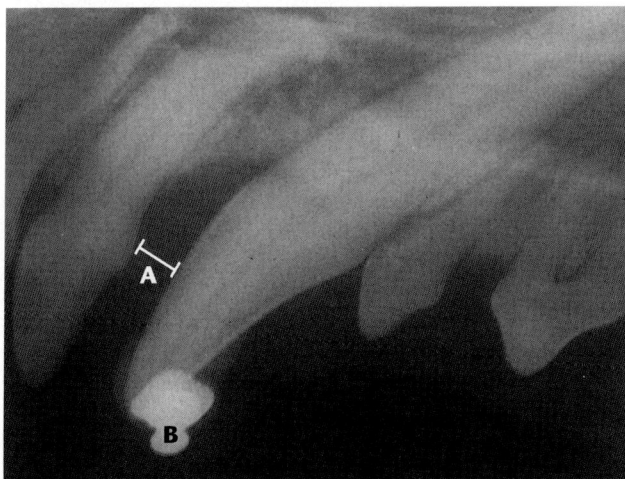

FIGURE 6.16

Contributing Author:
Thomas H. Kavanagh

Description: Same patient as in Figure 6.15, 2 weeks later. Elastics had been removed from the natural fissure of 208 and were instead attached to 309. It appears that the interproximal (208/209) iatrogenic gap is closing and furcation bone is remodeling. This is impossible to verify because of tube angulation and bisecting angle differences between Figures 6.14 and 6.16.

Points Identified:

A. Mesiobuccal root 208
B. Furcation/crestal bone 208
C. Distal root 208

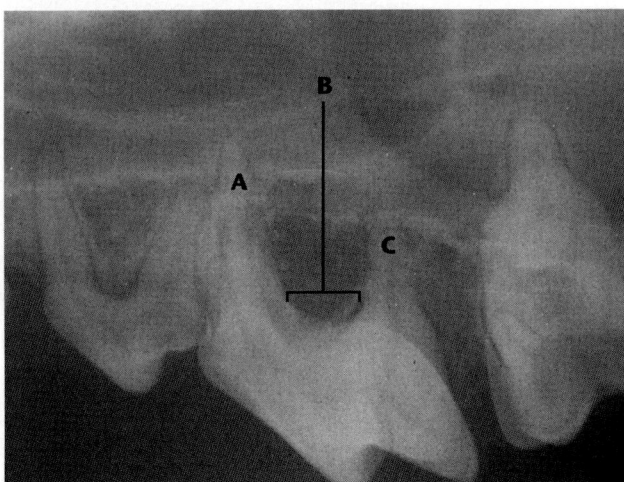

FIGURE 6.17

Contributing Author:

Thomas H. Kavanagh

Description: Same patient as in Figures 6.13–6.16. Increased radiolucency of mesial root apex lamina dura of 309, most likely secondary to rotation (intrusion of this apex) due to the elastic chain attached to the natural fissure. Note the minor furcation bone loss.

Points Identified: 309

A. Increased radiolucency of mesial root
B. Furcation bone loss
C. Ortho button/elastic chain attachment site
D. Artifact

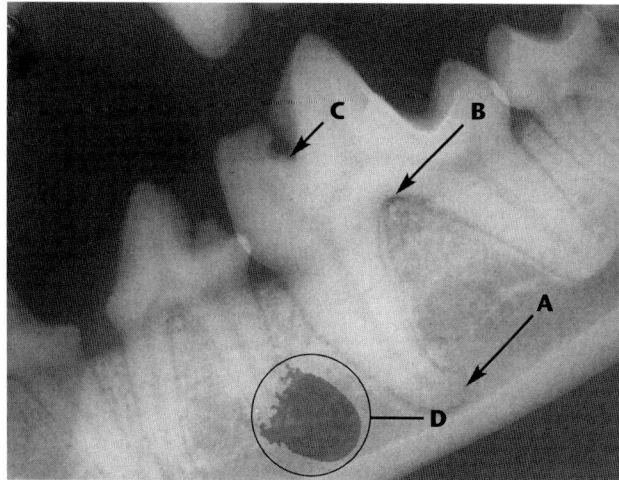

FIGURE 6.18

Contributing Author:

Thomas H. Kavanagh

Description: Same patient as shown in Figures 6.13–6.17. At the conclusion of operative orthodontics, greater superimposition of 204 and 205 is seen and adequate bony infiltration at the diastema 203/204 is seen. Note that the apex of 204 is normal. The bisecting angle projection shown is incorrect, with tooth elongation present. The beam was directed too perpendicular to the tooth axis. The long straight root is typical of mesioversion of canine teeth but distorted by bisecting angle in this film.

Points Identified:

A. 203
B. 204
C. Improper tooth elongation from incorrect bisecting angle technique

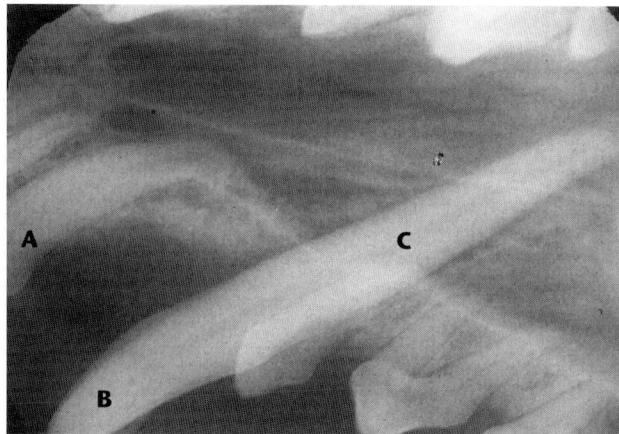

FIGURE 6.19

Contributing Author:

Thomas H. Kavanagh

Description: Same patient as shown in Figures 6.13–6.18. Conclusion of operation film shows that the 208 apex has remodeled, the gap between 208/209 has closed, and the furcation fill is near complete.

Points Identified: 208

A. Mesiobuccal root
B. Furcation
C. Distal root

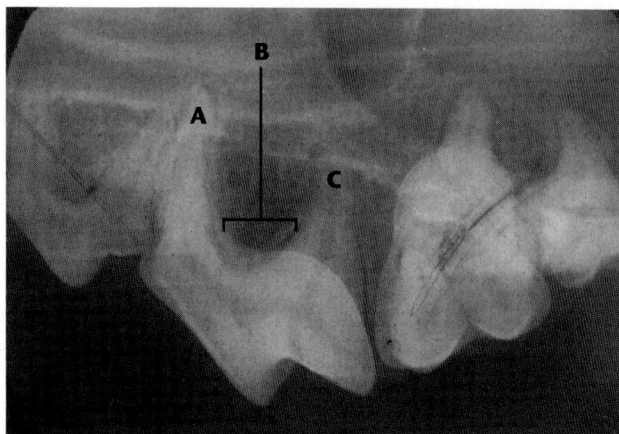

7 Canine Oral Neoplasia

Dr. Jamie G. Anderson
Dr. Anna Fong Revenaugh

INTRODUCTION

Epidemiology and Etiology

In the human population worldwide, an estimated 500,000 new cases of head and neck cancer occur annually.[1,2] In the dog, the oral and pharyngeal cavities represent the fourth most frequent site for the occurrence of malignant neoplasms.[3,4] Malignant and benign oral neoplasms combined account for 6.6 percent of all canine neoplasia.[5] The reported incidence rate of malignant oropharyngeal neoplasia is 20.4 cases per 100,000 dogs,[4,6–10] risk increasing with age. Males have a 2.4 times greater relative risk of developing oral neoplasms than females.[4] Specific breeds at risk for oral neoplasia include cocker spaniels, poodles, German shepherds, German shorthaired pointers, weimaraners, golden retrievers, and boxers.[7,8,10,11]

Oral neoplasms can be odontogenic or nonodontogenic in origin, and malignant or benign in behavior. An estimated 50 percent of oral neoplasms are malignant;[11,12,13] malignant melanoma, squamous cell carcinoma, and fibrosarcoma are the most common.[3,6,14] Larger breeds of dogs (>23 kg) have a greater tendency to develop fibrosarcomas (2.3:1) and squamous cell carcinomas (2:1); smaller breeds (<23kg) are more likely to have malignant melanomas (1.8:1).[10] Approximately 25 percent of canine oral neoplasms are benign tumors of periodontal origin, the epulides.[9,11,13] Oral neoplasms most commonly occur on the gingiva, followed by the buccal mucosa, the palate and the tongue.[6,7,8,10]

Epidemiologic data in human head and neck cancer patients incriminates alcohol and tobacco products as important risk factors.[15–19] Increasing evidence supports a viral contribution to development of head and neck and nasopharyngeal cancer.[20–24] The human papilloma virus and the Epstein-Barr virus are implicated, respectively. In the canine population, the factors responsible for oral cancer are largely undetermined.[8] Known factors include the self-limiting canine oral papillomatosis, caused by the oral papilloma virus and papovavirus.[25] A heavily polluted urban environment has been suggested as a risk factor for dogs with tonsillar squamous cell carcinoma.[26,27]

Clinical Signs

The clinical signs associated with oral masslike lesions may be similar for neoplasia, severe inflammation, or developmental anomalies. Signs referable to oral neoplasia include hemorrhage from the mouth, apparent pain or reluctance to eat, excessive salivation, fetid odor, tooth mobility or loss, and disturbance in oral/maxillofacial contour. Unfortunately, because of the relative infrequency with which the oral cavity is examined, oral neoplasms often grow quite large prior to detection. A visible mass may become ulcerated and necrotic as the neoplasm outgrows its blood supply and becomes secondarily infected.

Diagnosis and Clinical Staging

Early diagnosis and aggressive treatment are crucial in the management of oral malignancies. A complete physical and oral examination with a minimum clinical pathologic data base (complete blood count, chemistry panel, urinalysis) are requisite first steps in the diagnostic workup. The value of fine-needle aspirates and exfoliative cytology (although easy and noninvasive to collect) lies in the skill of the clinical pathologist. It is suggested that positive and negative cytologic diagnoses always be confirmed by histopathologic examination.[28] An incisional or excisional biopsy of the lesion is indicated to determine the definitive diagnosis. Attention to proper biopsy technique will minimize confusion about the histopathologic diagnosis.[29,30] Repeat biopsy evaluation is not uncommon and should be pursued if the degree of differentiation or histopathologic report (in general) does not coincide with the clinical picture.

Radiographs, CAT scanning or MRI are important adjuncts for determining the extent of local disease. Thoracic radiographs (three views) may be indicated, depending on the biologic behavior of the tumor. A 60 percent incidence of radiographically demonstrable bone invasion in canine malignant oropharyngeal neoplasia is reported.[31] A recent paper evaluated the radiologic assessment of fifty cases of oral neoplasms.[32] The radiologic appearance of bone involvement was defined and classified as destructive, productive, periosteal unstructured bone, or calcification. Sclerosis surrounding an area of bone destruction (seen commonly with malar abscessation) was not an apparent tumor associated feature. Radiologic evidence of bone involvement was apparent for 78 percent of fibrosarcomas, 82 percent of squamous cell carcinomas, 100 percent of malignant melanomas (*n*=3) and 87 percent of all malignant tumors. Malignant tumors showed a tendency to irregular or aggressive bone loss. Tumor associated dental disruption was evident in 60 percent of cases. Bone production or calcification was the predominant radiographic change seen in benign tumors. Excluding the ameloblastoma (because of its characteristic radiographic appearance), none of the radiographic changes were specific for a particular tumor type. It is important to note that the absence of detectable radiographic change does not rule out malignancy.

Clinical staging should be attempted. Criteria delineated by the World Health Organization TNM Classification for oral neoplasia are based on size and extent of primary tumor involvement, regional lymph node involvement, and the presence of distant metastasis.

Malignant Neoplasms

Malignant Melanoma

Malignant melanoma (MM) is the most common oral malignancy, representing approximately 33 percent of oral tumors.[6,7,8,10] The origin for the tumor is from melanocytes in the mucosal epithelium or in the superficial stroma of the gingiva.[33] The MM occurs most frequently in the gingival tissues, followed by the buccal mucosa, palate, and tongue.[6,7,8,10,11,33] A male predisposition to MM (1.4 to 6 times greater than females) has been variously reported,[3,4,6-10,11] and the mean age of occurrence is 11 years.[6,7,9,10] A breed predisposition to MM for dogs with heavily pigmented mucosal tissues, such as German shepherds and Cocker spaniels, is also reported.[4,6,7,9,11,34]

Malignant melanomas are rapidly growing tumors characterized by an aggressive course of early local growth and bone involvement and early metastasis to regional lymph nodes and pulmonary tissues.[10,14] Radiographically, MMs are most likely to demonstrate irregular bone destruction.[10,32] The prognosis for dogs with MM is poor.[10] Post-treatment, approximately 90 percent of animals die or are euthanatized due to recurrence or metastatic disease.[35,36] Evaluation of several factors including microscopic appearance, mitotic index, degree of pigmentation, intraoral tumor location, extent, and timing, or type of surgery has failed to elucidate important prognostic criteria for dogs with MM.[35,37]

Carcinoma

Carcinomas of the oral cavity are usually squamous cell carcinomas. Non-tonsillar squamous cell carcinoma is the second most common canine oral malignancy.[6-10] Common non-tonsillar sites in order of frequency include gingiva, buccal mucosa, lip, palate, and tongue. The mean age of occurrence for non-tonsillar tumors is 8–9.7 years.[6–8,10] Larger breed dogs (>23 kg) are predisposed by a 2:1 ratio.[10] Tonsillar squamous cell carcinomas have been reported to occur more frequently in urban settings with heavy pollution.[26,27] The disparate biologic behavior of tonsillar and non-tonsillar squamous cell carcinomas warrants emphasis. Squamous cell carcinomas spread by direct extension, invading and destroying mucosa, submucosa, muscle, and bone. As such, the clinical appearance is one of a rapidly growing, proliferative, ulcerated, and friable mass which may displace teeth.[38] Radiographically,

these tumors are most likely to demonstrate aggressive bone destruction.[32] Non-tonsillar tumors will spread to draining lymph nodes yet have a low tendency for distant metastasis.[6] Tonsillar squamous cell carcinomas are more aggressive; 98 percent show early metastasis to regional lymph nodes, and 63 percent show evidence of distant metastasis.[14] The clinical presentation for tonsillar tumors may also include signs referable to upper airway obstruction.[7,9,38] In general, non-tonsillar squamous cell carcinoma carries a better prognosis than MM or fibrosarcoma.[39] Four factors reported to have a significant association with survival post–radiation therapy for non-tonsillar squamous cell carcinoma include intraoral location, tumor recurrence, relative portal size, and age at diagnosis.[40]

Fibrosarcoma

Fibrosarcoma (FSA) is the third most frequent canine oral malignancy.[3,6,7,10-12,14,34] Fibrosarcomas are derived from connective tissue elements and therefore may arise within gingiva, bone, or periosteum. This tumor usually involves the gingiva (especially the maxilla between the canine and upper fourth premolar tooth[10]), followed by the palate, mucosa, and tongue, respectively.[6-8,10] Male dogs seem to be predisposed (1.4–2.0:1),[6-8,10] and the average age for tumor development is 7.5 years.[6,7,10] Grossly, these neoplasms are protruding, firm, smooth or nodular masses with fleshy pink or ulcerated areas. The biologic behavior of oral fibrosarcomas is characterized by moderately rapid, local invasion into adjacent soft tissue and bone, high rate of recurrence, and a diminished (but possible) capacity for distant metastasis[6,9,38] intermediate between MM and squamous cell carcinoma.[10] Radiographically, fibrosarcomas often show a brush border periosteal reaction.[32] Fibrosarcomas warrant a poor prognosis[6,10,14] due to aggressive local infiltration; surgical challenge if located on the palate, high rate of postsurgical recurrence; chemo-, immuno-, and radioresistance; and the tendency to metastasize. The degree of differentiation of gingival FSAs has not been born out as a prognostic factor associated with survival.[10]

Other less common malignant nonodontogenic oral tumors include lymphosarcoma, plasmacytoma, rhabdomyosarcoma, hemangiosarcoma, mastocytoma, and soft tissue osteosarcoma (mixed mesenchymal tumor).[38]

Benign Neoplasms

Epulides

The nomenclature of epulides in the dog has been variously reported.[41,42] The most widely accepted classification scheme describes three types of epulides, grouped together because they contain stroma that resembles normal periodontal ligament.[41] These benign tumors of periodontal origin include the fibromatous epulis, the ossifying epulis, and the locally destructive acanthomatous epulis.[41,43] A recent review has divided canine epulides into reactive lesions and peripheral odontogenic tumors.[42] In this review, epulis refers to a "non-specific, clinical designation for a focal growth on the gingiva." From this definition, reactive lesions include focal fibrous hyperplasia (fibrous epulis), pyogenic granuloma, peripheral giant cell granuloma (giant cell epulis), peripheral ossifying fibroma (calcifying fibrous epulis) and reactive exostosis (osteoma). Odontogenic tumors occurring on the gingiva are considered peripheral odontogenic tumors and include the fibromatous epulis (which encompasses the ossifying epulis[41] as a histologic variant[44]), the acanthomatous epulis, and the calcifying epithelial odontogenic tumor. Only the acanthomatous epulis is locally aggressive.[41] The acanthomatous epulis occurs with frequency in a wide age range of dogs, with the peak incidence around 10 years of age.[42] These pink, fibrous, nodular appearing masses have a predilection for the mandibular incisor and premolar region. On radiographic evaluation, varying degrees of osteolysis or osseous proliferation are evident.[45] Some benign tumors display a wispy periosteal reaction radiographically.[32] The biologic behavior of the acanthomatous epulis is similar to the human intraosseous ameloblastoma: destructive infiltration of the intertrabecular spaces of the cancellous bone and lack of metastatic potential.[42,46] The term canine acanthomatous ameloblastoma has been suggested to replace acanthomatous epulis, especially when the tumor arises intraosseously.[47]

Odontogenic Neoplasms

The classification of odontogenic neoplasms is based on the potential inductive effect one dental tissue has on another.[38] The dental laminar epithelium gives rise to these rare tumors.[9,33] As such, dental laminar neoplasms refer to tumors of dental tissue with a high degree of organization of dental features, such as the production of differentiated dentin and enamel.[48–50] The most common dental laminar neoplasm reported in dogs is the ameloblastoma.[13,32,51] The tumor appears as a gingival soft tissue mass which grows by expansion and results in loss or mobility of associated teeth.[13,32,48] The radiographic appearance reveals a multilocular or unilocular,[50,52] cystic or solid mass[33,50,52,53] with osteolysis around associated tooth roots.[48]

References

1. Boring CC, Squires TS, Tong T. Cancer statistics, 1992. *CA Cancer J Clin* 42:19-38 (1992).

2. Parkin DM, Laara E, Muir CS. Estimates of the worldwide frequency of sixteen major cancers in 1980. *Int J Cancer* 41:184-97 (1988).

3. Dorn CR, Taylor DO, Frye FL, et al. Survey of animal neoplasms in Alameda and Contra Cost counties, California. I. Methodology and description of cases. *J Natl Cancer Inst* 40:295-305 (1968).

4. Dorn CR, Taylor DO, et al. Survey of animal neoplasms in Alameda and Contra Costa counties, California. II. Cancer morbidity in dogs and cats from Alameda County. *J Natl Cancer Inst* 40:307-318 (1968).

5. Priester WA, McKay FW. The occurrence of tumors in domestic animals. *Natl Cancer Inst Monogr* 54:1-120 (1980).

6. Brodey RS. A clinical and pathologic study of 130 neoplasms of the mouth and pharynx in the dog. *Am J Vet Res* 21:787-812 (1960).

7. Cohen D, Brodey RS, et al. Epidemiologic aspects of oral and pharyngeal neoplasms in the dog. *Am J Vet Res* 25(109):1776-79 (1964).

8. Dorn CR, Priester WA. Epidemiologic analysis of oral and pharyngeal cancer in dogs, cats, horses, and cattle. *J Am Vet Med Assoc* 169(11):1202-6 (1976).

9. Gorlin RJ, Barron CN, et al. The oral and pharyngeal pathology of domestic animals. A study of 487 cases. *Am J Vet Res* 79(20):1032-61 (1959).

10. Todoroff RJ, Brodey RS. Oral and pharyngeal neoplasia in the dog: A retrospective survey of 361 cases. *J Am Vet Med Assoc* 175(6):561-71 (1979).

11. Vos JH, van der Gaag I. Canine and feline oral pharyngeal tumors. *J Vet Med (Series A)* 34:420-27 (1987).

12. Borthwick R, Else RW, Head KW. Neoplasia and allied conditions of the canine oropharynx. *Vet Annu* 22:248-69 (1982).

13. Richardson RC, Jones MA, Elliot GS. Oral neoplasms in the dog: A diagnostic and therapeutic dilemma. *Comp Cont Ed Pract Vet* 5(6):441-46 (1983).

14. Brodey RS. The biological behavior of canine oral and pharyngeal neoplasms. *J Sm Anim Pract* 11:45-53 (1970).

15. Decker J, Goldstein JC. Risk factors in head and neck cancer. *N Engl J Med* 306:1151-55 (1982).

16. Jacobs CD. Etiologic considerations for head and neck squamous cancers. In: Jacobs C, ed. *Carcinomas of the Head and Neck: Evaluation and Management.* Boston:Kluwer Academic, 1990, 265-82.

17. Winn DM, Blot WJ, McLaughlin JK, et al. Mouthwash use and oral conditions in the risk of oral and pharyngeal cancer. *Cancer Res* 51:3044-47 (1991).

18. Falk RT, Pickle LW, Brown LM, et al. Effect of smoking and alcohol consumption on laryngeal cancer risk in coastal Texas. *Cancer Res* 49:402-429 (1989).

19. Nam J, McLaughlin JK, Blot WJ. Cigarette smoking, alcohol and nasopharyngeal carcinoma: A case-control study among U.S. whites. *J Natl Cancer Inst* 84:619-22 (1992).

20. Shillitoe EJ, Greenspan D, Greenspan JS, et al. Antibody to early and late antigens of herpes simplex virus type 1 in patients with oral cancer. *Cancer* 54:266-73 (1984).

21. Watts SL, Brewer EE, Fry TL. Human papillomavirus DNA types in squamous cell carcinomas of the head and neck. *Oral Surg Oral Med Oral Pathol* 71:701-7 (1991).

22. Henle G, Henle W. Epstein-Barr virus-specific IgA serum antibodies as an outstanding feature of nasopharyngeal carcinoma. *Int J Cancer* 17:1-7 (1976).

23. de-Vathaire F, Sancho-Garnier H, de-The H, et al. Prognostic value of EBV markers in the clinical management of nasopharyngeal carcinoma (NPC): A multicenter follow-up study. *Int J Cancer* 42:176-81 (1988).

24. Young LS, Dawson CW, Clark D, et al. Epstein-Barr virus gene expression in nasopharyngeal carcinoma. *J Gen Virol* 69:1051-65 (1988).

25. Greene CE. *Clinical Microbiology and Infectious Diseases of the Dog and Cat.* Philadelphia:WB Saunders Co., 1984, 465-66.

26. Bostock DE. Comparison of canine oropharyngeal malignancy in various geographical locations. *Vet Rec* 114:341 (1984).

27. Reif JS, Cohen D. The environmental distribution of canine respiratory tract neoplasms. *Arch Environ Health* 2:136 (1971).

28. Roszel JF. University of Pennsylvania, School of Veterinary Medicine, Philadelphia. Personal communication. 1969.

29. Withrow SJ. Surgical management of cancer. *Vet Clin NA* 1(7):13-20 (1977).

30. Withrow SJ, Lowes N. Biopsy techniques for use in small animal oncology. *J Am Anim Hosp Assoc* 17(6):889-900 (1981).

31. White RA, Jefferies AR, Freedman LS. Clinical staging for oropharyngeal malignancies in the dog. *J Sm Anim Prac* 26:581-94 (1985).

32. Frew DG, Dobson JM. Radiological assessment of 50 cases of incisive or maxillary neoplasia in the dog. *J Sm Anim Prac* 33:11-18 (1992).

33. Dubielzig RR. Proliferative dental and gingival diseases of dogs and cats. *J Am Anim Hosp Assoc* 18:577-84 (1982).

34. Brodey RS. A clinico-pathological study of 200 cases of oral and pharyngeal cancer in the dog. *Gaines Vet Symp* 11:5 (1961).

35. Bostock DE. Prognosis after surgical excision of canine melanomas. *Vet Path* 16:32-40 (1979).

36. Bostock DE. The biological behavior of mastocytomas and melanomas in the dog. *Vet Ann* 20:124-28 (1980).

37. Harvey HJ, MacEwen EG, Braun D, et al. Prognostic criteria for dogs with oral melanoma. *J Am Vet Med Assoc* 178(6):580-82 (1981).

38. Head KW. Tumors of the alimentary tract. In: Moulton JE, ed, *Tumors in domestic animals*, 3rd Edition. Berkeley: University of California Press, 1990, 347-435.

39. Hoyt RF, Withrow SJ. Oral malignancy in the dog. *J Am Anim Hosp Assoc* 20:83–92 (1982).

40. Evans SM, Shofer F. Canine oral nontonsillar squamous cell carcinoma. Prognostic factors for recurrence and survival following orthovoltage radiation therapy. *Vet Rad* 29 (3):133-37 (1988).

41. Dubielzig RR, Goldschmidt MH, Brodey RS. The nomenclature of periodontal epulides in dogs. *Vet Pathol* 16:209-14 (1979).

42. Gardner DG. Epulides in the dog: A review. *J Oral Pathol Med* 25:32-37 (1996).

43. Gardner DG, Baker DC. Fibromatous epulis in dogs and peripheral odontogenic fibroma in human beings: Two equivalent lesions. *Oral Surg Oral Med Oral Pathol* 71:317-21 (1991).

44. Barker IK, Van Dreumel AA. The alimentary system. In: Jubb KF, Kennedy PC, Palmer N, eds. *Pathology of Domestic Animals*, Vol. 2, 3rd Edition. New York:Academic Press, 1985, 17-19.

45. Thrall DE, Goldschmidt MH, Biery DN. Malignant tumor formation at the site of previously irradiated acanthomatous epulides in four dogs. *J Am Vet Med Assoc* 178(2):127-32 (1981).

46. Gardner DG. Canine acanthomatous epulis. The only common spontaneous ameloblastoma in animals. *Oral Surg Oral Med Oral Pathol* 79:612-15 (1995).

47. Gardner DG, Baker DC. The relationship of the canine acanthomatous epulis to ameloblastoma. *J Comp Pathol* 108:47-55 (1993).

48. Langham RF, Mostosky UV, Schirmer RG. Ameloblastic odontoma in the dog. *Am J Vet Res* 30:1873-76 (1969).

49. Dubielzig RR, Thrall DE. Ameloblastoma and keratinizing ameloblastoma in dogs. *Vet Pathol* 19:596-607 (1982).

50. Gorlin RJ, Meskin LH, Brodey R. Odontogenic tumors in man and animals: Pathologic classification and clinical behavior—A review. *Ann NY Acad Sci* 108:722-71 (1963).

51. Clark JJ, Chaudhry AP. The oral pathology of domesticated animals. *Oral Surg Oral Med Oral Pathol* 11:500-35 (1958).

52. Gorlin RJ, Chaudhry AP, Pindborg JJ. Odontogenic tumors: Classification, histopathology and clinical behavior in man and domesticated animals. *Cancer* 14:73 (1961).

53. Bostock DE, White RA. Classification and behavior after surgery of canine 'epulides'. *J Comp Path* 97:197-206 (1987).

X-RAY PLATES AND SLIDES

FIGURE 7.1

Contributing Authors:
Anna Fong Revenaugh and Jamie G. Anderson

Description: Fibromatous epulis. Fibromatous epuli are benign oral tumors. This radiograph shows the characteristics of this type of tumor. A well demarcated soft tissue mass is seen surrounding the lower right first premolar. There is no associated bony change.

Points Identified:

A. Area of protuberant soft tissue mass

Diagnostic Keys: Soft tissue mass without associated bony change.

Common Errors: Superimposition of the mental foramen of the mandible can sometimes resemble periapical osteolysis. May be responsible for misdiagnosis of periapical abscess or invasion of tumor into bone.

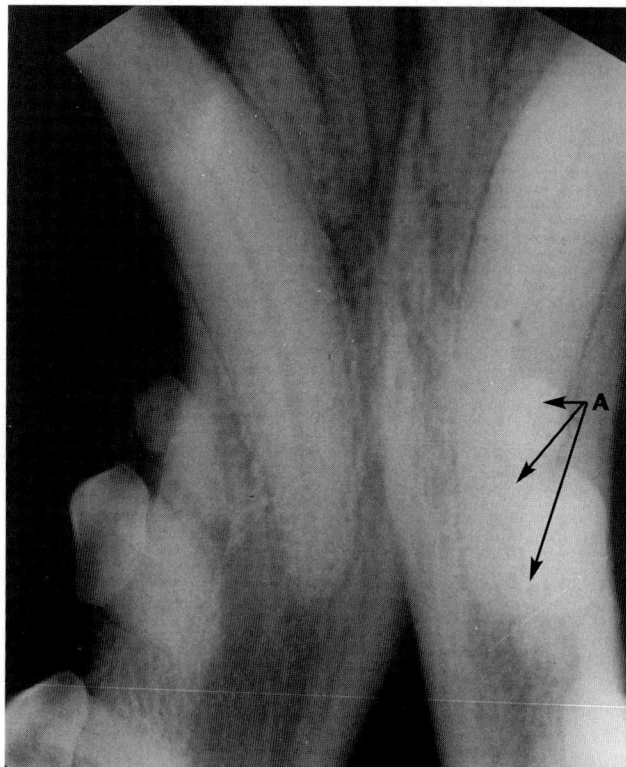

FIGURE 7.2

Contributing Authors:

Anna Fong Revenaugh and Jamie G. Anderson

Description: This soft tissue mass extending from the gingival margin of the right upper canine tooth and first premolar clinically resembled gingival hyperplasia. Radiographs show no evidence of bony involvement adjacent to the mass. The characteristics seen on histopathology, including a central area of mineralized osteoid, diagnosed this lesion as an ossifying epulis.

Points Identified:

A. Soft tissue mass adjacent to the right upper canine tooth
B. Mineralization within the soft tissue mass

Diagnostic Keys: Gingival soft tissue mass with mineralization. No associated bony destruction.

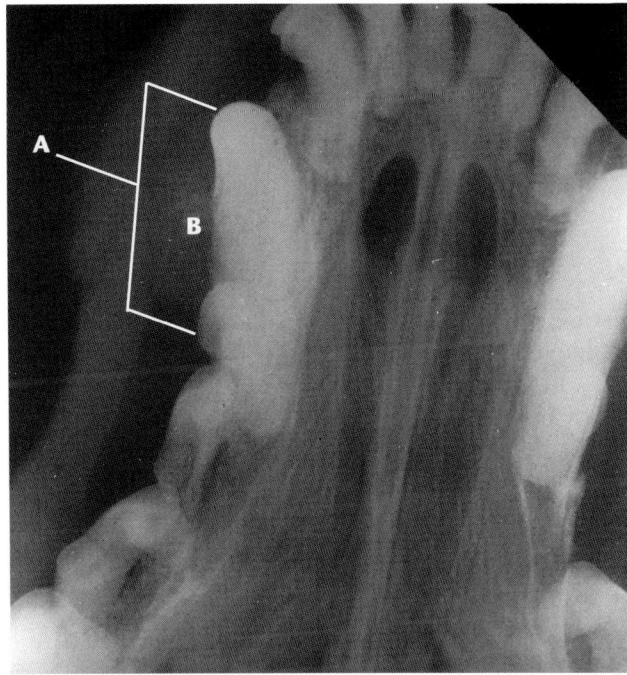

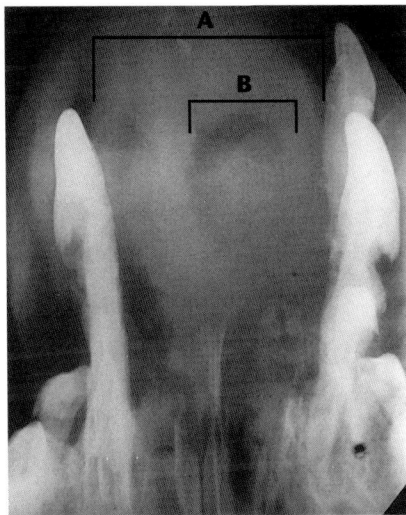

A

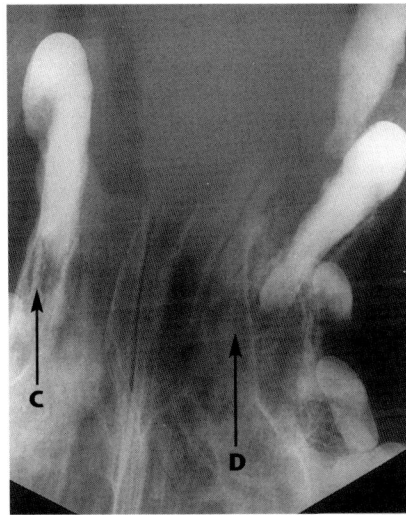

B

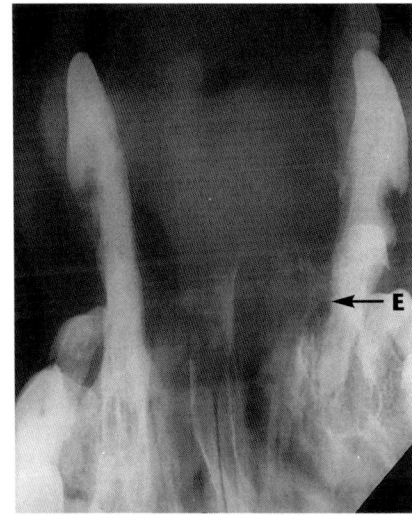

C

FIGURE 7.3

Contributing Authors:

Anna Fong Revenaugh and Jamie G. Anderson

Description: Acanthomatous epulis. Acanthomatous epuli are locally invasive periodontal neoplasms that do not metastasize. This case demonstrates how aggressive these tumors can behave. The soft tissue tumor has caused massive destruction of the incisive and maxillary bones. There is tooth lysis, disruption, and loss. There is the possibility of malignant transformation of this particular tumor, as this dog was treated with radiation therapy 7 years ago. However, histopathology of the lesion was consistent with an acanthomatous epulis. The nasal cavity involvement, seen as decreased turbinate detail, may be secondary to the previous radiation therapy.

Points Identified:

A. Very large soft tissue mass involving the maxilla rostral to the second premolars

B. Massive destruction of the incisive and maxillary bones
C. Tooth lysis, loss and disruption
D. Loss of turbinate detail
E. Dystrophic mineralization within the soft tissue mass

Diagnostic Keys: Soft tissue mass. Locally invasive.

FIGURE 7.4

Contributing Authors:

Anna Fong Revenaugh and Jamie G. Anderson

Description: Acanthomatous epulis. Among the epulides, only the acanthomatous epulis is locally invasive. This particular tumor has destroyed the rostral maxilla and incisive bones. A bulbous soft tissue mass, with amorphous mineralization, can be seen extending from the rostral maxilla.

Points Identified:

A. Marked destruction of the incisive and maxillary bones with associated tooth loss and soft tissue mass with mineralization

B. Periodontal disease with furcation pathology

Diagnostic Keys: Soft tissue mass with mineralization. Bone destruction.

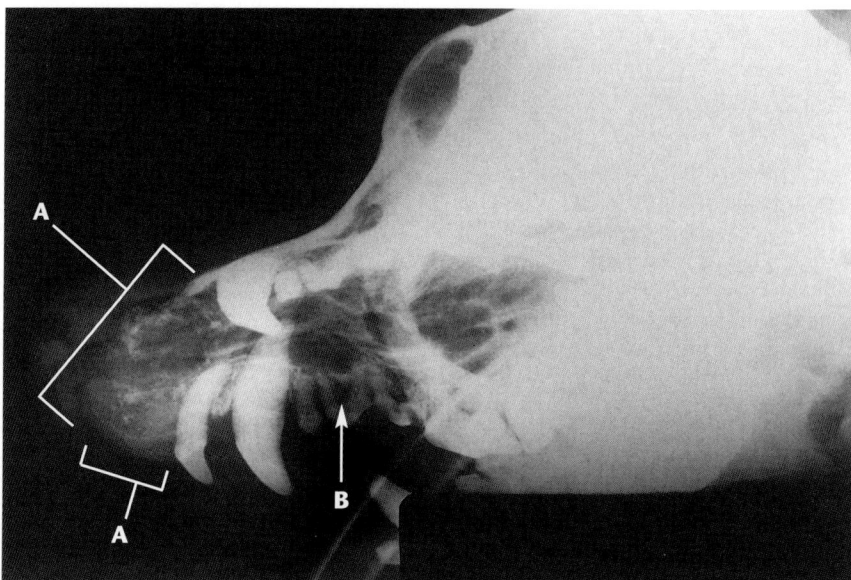

FIGURE 7.5

Contributing Authors:

Anna Fong Revenaugh and Jamie G. Anderson

Description: Acanthomatous epulis. Another example of the aggressive destructive/productive process that accompanies this tumor type.

Points Identified:

A. Soft tissue mass involving the rostral mandible

B. Interrupted periosteal proliferation showing spicules of new bone in a "palisading" formation

C. Moth-eaten osteolysis of the rostral mandible

D. Displacement of central incisor

E. Area of tooth loss

Diagnostic Keys: Soft tissue mass. Osteolysis. Interrupted periosteal production.

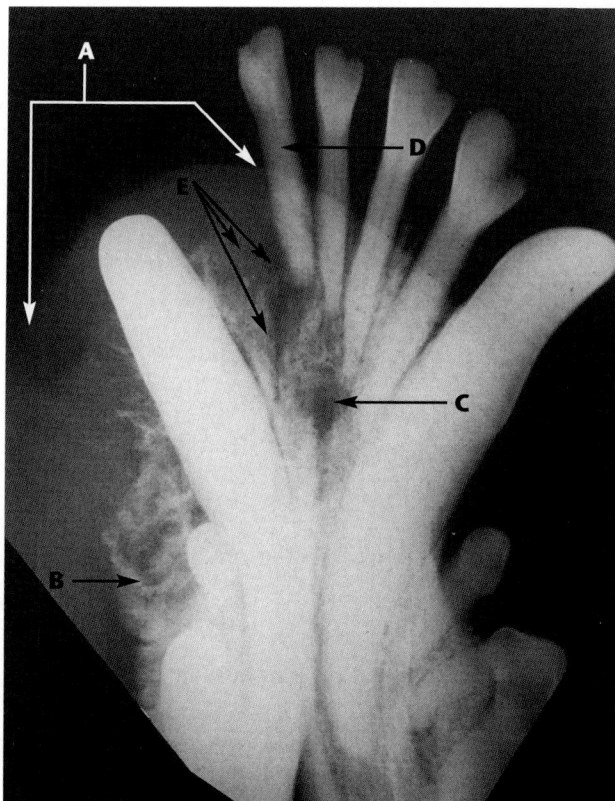

FIGURE 7.6

Contributing Authors:
Anna Fong Revenaugh and Jamie G. Anderson

Description: Acanthomatous epulis. CT scan of maxillary mass. Large soft tissue mass with massive destruction of the incisive bone and hard palate. Destruction of the nasal turbinates caudal to the mass may be due to previous radiation therapy.

Points Identified:

A. Massive osteolysis of the incisive bone and hard palate
B. Nasal turbinate destruction
C. Deviation and disruption of the vomer and nasal septum

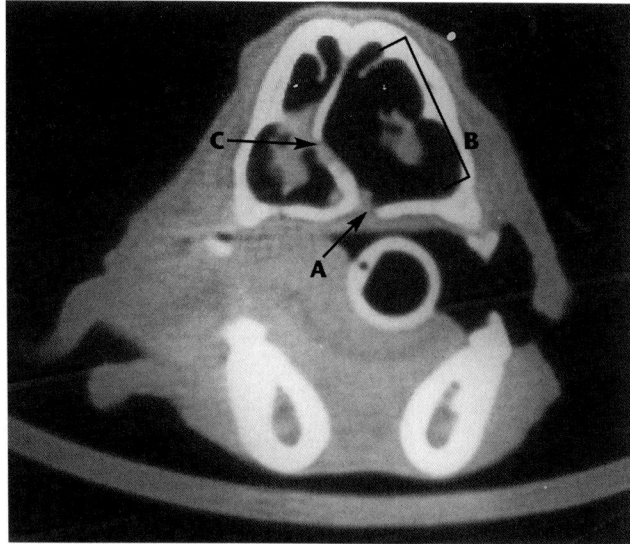

FIGURE 7.7

Contributing Authors:
Anna Fong Revenaugh and Jamie G. Anderson

Description: Acanthomatous epulis. This presentation of an acanthomatous epulis could easily be mistaken for a more malignant tumor type. Interrupted periosteal production and moth-eaten osteolysis radiographically resemble osteosarcoma (see Figure 7.10) or squamous cell carcinoma (see Figure 7.11).

Points Identified:

A. Large soft tissue mass adjacent to the left upper canine tooth
B. Moth-eaten osteolysis of alveolar bone
C. Interrupted spiculated periosteal production

Diagnostic Keys: Soft tissue mass. Alveolar bony lysis. Interrupted periosteal proliferation.

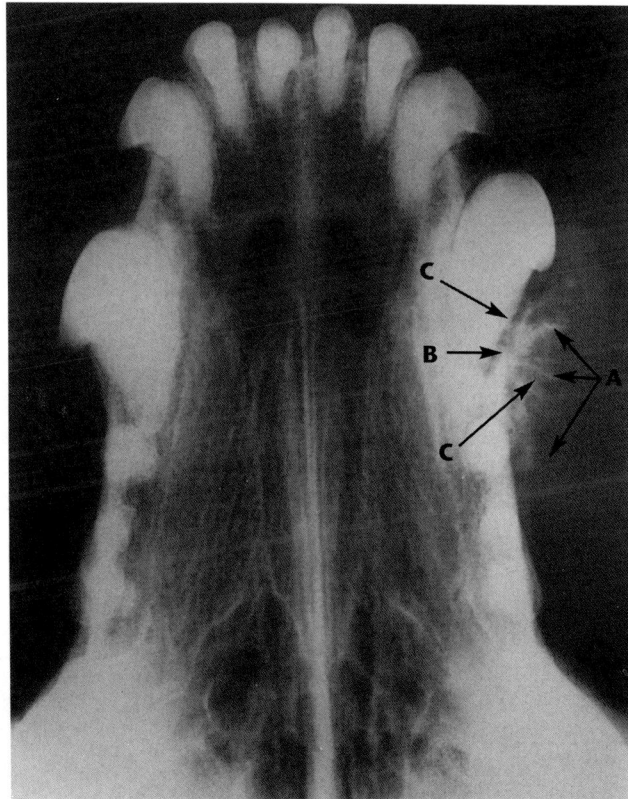

FIGURE 7.8

Contributing Authors:
Anna Fong Revenaugh and Jamie G. Anderson

Description: Papillary squamous cell carcinoma. This radiograph of a papillary squamous cell carcinoma demonstrates an unusual appearing expansile destructive lesion involving the maxilla. The expansile nature of this tumor has caused displacement of teeth and disruption of the palatine compacta. A multilobulated soft tissue mass extends from the canine tooth to the right upper third premolar.

Points Identified:

A. Large soft tissue mass with dystrophic mineralization extending from the right upper canine tooth to the third premolar
B. Expansile appearing destruction of the maxilla
C. Possible nasal involvement with vomer disruption

Diagnostic Keys: Multilobulated soft tissue mass with dystrophic mineralization. Invasion of bone; expansile appearance. Teeth disrupted, resorbed, displaced.

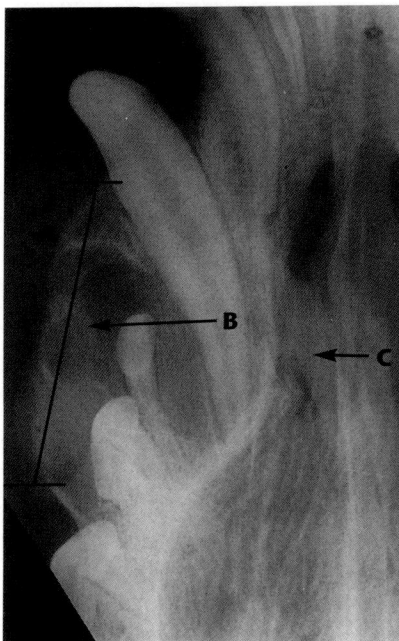

FIGURE 7.9

Contributing Authors:
Anna Fong Revenaugh and Jamie G. Anderson

Description: Papillary squamous cell carcinoma. (See x-ray, Figure 7.8.)

(See also color plate.)

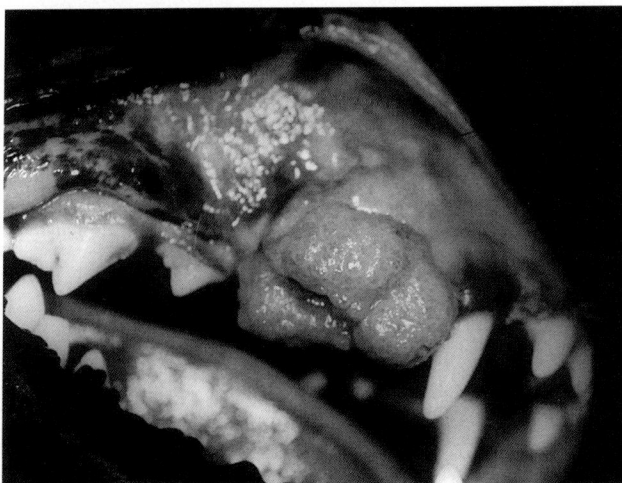

FIGURE 7.10

Contributing Authors:
Anna Fong Revenaugh and Jamie G. Anderson

Description: Osteosarcoma. This oral mass with bone involvement is an example of osteosarcoma. The radiographic presentation is similar to that seen with osteosarcoma of the extremities. Interrupted periosteal new bone formation associated with permeative and coalescing moth-eaten bone lysis is seen to involve the right hemimandible.

Points Identified:

A. Soft tissue mass extending along the right hemimandible from the first premolar to the first molar
B. Interrupted periosteal proliferation along the axial and abaxial cortices of the right hemimandible; spiculated new bone
C. Moth-eaten osteolysis from 405 to 409
D. Tooth root destruction, displaced and lost teeth.

Diagnostic Keys: Soft tissue mass. Active aggressive destructive and productive change.

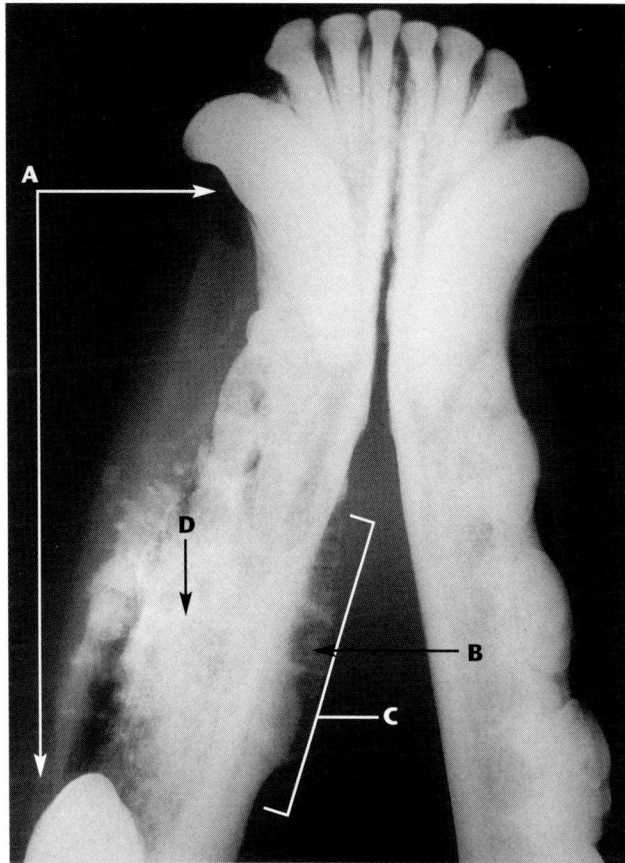

FIGURE 7.11

Contributing Authors:
Anna Fong Revenaugh and Jamie G. Anderson

Description: Squamous cell carcinoma. This radiograph of a squamous cell carcinoma shows a large gingival mass extending from the left upper canine tooth to the second premolar. There has been associated bone destruction and displacement of the first premolar. Interrupted periosteal proliferation with spicules of new bone is typical of an active and aggressive lesion.

Points Identified:

A. Soft tissue mass adjacent to the left upper canine tooth and second premolar
B. Destruction of the maxillary bone around the canine tooth and first premolar
C. Periosteal new bone production
D. Loosened and displaced left upper first premolar

Diagnostic Keys: Soft tissue mass. Bone invasion and destruction. Interrupted periosteal proliferation.

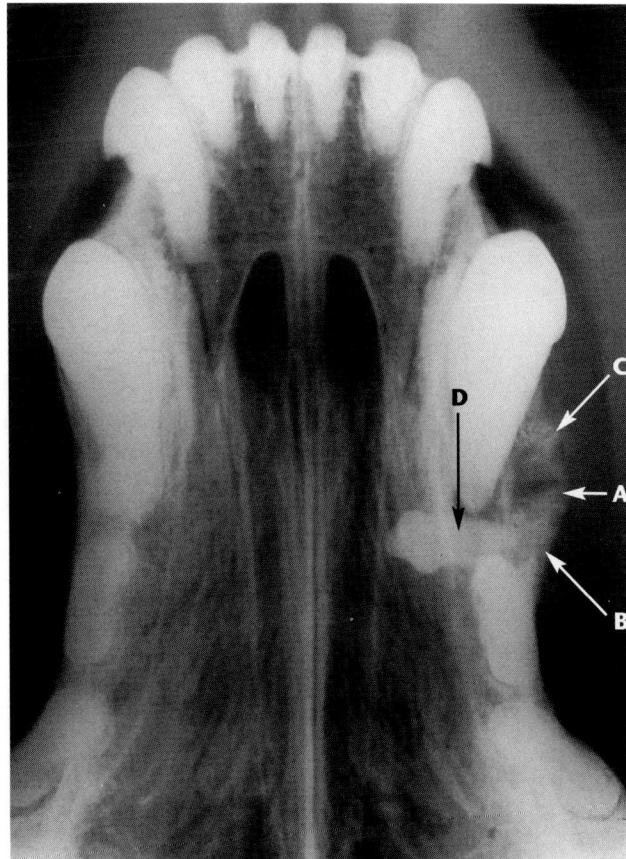

FIGURE 7.12

Contributing Authors:

Anna Fong Revenaugh and Jamie G. Anderson

Description: Fibrosarcoma. One-month history of a left maxillary gingival mass. Radiographs and CT scan showed alveolar bone loss and periapical lysis involving the maxilla around the first through third premolars. A soft tissue mass extended across this area. A partial maxillectomy was performed. Histopathology revealed fibrosarcoma. These radiographs and CT results should be compared with examples of periodontal disease included in this chapter. The similarities point out the difficulties in diagnosis and the need for biopsy.

Points Identified:

A. Soft tissue mass extending from 205 to 207
B. Decreased alveolar bone density
C. Lucencies around the roots of 206 and 207

Diagnostic Keys: Soft tissue mass. Associated alveolar bone loss.

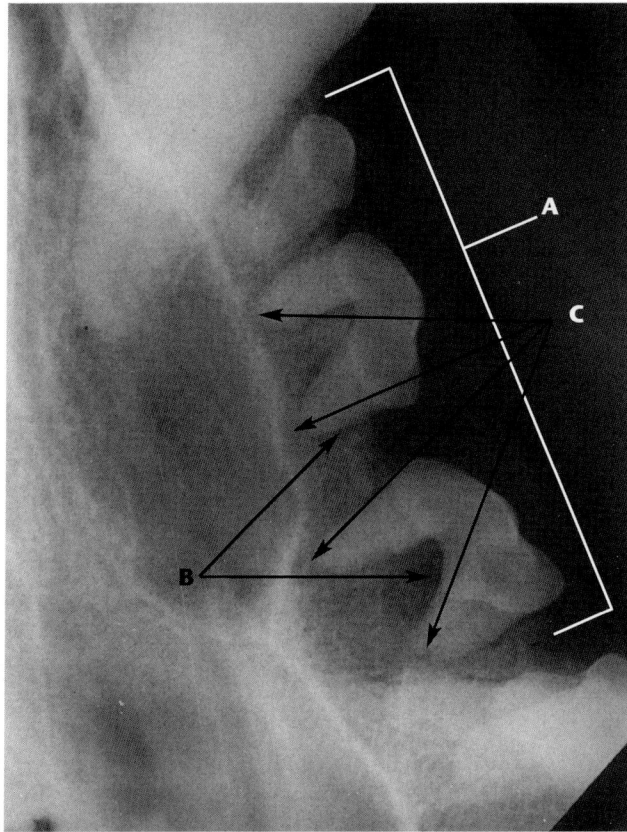

FIGURE 7.13

Contributing Authors:

Anna Fong Revenaugh and Jamie G. Anderson

Description: Fibrosarcoma CT scan. 1.5 mm transverse slices were obtained through the area of interest. Increased soft tissue thickness is seen adjacent to the left maxilla. Periapical alveolar bone lysis is identified surrounding the roots of the first and third premolars. The second premolar has been removed.

Points Identified:

A. Soft tissue mass
B. Alveolar bone lysis surrounding 207

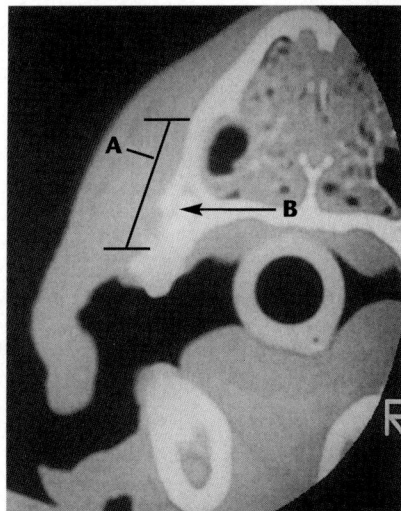

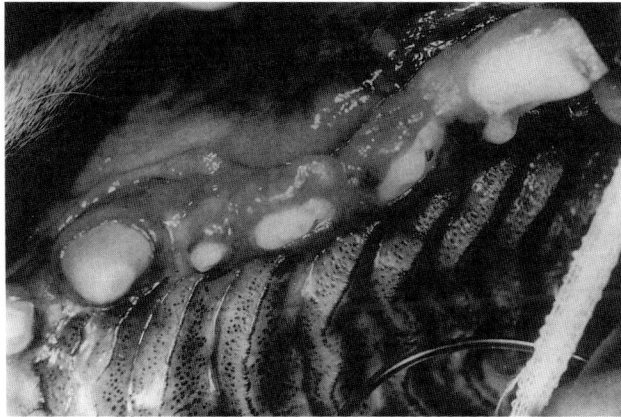

FIGURE 7.14

Contributing Authors:
Anna Fong Revenaugh and Jamie G. Anderson

Description: Fibrosarcoma (see x-ray, Figure 7.12; CT scan, Figure 7.13).

(See also color plate.)

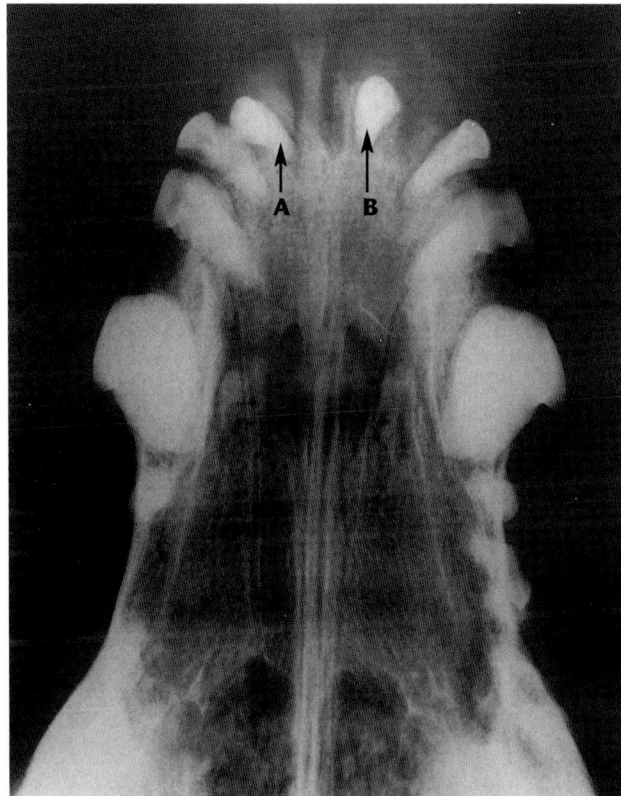

FIGURE 7.15

Contributing Authors:
Anna Fong Revenaugh and Jamie G. Anderson

Description: Fibrosarcoma. This case of oral fibrosarcoma shows how the tumor will displace the teeth as the mass enlarges and invades. Minimal osteolysis seen around the roots of the incisors may be a combination of tumor invasion and periodontal disease. Maxillary fibrosarcomas tend to be benign appearing microscopically, but are locally destructive and difficult to treat.

Points Identified:

A. Large well circumscribed soft tissue mass surrounding the upper incisor teeth
B. Mass can be seen causing abaxial displacement of the central incisors

Diagnostic Keys: Soft tissue mass that causes tooth displacement. Minimal alveolar bone loss.

FIGURE 7.16

Contributing Authors:

Anna Fong Revenaugh and Jamie G. Anderson

Description: Plasmacytoma. This dog had a 6-month history of an enlarging oral mass that was diagnosed as a plasmacytoma. Extramedullary plasmacytomas have been reported in the skin, oral cavity, and gastrointestinal tract of the dog. Most cutaneous plasmacytomas are benign and are cured with surgical excision. This radiograph reveals a mild amount of alveolar bone loss adjacent to the mass.

Points Identified:

A. Soft tissue mass on the lingual aspect of the right lower canine tooth and lateral incisor

Diagnostic Keys: Well defined soft tissue mass. Minimal bony involvement.

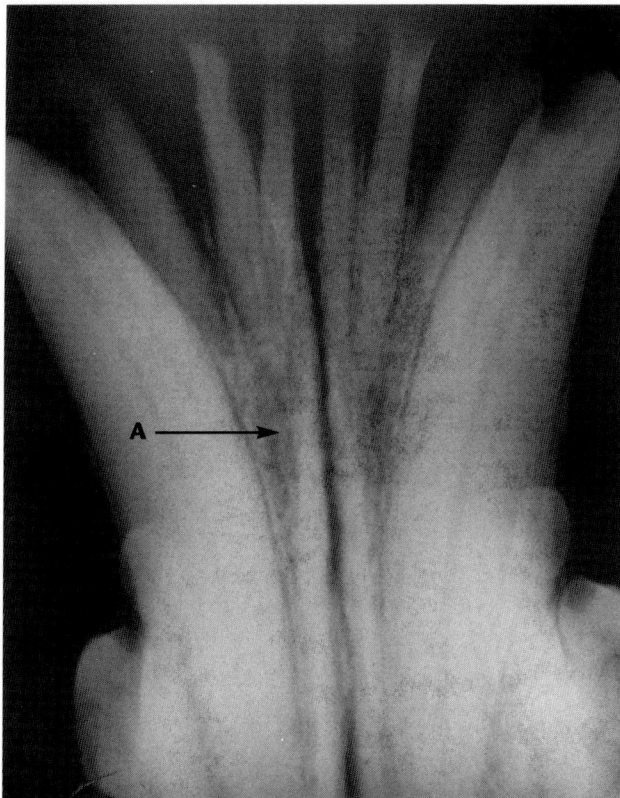

FIGURE 7.17

Contributing Authors:

Anna Fong Revenaugh and Jamie G. Anderson

Description: Plasmacytoma prior to mandibulectomy. (See x-ray, Figure 7.16.)

(See also color plate.)

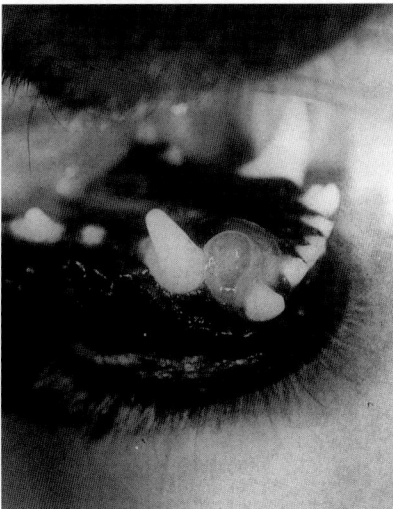

FIGURE 7.18

Contributing Authors:
Anna Fong Revenaugh and Jamie G. Anderson

Description: Ameloblastoma. This unusual appearing lesion is an ameloblastoma. Ameloblastomas are tumors of odontogenic epithelium. Unlike ameloblastic odontomas, they have no inductive effect on the surrounding connective tissue to form dental structures. These tumors are locally invasive and rarely metastasize. There is radiographic evidence of destruction of the right rostral hemimandible. The destructive process is cavitary and fairly well marginated, suggesting a less aggressive or slower growing lesion. The history relates that the right lower canine tooth never erupted. It is seen here displaced caudally.

Points Identified:

A. Soft tissue mass around the right rostral hemimandible
B. Dystrophic mineralization within the mass
C. Destruction of the rostral hemimandible to the level of the fourth premolar
D. Displaced incisors
E. Unerupted and displaced right lower canine tooth

Diagnostic Keys: Soft tissue mass with mineralization. Tumor invasion of bone; less aggressive appearance to lysis.

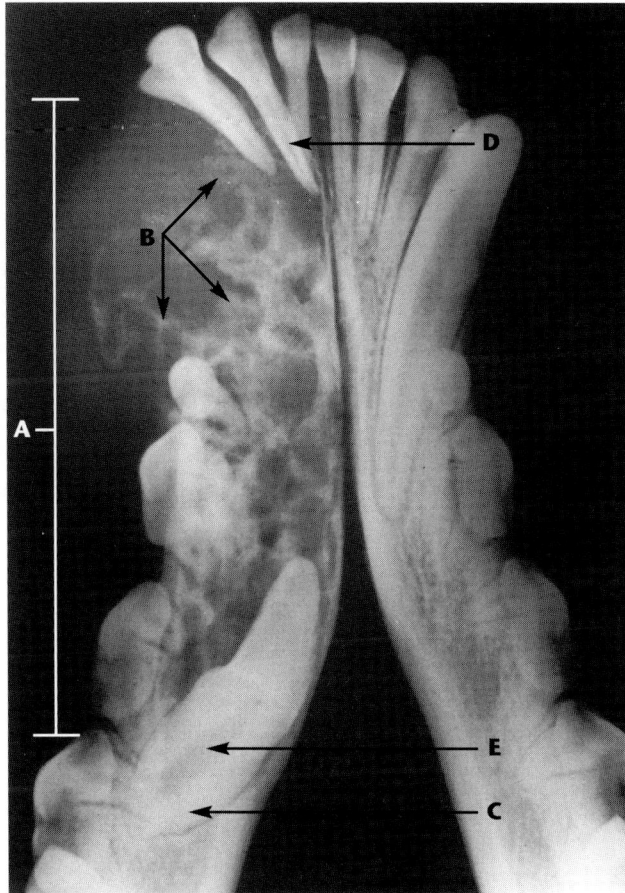

FIGURE 7.19

Contributing Authors:

Anna Fong Revenaugh and Jamie G. Anderson

Description: Melanoma. This Labrador retriever presented for a mandibular mass that had doubled in size over a 1-week period. Histopathology revealed a malignant melanoma. Radiographs taken at that time show marked bone destruction of the left hemimandible. The teeth surrounded by the mass are also being destroyed. The smooth continuous periosteal reaction along the ventral margin of the mandible belies the aggressive nature of this tumor. Oral melanomas are very malignant.

Points Identified:

  A. Soft tissue mass extending from the incisors to the first premolar
  B. Displacement and lysis of 307
  C. Marked bone destruction
  D. Ventral smooth periosteal bone formation

Diagnostic Keys: Soft tissue mass. Bone invasion; osteolysis.

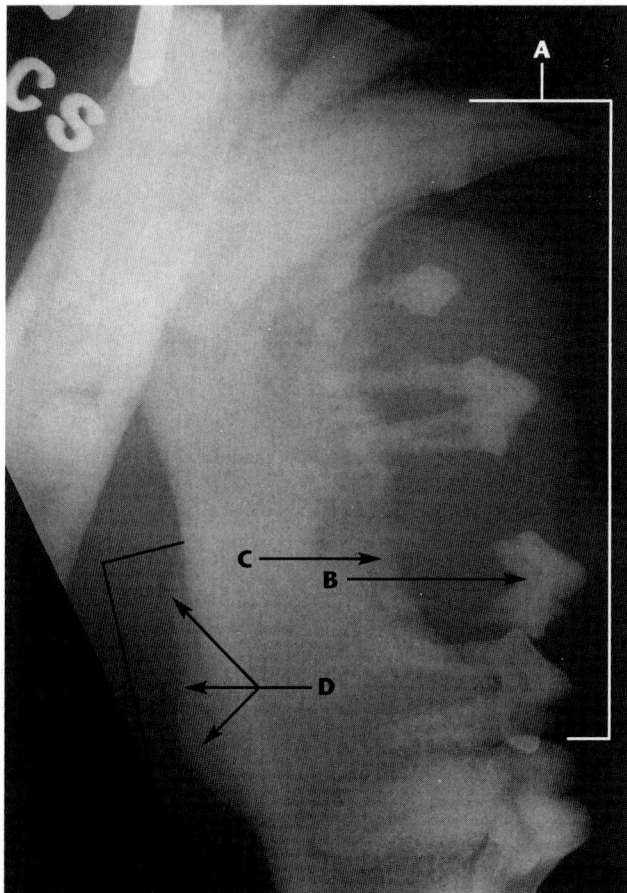

FIGURE 7.20

Contributing Authors:

Anna Fong Revenaugh and Jamie G. Anderson

Description: Tooth root abscess. This aged Doberman presented with a swollen right maxilla, enlarged right peripheral lymph nodes, and vestibular signs. Radiographs and CT findings were highly suspect for neoplasia. Radiographs revealed marked alveolar bone lysis surrounding the right upper fourth premolar. The tooth roots were showing evidence of lysis. CT scan substantiated the radiographic findings. Resection of the maxilla was performed. Histopathology diagnosed a tooth root abscess. Radiographic similarities to case shown in Figures 7.12 and 7.13 of a fibrosarcoma are striking.

Points Identified:

  A. Alveolar bone lysis 108
  B. Tooth root resorptive changes (distal root 108)

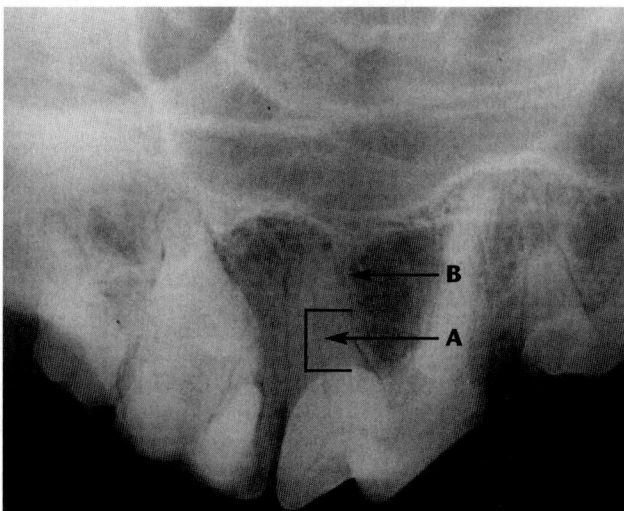

FIGURE 7.21

Contributing Authors:

Anna Fong Revenaugh and Jamie G. Anderson

Description: Toot root abscess CT scan. 1.5 mm transverse slices obtained through the region of interest revealed soft tissue swelling on the lateral aspect of the right maxilla. A destructive bone lesion is identified in the area of the fourth premolar. Periosteal proliferation is also seen in this region.

Points Identified:

   A. Soft tissue swelling on lateral aspect of right maxilla
   B. Bony destruction in the area of the fourth premolar
   C. Periosteal proliferation along the right maxilla

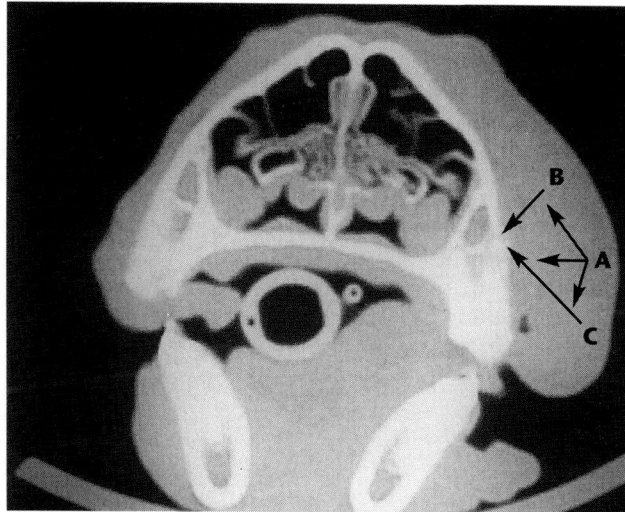

FIGURE 7.22

Contributing Authors:

Anna Fong Revenaugh and Jamie G. Anderson

Description: Periodontitis. Significant alveolar bone loss is seen around the mandibular and maxillary incisors and right upper premolar 108. Extensive lobulated soft tissue swelling is identified on all gingival surfaces. These radiographic findings represent gingival hyperplasia and periodontal disease secondary to chronic dental disease.

Points Identified:

   A. Gingival hyperplasia
   B. Alveolar bone loss involving the maxilla third and fourth premolars
   C. Horizontal and vertical bone loss (incisor)
   D. Deviation of the vomer with decreased turbinate detail: characteristic of brachycephalic breeds

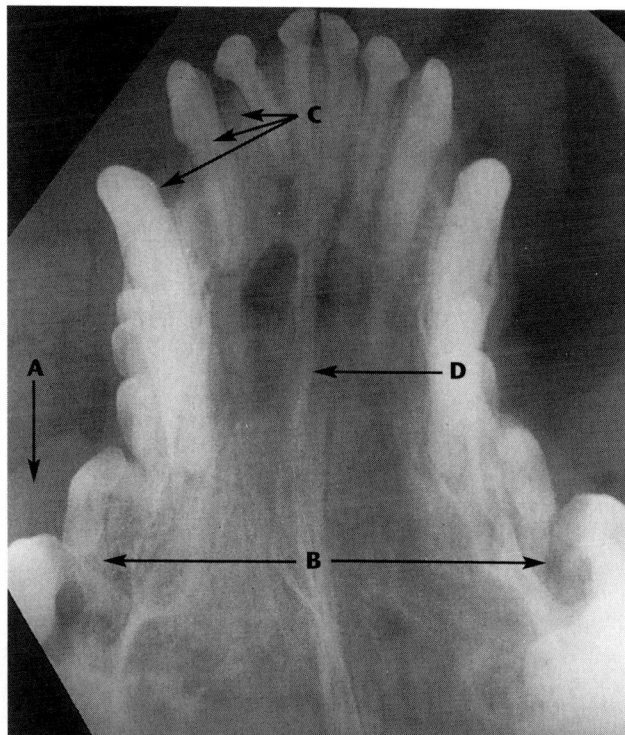

FIGURE 7.23

Contributing Authors:

Anna Fong Revenaugh and Jamie G. Anderson

Description: Stomatitis. This patient presented with a 9 × 10 mm ulcerated soft tissue mass on the buccal aspect of the gingiva on the right rostral maxilla. Radiographs show the soft tissue mass with associated interdental alveolar bone loss. Focal periapical lucency is noted around the right lateral incisor. Sections from the maxilla revealed this to be a severe, chronic, pleocellular stomatitis.

Points Identified:

A. Soft tissue mass adjacent to the right lateral incisor and canine tooth
B. Interdental alveolar bone loss
C. Focal periapical lysis

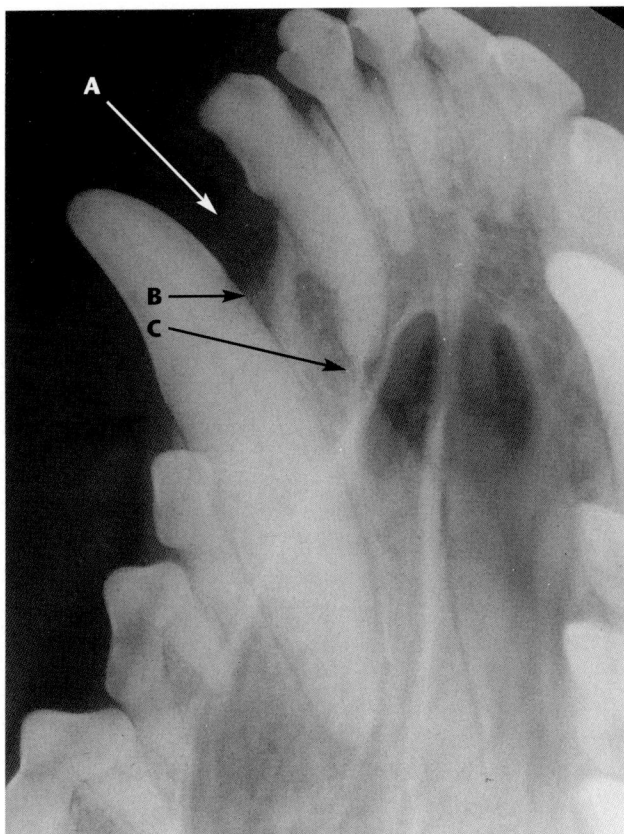

A

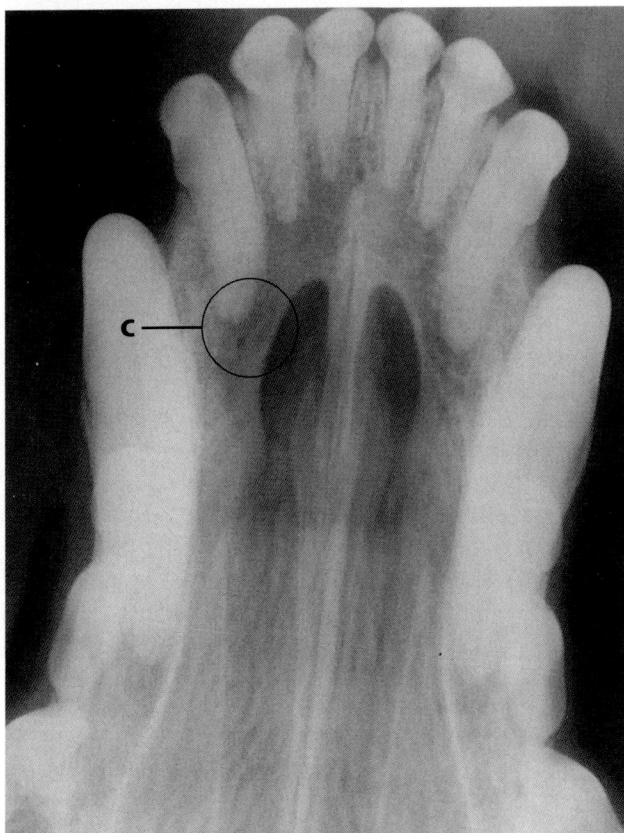

B

FIGURE 7.24

Contributing Authors:
Anna Fong Revenaugh and Jamie G. Anderson

Description: Pleocellular stomatitis, right rostral maxilla (see x-rays, Figure 7.23).

(*See also color plate.*)

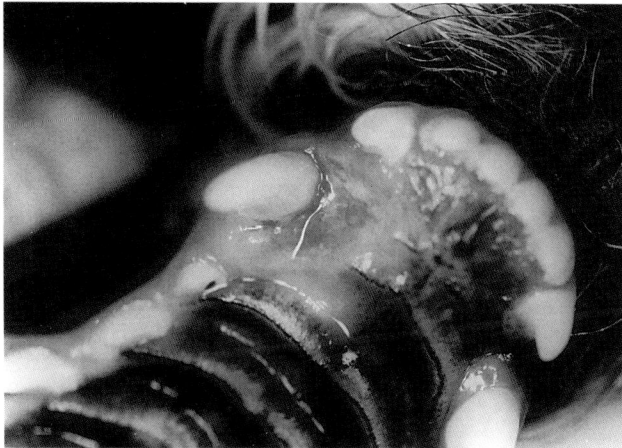

FIGURE 7.25

Contributing Authors:
Anna Fong Revenaugh and Jamie G. Anderson

Description: Periodontal disease. This dog presented with a history of a slowly enlarging right mandibular mass of 6-month duration. Radiographs show an area of alveolar bone lysis surrounding the roots of the fourth premolar. Smooth periosteal reaction and bony sclerosis represent chronic change. The tooth roots show resorption. Histopathology following biopsy revealed periodontal disease.

Points Identified:

A. Osteolysis of the mandible surrounding the distal root of the fourth premolar

B. Condensing osteitis

C. Smooth periosteal reaction

D. Tooth root resorption

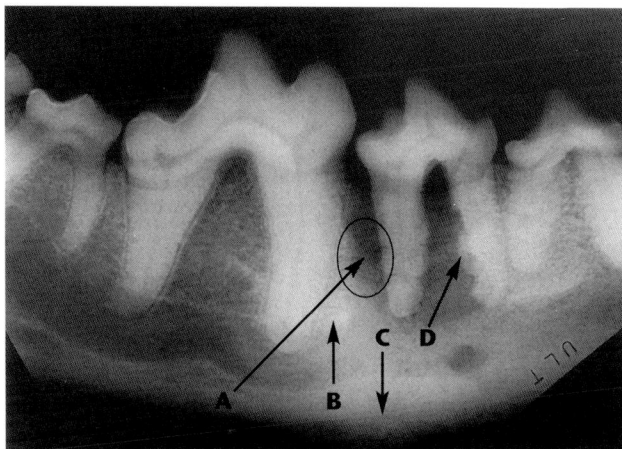

FIGURE 7.26

Contributing Author:
Anna Fong Revenaugh and Jamie G. Anderson

Description: Periodontal disease, right mandible (see x-ray, Figure 7.25).

(*See also color plate.*)

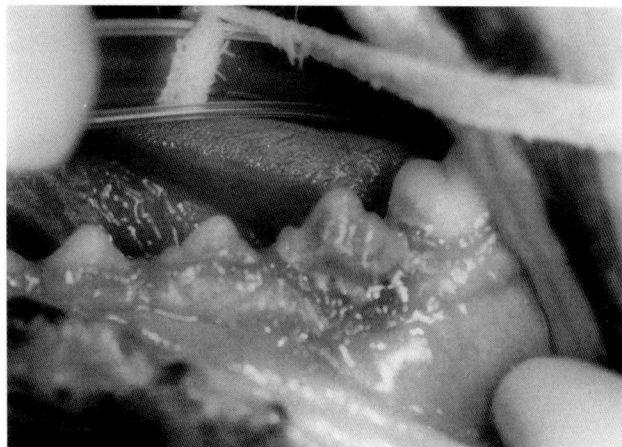

FIGURE 7.27

Contributing Author: Richard Esquivel

Description: Odontoma. Complex odontoma in a 9-month-old male Great Dane. An odontoma is a develomental anomaly consisting of a calcified mass of enamel, dentin, and cementum that may or may not resemble a tooth.

Points Identified:

A. Massive proliferation of tumor
B. Multiple small partially developed abnormal teeth.

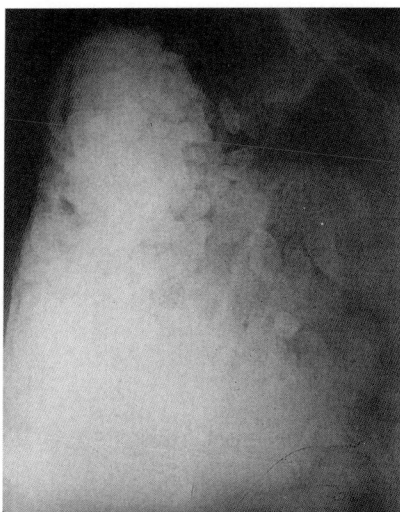

A

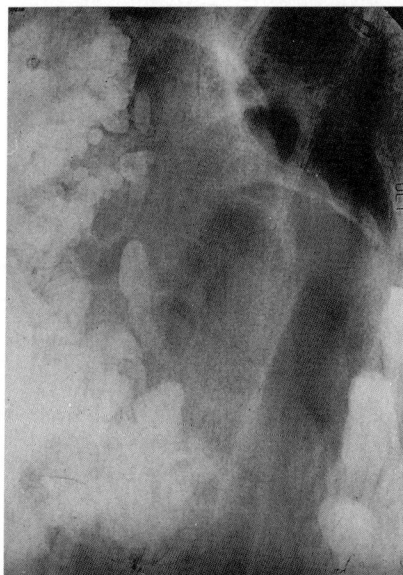

B

8 Canine Oral Trauma

Dr. Ben H. Colmery III

INTRODUCTION

Radiographic evaluation of oral trauma is essential for effective treatment planning. While extraoral "scout films" give an overall impression of the extent of hard tissue trauma experienced by the animal, intraoral films are critical for evaluation of tooth root and periodontal injury.

Intraoral radiographic interpretation or oral injury must include:

1. Status of major blood supply to fracture sites,
2. Status of cortical bone in mandible or maxilla,
3. Status of blood supply to individual teeth,
4. Status of alveolus of teeth in fracture sites,
5. Status of individual roots and crowns of teeth, and
6. Status of periodontal health at fracture sites and in general.

The advantage of intraoral dental films is that they give high detail information in a very short period of time. Intraoperative evaluation of fracture repair is easily accomplished with chairside developers and moveable dedicated dental x-ray machines.

Perhaps the most important observation to make while examining dental films of recent oral trauma is the animal's periodontal health. A firm understanding of periodontal lesions is necessary to properly distinguish between pre-existing oral pathology and acute oral trauma. Too many times treatment planning for fracture repair misses the predisposing periodontal lesions that precipitated the fracture, thus ensuring a nonhealing repair.

In addition, monitoring postoperative fracture healing, paying particular attention to endodontic and periodontic health of teeth at the fracture site, is important. If the fracture involves the alveolus of a tooth, radiographic monitoring of the affected tooth is essential. Any evidence of bone resorption or periodontal disease must be addressed. Likewise, apical disease indicating pulpal death must not be ignored. Quite often teeth are endodontically compromised but are needed for fracture stabilization. Without proper endodontic therapy and monitoring of tooth fractures, healing will not occur.

X-RAY PLATES

FIGURE 8.1

Contributing Author: Ben H. Colmery III

Description: Anterior maxillary midline fracture.

Points Identified:

A. Open midline
B. Fractured vomer

Diagnostic Keys: Displacement incisal symphysis.

Common Errors: Overlooking fractured vomer.

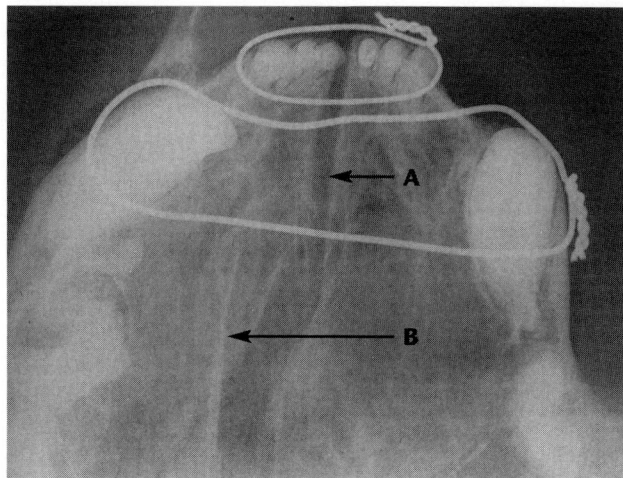

FIGURE 8.2

Contributing Author: Ben H. Colmery III

Diagnosis: Symphyseal separation—feline.

Points Identified:

A. Simple separation, Grade III
B. Class IV fracture, G.V. Black*

Common Errors: Overlooking vertical bone loss incisors. Overlooking Class IV defect of the left canine.

---

*G.V. Black Classification System—Class IV—a lesion at proximal surface of an incisor or canine tooth that involves an incisal edge.

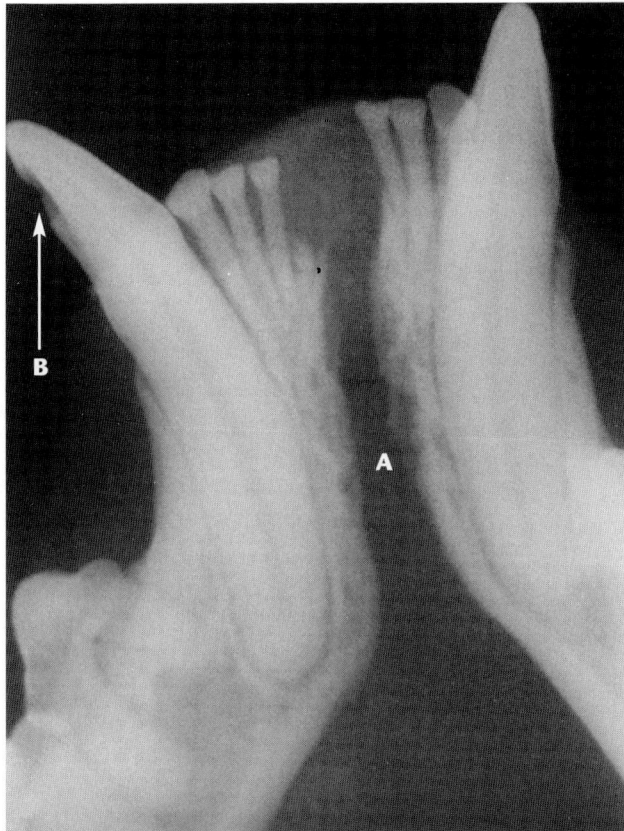

FIGURE 8.3

Contributing Author: Ben H. Colmery III

Description: Fractured mandible (anterior).

Points Identified:

A. Transverse alveolar fracture, apex of canine tooth

Diagnostic Keys: Exposed apical end.

Common Errors: Overlooking potential endodontic complications.

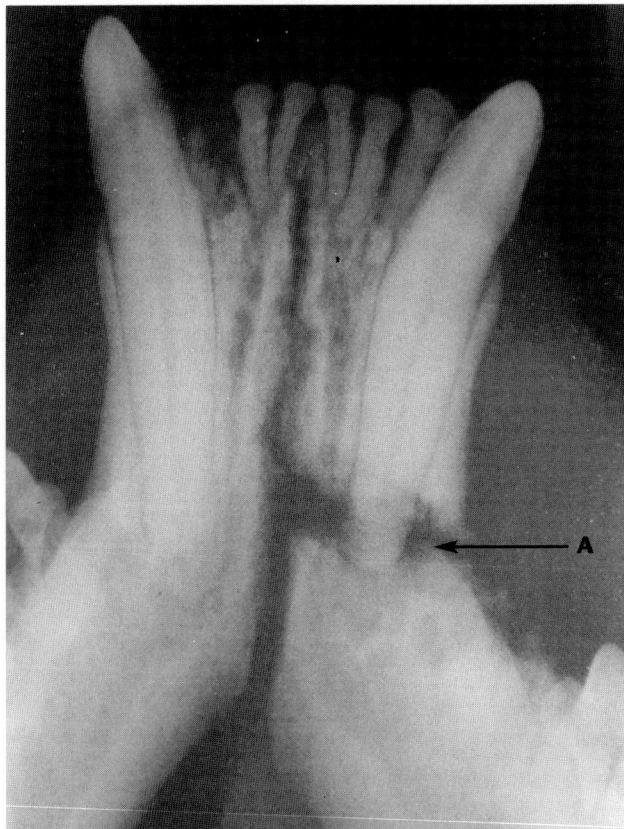

FIGURE 8.4

Contributing Author: Ben H. Colmery III

Description: Oblique anterior mandible.

Points Identified:

A. Open apex canines
B. Open apex lateral incisor
C. Partial alveolar fracture

Diagnostic Keys: Immature teeth. Intact but immature symphysis.

Common Errors: Overlooking exposed lateral incisor apex.

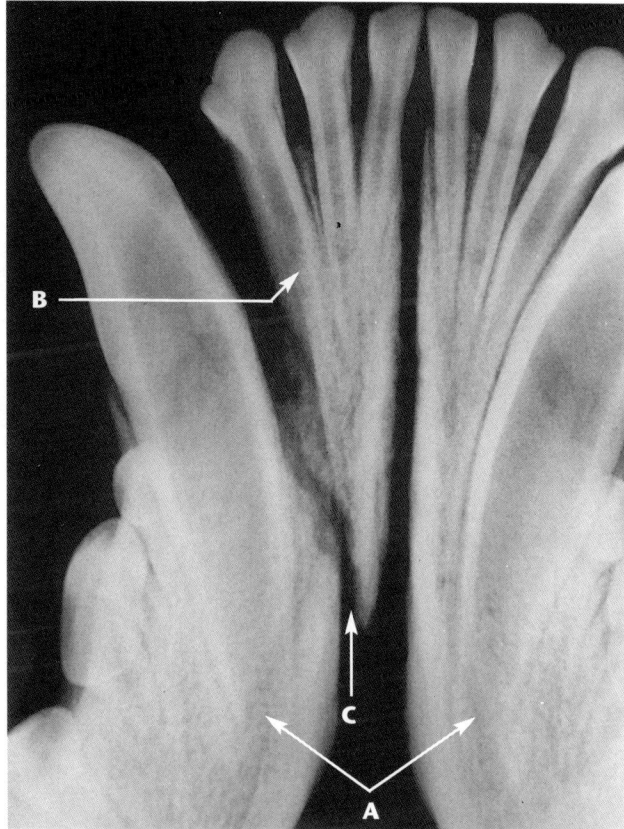

FIGURE 8.5

Contributing Author: Ben H. Colmery III

Description: Oblique rostral mandibular fracture.

Points Identified:

A. Fracture mesial root of second premolar
B. Avulsed apex of canine tooth
C. Alveolar fracture of first premolar

Common Errors: Overlooking alveolar fracture of first premolar.

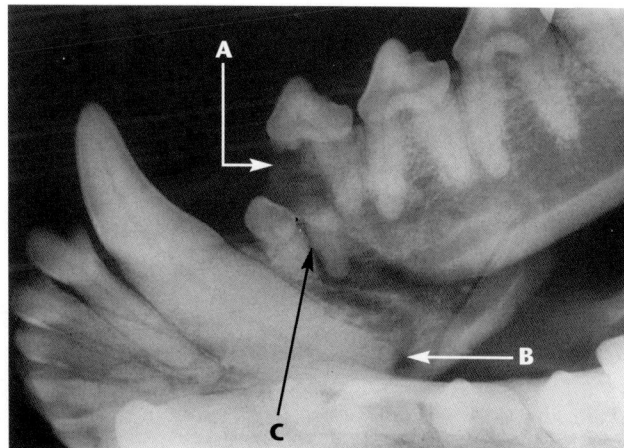

FIGURE 8.6

Contributing Author: Ben H. Colmery III

Description: Oblique fracture of anterior mandible.

Points Identified:

   A. Combined periodontal/endodontal lesion, second premolar
   B. Infrabony pocket, canine
   C. Oblique fracture

Common Errors: Overlooking extent of pre-existing periodontal disease.

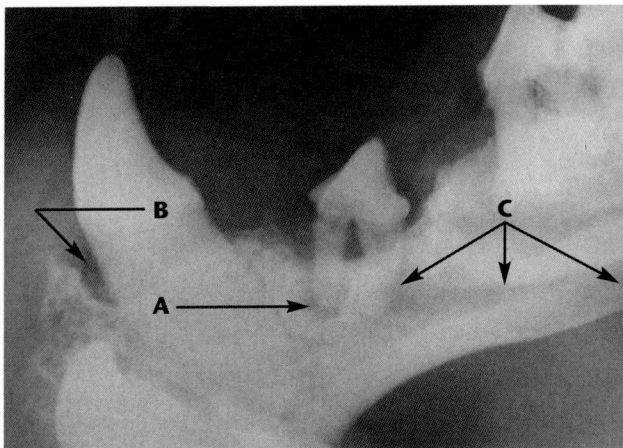

FIGURE 8.7

Contributing Author: Ben H. Colmery III

Description: Interoperative film.

Points Identified:

   A. Reduction of fracture line
   B. Complete extraction of fourth premolar

Diagnostic Keys: Reduced fracture.

Common Errors: Overlooking pathology of fourth premolar.

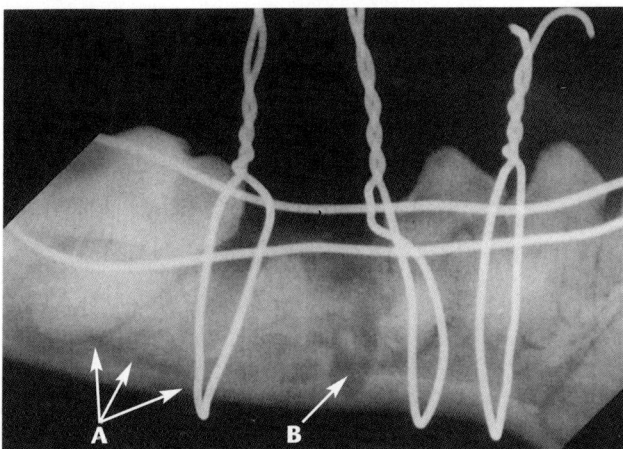

FIGURE 8.8

Contributing Author: Ben H. Colmery III

Description: 12-week postoperative mandibular fracture repair (see Figure 8.7).

Points Identified:

   A. Fracture site

Diagnostic Keys: Healed mandibular bone.

Common Errors: Mistaking loss of density of distal apex of third premolar as pathologic. In this case, it is due to loss of bone mass from bone fragments when fractured.

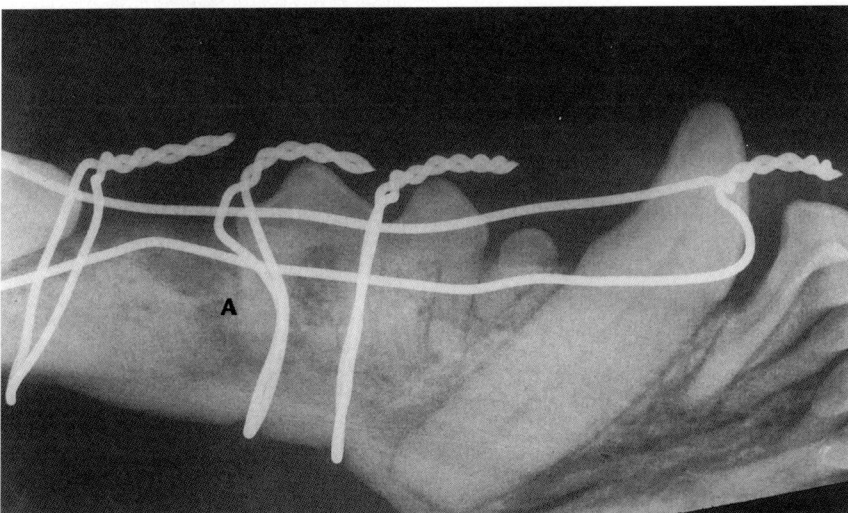

FIGURE 8.9

Contributing Author: Ben H. Colmery III

Description: 12 weeks postoperative (see Figures 8.7, 8.8).

Points Identified: Wire removed from fracture site.

    A. Partial wire removal from fracture site
    B. Healthy apex of distal root, third premolar

Diagnostic Keys: Cerclage wire dimple cortical bone.

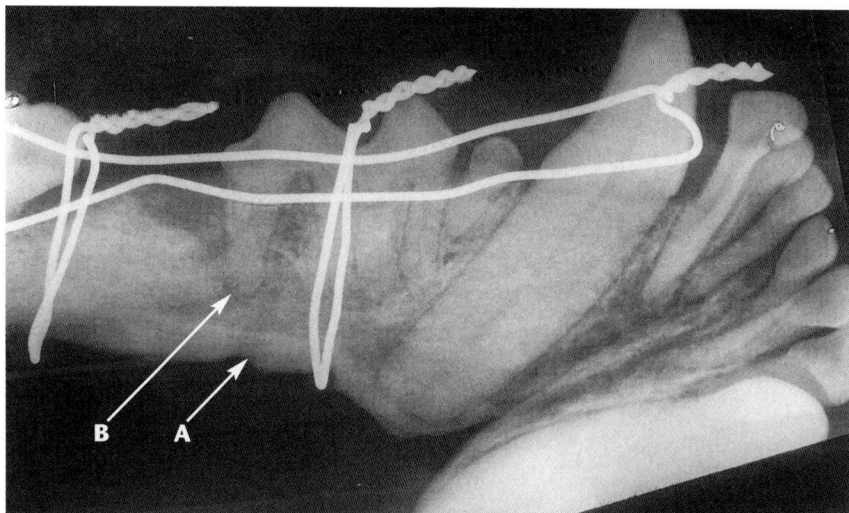

FIGURE 8.10

Contributing Author: Ben H. Colmery III

Description: 12 weeks postoperative (see Figures 8.7–8.9).

Points Identified: All wires removed.

Diagnostic Keys: Healed bone.

Common Errors: Distal root mandibular third premolar healthy.

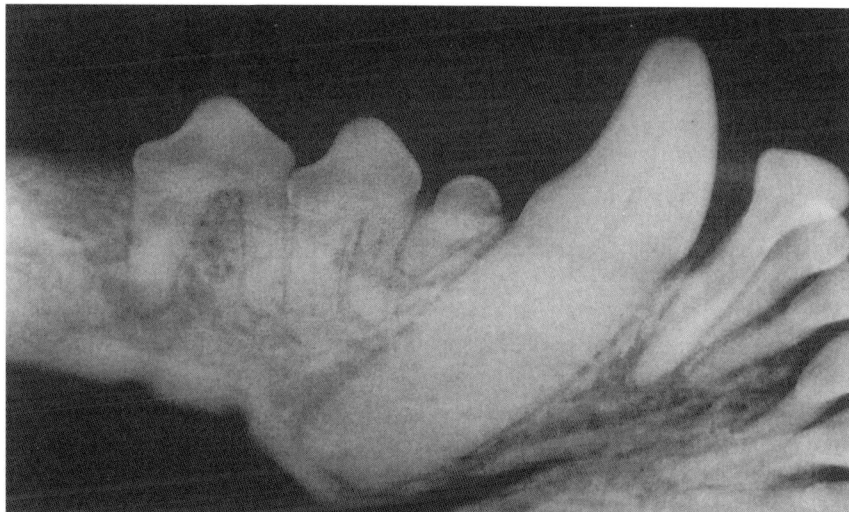

FIGURE 8.11

Contributing Author: Ben H. Colmery III

Description: Midbody fracture edentulous mandible.

Points Identified: Periosteal reaction to chronic inflammation of anterior mandible.

Diagnostic Keys: Thinning of cortical bone.

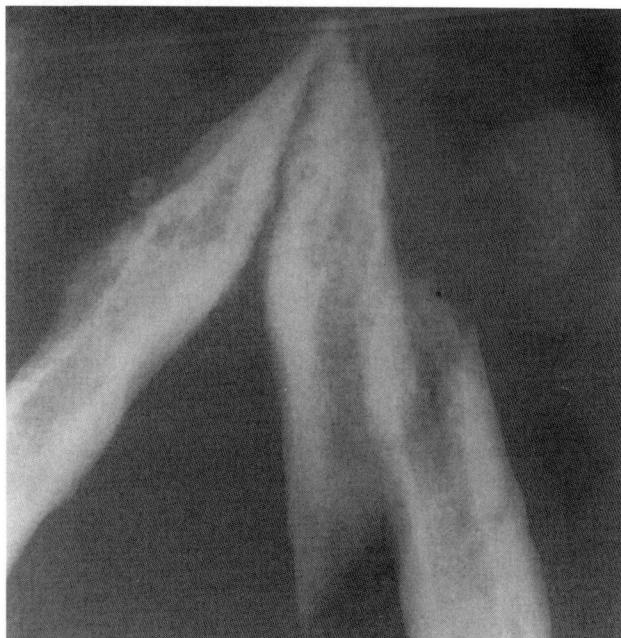

FIGURE 8.12

Contributing Author: Ben H. Colmery III

Description: Midbody pathologic fracture of the mandible.

Points Identified:

A. Midbody vertical fracture at level of distal root of fourth premolar
B. Class V lesion mesial surface mandibular first molar, G.V. Black*
C. Infrabony pocket, distal root, third premolar

Diagnostic Keys: Cortical bone.

Common Errors: Overlooking vertical bone loss of mandibular first molar.

---

*G.V. Black Classification System—Class V—a lesion on facial lingual, labial, or buccal surface at gingival third of tooth.

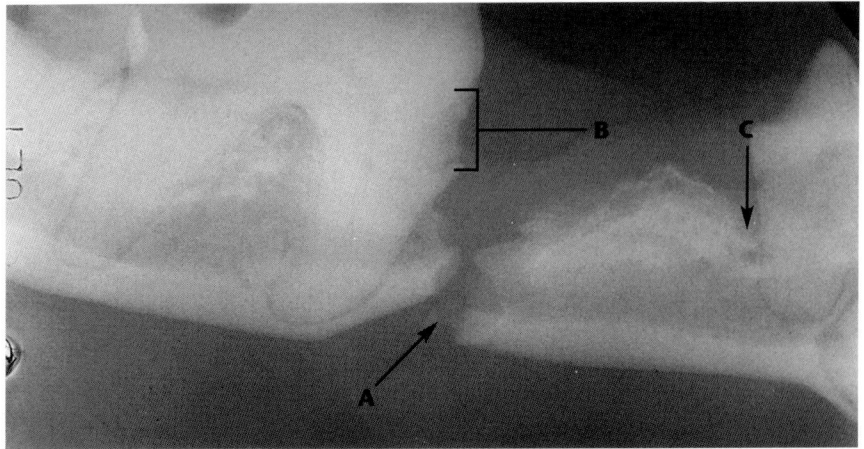

FIGURE 8.13

Contributing Author: Ben H. Colmery III

Description: Oblique alveolar fracture, midmandible.

Points Identified:

A. Open apex—immature teeth
B. Exposed root/alveolus mesial root of first molar

Common Errors: Mistaking open apices for apical pathology.

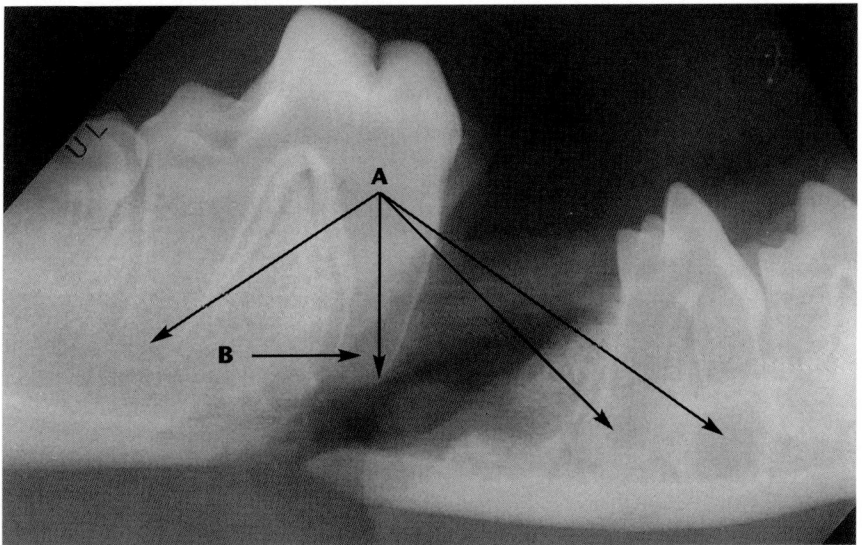

FIGURE 8.14

Contributing Author: Ben H. Colmery III

Description: Oblique distal fracture, mandible.

Points Identified:

A. Exposed pulp, first molar

Diagnostic Keys: Multiple fragments at fracture site.

Common Errors: Missing alveolar fracture at mesial root of second molar. Missing (or ignoring) exposed pulp mandibular first molar.

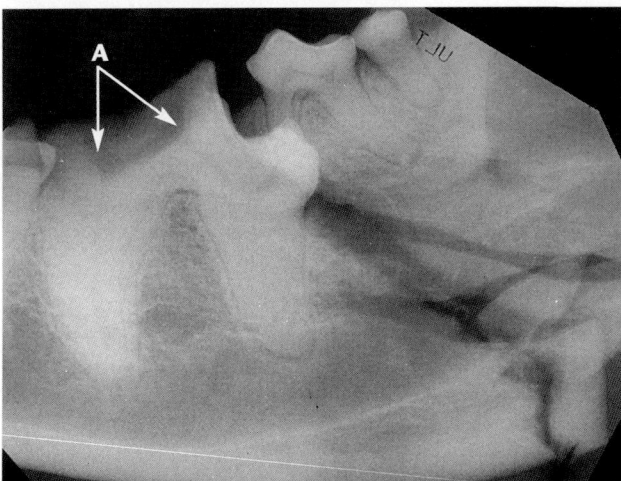

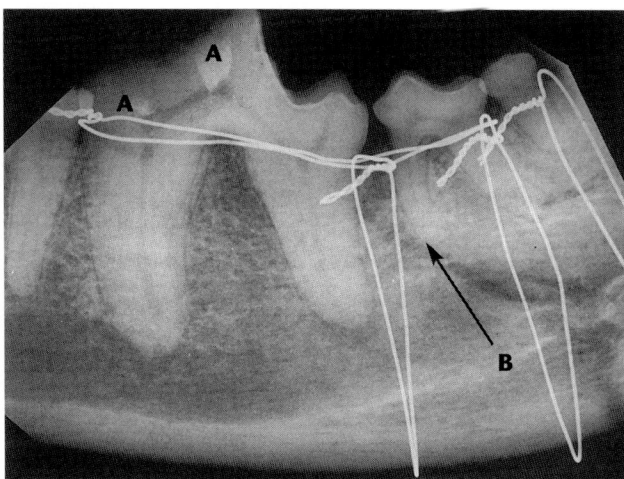

FIGURE 8.15

Contributing Author: Ben H. Colmery III

Description: Immediate postoperative, oblique distal fracture of the mandible (see Figure 8.14).

Points Identified:

A. Exposed pulp, mandibular first molar with pulpotomy therapy
B. Exposed apex mesial root, mandibular second molar

Common Errors: Ignoring endodontic complications (i.e., mandibular first and second molars).

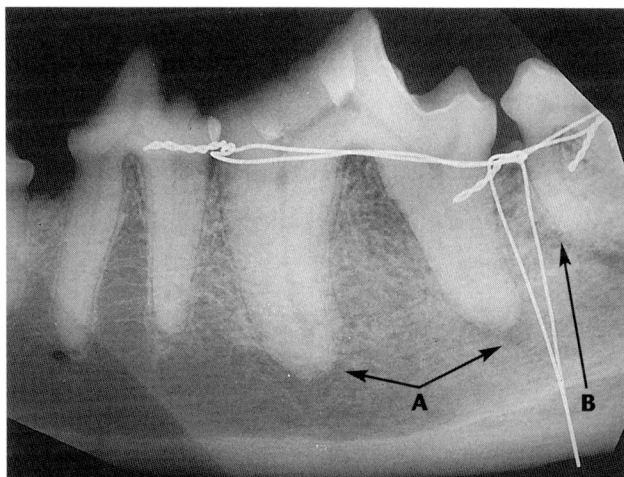

FIGURE 8.16

Contributing Author: Ben H. Colmery III

Description: 12 weeks postoperative, oblique distal fracture, mandible (see Figures 8.14 and 8.15).

Points Identified:

A. Early apical disease, endodontic pulpotomy failure
B. Healing apex mesial root, mandibular second molar

Diagnostic Keys: Healing fracture site.

Common Errors: Ignoring impending failure of pulpotomy therapy.

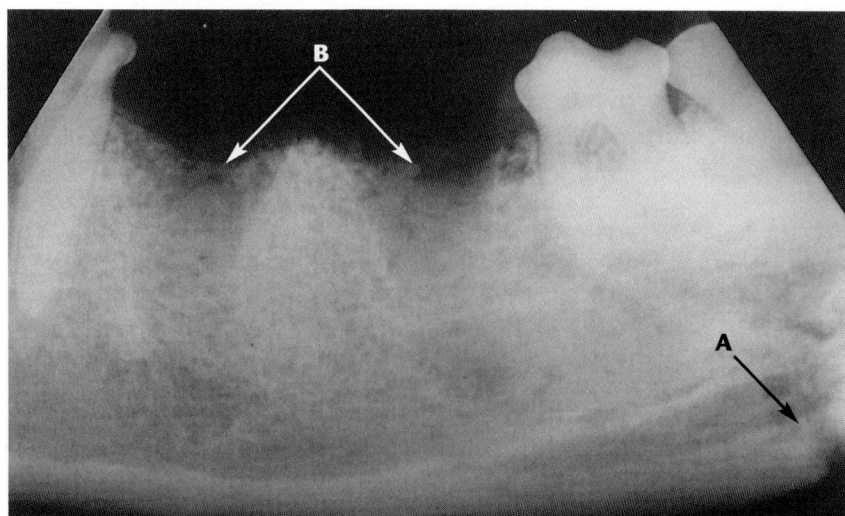

FIGURE 8.17

Contributing Author: Ben H. Colmery III

Description: Healed fracture site, oblique distal fracture of mandible (see Figures 8.14–8.16).

Points Identified: Healed fracture site; postextraction, mandibular first molar. (Owner declined conventional endodontic therapy.)

A. Healed fracture site
B. First molar extraction site

FIGURE 8.18

Contributing Author: Ben H. Colmery III

Description: Pathologic mandibular fracture.

Points Identified:

A. A pathologic fracture of furcation through mesial root of first molar with minimal displacement

Diagnostic Keys: Bone loss and apical exposure distal root mandibular first molar.

Common Errors: Overlooking the extent of periodontitis of the mandibular first molar. Overlooking need to radiograph tooth prior to extraction.

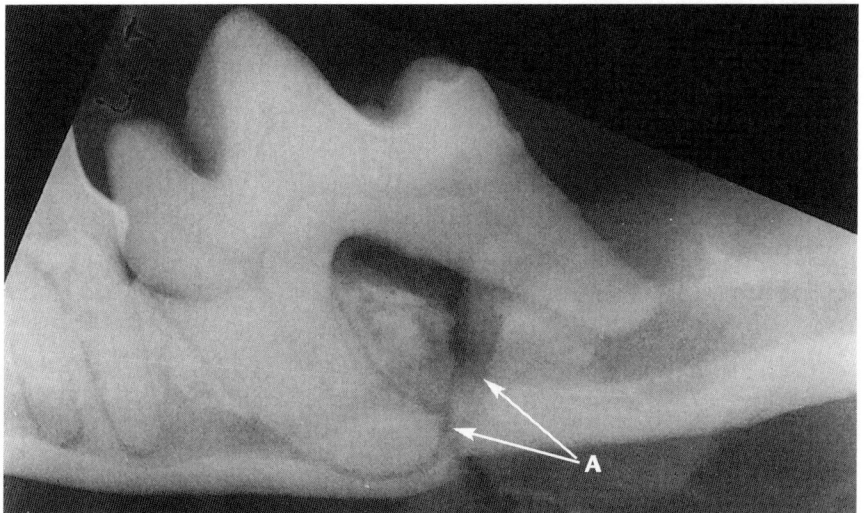

FIGURE 8.19

Contributing Author: Ben H. Colmery III

Description: Vertical fracture midbody mandible.

Points Identified:

A. Distal root apex, mandibular first molar, exposed by fracture

Common Errors: Overlooking exposed apical end.

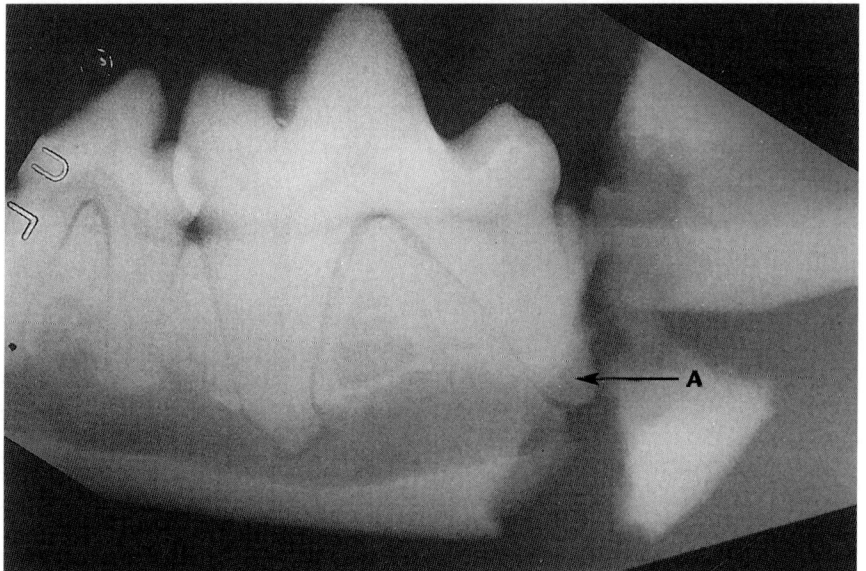

FIGURE 8.20

Contributing Author: Ben H. Colmery III

Description: Vertical fracture midbody mandible, immediate postoperative (see Figure 8.19).

Points Identified:

A. Reduced fracture line

Diagnostic Keys: Closed fracture lines apex of first molar distal root.

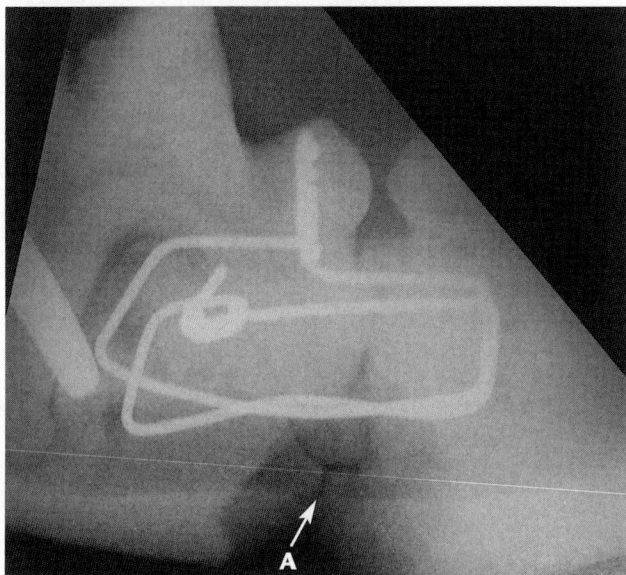

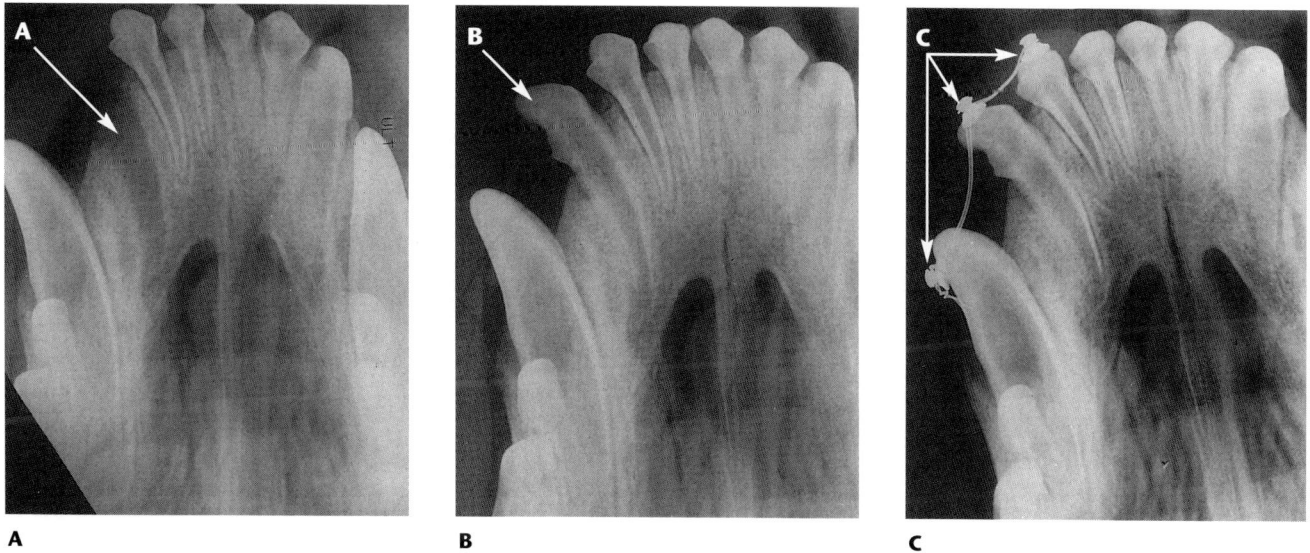

A

B

C

FIGURE 8.21

Contributing Author:
Donald H. DeForge

Description: Avulsion 103.

Points Identified:

A. 103, alveolus with avulsed tooth missing

B. 103, replacement of avulsed tooth shown in view A
C. 103, orthodontic buttons on 102/103/104 with 30 gauge wire base for acrylic splinting

Note: Radiographic image appears to show buttons being placed on incisal edge of teeth. In actuality, buttons are placed on midfacial crown surface.

Diagnostic Keys: An avulsion is a separation of a tooth from its alveolus. In the case shown below, the ideal conditions occurred. The owner brought the avulsed tooth for reimplantation, in a milk bath, within 2 hours of traumatic avulsion.

Common Errors: Client should be informed of complications of reimplantation and need for potential endodontic care.

FIGURE 8.22

Contributing Author: Ben H. Colmery III

Description: Interoperative film—avulsed left canine 104.

Points Identified: Anterior maxillar fracture. Fracture courses along palatine fissure mesiodistally to the right of the midline with a 90 degree deviation behind the palatine fossa to 104.

A. Fracture lines
B. 104

Common Errors: Overlooking the extent of the fracture lines.

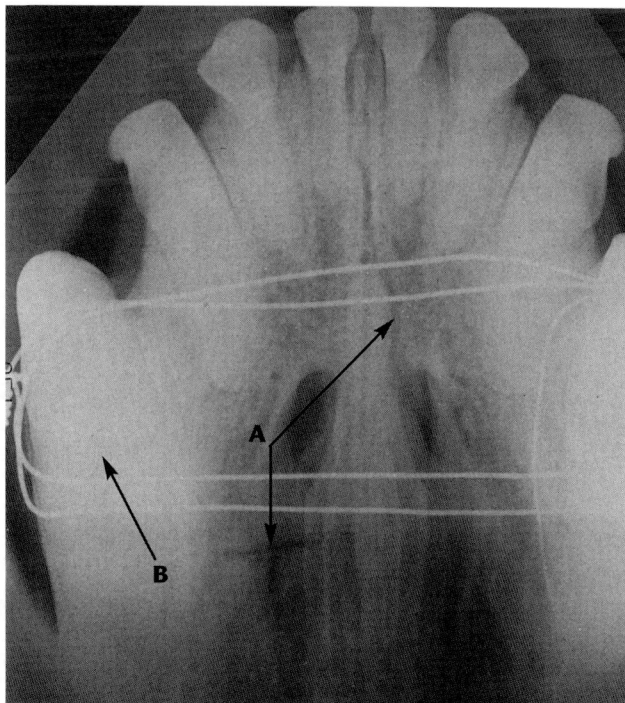

PART TWO   **Feline**

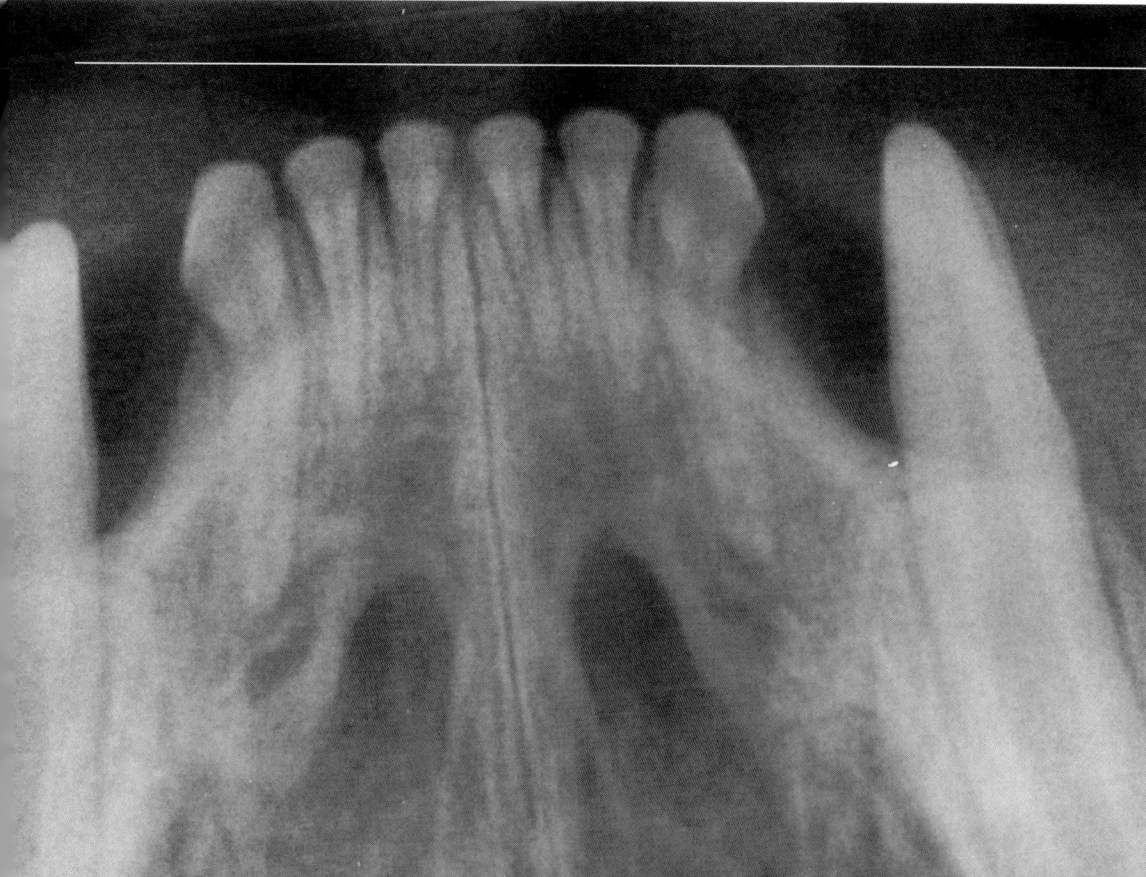

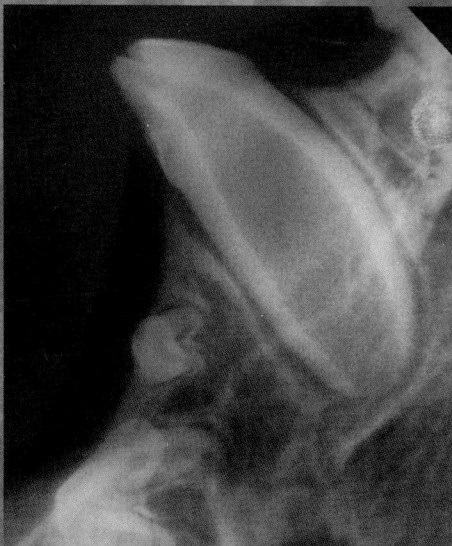

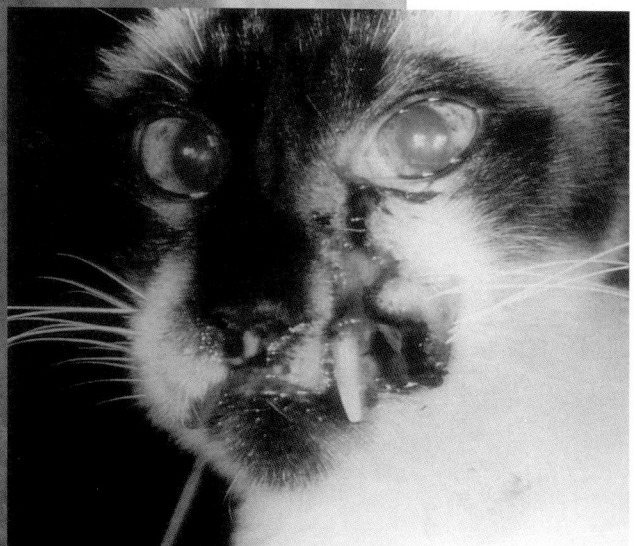

9 Normal Feline Oral Radiographic Anatomy

Dr. Mary Suzanne Aller

INTRODUCTION

This chapter reviews the normal anatomical structures and landmarks seen on dental radiographs of the cat as well as the changes that occur during maturation and aging. Various views of the temporomandibular joint are also presented.

The Dentition

The cat normally has thirty adult teeth, all of which usually exhibit clinical emergence by 6 months of age, although the roots are not completely formed until later. In each maxillary quadrant there are three incisors, a canine, three premolars, and a molar. In each mandibular quadrant there are three incisors, a canine, two premolars, and a molar. Using the anatomical shorthand designating incisors as "I," canines as "C," premolars as "P," and molars as "M," the dental formula of the cat is expressed as a series of fractions with the maxillary quadrant designated as the numerator and the mandibular quadrant as the denominator:

$$2 \, (\, I3/3 + C1/1 + P3/2 + M1/1 \,) = 30 \text{ teeth}$$

When referring to a particular tooth, note that the maxillary premolars are numbered 2, 3, and 4, while the mandibular premolars are numbered 3 and 4. Conventional anatomical nomenclature for dentition dictates a number designation based on the position of the teeth relative to the carnassial teeth. The maxillary carnassial tooth is the fourth premolar, so the teeth preceding it in the arch are numbered accordingly. The mandibular carnassial tooth is the first molar, so the tooth immediately preceding it in the arch is designated the fourth premolar, and again the preceding tooth is numbered accordingly. The modified Triadan system is another commonly used nomenclature system and designates the quadrant and tooth position by a number code. Quadrants are designated by 100s, 200s, 300s, or 400s, and the teeth are assigned particular numbers within the quadrant according to their position. For example, the maxillary right canine tooth number assignment is 104.[1,2,3,4] (See Figure 9.1.)

FIGURE 9.1

Schematic diagram of feline dental anatomy and corresponding anatomical and Modified Triadan System nomenclature.

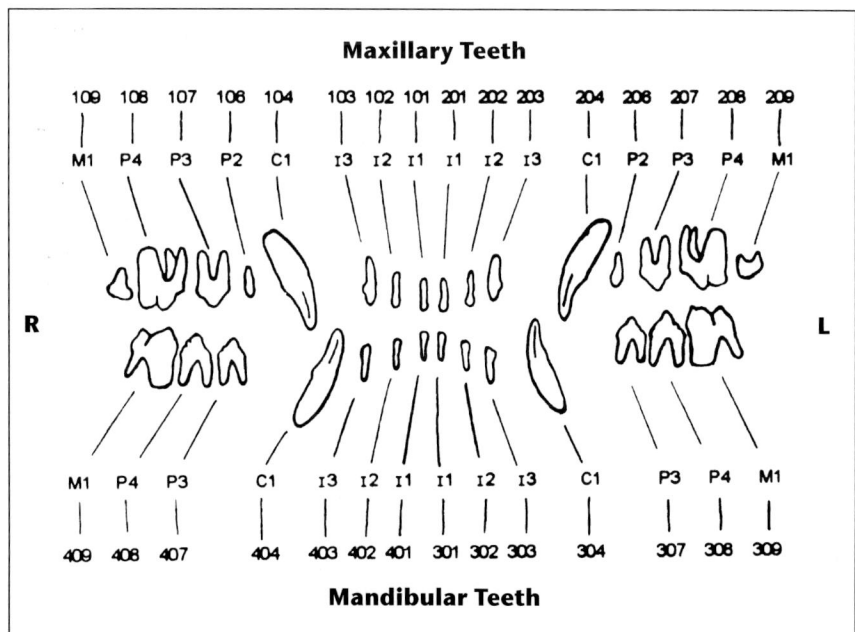

Knowing the normal root structures for each tooth is important for the recognition of congenital anomalies and helps to identify which teeth are present, missing, ectopic, or supernumerary. Familiarity with the root numbers, form, and positions will also aid in the performance of extractions and root retrieval when indicated. Incisors, canines, and the maxillary second premolar are single-rooted teeth. Although sometimes the maxillary second premolar exhibits two roots that are fused together. The maxillary third premolar, the mandibular third and fourth premolars, and the molars exhibit two roots each. The maxillary fourth premolar is the only three-rooted tooth in the cat, with mesiopalatal, mesiobuccal, and distal roots. Note that the roots are not necessarily symmetrical in size or shape. The distal root of the maxillary fourth premolar is much broader than the mesial roots. Likewise, the mesial root of the mandibular molar is much broader and often longer than its distal root. The root structure of the maxillary molar is normally quite small and short, and thus difficult to accurately evaluate radiographically. Usually two short roots are discernible anatomically after extraction, but variable root numbers or forms are not unusual for the maxillary molar. Occasionally, its roots are fused into a relatively large single root structure.[1,2,3] (See Figure 9.1 and Table 9.1.)

Table 9.1. Numbers of roots per tooth in the permanent dentition of the cat

Tooth	Maxillary	Mandibular
Incisor	1	1
Canine	1	1
Second premolar	1	–
Third premolar	2	2
Fourth premolar	3	2
Molar	2	2

Basic Dental Anatomy

The enamel, dentin, cementum, and lamina dura are radiopaque, while the pulp cavity and periodontal ligament are radiolucent. Teeth are divided topographically into regions called the crown, neck, and root. The crown is that part of the tooth exposed to the oral cavity and is covered with an outermost layer of radiopaque enamel. The root portion is that part of the tooth that resides in the alveolus and is covered with an outer layer of cementum that is radiographically indistinguishable from dentin. Beneath the enamel and cementum is the radiopaque dentin, which comprises most of the tooth and encases the radiolucent vessels and nerves of the pulp. The junction of the crown and the root is referred to as the cementoenamel junction or neck. The point at which the roots branch in multirooted teeth is called the furcation, which in cats is very close to the cementoenamel junction. The tooth resides in a bony alveolar socket suspended by the periodontal ligament that connects the root cementum to the surrounding bone. The periodontal ligament space appears as a uniformly narrow radiolucent space between the root and alveolar bone. The alveolus is lined with specialized cortical bone that appears as a radiopaque line of fairly uniform thickness called the lamina dura. The lamina dura is contiguous with the crestal bone. Ideally, the alveolar bone should extend to the cementoenamel junction.[5,6,7]

Anatomical Landmarks and Artifacts

There are several normal anatomical structures that serve as landmarks or produce anatomical artifacts on the dental radiograph.

Radiolucent anatomical structures of the mandible are the mandibular canal, the mental foramina, and the mandibular symphysis. The mandibular canal houses the inferior alveolar vessels and nerves supplying the mandibular teeth and is a radiolucent tubular structure paralleling the ventral border of the mandible. The roots of the mandibular teeth often appear to project into the canal. The mental foramina can be seen as radiolucent oval or round defects in the mandible. The cranial mental foramen is in the incisor area, the middle mental foramen is at the level of the mandibular canine root, and the caudal mental foramen is at the level of the third premolar. In the cat, the middle and caudal mental foramina are often visualized and can give the false impression of pathological periapical lucencies when superimposed over a tooth root. Retaking the radiograph from a different angle will show that the foramen will shift position in relation to the tooth whereas a true periapical lucency will maintain its association with the root. The mandibular symphysis is a fibrous joint joining the two halves of the mandible rostrally and presents as a narrow irregularly contoured radiolucent line, sometimes also containing some radiopaque tissue.[5,6,7,8]

Cervical burnout is an artifact that makes the neck of feline teeth appear relatively more radiolucent than neighboring structures, especially in mandibular views, and must be differentiated from resorptive lesions. The cervical region of the crown not covered by alveolar bone has relatively less mass penetrated by the x-ray beam, resulting in a radiolucent collar visualized at the cementoenamel junction. Radiolucent defects due to cervical burnout disappear on other views of different horizontal angulations, whereas cervical defects due to resorption will persist in each view.[7,9]

Maxillary radiolucent anatomical structures include the palatine fissures and the infraorbital foramen. The palatine fissures are large paired openings in the incisive bone through which the palatine vessels and the nasopalantine ducts course. The infraorbital foramen, through which the infraorbital vessels and nerve travel, is found where the zygomatic arch joins the maxilla. The infraorbital foramen is sometimes seen as a large oval radiolucency superimposed over the maxillary third premolar or mesial fourth premolar apices, but usually is obscured by the mass of the zygomatic bone. Because the radiopaque zygomatic bone accentuates the relative radiolucency of the skull on either side of the arch at the level of the infraorbital foramen, an artifactual periapical radiolucency of the third and fourth premolars is often apparent.[5,6,7,8]

Maxillary radiopaque anatomical landmarks include the zygomatic bone, the attachment of the palatal bones, and the nasal septum. In lateral views, the zygomatic bone is a bony arch often superimposed over the maxillary fourth premolar, obscuring detail. Achieving adequate visualization of the maxillary fourth premolar in the cat often requires elongation of the radiographic image. The point where the bones of the palate join the maxillary bones forms a region of very dense compact bone, seen as a thin radiopaque undulating line superimposed over the roots of the maxillary teeth in lateral view radiographs. This white line will change position slightly depending on the vertical angulation of the beam. The nasal septum is seen as a radiopaque structure bisecting the nasal cavity in dorsoventral views.[5,6,7,8]

Maturation and Aging

After the teeth have erupted, completion of root formation occurs. The majority of teeth exhibit radiographic closure of the apical foramen by a year of age, although formation of the apical delta may not be truly anatomically complete until later. The apical delta is a grouping of small apical perforations allowing passage of the pulp vessels and nerve into the tooth and is not radiographically visible unless delineated by endodontic filling materials. The odontoblasts lining the pulp chamber and root canal continuously deposit dentin during the life of the cat, so that the pulp cavity and root canal become progressively more narrow and shorter with time. As the cat ages, the trabecular bone surrounding the teeth becomes more dense and radiographically presents a more coarse and increasingly radiopaque pattern that obscures the lamina dura. Some slight regression or blunting of the crestal bone is also considered normal with age and must be differentiated from periodontal disease.[5,6,7](See Table 9.2.)

Temporomandibular Joint

The temporomandibular joint is found where the mandibular condyles articulate in the mandibular fossa of the zygomatic process of the temporal bone. In the cat, the temporomandibular joint is difficult to evaluate radiographically because of its very narrow joint space and the superimposition of neighboring structures. Locating the joint on a radiograph is challenging, but generally it is most easily found using the tympanic bullae as landmarks. On lateral and oblique views, the joint is located just rostral to the tympanic bulla. On rostrocaudal open mouth and dorsoventral views, the joint is just rostral and lateral to the tympanic bulla where the zygomatic process extends from the skull. Several different positioning techniques are required to eliminate superimposition and render useful radiographs. Comparative studies can be made with the mouth open and closed in any view to evaluate joint function.[8,10,11,12]

References

1. Boyd JS, Paterson C, and May AH. *Color Atlas of Clinical Anatomy of the Dog and Cat*. Philadelphia:Mosby Year Book, 1991, 17–30.

2. Harvey CE. *Veterinary Dentistry* Philadelphia:WB Saunders, 1985, 11–22.

3. Orsini P and Hennet P. Anatomy of the mouth and teeth of the cat. In: Harvey CE, ed. *The Veterinary Clinics of North America: Feline Dentistry*, vol 22, no 6. Philadelphia:WB Saunders, 1992, 1265–77.

4. Holmstrom SE, Frost P, and Gammon RL. *Veterinary Dental Techniques*. Philadelphia:WB Saunders, 1992, 2–13.

5. Zontine WJ. Dental radiographic technique and interpretation. In: *The Veterinary Clinics of North America: Radiology*, vol 4, no 4. Philadelphia:WB Saunders, 1974, 741–62.

6. Zontine WJ. Canine dental radiology: radiographic technique, development, and anatomy of teeth. *J Am Vet Radiol Soc* 16:75–82 (1975).

7. Harvey CE and Flax BM. Feline oral-dental radiographic examination and interpretation. In: Harvey CE, ed. *The Veterinary Clinics of North America: Feline Dentistry*, vol 22, no 6. Philadelphia:WB Saunders , 1992, 1279–95.

8. Schebitz H and Wilkens H. *Atlas of Radiographic Anatomy of the Dog and Cat*, 4th Edition. Philadelphia:WB Saunders 1986, 30–31, 154–165.

9. Razmus TF. Caries, periodontal disease, and periapical changes. In: Miles DA and Van Dis ML, eds. *The Dental Clinics of North America: The Clinical Approach to Radiological Diagnosis*, vol 38, no 1. Philadelphia:WB Saunders, 1994, 13–31.

10. Thrall DE. *Textbook of Veterinary Diagnostic Radiology*, 2nd edition. Philadelphia:WB Saunders 1994, 35–38.

11. Ticer JW. *Radiographic Technique in Veterinary Practice*, 2nd edition. Philadelphia:WB Saunders, 1984, 231–59.

12. Douglas SW, Herrtage ME, and Williamson HD. *Principles of Veterinary Radiography*, 4th Edition. Philadelphia:Balliere Tindall, 1987, 177–93.

Table 9.2. Radiographic features of maturation and aging

Tooth	Bone
Root formation and apical closure	Increased trabecular bone density
Internal dentin deposition	Indistinct lamina dura
Increased thickness of dentinal wall	Slight regression of alveolar crest
Root canal constriction	

FIGURE 9.2

Contributing Author:
Mary Suzanne Aller

Description: Radiographic dental anatomy of feline mandibular teeth. Lateral view, parallel technique, intraoral.

Points Identified:

A. Pulp horns   E. Apex
B. Pulp chamber   F. Lamina dura
C. Cementoenamel   G. Alveolar crest
    junction   H. Furcation
D. Root canal

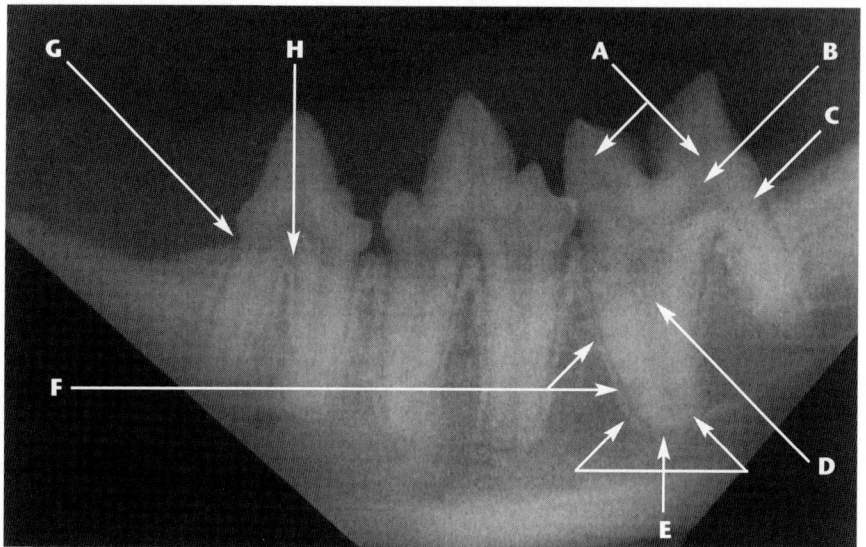

Anatomical Structures and Landmarks of the Feline Mandible

FIGURE 9.3

Contributing Author:
Mary Suzanne Aller

Description: Feline mandibular teeth. Lateral view, parallel technique, intraoral.

Points Identified:

A. Middle mental foramen
B. Caudal mental foramen
C. Mandibular canal
D. Molar
E. Summation image of fourth premolar and molar
F. Premolars

Common Errors: Note the cervical burnout of especially the fourth premolar. It can be confused with resorptive lesions.

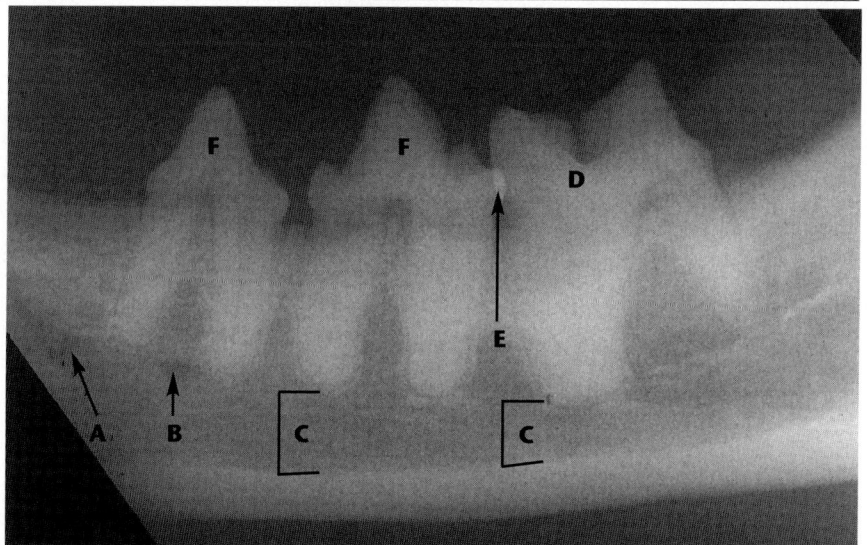

FIGURE 9.4

Contributing Author:
Mary Suzanne Aller

Description: Anterior mandibular teeth. Ventrodorsal oblique view, bisecting angle technique, intraoral.

Points Identified:

A. Mandibular symphysis
B. Canines
C. Incisors

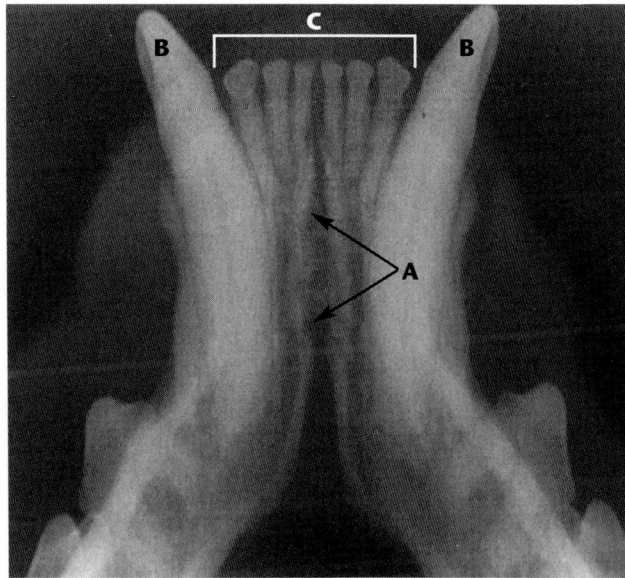

Anatomical Structures and Landmarks of the Feline Maxilla

FIGURE 9.5

Contributing Author:
Mary Suzanne Aller

Description: Feline maxillary teeth. Dorsoventral oblique view, bisecting angle technique, intraoral.

Points Identified:

A. Incisors
B. Canines
C. Palatine fissures
D. Vomer bone, lower portion of nasal septum

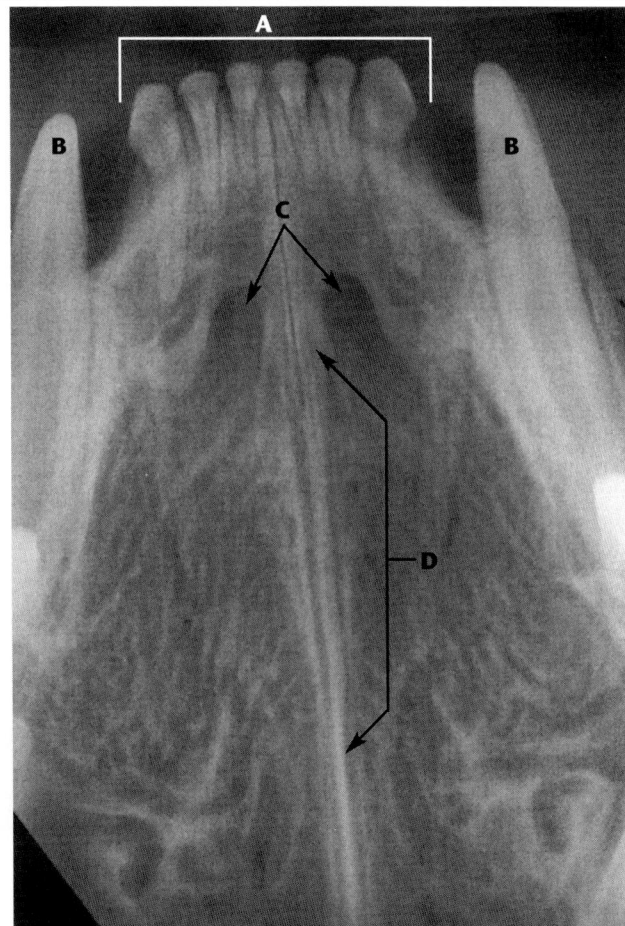

FIGURE 9.6

Contributing Author:
Mary Suzanne Aller

Description: Maxillary teeth. Mesiodistal lateral oblique view, bisecting angle technique, intraoral. Dry skull specimen with barium suspension in the infraorbital foramen.

- A. Zygomatic bone
- B. Barium-filled infraorbital foramen
- C. "White line," confluence of maxillary bones and palate
- D. Canine
- E. Premolars
- F. Molar

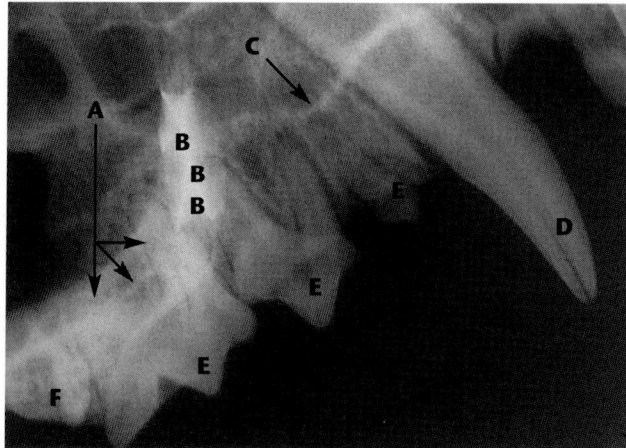

FIGURE 9.7

Contributing Author:
Mary Suzanne Aller

Description: Maxillary teeth. Mesiodistal lateral oblique view, bisecting angle technique. Clinical specimen shown in Figure 9.6 (without barium).

Points Identified:

- A. Zygomatic bone
- B. Infraorbital foramen
- C. Canine
- D. Premolars
- E. Molar superimposed over premolar

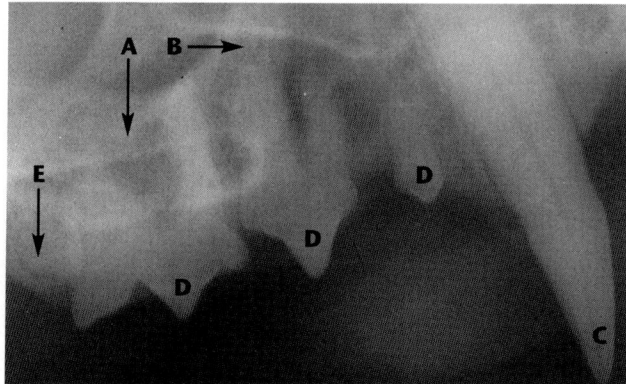

FIGURE 9.8

Contributing Author:
Mary Suzanne Aller

Description: Lateral oblique of maxillary canine tooth. Bisecting angle technique, intraoral. Dry skull specimen with barium suspension in the infraorbital foramen.

Points Identified:

- A. Palatine fissure
- B. "White line," confluence of the bones of the palate and the maxillary bones
- C. Zygomatic bone superimposed over fourth premolar
- D. Barium-filled infraorbital foramen

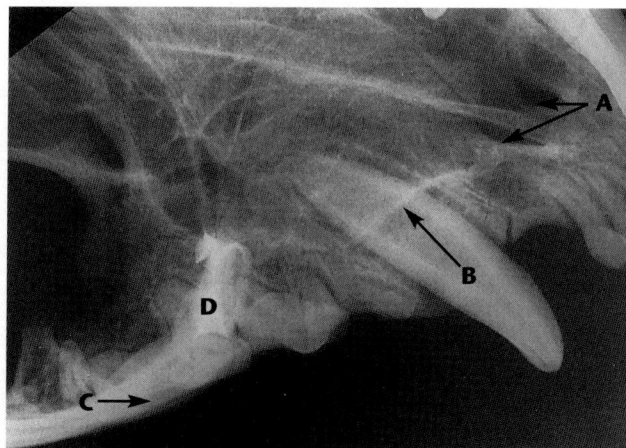

FIGURE 9.9

Contributing Author:
Mary Suzanne Aller

Description: Maxillary canine. Lateral oblique view, bisecting angle technique (fore-shortened premolars), intraoral. Clinical specimen shown in Figure 9.8 (without barium).

Points Identified:

  A. "White line," confluence of the bones of the palate and the maxillary bones
  B. Infraorbital foramen
  C. Zygomatic arch

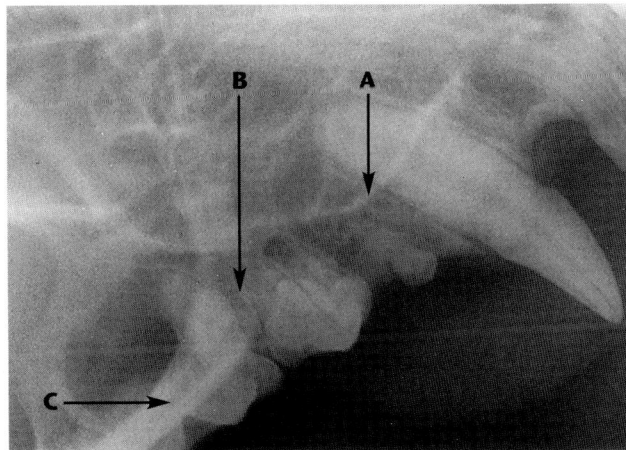

FIGURE 9.10

Contributing Author:
Mary Suzanne Aller

Description: Maxillary premolars. Dorso-ventral view, parallel technique, intraoral. Dry skull specimen with barium suspension in the infraorbital foramen.

Points Identified:

  A. Palatine fissures
  B. "White line," confluence of maxillary bones and bones of the palate
  C. Canine
  D. Premolars
  E. Barium-filled infraorbital foramen
  F. Zygomatic bone

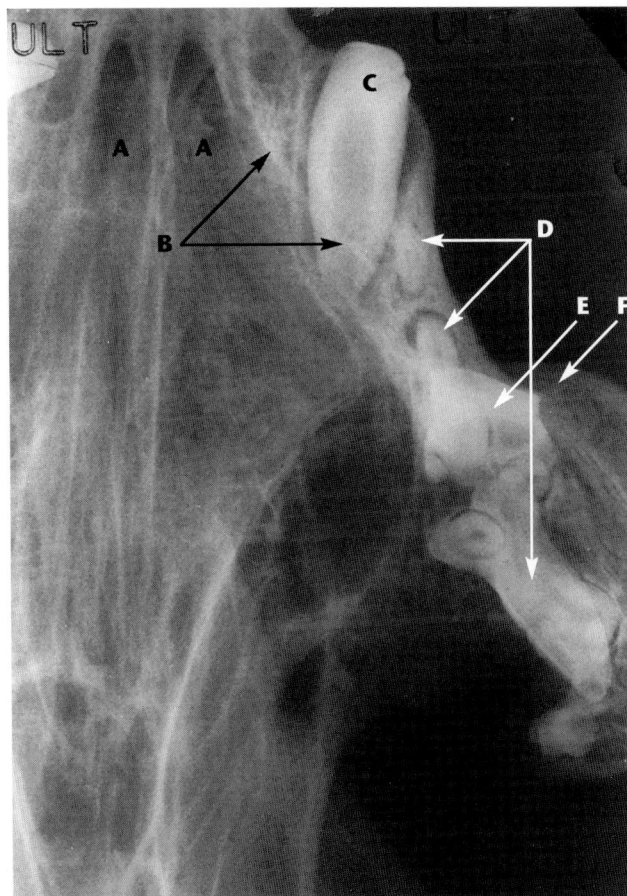

FIGURE 9.11

Contributing Author:

Mary Suzanne Aller

Description: Maxillary premolars. Dorso-ventral view, parallel technique, intraoral. Clinical specimen shown in Figure 9.10 (without barium).

Points Identified:

- A. Canine
- B. Premolars
- C. Mesiobuccal root of fourth premolar
- D. Mesiopalatal root of fourth premolar
- E. Distal root of fourth premolar
- F. Molar
- G. Lamina dura

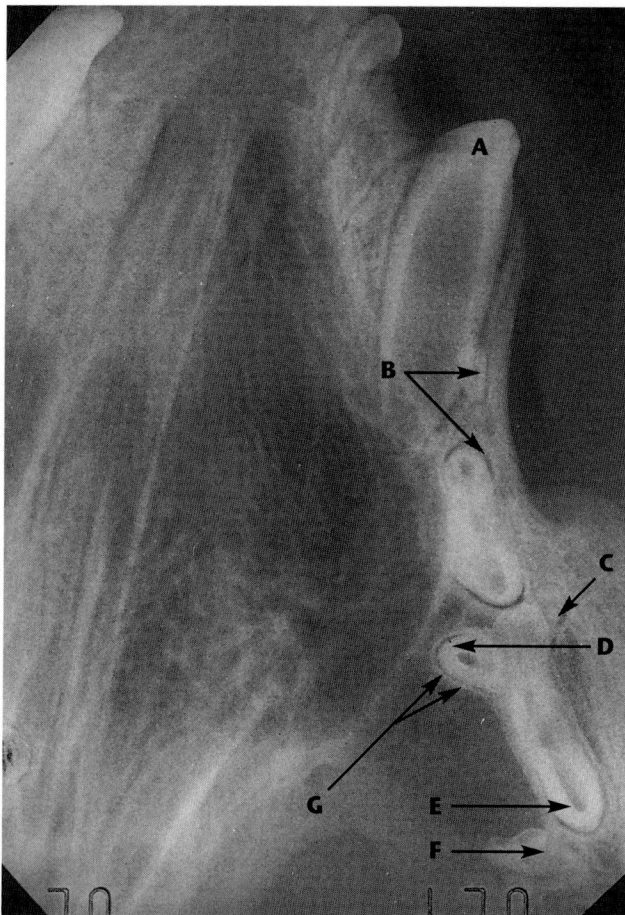

FIGURE 9.12

Contributing Author:

Mary Suzanne Aller

Description: Distomesial lateral oblique, bisecting angle technique, intraoral. Dry skull specimen with barium suspension in the infraorbital foramen.

Points Identified:

- A. "White line," confluence of bones of the palate and maxilla
- B. Barium-filled infraorbital foramen
- C. Zygomatic bone
- D. Premolars
- E. Molar

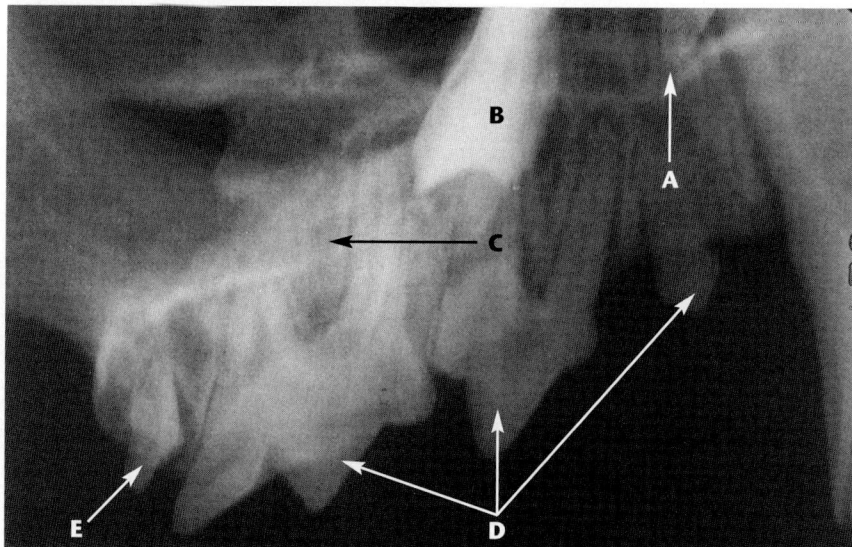

FIGURE 9.13

Contributing Author:
Mary Suzanne Aller

Description: Distomesial lateral oblique view, bisecting angle technique, intraoral. Clinical specimen shown in Figure 9.12 (without barium).

Points Identified:

A. "White line," confluence of bones of the palate and maxilla
B. Infraorbital foramen
C. Zygomatic bone
D. Molar
E. Premolars

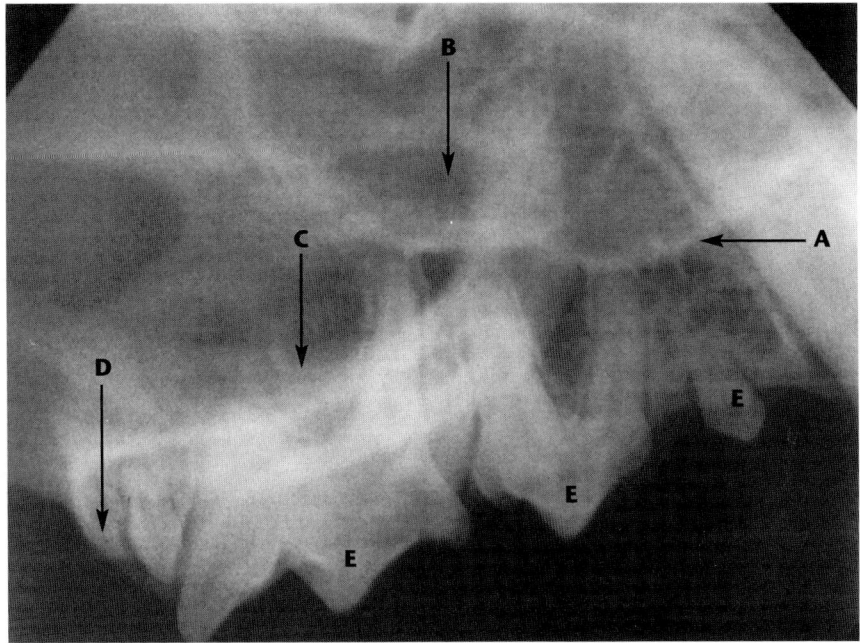

Maturation and Aging of the Feline Teeth

In the following x-rays (Figures 9.14–9.20), please note the tooth and bone changes with age in each series.

FIGURE 9.14

Contributing Author:
Mary Suzanne Aller

Description: Feline mandibular canine, premolars, and molar. Lateral oblique view, bisecting angle technique, intraoral. Note that this view allows visualization of the bone between the canine and the third premolar, an area often missed by the parallel technique.

Points Identified: Feline maturation/ aging series.

A. Adolescent (6–8 months old)
B. Young adult (1–2 years old)
C. Mature adult (6–10 years old)

Common Errors: Mandibular premolars and molar slightly foreshortened. Errors of foreshortening or elongation are common in this view.

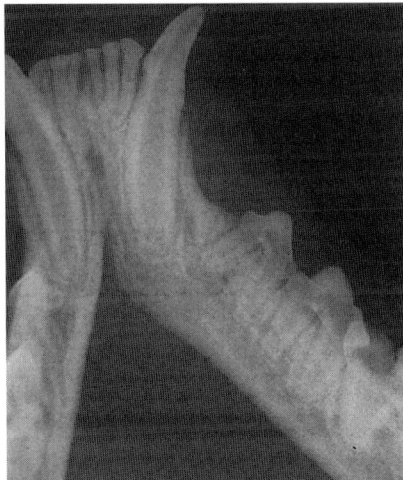

A

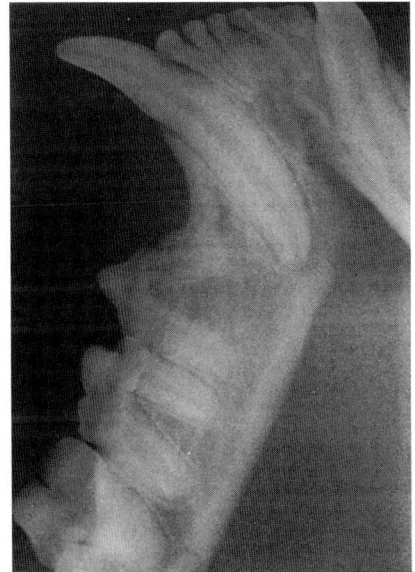

B

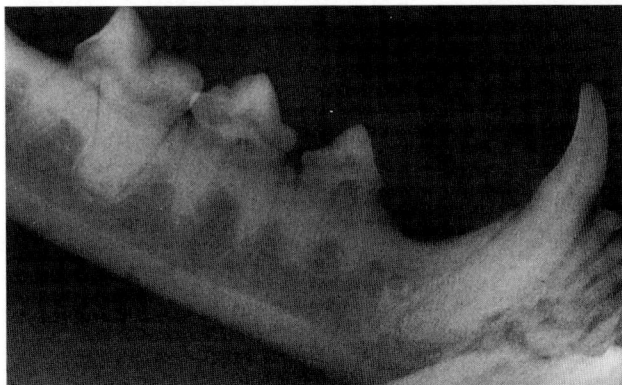

C

FIGURE 9.15

Contributing Author:
Mary Suzanne Aller

Description: Feline mandibular incisors and canine. Ventrodorsal oblique view, bisection angle technique, intraoral.

Points Identified: Feline maturation/aging series.

  A. Adolescent (6–8 months)
  B. Young adult (1–2 years old)
  C. Mature adult (6–10 years old)

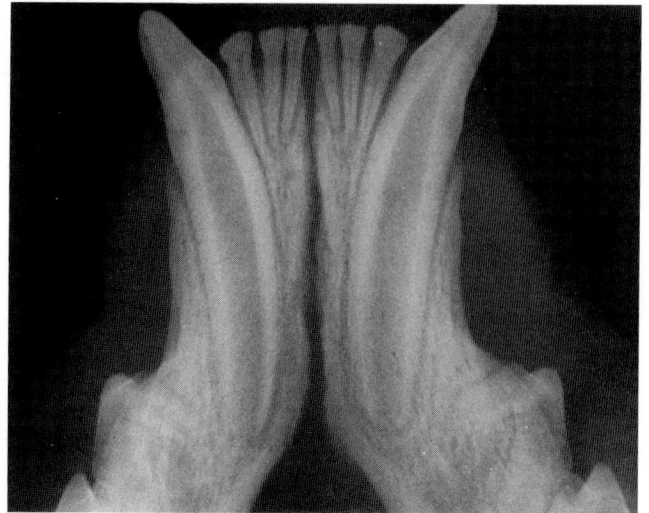

A

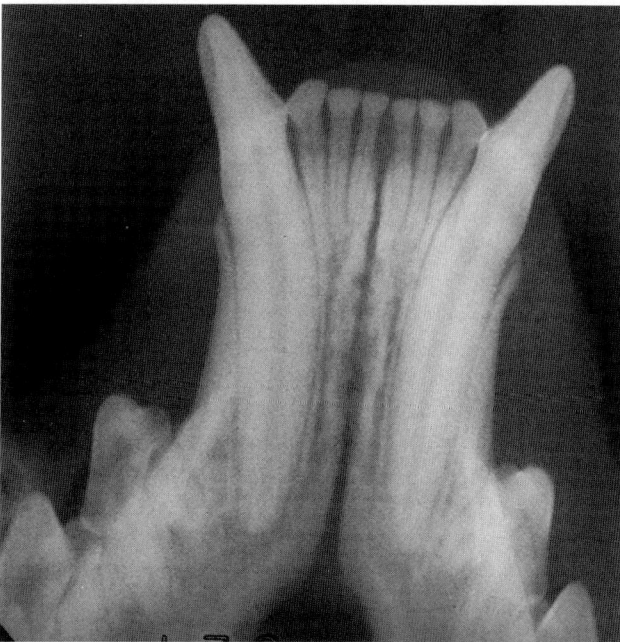

B

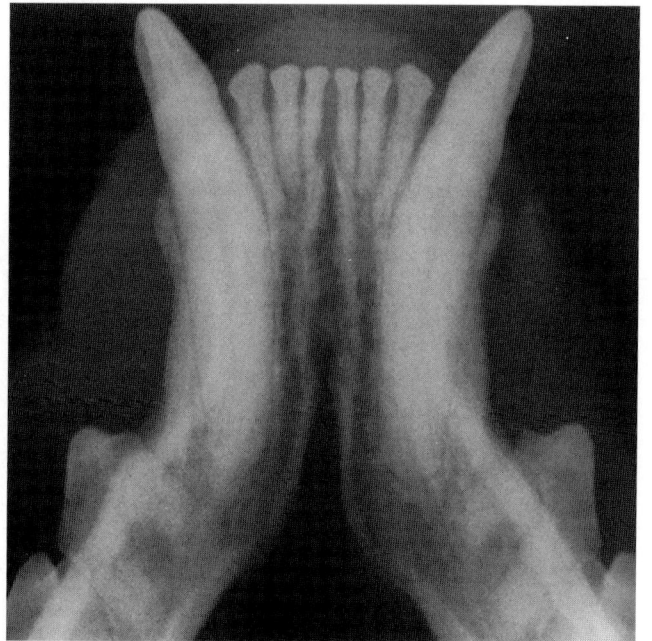

C

FIGURE 9.16

Contributing Author:
Mary Suzanne Aller

Description: Feline mandibular premolars and molars. Lateral view, parallel technique, intraoral.

Points Identified: Feline maturation/ aging series.

- A. Adolescent (6–8 months old)
- B. Young Adult (1–2 years old)
- C. Mature adults (6–10 years old)

Common Errors: C. Note the cervical burnout sometimes confused with resorptive lesions.

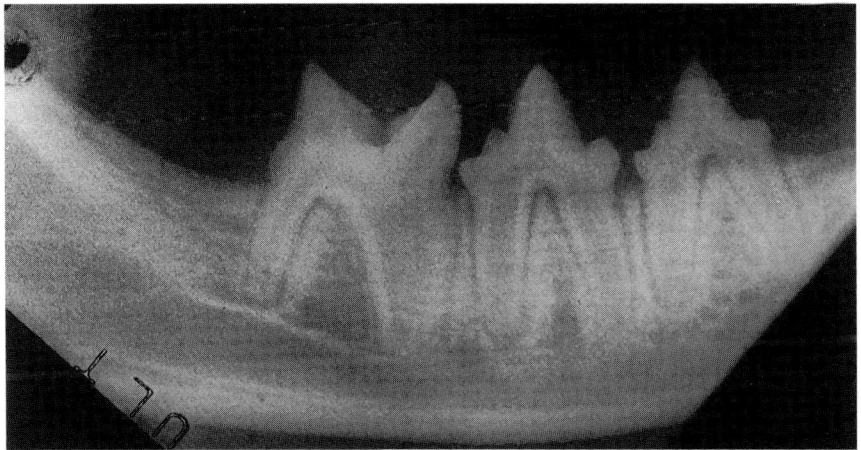

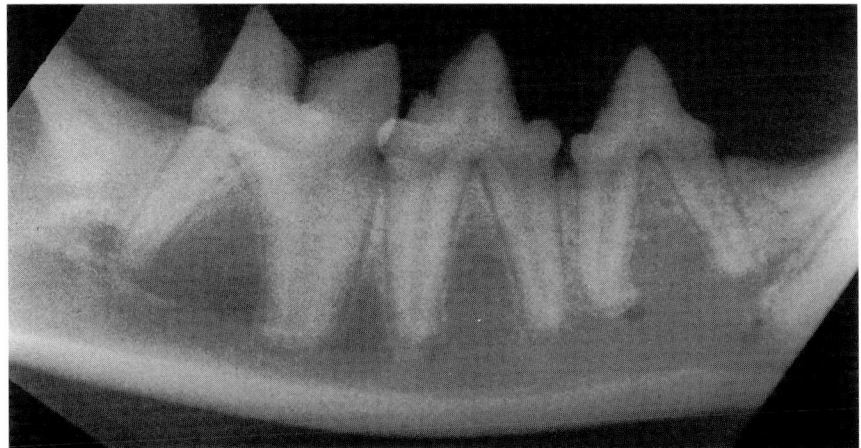

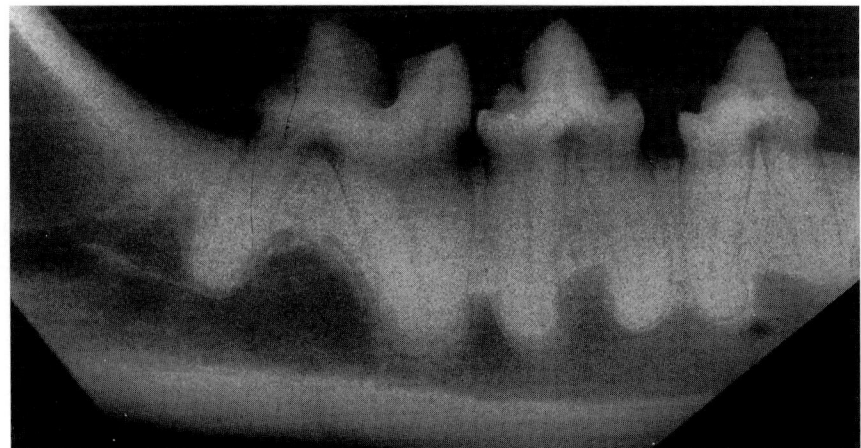

A

B

C

FIGURE 9.17

Contributing Author:
Mary Suzanne Aller

Description: Feline maxillary incisors. Dorsoventral oblique view, bisection angle technique, intraoral.

Points Identified: Feline maturation/aging series.

    A. Adolescent (6–8 months old)
    B. Young adult (1–2 years old)
    C. Mature adult (6–10 years old)

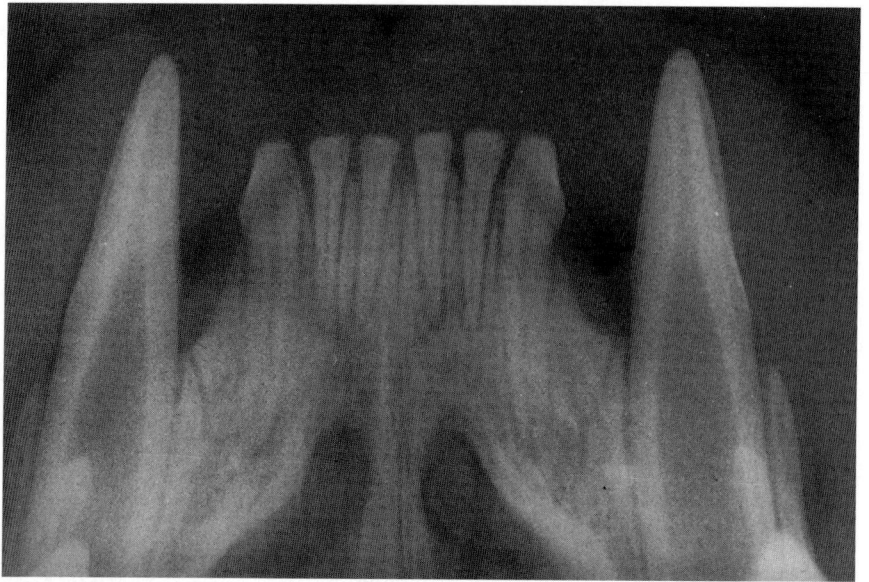

A

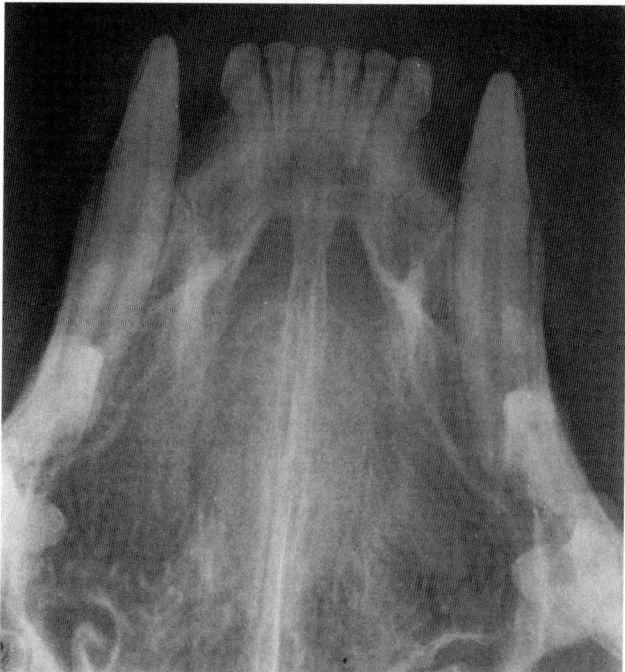

B

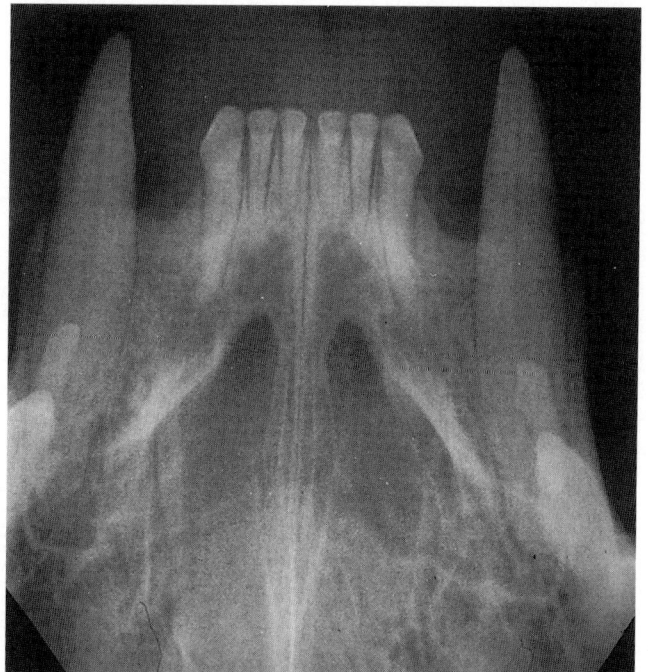

C

FIGURE 9.18

Contributing Author:

Mary Suzanne Aller

Description: Feline maxillary canine. Lateral oblique view, bisecting angle technique, intraoral.

Points Identified: Feline maturation/ aging series.

A. Adolescent (6–8 months old)
B. Young adult (1–2 years old)
C. Mature adult (6–10 years old)

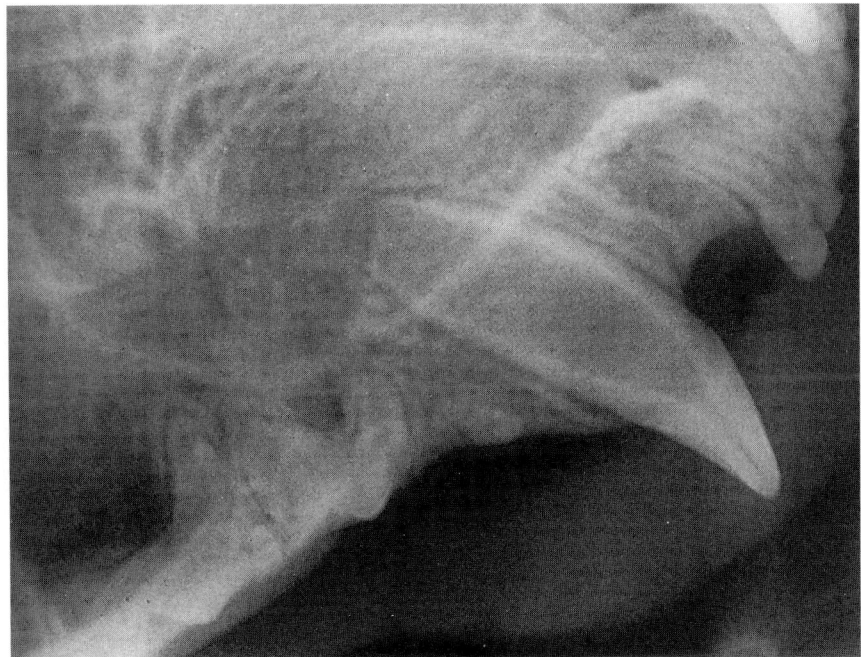

A

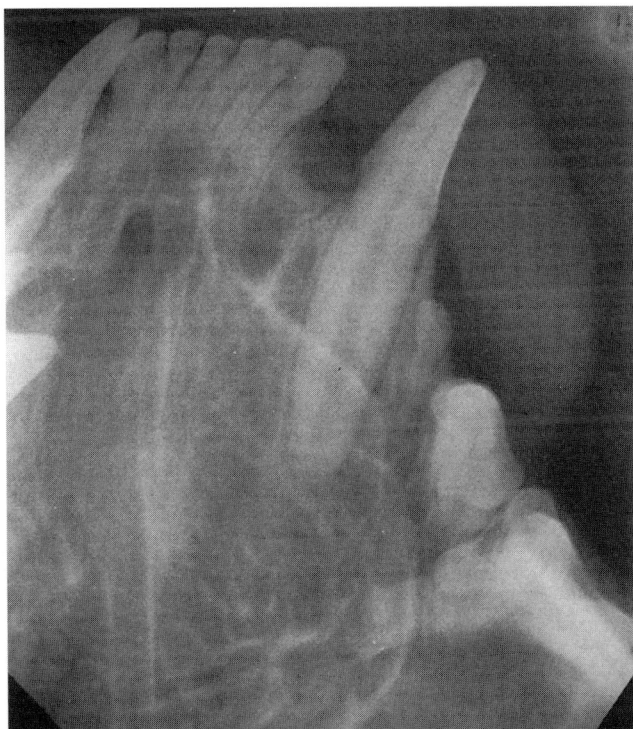

B

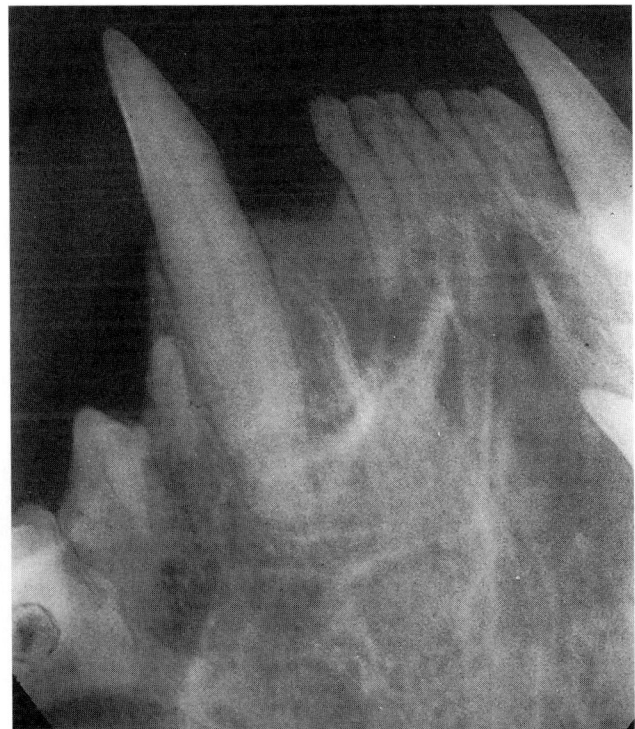

C

FIGURE 9.19

Contributing Author:
Mary Suzanne Aller

Description: Feline maxillary premolars and molar. Mesiodistal lateral oblique view, bisecting angle technique, intraoral.

Points Identified: Feline maturation/aging series.

A. Adolescent (6–8 months old)
B. Young adult (1–2 years old)
C. Mature adult (6–10 years old)

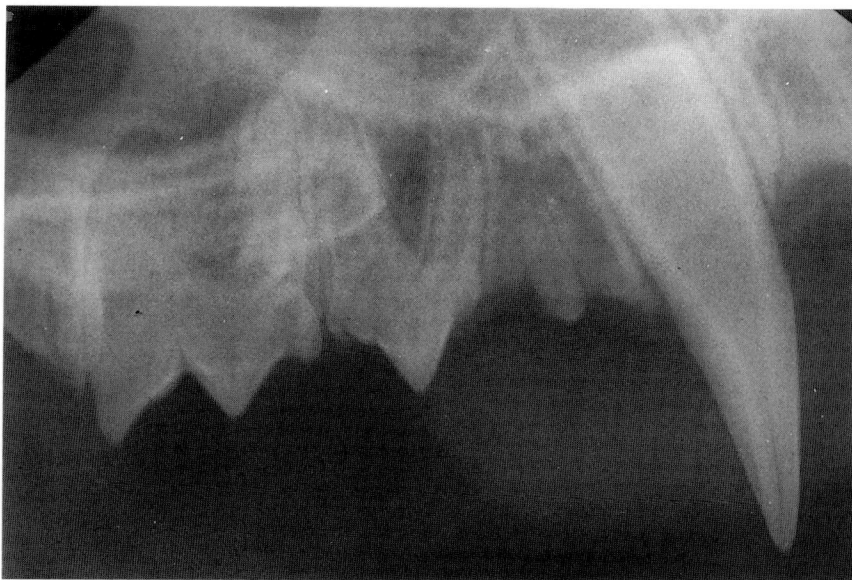

A

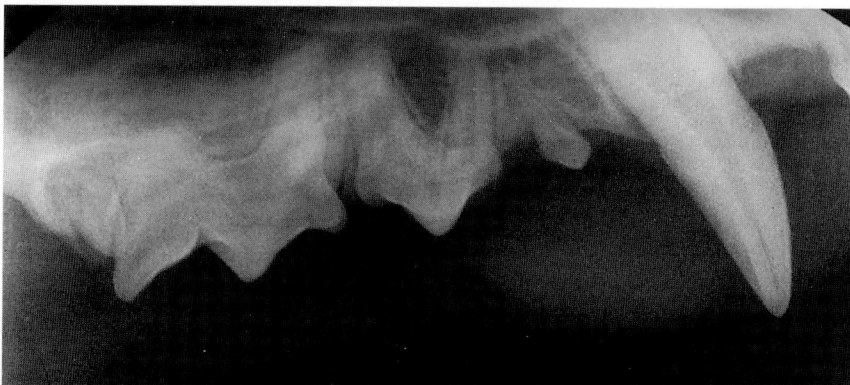

B

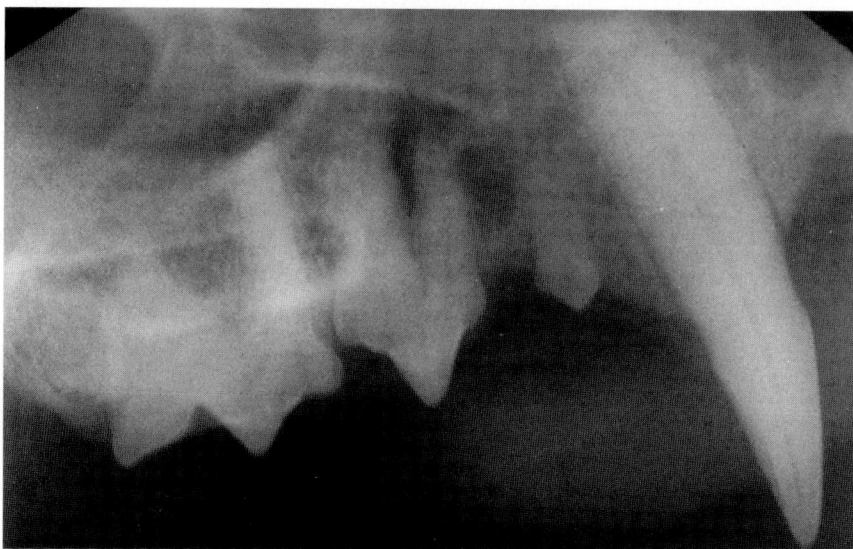

C

FIGURE 9.20

Contributing Author:

Mary Suzanne Aller

Description: Feline maxillary premolars and molar. Distomesial lateral oblique view, bisecting angle technique, intraoral.

Points Identified: Feline maturation/aging series.

A. Adolescent (6–8 months old)
B. Young adult (1–2 years old)
C. Mature adult (6–10 years old)

Common Errors: A. Note the infraorbital foramen over the distal root of the third premolar. C. Note the infraorbital foramen.

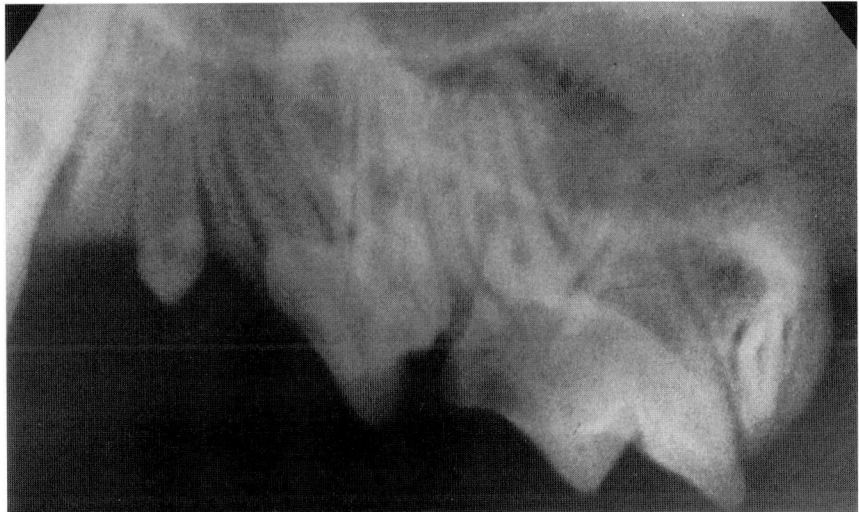

A

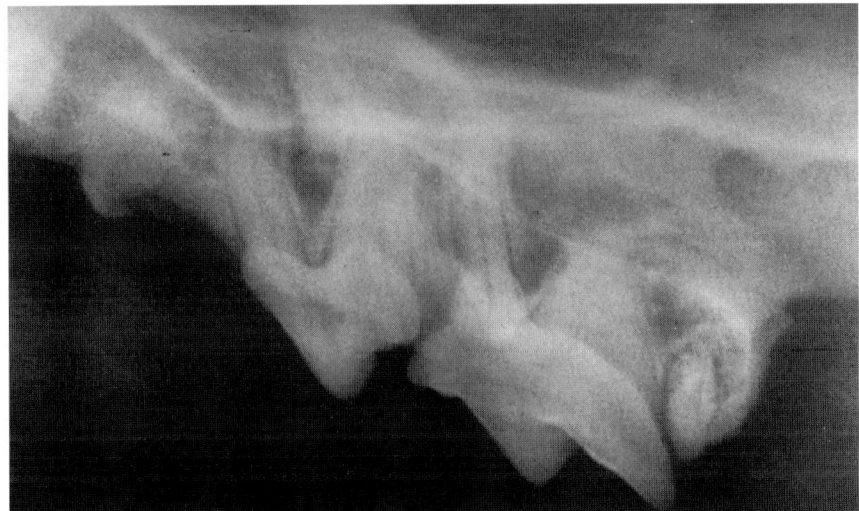

B

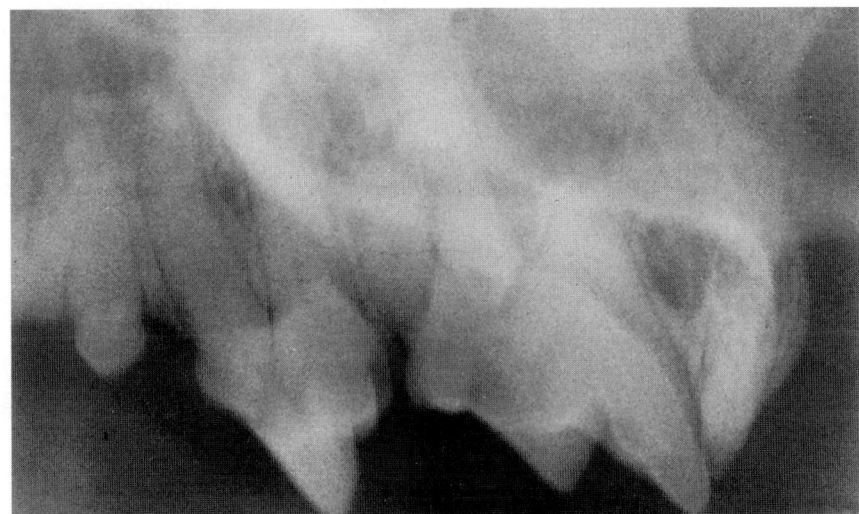

C

Views of Temporomandibular Joint

FIGURE 9.21

Contributing Author:
Mary Suzanne Aller

Description: Temporomandibular joint. Lateral view, parallel technique, extraoral.

Points Identified:

A. Angular process of the mandible
B. Mandibular condyles (TMJ)
C. Tympanic bullae
D. Hyoid apparatus
E. Endotracheal tube

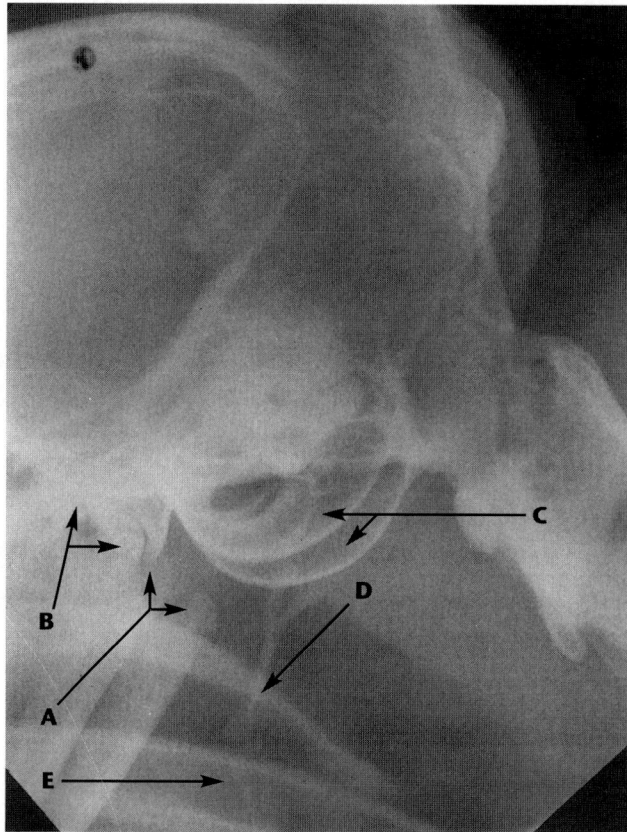

FIGURE 9.22

Contributing Author:
Mary Suzanne Aller

Description: Temporomandibular joint. Dorsoventral view, parallel technique, extraoral.

Points Identified:

A. Coronoid process of the mandible
B. Mandibular condyles
C. Angular process of the mandible
D. Zygomatic process of the temporal bone
E. Tympanic bullae

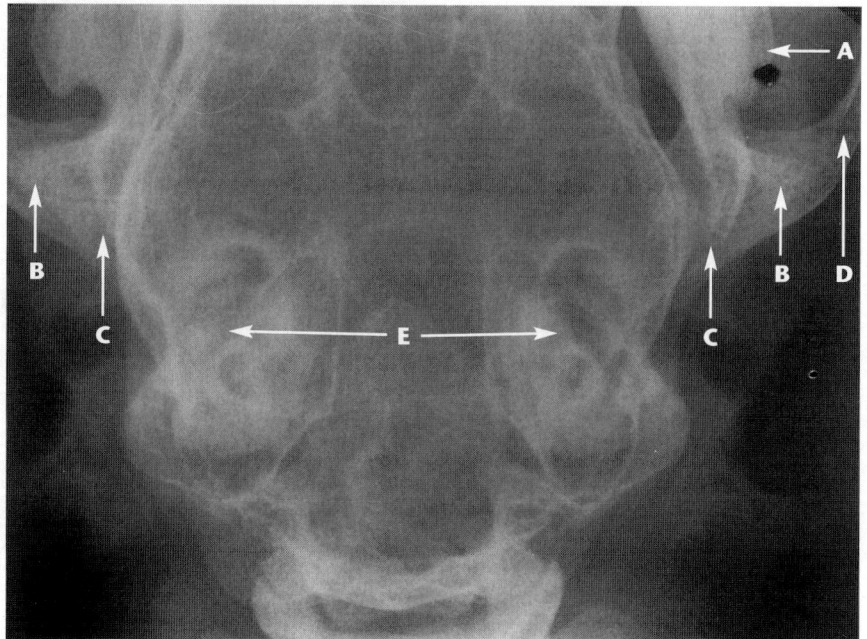

FIGURE 9.23

Contributing Author:
Mary Suzanne Aller

Description: Temporomandibular joint. Dorsoventral oblique view, parallel technique, extraoral.

Points Identified:

A. Tympanic bullae
B. Mandibular condyle
C. Coronoid process of the mandible
D. Hyoid apparatus

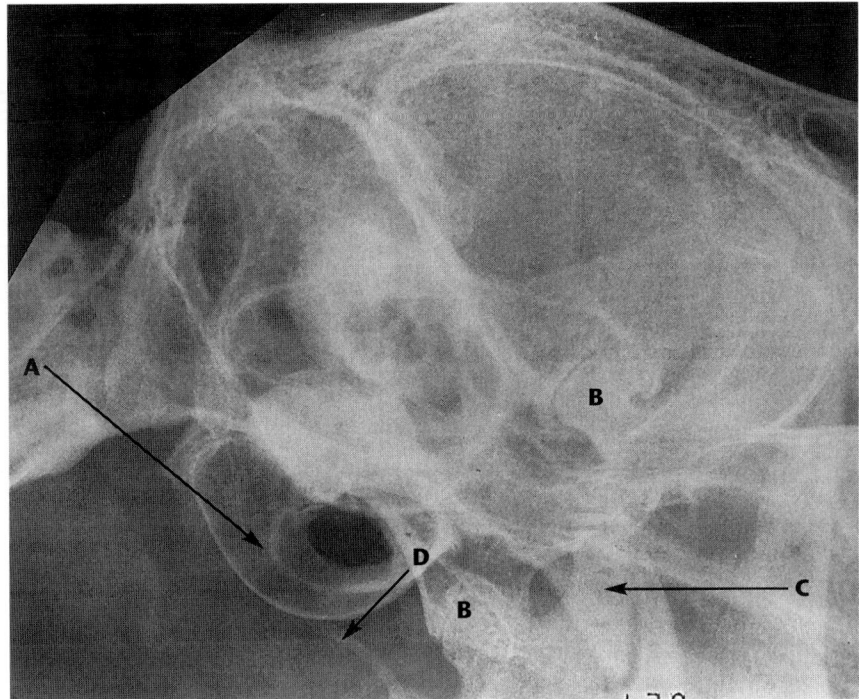

FIGURE 9.24

Contributing Author:
Mary Suzanne Aller

Description: Temporomandibular joint. Ventrodorsal oblique view, parallel technique, extraoral.

Points Identified:

A. Tympanic bullae
B. Hyoid apparatus
C. Mandibular condyles
D. Angular process of the mandible

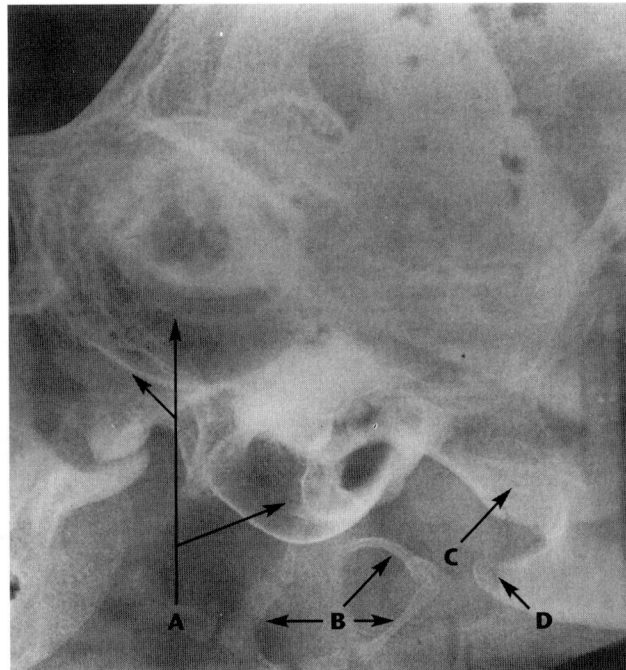

FIGURE 9.25

Contributing Author:
Mary Suzanne Aller

Description: Temporomandibular joint. Rostrocaudal open mouth view, parallel technique, extraoral.

Points Identified:

A. Tympanic bullae
B. Body of the mandible
C. Mandibular condyle
D. Zygomatic process of the temporal bone

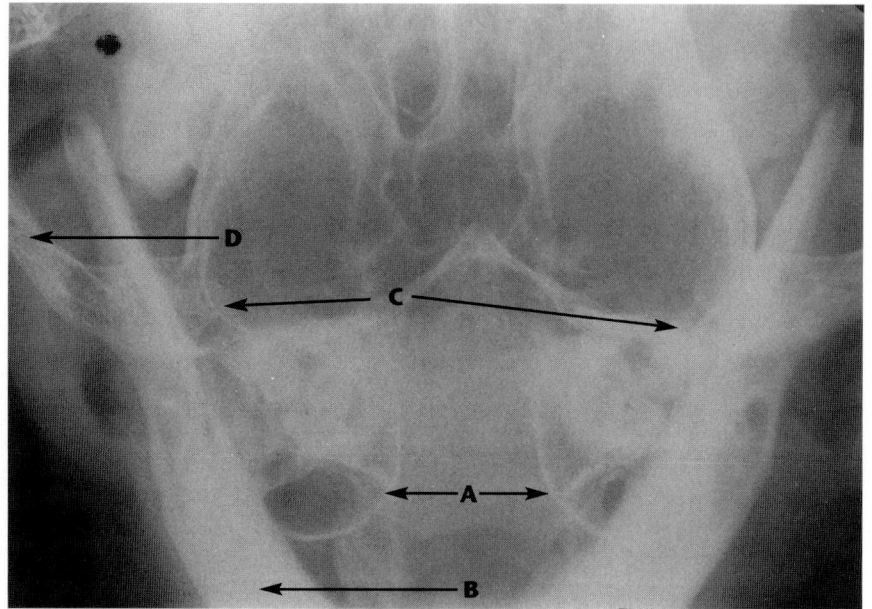

10 Feline Pedodontics

Dr. Heidi B. Lobprise
Dr. Ayako Okuda

INTRODUCTION

As veterinary dentistry continues to evolve, feline pedodontics will become critical in the better understanding of feline oral pathology. Odontoclastic resorptive lesions, stomatitis, and periodontal disease will be viewed through a continuum from postnatal dental development to maturity. Before the abnormal can be understood, it is important to understand the normal development of feline pedodontic oral and dental radiography and what physiological processes are occurring at each stage.

This chapter looks at intraoral radiographs from developing kittens. The time line starts at late fetal development and continues up to 1 year of age. The sequential images show the progression of tooth development of deciduous teeth as well as the permanent teeth as they mature and erupt.

Occasional instances of abnormal findings, such as aberrant dentition with missing teeth, or trauma to the oral cavity, may require radiographs for full evaluation. While not much can be done for missing teeth, the area can be examined for unerupted teeth. Fractures of immature permanent teeth at times can benefit from special procedures to deal with structures that are not fully mature, such as an open apex.

A tooth is a living functional organ. This chapter radiographically emphasizes that tooth development is a continual process. The primary dentition leads to mixed dentition and eventually progresses to permanent tooth structure. The normal deciduous and permanent dental formula, the number of roots normally found for each type of tooth, and the normal eruption times for the various deciduous and permanent teeth in the feline are shown below.

The deciduous and permanent dental formula of the feline:

Primary (deciduous)
    2 × (3/3 Incisor − 1/1 Canine − 3/2 Premolar)
Permanent
    2 × (3/3 Incisor − 1/1 Canine − 3/2 Premolar − 1/1 Molar)

Number of tooth roots in the feline:

Incisor− 1
Canine− 1
Maxillary teeth
    2nd premolar− 1
    3rd premolar− 2
    4th premolar− 3
    1st molar− 3 (clinically difficult to identify)
Mandibular teeth
    3rd premolar− 2
    4th premolar− 2
    1st molar− 2

Eruption times of primary deciduous and permanent teeth in the feline

Teeth	Primary (deciduous) (in weeks)	Permanent (in weeks)
Incisors	2–4	11–16
Canines	3–4	12–20
Premolars	3–6	16–24
Molars	−	20–24

FIGURE 10.1

Contributing Author: Heidi B. Lobprise

Description: Feline, 1½ months old. Rostral maxilla (view A) and rostral mandible (view B). Presence of erupted deciduous teeth. Early indication of presence of permanent tooth buds (radiolucency) ventral and lingual to some deciduous teeth (central incisors, canines, mandibular premolars) especially in the mandible are difficult to identify. Mandibular first molar tooth buds are visible.

Points Identified:

A. Mandibular first molar tooth buds (view B)

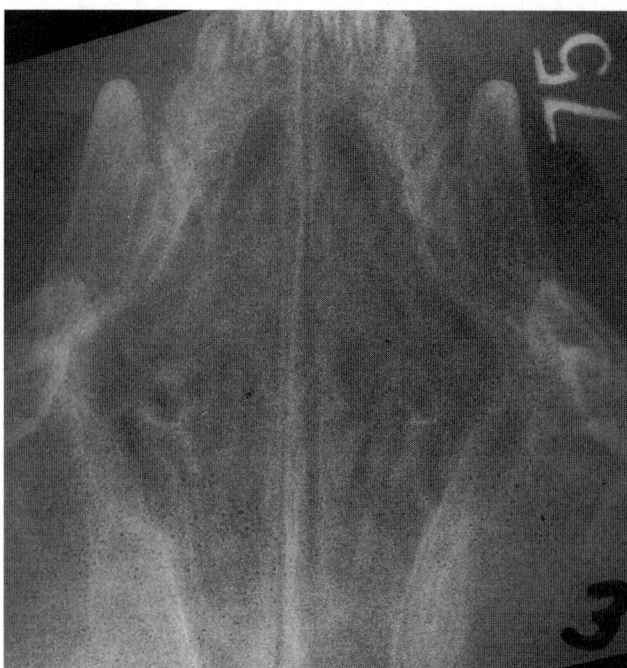

A

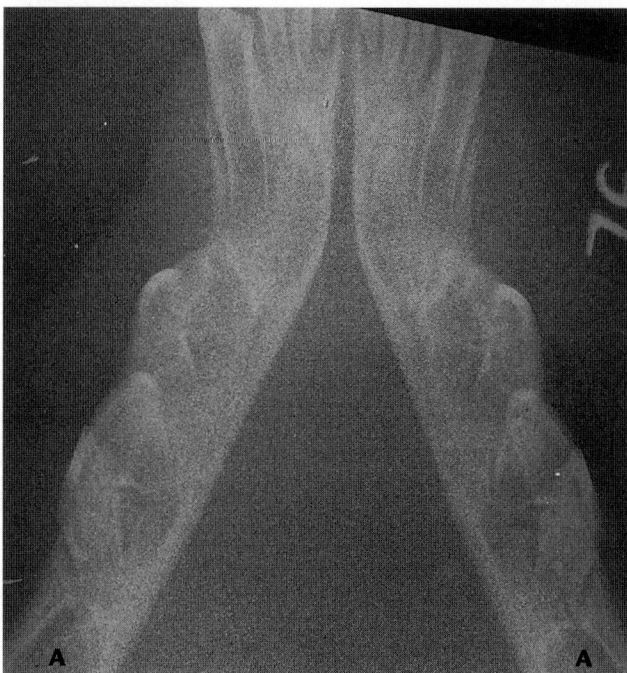

B

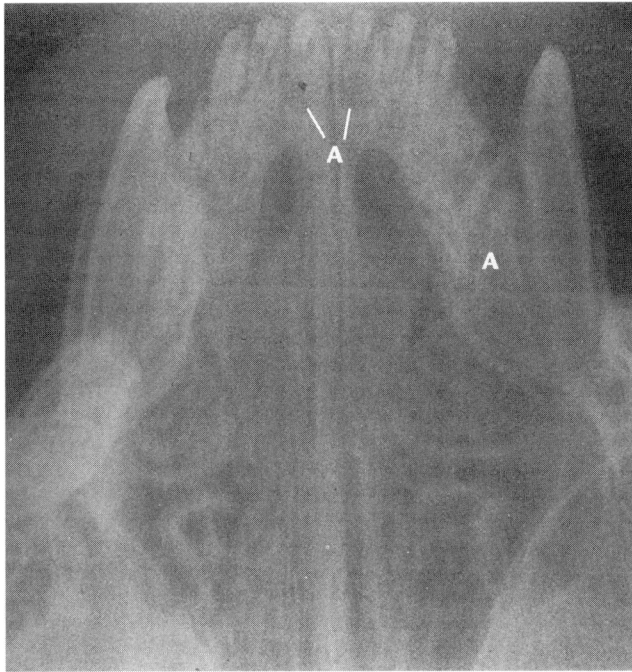

A

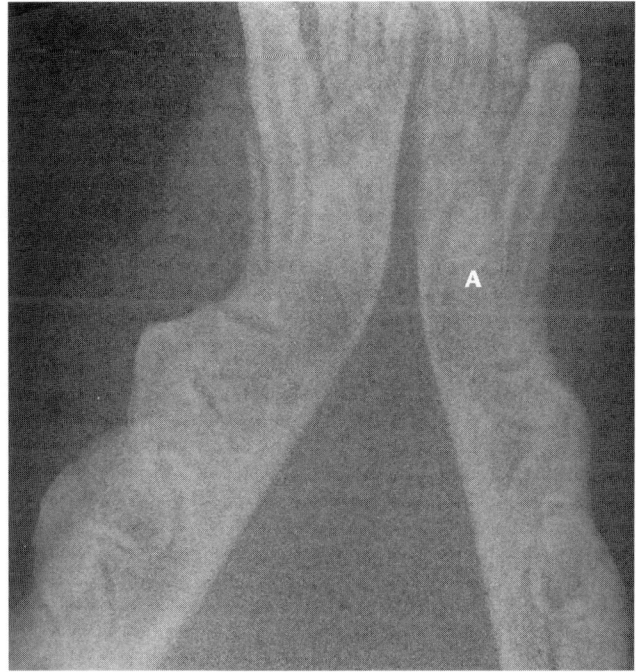

B

FIGURE 10.2

Contributing Author: Heidi B. Lobprise

Description: Feline, 2 months old. Rostral maxilla (view A), rostral mandible (view B), and mandibular arcade (view C).

Points Identified:

A. Permanent tooth bud

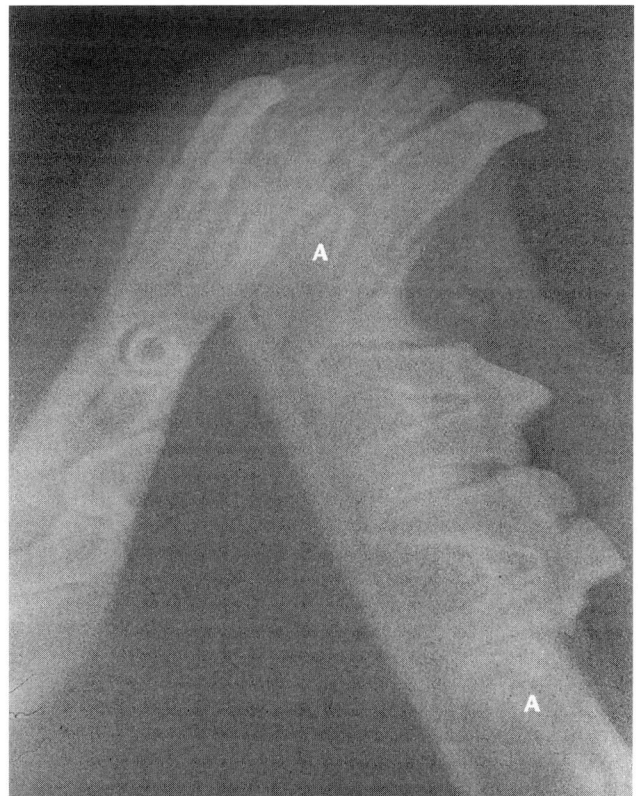

C

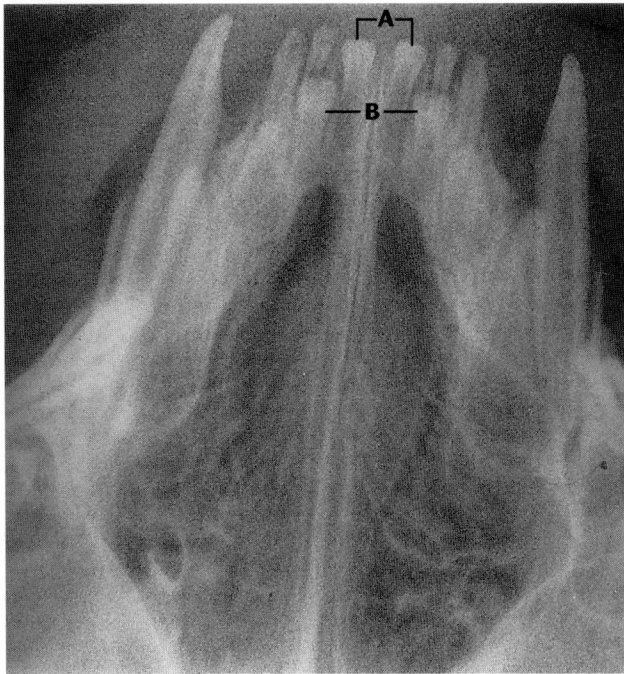

A

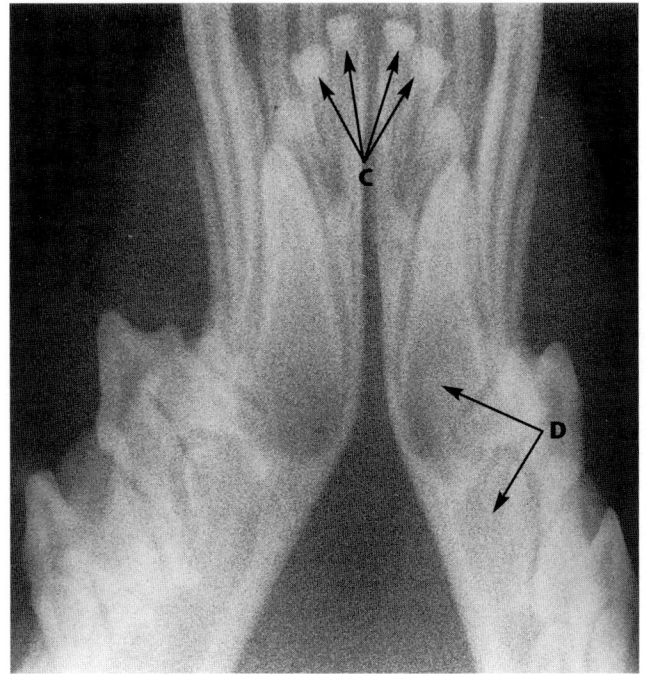

B

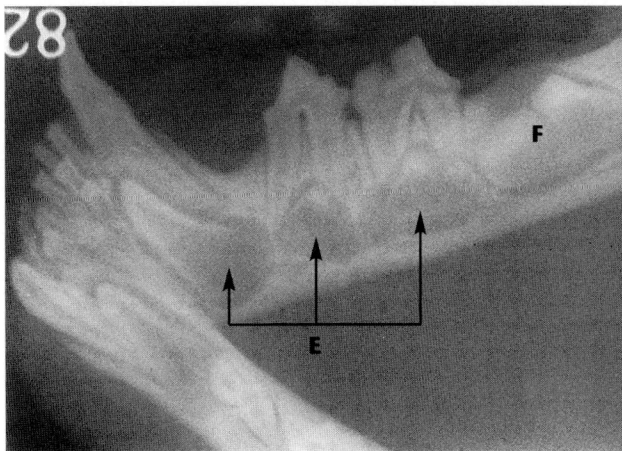

C

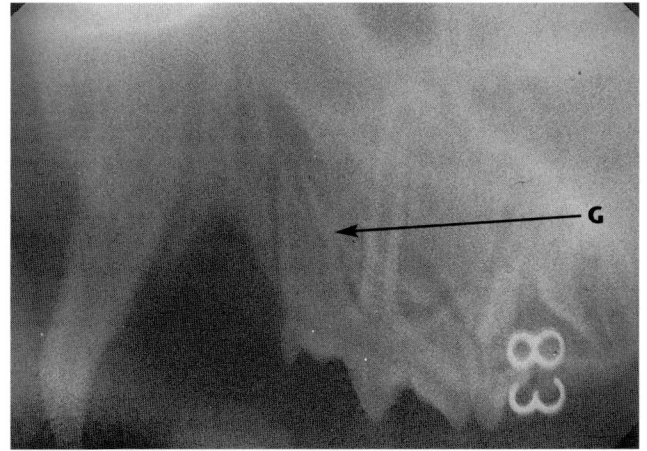

D

FIGURE 10.3

Contributing Author: Heidi B. Lobprise

Description: Feline, 3 months old. Rostral maxilla (A), rostral mandible (B), mandibular arcade (C), and maxillary arcade (D).

Points Identified: Note significant permanent tooth bud formation.

A. Permanent central incisors erupted
B. Intermediate incisors beginning to erupt
C. Permanent central and intermediate incisors beginning to erupt
D. Tooth bud formation progressing
E. Maturation of permanent tooth buds

F. First molar approaching eruption time
G. Premolar tooth buds visible

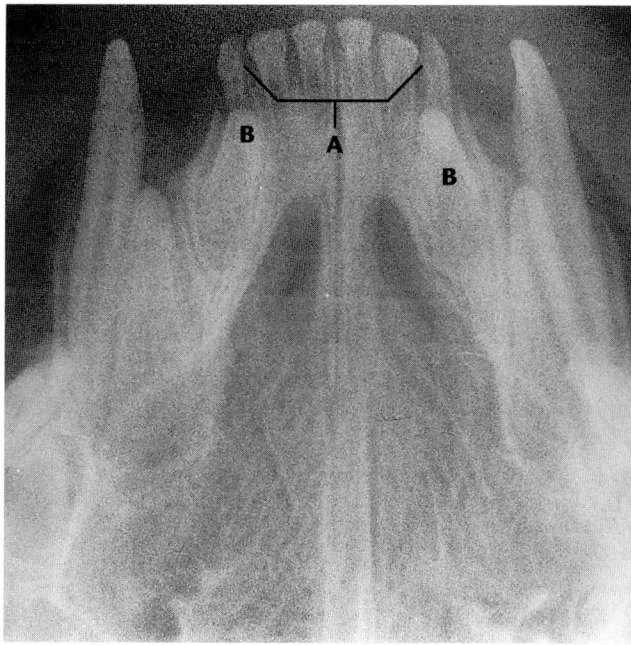

A

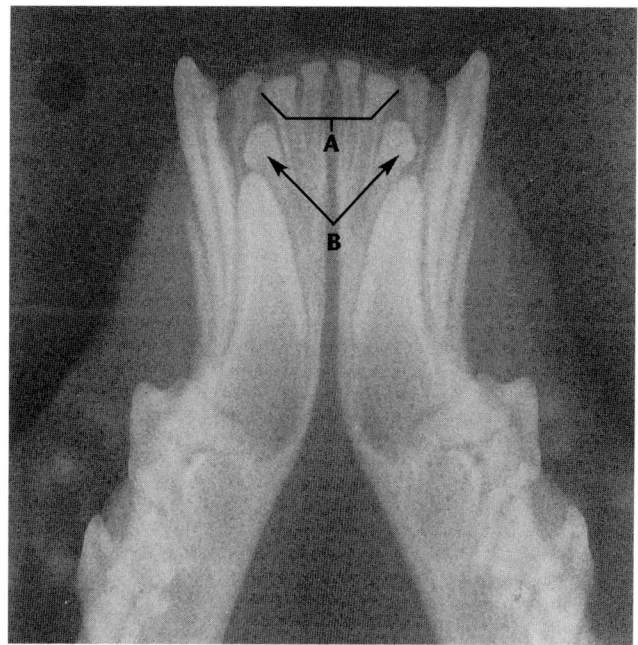

B

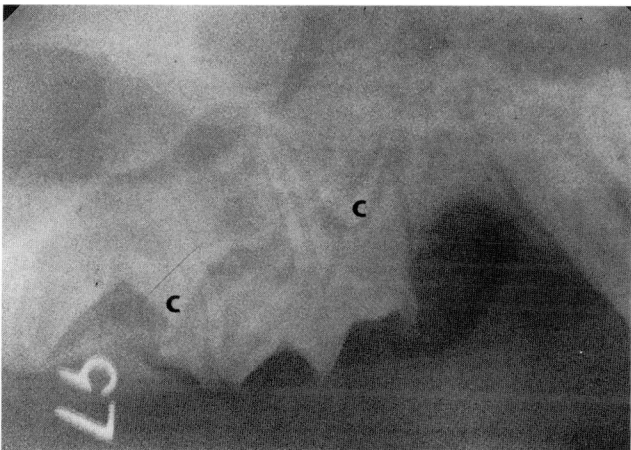

C

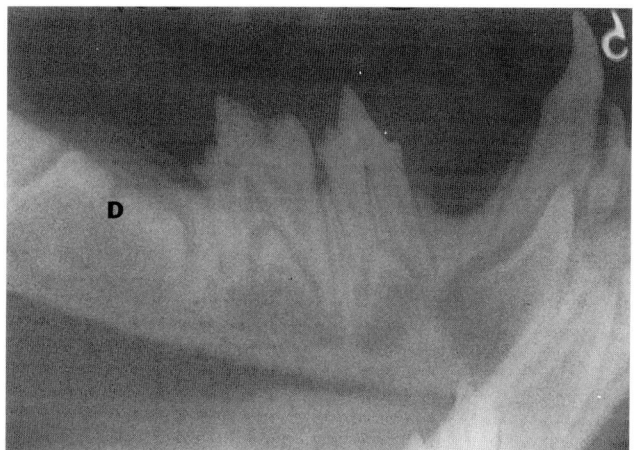

D

FIGURE 10.4

Contributing Author: Heidi B. Lobprise

Description: Feline, 3½ months old. Rostral maxilla (view A), rostral mandible (view B), maxillary arcade (view C), and mandibular arcade (view D).

Points Identified:

A. Permanent central and intermediate incisors erupted
B. Corner incisors not yet erupted
C. Permanent premolars developing
D. Permanent molar beginning to erupt

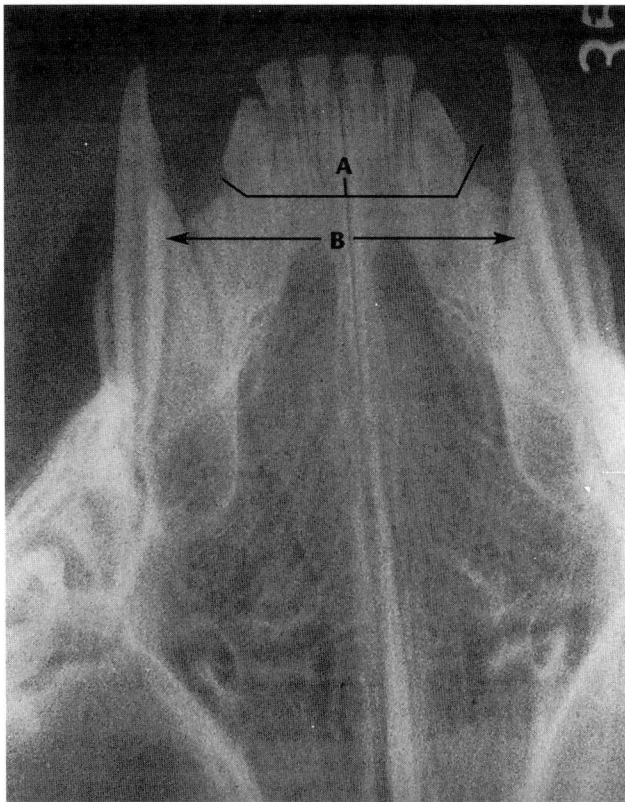

A

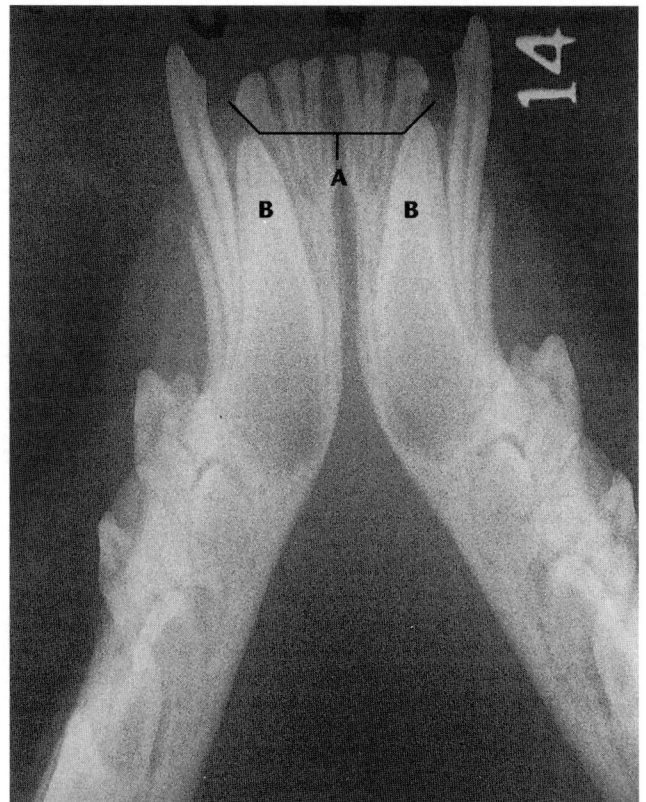

B

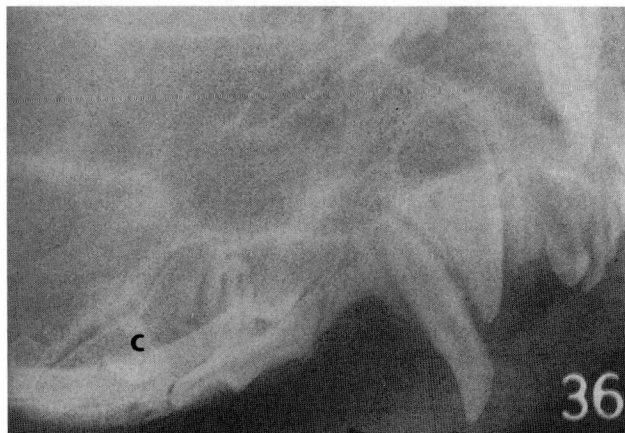

C

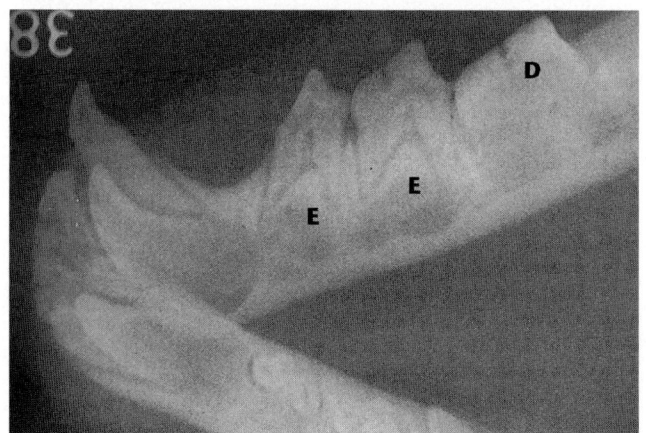

D

FIGURE 10.5

Contributing Author: Heidi B. Lobprise

Description: Feline, 4 months old. Rostral maxilla (view A), rostral mandible (view B), maxillary arcade (view C), and mandibular arcade (view D).

Points Identified:

A. All incisors erupted
B. Permanent canine tooth buds nearing eruption
C. Maxillary fourth premolar nearing eruption
D. Molar erupting
E. Premolar bud development

FIGURE 10.6

Contributing Author: Heidi B. Lobprise

Description: Feline maxilla, 5 months old.

Points Identified: Eruption of canines with retained maxillary deciduous canines (504, 604). All premolar roots immature and open. Note permanent 106/206 and 109/209 with no deciduous counterparts.

A. 104
B. 106
C. 107
D. 108
E. 109
F. 507
G. 504

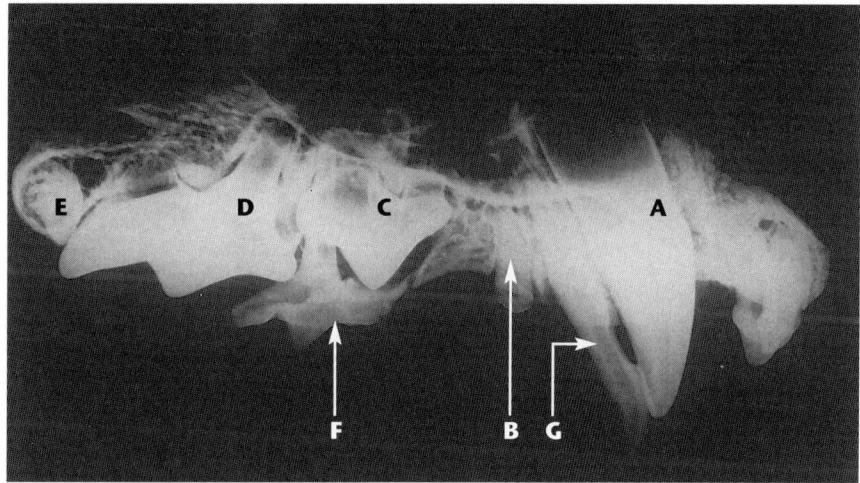

FIGURE 10.7

Contributing Author: Heidi B. Lobprise

Description: Feline, 5 months old.

Points Identified: Mandibular permanent 304, 307, 308, 309. Note large open apices. Also note deciduous 707 and 708 above their permanent counterparts.

A. 304
B. 307
C. 308
D. 309
E. 708
F. 707

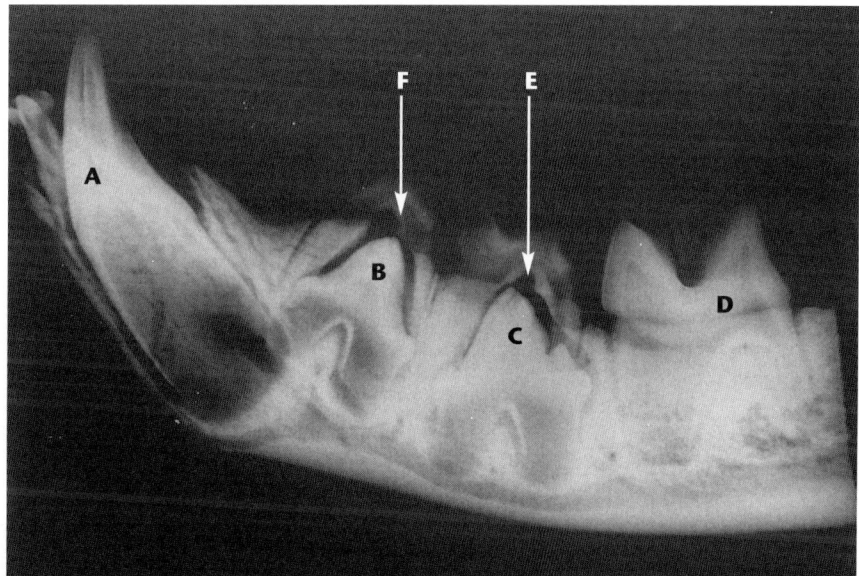

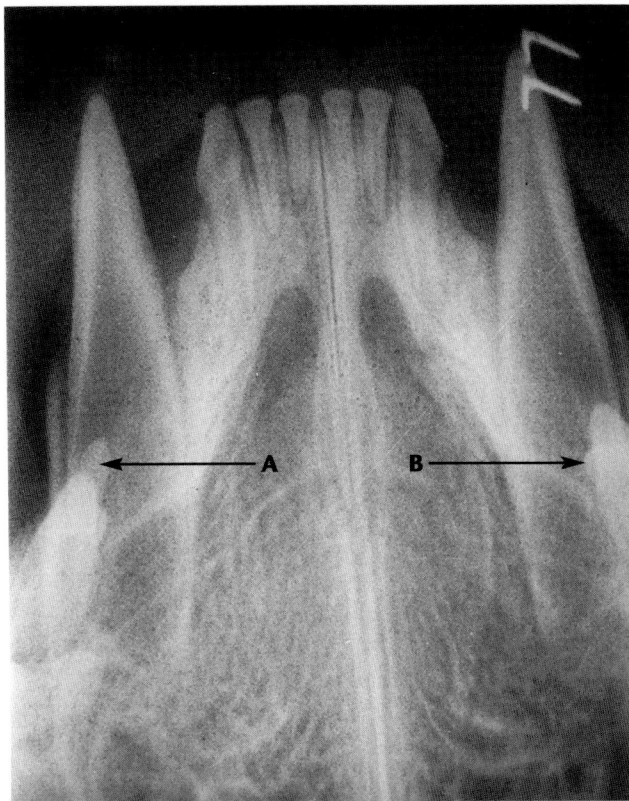

A

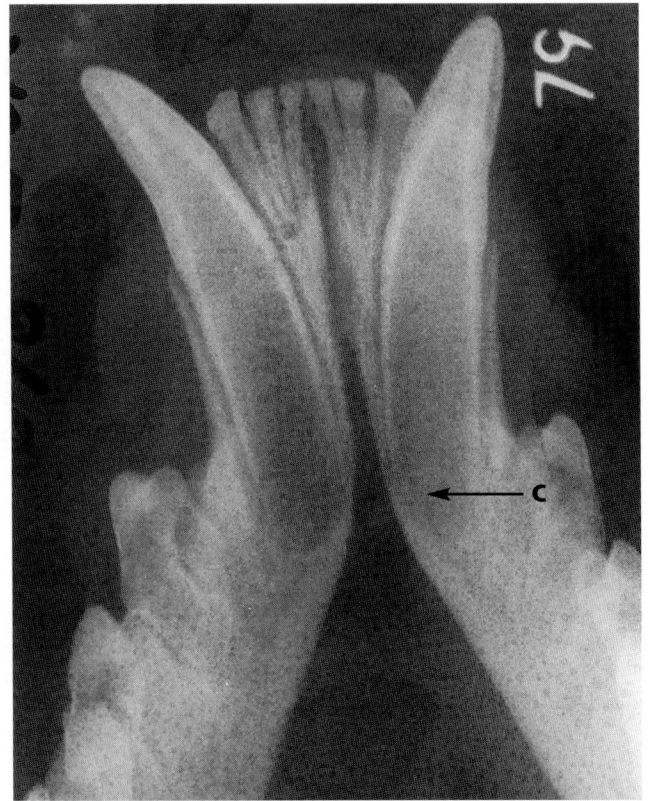

B

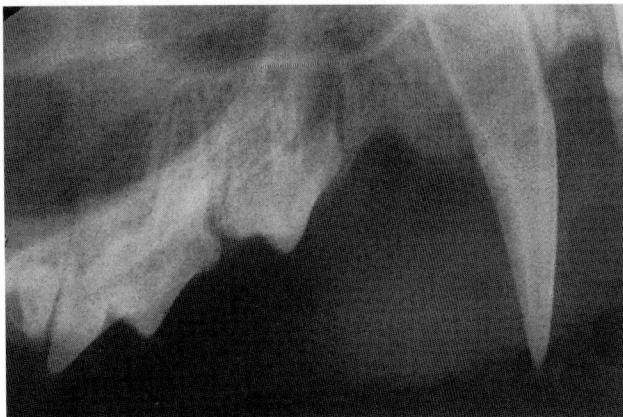

C

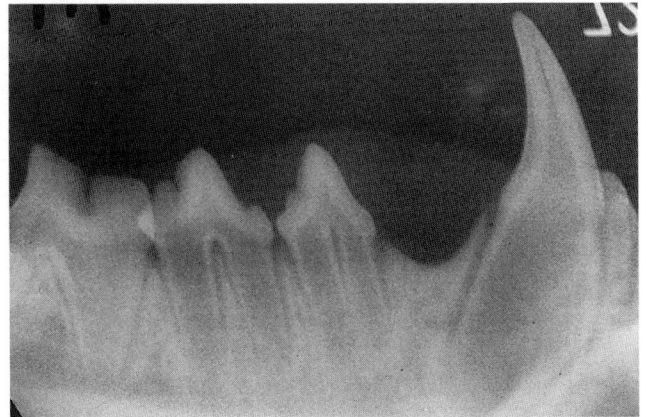

D

FIGURE 10.8

Contributing Author: Heidi B. Lobprise

Description: Feline, 6 months old (at 9-19-94). Rostral maxilla (view A), rostral mandible (view B), maxillary arcade (view C), and mandibular arcade (view D).

Points Identified: All permanents erupting at various stages of root maturation. This is the only kitten of five with one of the maxillary third premolars (206) detectable.

A. 106
B. 206
C. Blunderbuss apex

FIGURE 10.9

Contributing Author: Heidi B. Lobprise

Description: Sequential films, feline mandible. From 5–6 months to approximately 1 year.

Points Identified: Progression of tooth maturation showing eruption, root closure, and dentinal wall thickening.

A. 5 months
B. 9 months
C. 12 months

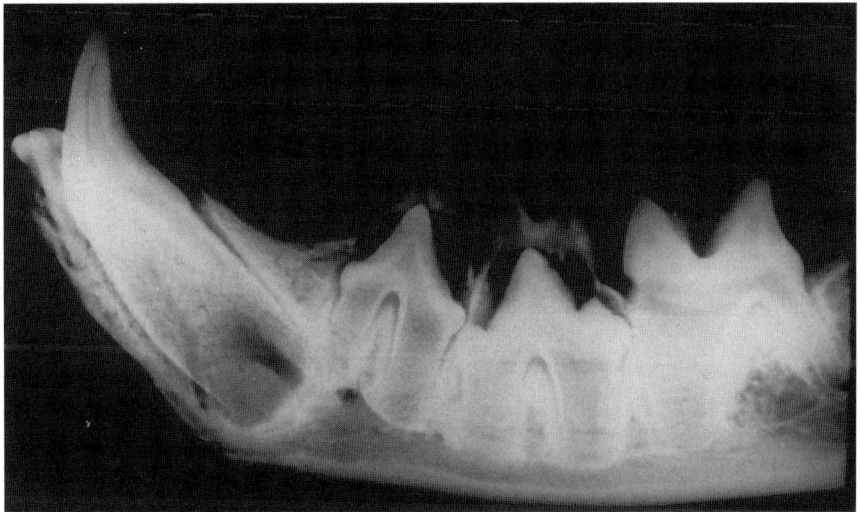
A

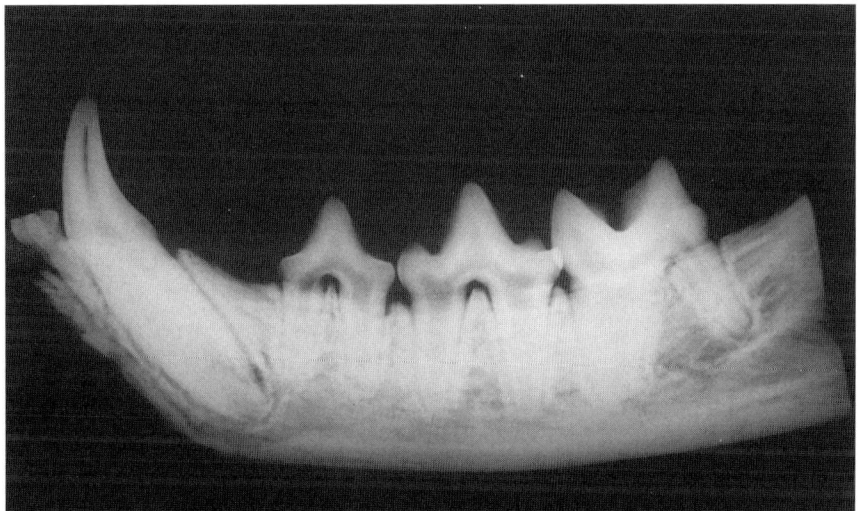
B

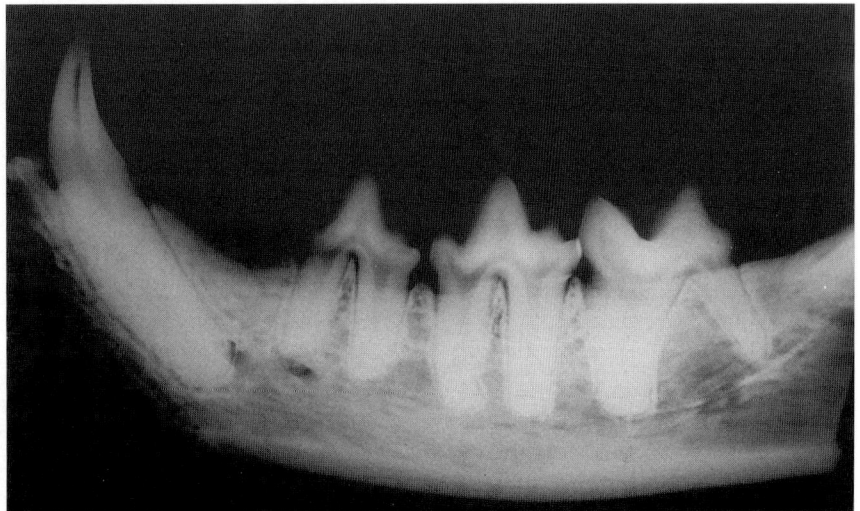
C

FIGURE 10.10

Contributing Author: Heidi B. Lobprise

Description: Sequential films, feline maxilla. From 5–6 months to approximately 1 year.

Points Identified: Progression of tooth maturation showing eruption, root closure, and dentinal wall thickening.

A. 5 months
B. 9 months
C. 12 months

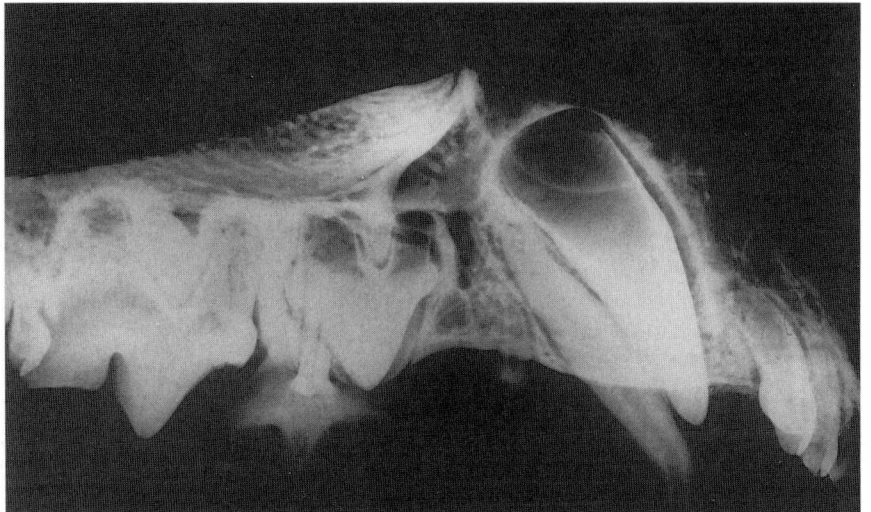

A

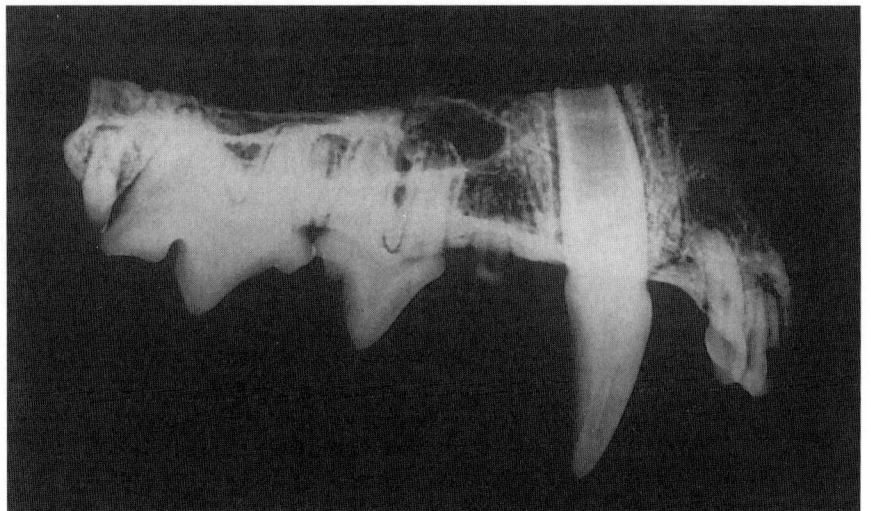

B

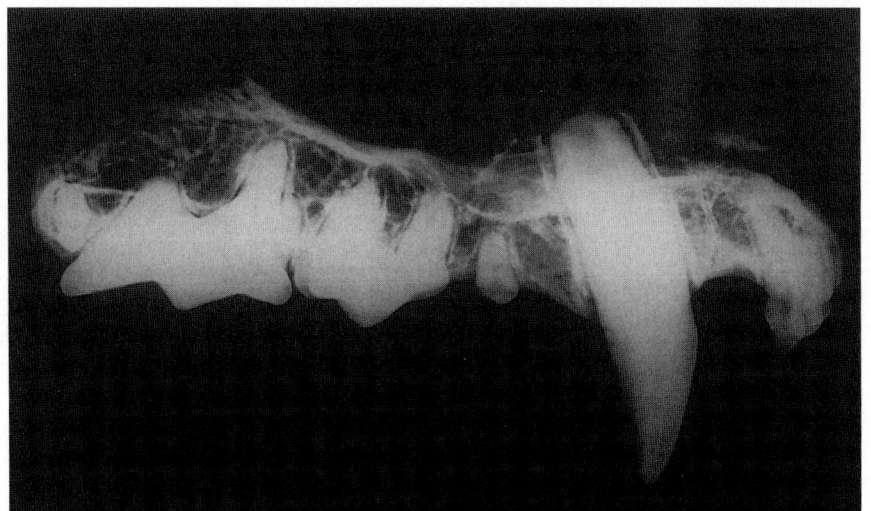

C

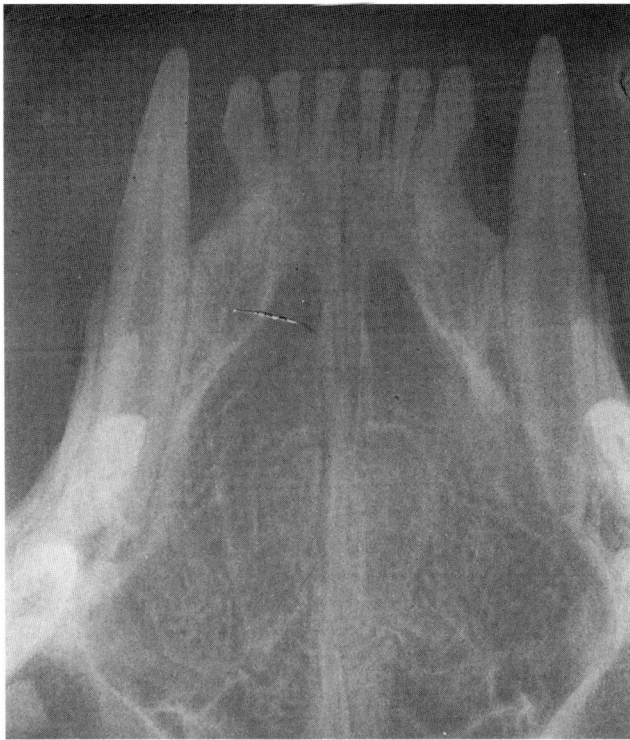

A

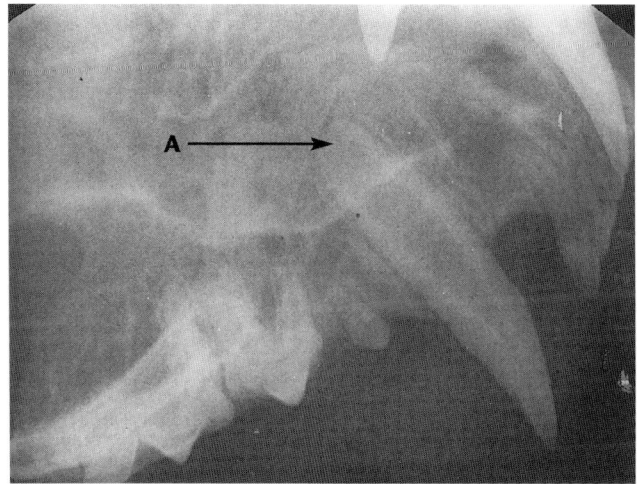

B

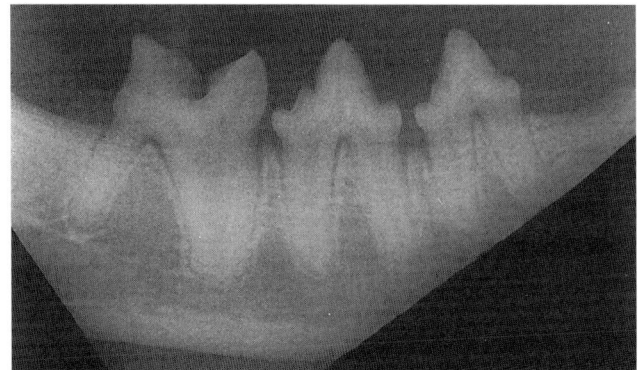

D

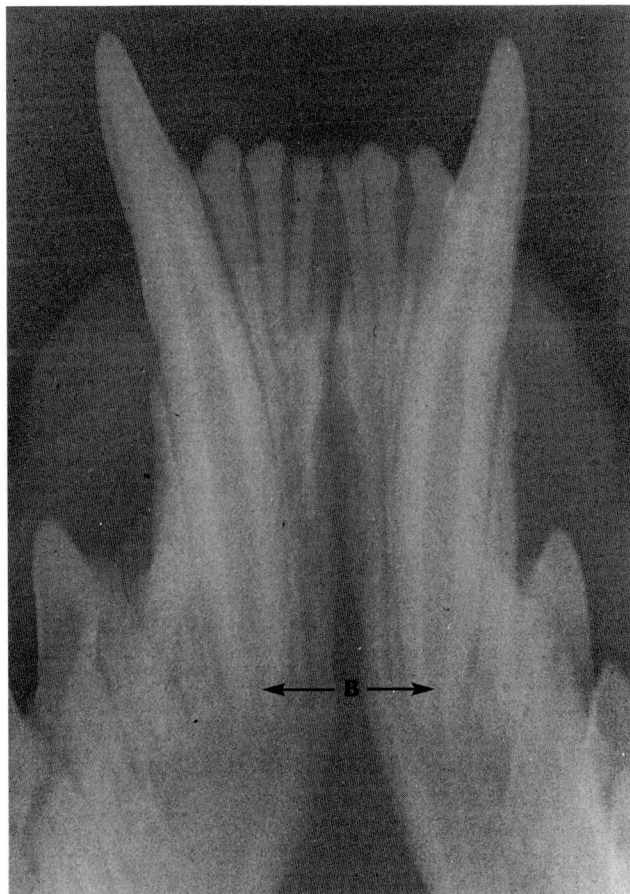

C

FIGURE 10.11

Contributing Author: Heidi B. Lobprise

Description: Feline, 11 months old. Teeth demonstrate wide canals with root maturation of incisors, premolars and molars. Apices of canines still open to some degree (closure not complete). Rostral maxilla (view A), maxillary arcade (view B), rostral mandible (view C), and mandibular arcade (view D).

Points Identified: Note maturing incisors and wide canine canals in view A, incomplete canine root closure in view B, nearly complete canine root closure in view C, and complete root closure in premolars and molar in view D.

    A. Incomplete root closure (canine)
    B. Nearly complete root closure (canines)

Common Errors: Note artifact, left side of view A (scratched film).

FIGURE 10.12

Contributing Author: Heidi B. Lobprise

Description: Anterior maxilla, 1-year-old feline.

Points Identified: Normal permanent incisors present. No evidence of permanent canines; no evidence of alveolar development to indicate canines were once present then subsequently lost.

    A. Permanent incisors
    B. Permanent canines missing

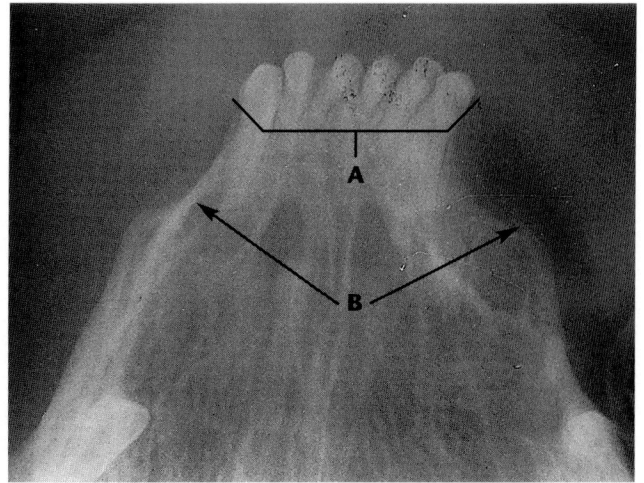

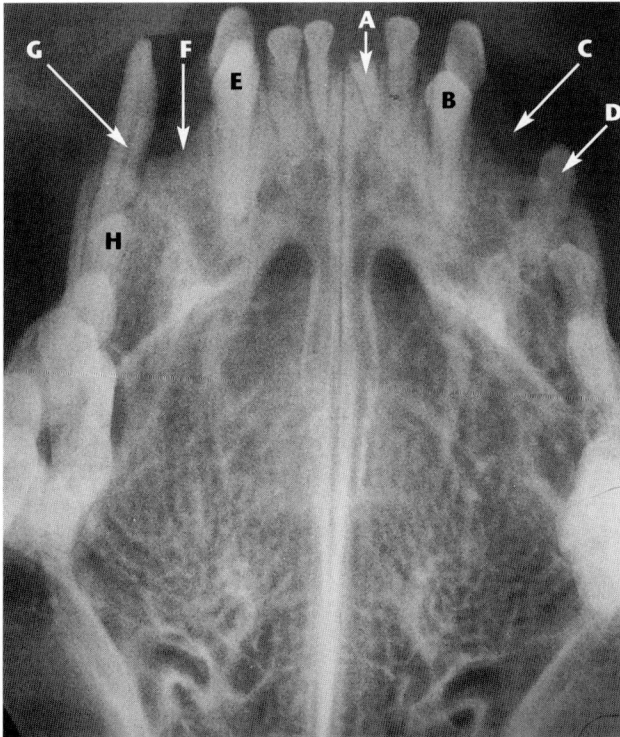

A

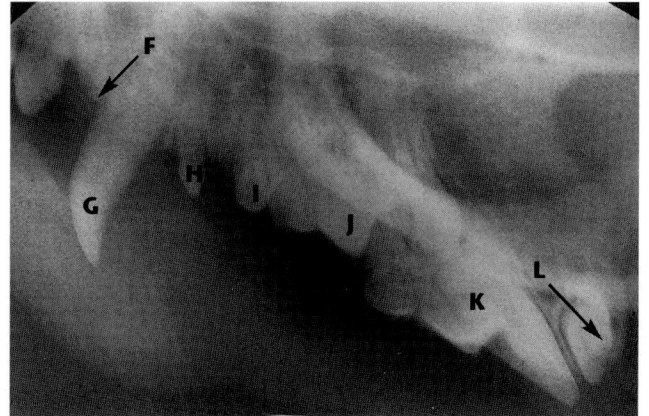

B

FIGURE 10.13

Contributing Author: Heidi B. Lobprise

Description: Abnormal dentition, 1-year-old feline. Anterior maxilla (view A) and maxillary arcade (view B).

Points Identified: Note supernumerary teeth S103, S106, S203, and S206; retained 604; and missing 104 and 204.

    A. 101, fractured crown, retained root
    B. S103
    C. 104 (missing)
    D. S106
    E. S203
    F. 204 (missing)
    G. 604 (retained)
    H. S206
    I. 206
    J. 207
    K. 208
    L. 209

FIGURE 10.14

Contributing Author: Heidi B. Lobprise

Description: Anterior maxilla, 10-month-old feline. Root canal of fractured 104 filled with calcium hydroxide to stimulate apexification (hard tissue closure) of open apex (immature).

Points Identified:

A. 104, fractured crown (Class VI fracture)
B. Filled root
C. Artifact

Common Errors: Artifact (scratched film).

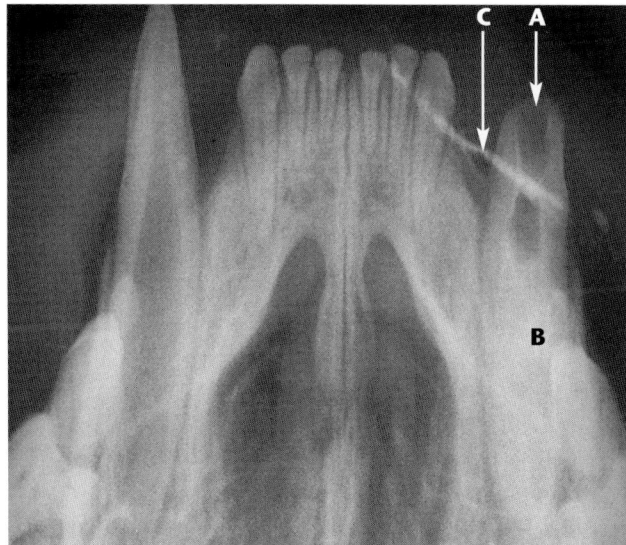

11 Feline Endodontics

Dr. James M.G. Anthony   *Dr. Ayako Okuda*
Dr. Sandra Manfra Marretta

INTRODUCTION

Endodontics involves those dental procedures which are necessary to treat and preserve the dental pulp and periapical tissues and the resultant functional normalcy of the tooth.

In the feline, as in other species, the pathology of endodontal disease left untreated can lead to pain and eventual loss of the affected teeth. With dental radiology and proper identification of pathology, proper treatment can remove the pain and give excellent long-term results. Below is a list of feline endodontal findings in this chapter.

1. Acute apical periodontitis
2. Periapical granuloma/cyst
3. Radicular cyst
4. Pulp stone
5. External root resorption
6. Apical root resorption
7. Internal resorption
8. Deciduous teeth
9. Endodontic system of a young feline (open apex)
10. Endodontic system of a mature tooth (older feline)
11. Mental foramen
12. Endodontic treatment
    A. Apical puff
    B. Premolar conventional endodontics
    C. Molar conventional endodontics
    D. Apexification
    E. Obturation voids
13. Endo-perio lesion

FIGURE 11.1

Contributing Author:
James M.G. Anthony

Description: Apical periodontitis. An apical radiolucency with poorly defined irregular margins is characteristic of an apical abscess. The lamina dura is lost between the root apex and the apical lesion. With time the lesion enlarges.

Points Identified: Note radiolucent area around the root apex. Also note overfill of obturation material with gutta percha extending beyond the apex.

    A. Radiolucent area at root apex
    B. Overfill of obturation material

Diagnostic Keys: Irregular margin of periapical radiolucency.

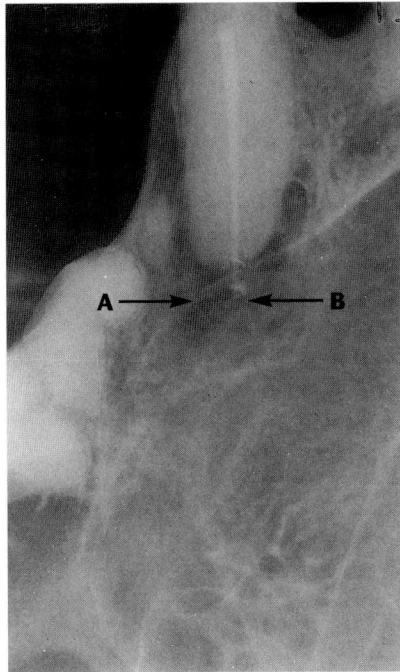

FIGURE 11.2

Contributing Author:
James M.G. Anthony

Description: Periapical granuloma/cyst. A thickened periodontal ligament space at the periapical area is the earliest radiological sign noted in the periapical granuloma/cyst. Hyperostosis is present (exostosis) in many cases such as this.

Points Identified: The periapical granuloma/cyst, the radicular cyst, and acute apical periodontitis cannot always be radiologically differentiated. Definitive differentiation is only possible with histologic examination.

    A. Periapical granuloma/cyst

Diagnostic Keys: Examine for oval cyst-like periodontal ligament space with ill defined margins.

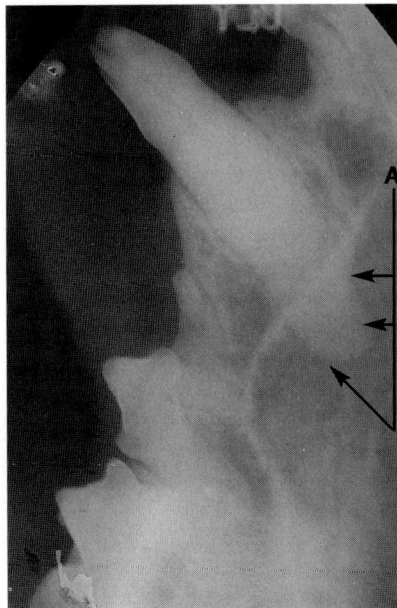

A

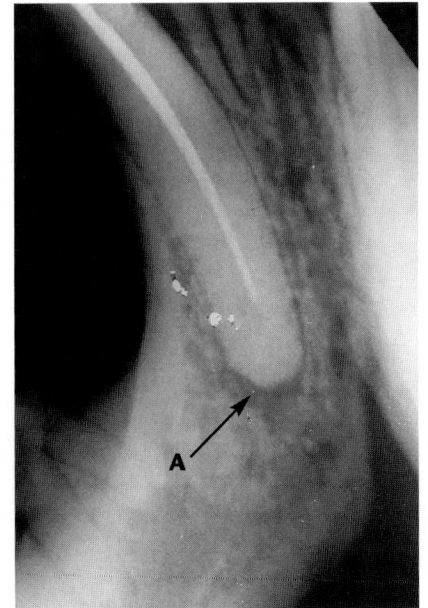

B

FIGURE 11.3

Contributing Author:
James M.G. Anthony

Description: Radicular cyst (apical periodontal cyst, periapical cyst, dental cyst).

Points Identified: Note the apical resorption with exostosis. The periapical radiolucent area is well defined.

    A. Apical resorption with osteolytic changes

Diagnostic Keys: Note the well-defined radiolucent area of the periapical area.

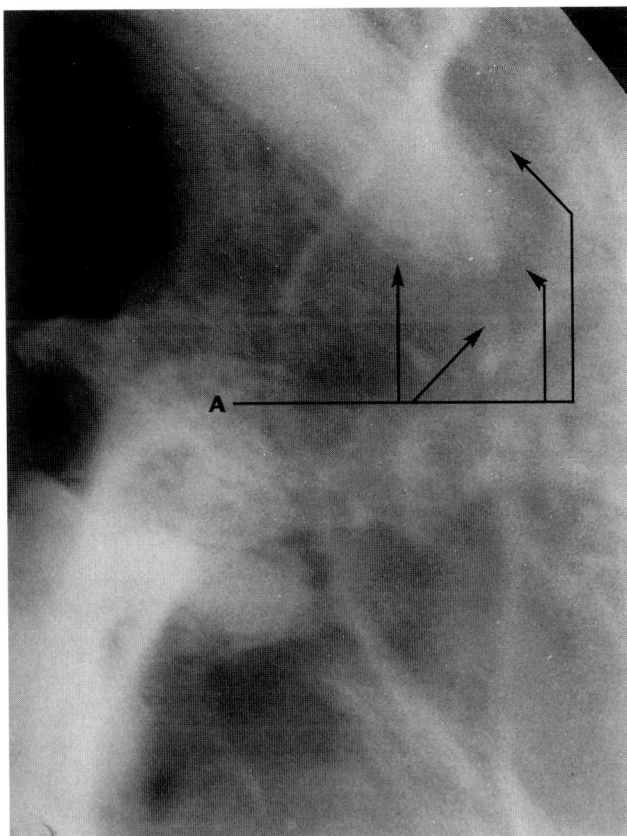

FIGURE 11.4

Contributing Author: Ayako Okuda

Description: Endodontic pulp calcifications.

Points Identified: Note the pulp calcifications in mid-pulp. Apical root resorption is also present.

    A. Pulp calcifications
    B. Root resorption

Diagnostic Keys: Pulp stones are usually round masses within the endodontic system. These masses can be nonattached (free denticle) or attached to the dentinal wall (adherent denticle) and are difficult to visualize.

Common Errors: Foreign bodies and internal root resorption.

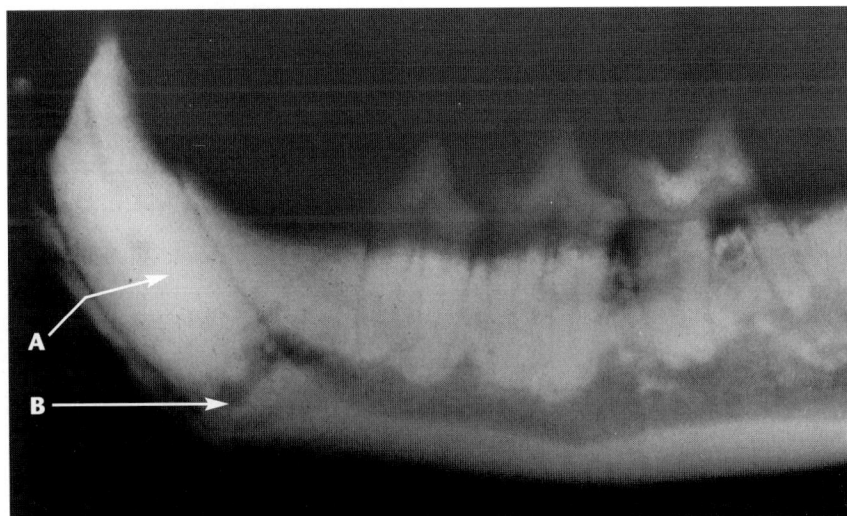

FIGURE 11.5

Contributing Author:
James M.G. Anthony

Description: Root resorption with periapical destruction.

Points Identified: Note the slightly ragged and blunted root apex with significant loss of tooth root. Normal root contours are missing.

    A. Blunted root apices with significant root loss

Diagnostic Keys: The crest of the alveolar bone next to the radiolucent area is resorbed and the periodontal ligament space is widened. The area that is resorbed has an ill-defined border.

Common Errors: Deciduous tooth resorption should never be confused with external odontoclastic root resorption. Always radiograph the contralateral tooth if this is a question.

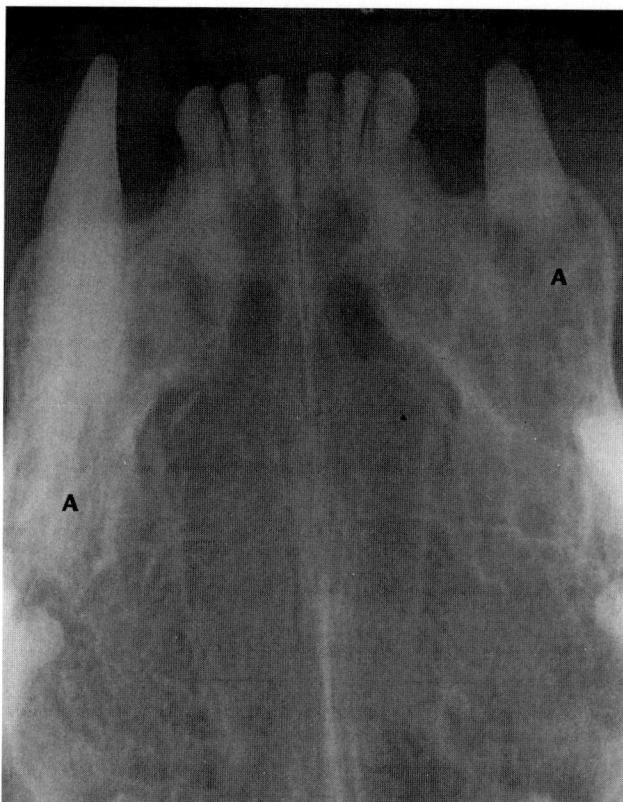

FIGURE 11.6

Contributing Author:
James M.G. Anthony

Description: Internal resorption.

Points Identified: Note the oval central radiolucent area in the endodontic system of the apical third of the root.

    A. Radiolucent area within pulp of canine

Diagnostic Keys: A round or oval radiolucent area in the central portion of the tooth is visualized within the pulp, but does not include the external surface of the tooth. With time, internal resorption can lead to perforation of the tooth's external surface.

Common Errors: Confusion of internal resorption with normal anatomical structures such as foramina overlap.

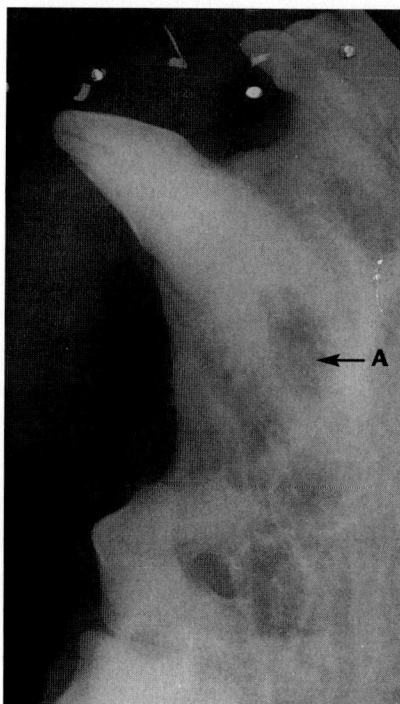

FIGURE 11.7

Contributing Author:

James M.G. Anthony

Description: Deciduous tooth endodontic system.

Points Identified: Note the thin enamel layer, thin dentinal wall, and long narrow roots in deciduous teeth 504, 507, and 508. Also note developing adult dentition tooth buds 104, 107, 108.

A. 104	E. 504
B. 106	F. 507
C. 107	G. 508
D. 108	H. Pulp canal

Diagnostic Keys: Deciduous teeth have thin enamel and dentin layers with long narrow roots and a crown-to-root ratio greater than in adult dentition.

Common Errors: Adult dentition.

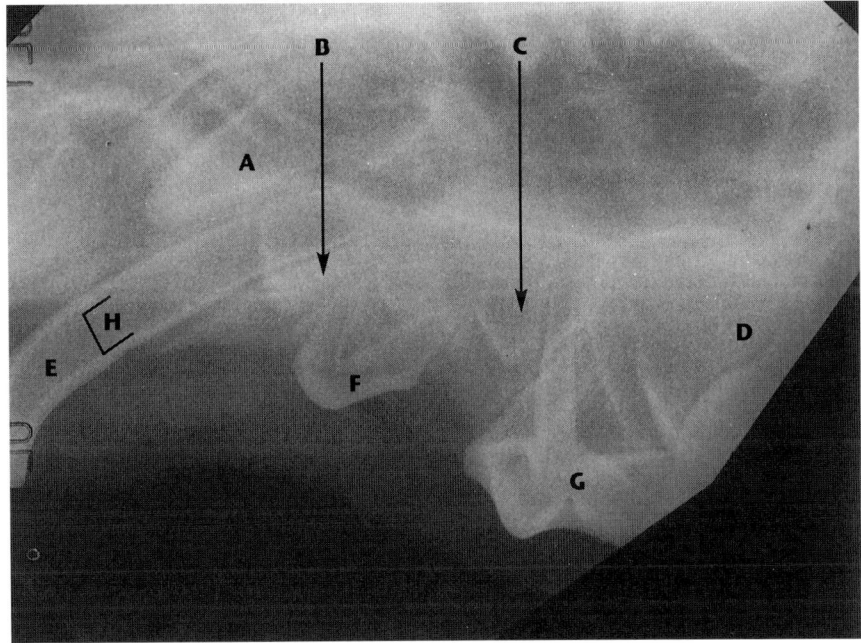

FIGURE 11.8

Contributing Author:

James M.G. Anthony

Description: Open apex.

Points Identified: Note that the apex is not completely closed. In immature dentition a larger endodontic system is visible in comparison to other dentition.

A. Open apex, canine tooth

Diagnostic Keys: The apex is not completely closed, allowing the endodontic system to communicate directly with the periapical area.

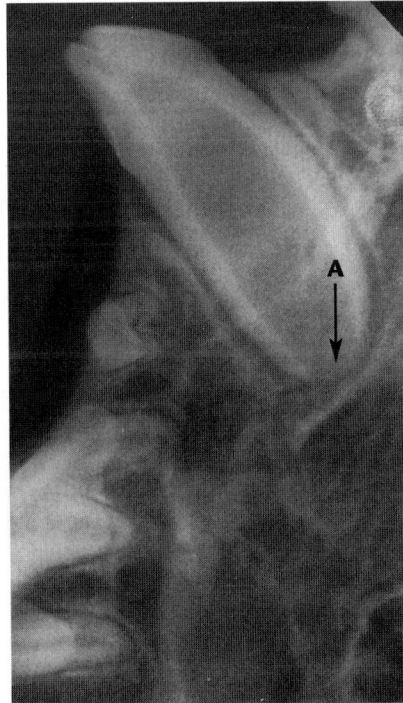

FIGURE 11.9

Contributing Author:

James M.G. Anthony

Description: Endodontic system of a mature feline.

Points Identified: Note the long thin endodontic system, closed apex, and thick dentin layer. This is characteristic of a mature feline's endodontic system.

    A. Long thin root canal
    B. Closed apex
    C. Thick dentin layer

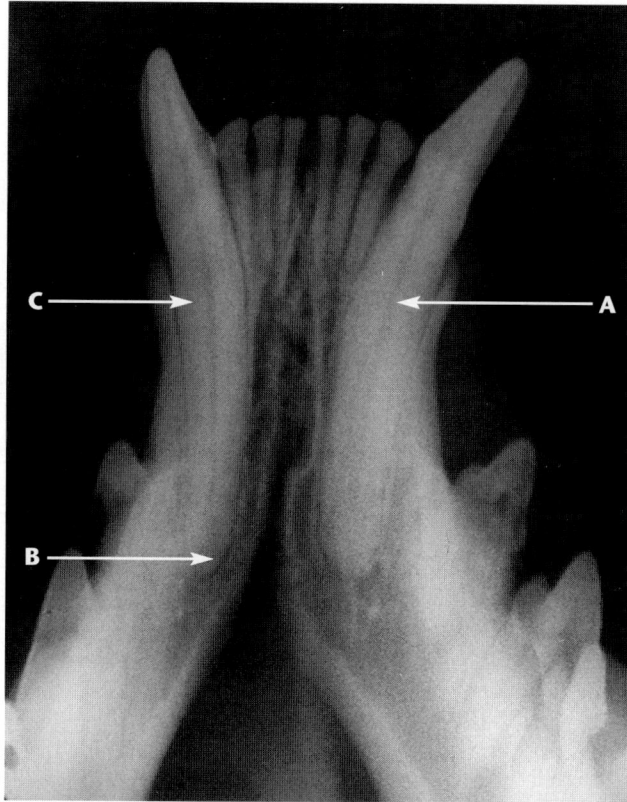

FIGURE 11.10

Contributing Author: Ayako Okuda

Description: Middle mental foramina (confusion with endodontic disease).

Points Identified: Note the round radiolucent area in conjunction with the apex of 104.

    A. 104
    B. Middle mental foramen
    C. Caudel mental foramen
    D. Retained tooth roots

Diagnostic Keys: The middle mental foramen is located in proximity to the apices of the canine and premolar teeth. It is an oval-shaped lucency through which the mental nerve, artery, and vein pass. Taking multiple oblique views will reveal that the lucency is not associated with the apex of the tooth.

Common Errors: Radicular cyst and periapical granuloma.

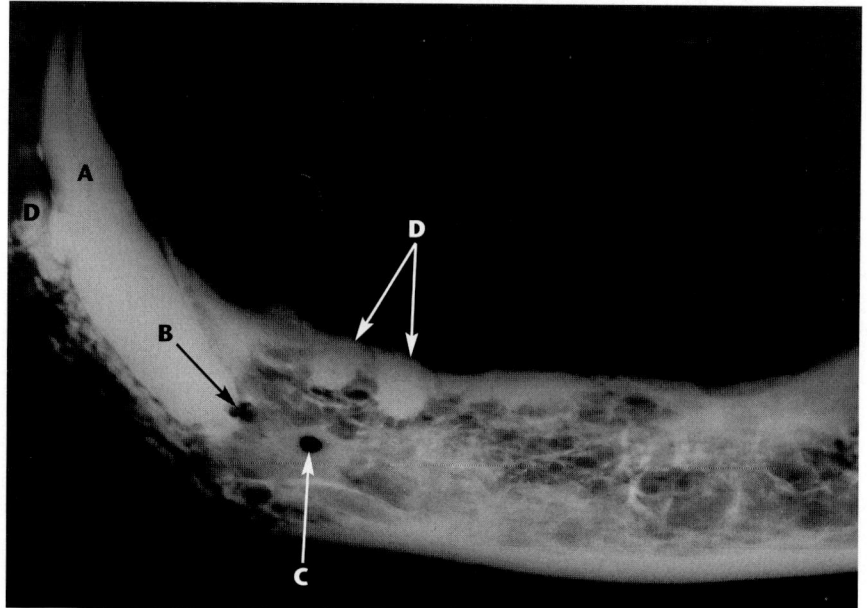

FIGURE 11.11

Contributing Author:
James M.G. Anthony

Description: Hypercementosis is excess deposition of cementum around a tooth root.

Points Identified:

A. Note radiodense thickening of the apical portion of the root, with the apical lesion blending with the periodontal ligament space
B. Also notice the diffuse bony sclerotic image surrounding the apex (condensing osteitis)

Diagnostic Keys: It is characteristic for a widened root apex (bulbous in shape) with a widened periodontal ligament space to blend into the lesion at the apex.

Common Errors: Cementoma. External resorption (above the lesion) creates a false zone of cementum apical enlargement.

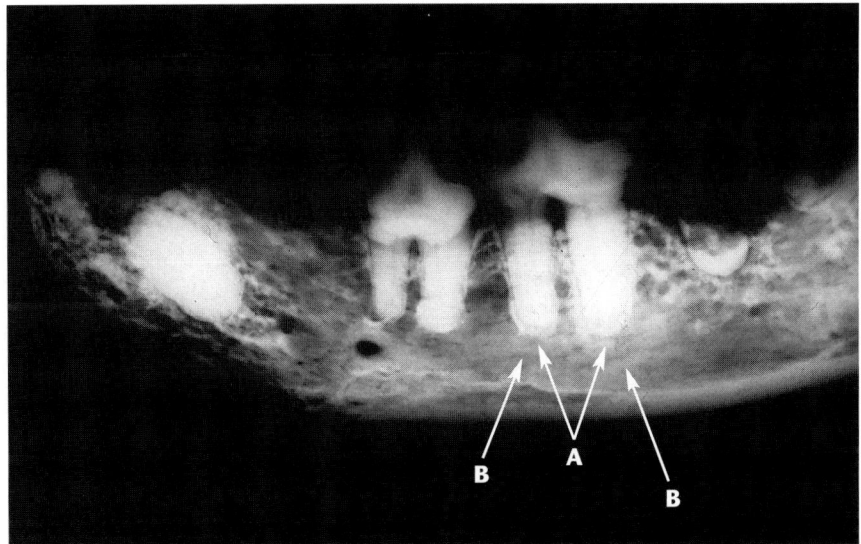

FIGURE 11.12

Contributing Author:
James M.G. Anthony

Description: Endodontic treatment 104 in feline with an apical puff.

Points Identified: Note a small amount of lining cement material extended beyond the apex in the periapical area.

A. Lining cement in periapical area

Diagnostic Keys: The apical puff has the same radiodensity as the lining cement and filling material in the endodontic system and has been extended beyond the apex of the tooth. Usually, periapical extrusions of lining cement are round or oval in shape. Overextension of gutta percha material usually forms a sharp point or curve. The final differentiation is only possible at the 6–12 month endodontic follow-up x-ray appointment. At that time, the overextension of lining cement would be resorbed and gutta percha would be present.

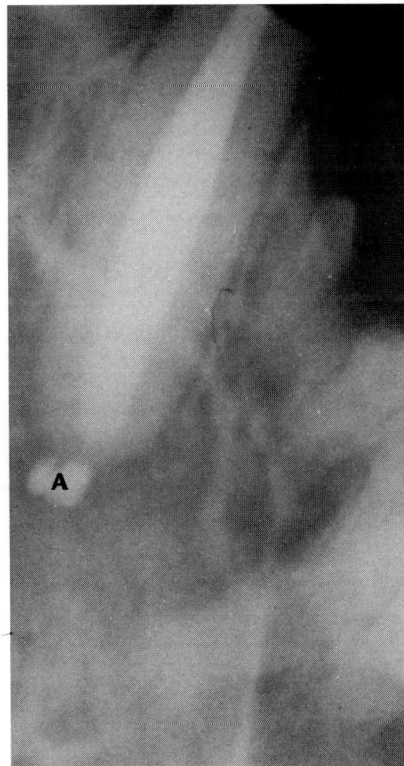

FIGURE 11.13

Contributing Author:
James M.G. Anthony

Description: Endodontic treatment (conventional).

Points Identified: View A: K-file placement (304 and 404) for measurement of endodontic system working length with endo-stop. The file is placed to the tip of the apex of the endodontic system. The endo-stop is positioned against the access site. The measurement from endo-stop to apex is the working length.

    A. 304
    B. 404
    C. Endo-stop

View B: The endodontic system is completely filled with lining cement and gutta percha after instrumentation and shaping of the endodontic system.

Diagnostic Keys: It is difficult to distinguish the working length on x-ray with files smaller than size 15. Use endo-stops and magnification to look for bending of the file tip. The tip of the file should rest at the base of the endodontic system. On final obturation, there should be no lucent areas, and the filling material should be of the same density throughout the endodontic system. Follow the wall along the endodontic system looking for voids. The apical one-third must be completely sealed.

Common Errors: Obturating too short or too long with voids and lack of uniform density of the filling material throughout the endodontic system are common mistakes to be avoided.

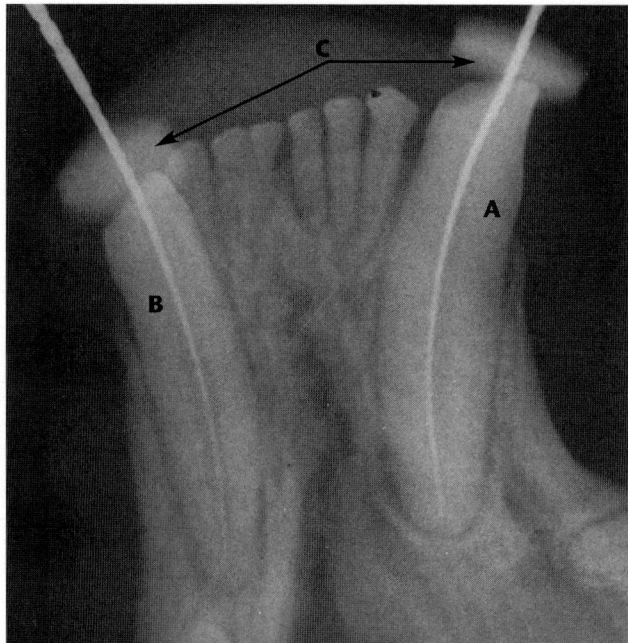

A

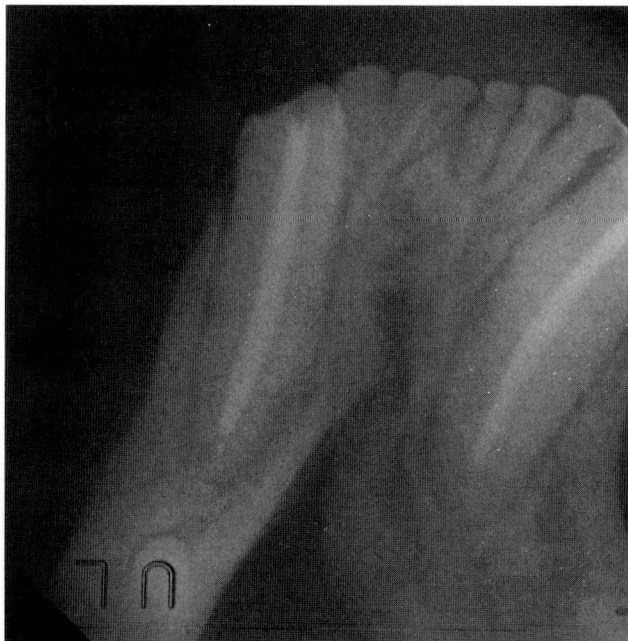

B

FIGURE 11.14

Contributing Author:

James M.G. Anthony

Description: Endodontic treatment of pre-molar (207) with diffuse narrowing of the distal root.

Points Identified: Note the obturation of the endodontic system of 207 with amorphous unorganized radiopaque calcification within the pulp space of the distal root. Sclerosing osteomyelitis is present at the mesial root apex of 207.

    A. 207, distal root, radiopaque calcification

    B. 207, mesial root, osteolysis

Diagnostic Keys: This tooth must be followed very closely radiographically. Apicoectomy or exodontal care may be necessary if conventional endodontics fails in this patient.

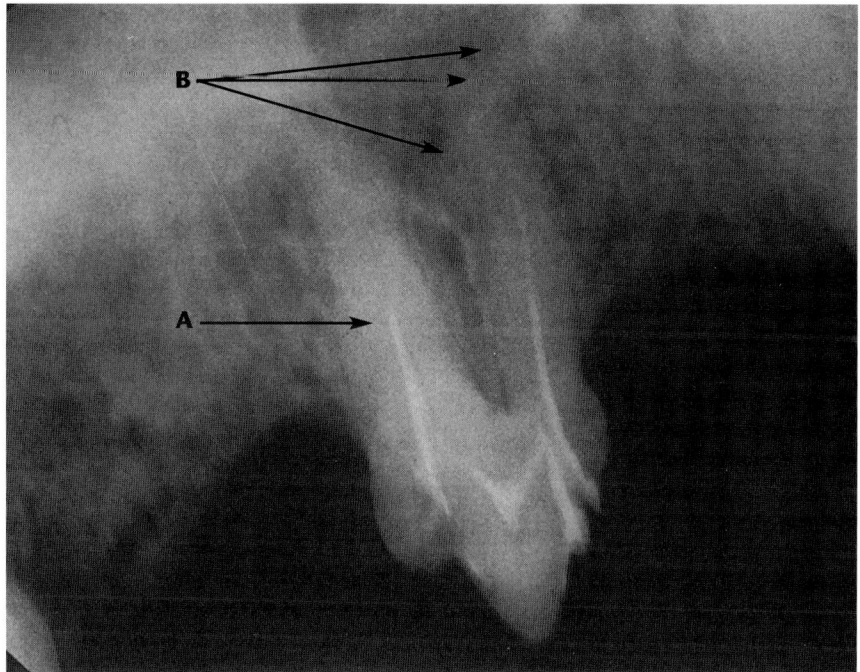

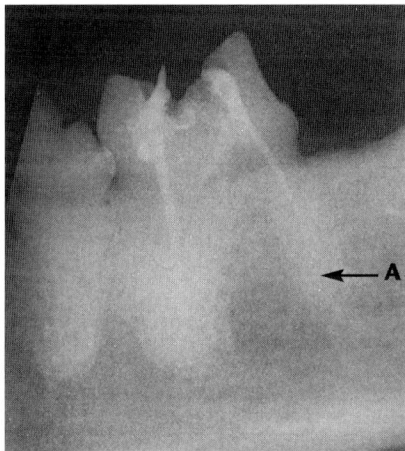

FIGURE 11.15

Contributing Author:

James M.G. Anthony

Description: Conventional endodontic treatment of molar (309) with ankylosis.

Points Identified: Note the completely closed endodontic system in an older feline with ankylosis of the distal root.

    A. 309, distal root

Diagnostic Keys: Loss of the radiolucent line that represents the periodontal ligament, mild sclerosis of the bone, and apparent blending of the bone with the tooth root are characteristic of ankylosis. This tooth must be followed very closely radiographically. Apicoectomy or exodontal care may be necessary if conventional endodontics fails in this patient.

FIGURE 11.16

Contributing Author:

James M.G. Anthony

Description: Endodontic treatment, apexification.

Points Identified: Endodontic system completely filled with a uniform density of $Ca(OH)_2$ plus barium sulfate to the open apex. Barium sulfate is added to make the $Ca(OH)_2$ radiopaque.

    A. Filled root canal with open apex

Diagnostic Keys: The filling material is not as dense as gutta percha. Recall radiographs at 6 months are essential for further treatment plans.

Common Errors: Failure to follow tooth radiographically.

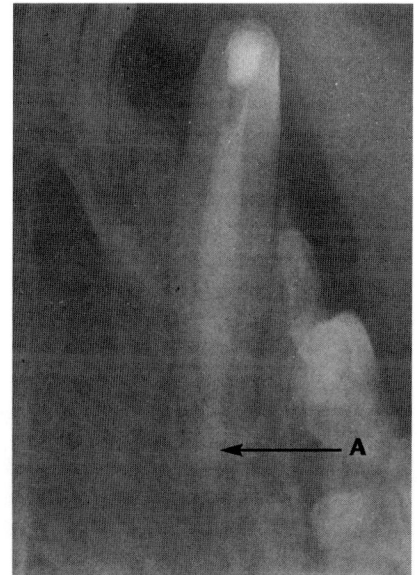

FIGURE 11.17

Contributing Author:
James M.G. Anthony

Description: Endodontic debridement complications.

Points Identified: This appearance can be caused by inappropriate debridement of canal with ledging. The important point is an imperfect apical debridement and subsequent obturation will lead to failure.

    A. Incomplete fill, 104

Diagnostic Keys: Take oblique radiographs to get a three-dimensional image of the endodontic system, and always look for the unexpected.

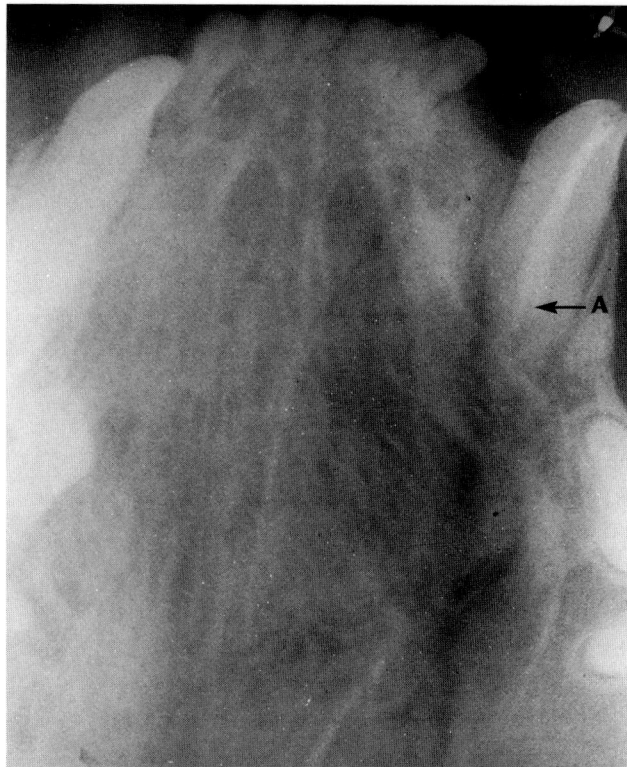

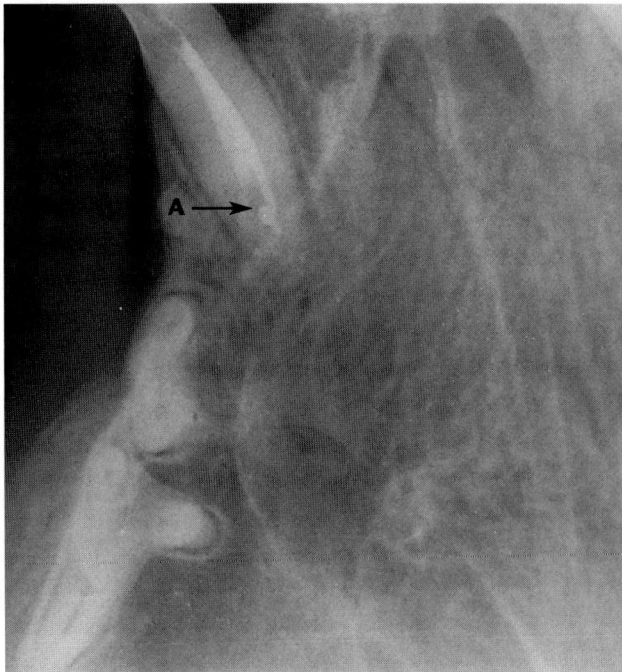

A

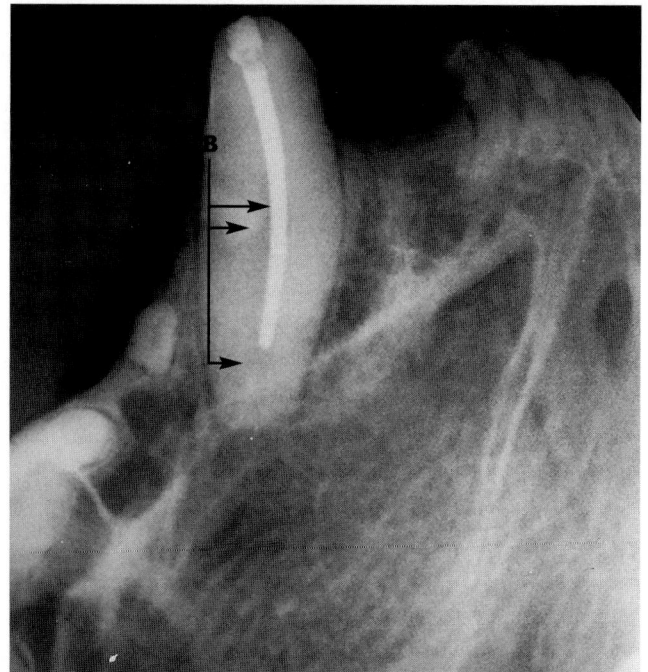

B

FIGURE 11.18

Contributing Author:
James M.G. Anthony

Description: Obturation voids 104 and 204.

Points Identified:

    A. Pigtail master cone with incomplete filling of the apex, 104

    B. Voids on lateral walls and apex of the endodontic system, 204

Diagnostic Keys: Look for lucent areas and/or incomplete filling material density between the filling material and the walls of the endodontic system.

12 Feline Oral Neoplasia

Dr. Eva M. Sarkiala-Kessel
Dr. Anna Fong Revenaugh

INTRODUCTION

Approximately 90 percent of feline oral tumors are malignant[1] Oral tumors occur in 0.5 percent of the cat population.[2] Squamous cell carcinoma (SCC) accounts for more than 70 percent of all oral neoplasms in cats.[1,3] Fibrosarcoma, the second most common malignant oral tumor in cats, occurs only occasionally.[1,3] Benign oral tumors are rare in cats. Tumor types show no gender predisposition. The most common locations of feline oral tumors are the gingiva and the ventral aspect of the tongue. Non-neoplastic oral lesions, such as eosinophilic granulomas, inflammatory lesions, and nasopharyngeal polyps, can mimic tumors. Mandibular swelling and osteomyelitis secondary to severe dental disease may be difficult to distinguish from malignant tumors without biopsy and histopathology.[4]

Clinical and Radiological Signs

The clinical signs of cats with oral neoplasia typically involve excessive salivation, facial swelling, increased mobility or loss of teeth, halitosis, oral hemorrhage and dysphagia.[5,6] Frequently, when a cat exhibits one or more of these signs the tumor is already well advanced. Loose teeth and gingival proliferation secondary to early neoplasia are often mistaken for dental disease. The opposite is true as well. A thorough oral examination should accompany the routine physical examination, especially in older animals.

Skull radiographs are indicated in all animals in which an oral tumor is suspected. Radiographic evidence of bone involvement may not be apparent. Thirty percent or more of existing bone must be destroyed before osteolysis is manifested radiographically.[3,7] The risk of pulmonary metastasis from oral neoplasias is rare, except in the case of oral melanoma and tonsillar carcinoma.[8] Thoracic radiographs are nonetheless essential for prognosis and staging. Radiographic signs of oral neoplasias include osteolysis as well as periosteal and tumor new bone production. Bone destruction can be described as either geographic, moth-eaten, or permeative, depending on aggressiveness. Neoplasias such as squamous cell carcinoma will cause a soft tissue mass and frequently invade adjacent bone. Oral neoplasias such as ameloblastoma can be seen to invade the nasal cavity.[9] High detail intraoral radiographs would be helpful in these cases to survey for nasal cavity pathology. Teeth may be displaced, loosened, deformed, resorbed, or lost. Pathologic fractures occur through areas of bony destruction. More ag-

gressive tumors, such as osteosarcoma, will exhibit an interrupted type of periosteal proliferative reaction. Patterns of osteoproliferation include the lamellated, spiculated, and amorphous patterns.

Benign Tumors

Inductive fibroameloblastoma has been reported to occur in young cats. These tumors commonly involve the maxilla adjacent to the canine tooth.[10–12] Ameloblastic fibroma is characterized radiographically by multiloculated radiolucent areas and resorption of tooth roots.[11,13,14] Fibroameloblastomas are tumors with both ameloblastic epithelium and dental pulp-like stroma. Reported radiographs of these tumors revealed varying degrees of infiltration and bone destruction.[13] Other benign oral tumors include fibropapilloma, fibroma, myxoma, epulis, ligual hemangioma and calcifying epithelial odontogenic tumors (amyloid-producing odontogenic tumors).[1,15–17] Osteoma is a mass of abnormally dense normal bone. Radiographically they are well circumscribed and very sclerotic.

Malignant Tumors

Squamous Cell Carcinoma (SCC)

A common location for SCC is the gingiva adjacent to the upper and lower premolars and molars. Involvement of the subgingival area, caudally from the frenulum, can cause difficulties in moving the tongue.[3,18] Gingival SCC is more aggressive locally in cats than in dogs.[19] Metastasis is infrequent with oral SCC, but it is locally invasive.[20] The majority of cats die or are euthanatized because of complications due to local tumor growth. Tonsillar SCC is rare in cats.[21]

Fibrosarcoma

Fibrosarcoma is the second most common feline oral-pharyngeal cancer. It frequently appears on the gingivae.[20] It is characteristically firm, smooth, and broad based. Fibrosarcoma invades local tissues rapidly, causing bone destruction.[6] Surgical en bloc resection with wide and deep margins is necessary to prevent local recurrence. Like SCC, fibrosarcoma appears to be more aggressive and destructive in cats than in dogs.[19] Metastasis occurs late in the course of the disease.

Malignant Melanoma

In contrast to dogs, melanomas involving the oral cavity of cats are rare. Oral melanomas are highly malignant and metastasize early.[3,22] In a report of five cats,[22] the most common location was the maxilla, followed by the mandible and palate. Wide surgical excision is the most effective treatment if the tumor is small. With all treatment methods the prognosis is unfavorable.

Other Malignant Tumors

Oral lymphosarcoma is often part of a multifocal cutaneous lymphosarcoma.[3] Chemotherapy is the main option for treatment, but the prognosis is poor. Tonsillar lymphosarcoma can be treated by surgery, but it also carries a poor prognosis. Localized lymphoma rarely affects the feline maxilla or mandible.[23] Osteosarcoma, hemangiosarcoma, neurofibrosarcoma, lymphohistiocytic sarcoma, myxosarcoma, mast cell tumor, and giant cell tumor are uncommon feline oral tumors.[3]

Conclusion

It is imperative that the veterinary dentist and clinician realize that feline oral neoplasia is not definitively diagnosed by radiology alone. Radiology must be coupled with a clinical impression, and a final diagnosis is made with biopsy and histopathologic identification. The histopathology must be read at a laboratory with pathologists trained in oral pathology of the feline.

References

1. Vos JH, van der Gaag I. Canine and feline oral-pharyngeal tumors. *J Vet Med* A 34, 420–27 (1987).

2. Dorn CR, Reiester WA. Epidemiological analyses of oral and pharyngeal cancers in dogs, cats, horses and cattle. *J Am Vet Med Assoc* 169:1202–6 (1976).

3. Harvey CE, Emily PP. Oral neoplasms. In *Small Animal Dentistry*. Philadelphia:Mosby, 1993, 297–311.

4. Kapatkin AS, Manfra Marretta S, Patnaik AK, Burk R, Matus RE. Non-malignant mandibular swellings in cats. *Vet Surgery* 19:69 (1990).

5. Postorino Reeves NC, Turrel JM, Withrow SJ. Oral squamous cell carcinoma in the cat. *J Am Anim Hosp Assoc* 29:369–80 (1993).

6. Howard PE. Neoplasms of the maxilla and mandible. In: Birchard SJ, Sherding RG, eds. *Saunders Manual of Small Animal Practice*. Philadelphia:W.B. Saunders, 1994, 957–64.

7. Kealy, JK. Bones and joints. In: *Diagnostic Radiology of the Dog and Cat*, 2nd edition, Philadelphia: WB Saunders, 1987, 312.

8. Theilen GH, Madewell BR. Tumors of the digestive tract. In: *Veterinary Cancer Medicine*, 2nd edition. Philadelphia:Lea and Febiger, 1987, 499–528.

9. Quigley PJ, Leedale, AH. Tumors involving bone in the domestic cat: a review of 58 cases. *Vet Pathol* 20:670 (1983).

10. Dubielzig RR. Proliferative dental and gingival diseases of dogs and cats. *J Am Anim Hosp Assoc* 18:577–84 (1982).

11. Poulet FM, Valentine BA, Summers, BA. A survey of epithelial odontogenic tumors and cysts in dogs and cats. *Vet Pathol* 29:369–80 (1992).

12. Withrow SJ. Tumors of the gastrointestinal system. In: *Clinical Veterinary Oncology*. Withrow SJ, MacEwen EG, eds. Phildelphia:Lippincott, 1989.

13. Holzworth, J. Tumors and tumor–like lesions. In: Holzworth, J., ed. *Diseases of the Cat*. Philadelphia:WB Saunders, 1987, 486–87.

14. Dernell WS, Hullinger GH. Surgical management of ameloblastic fibroma in the cat. *J Small Animal Pract* 35:35–38 (1994).

15. Crow SE, Pulley LT, Wittenbrock TP. Lingual hemangioma in a cat. *J Amer Anim Hosp Assoc* 1981, 17:71–74.

16. Walsh KM, Denholm LJ, Cooper BJ. Epithelial odontogenic tumors in domestic animals. *J Comp Path* 97:503–21 (1987).

17. Gardner DG, Dubielzig RR, McGee EV. The so-called calcifying epithelial odontogenic tumour in dogs and cats (amyloid-producing odontogenic tumour). *J Comp Path* 111:221–30 (1994).

18. Young PL. Squamous cell carcinoma of the tongue of the cat. *Aust Vet J* 54:133–34 (1978).

19. Harvey HJ. Oral tumors. In: Brown NO, guest ed. *Veterinary Clinics of North America: Small Animal Practice. Clinical Veterinary Oncology*. Philadelphia:WB Saunders, 1985, 493–500.

20. Cotter SM. Oral pharyngeal neoplasms in the cat. *J Amer Anim Hosp Assoc* 17:917–20 (1981).

21. Dobson JM, White RAS. Oral tumors in dogs and cats. *Practice* 12:135–46 (1990).

22. Patnaik AK, Mooney S. Feline melanoma: A comparative study of ocular, oral, and dermal neoplasms. *Vet Pathol* 1988, 25, 105–12.

23. Elmslie RE, Ogilvie GK, Gillette EL, McChesney-Gillette S. Radiotherapy with and without chemotherapy for localized lymphoma in 10 cats. *Vet Radiology* 32:277–80 (1991).

X-RAY PLATES AND SLIDES

Calcifying Epithelial Odontogenic Tumors

FIGURE 12.1

Contributing Authors:
Anna Fong Revenaugh
and Eva M. Sarkiala-Kessel

Description: Radiograph of a calcifying epithelial odontogenic tumor showing a well defined soft tissue mass at the level of the right upper third premolar. There is mineralization within the mass. This appearance is different from the honeycombed, ill defined lesion described in humans. The lysis of alveolar bone and widened cementoenamel junction around the third and fourth premolars is due to periodontal disease.

Points Identified:

A. Well defined soft tissue mass at the level of the right upper third premolar
B. Dystrophic mineralization within the mass
C. Alveolar bone lysis and widening of the cementoenamel junction around the canines secondary to periodontal disease
D. Lysis of the third premolar

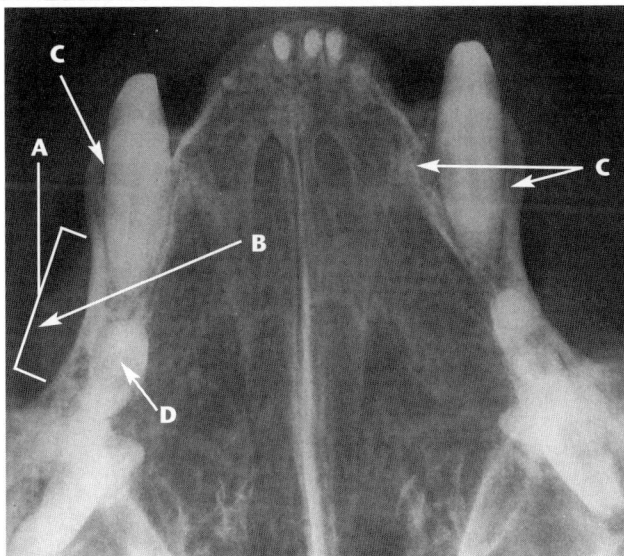

Diagnostic Keys: Soft tissue mass with mineralization. Well defined, clearly marginated mass. Locally invasive.

FIGURE 12.2

Contributing Authors:
Anna Fong Revenaugh
and Eva M. Sarkiala-Kessel

Description: Calcifying epithelial odontogenic tumor. This well defined tumor with a smooth surface extends from the distal gingival of the left upper canine tooth to the mesial part of the upper fourth premolar and dorsally along the buccal gingiva.

Common Errors: Calcifying epithelial odontogenic tumor may look like an epulis.

(See also color plate.)

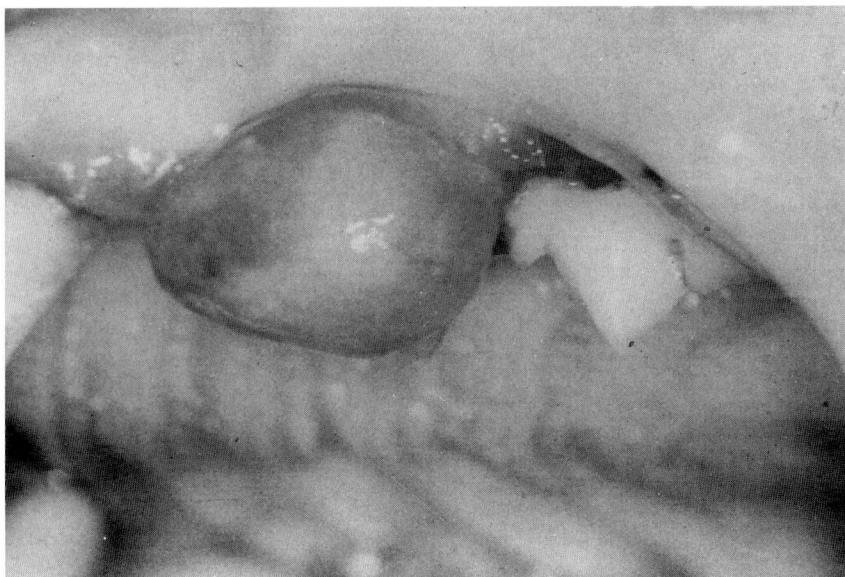

Osteomas

FIGURE 12.3

Contributing Authors:
Anna Fong Revenaugh
and Eva M. Sarkiala-Kessel

Description: Osteoma, a hard bulging mass under the left buccal mucosa between the distal part of the upper and lower dental arcades.

Points Identified:

A. Bulging mass under left buccal mucosa

Diagnostic Keys: Hard, well defined mass.

(*See also color plate.*)

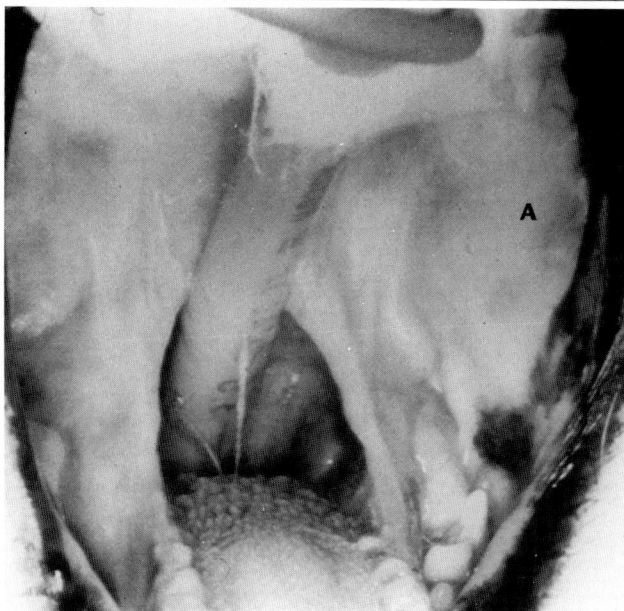

FIGURE 12.4

Contributing Authors:
Anna Fong Revenaugh
and Eva M. Sarkiala-Kessel

Description: The left buccal mucosa over the mass shown in Figure 12.3 has been incised and a hard, well defined osteoma is seen.

Diagnostic Keys: Hard, well defined mass.

(*See also color plate.*)

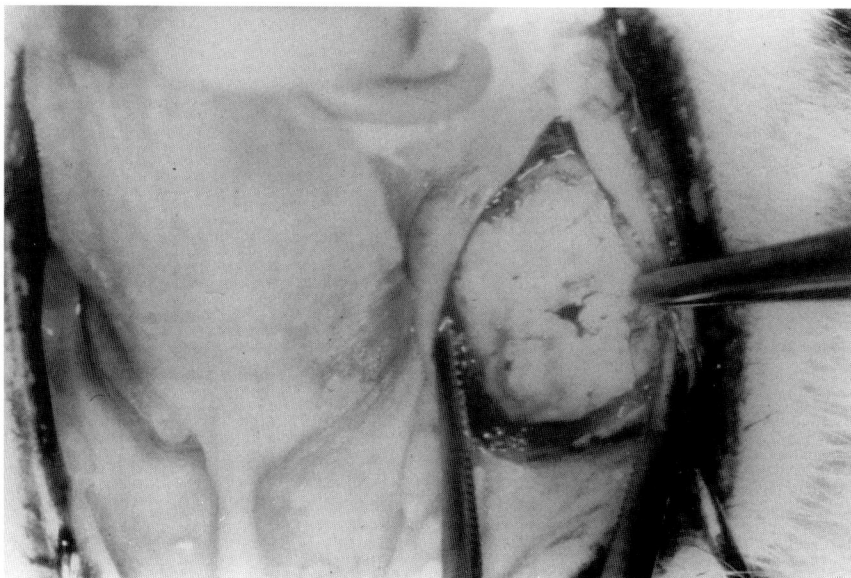

Squamous Cell Carcinomas

FIGURE 12.5

Contributing Authors:
Anna Fong Revenaugh
and Eva M. Sarkiala-Kessel

Description: Squamous cell carcinoma. Marked destruction of the rostral maxilla and incisive bone. Associated tooth loss, tooth erosion, and destruction of the rostral vomer. Turbinate destruction and patchy opacities indicative of nasal cavity involvement. Coarse trabecular pattern secondary to the loss of the fine, small trabeculae. No significant periosteal or new tumor bone formation evident.

Points Identified:

A. Poorly marginated, severely osteolytic lesion involving the incisive bone and rostral maxilla, squamous cell carcinoma

B. Destructive process has caused tooth loss, erosion, loosening and displacement

C. Destruction of the rostral vomer

D. Nasal cavity involvement with turbinate destruction

Diagnostic Keys: Severely lytic, poorly marginated lesion.

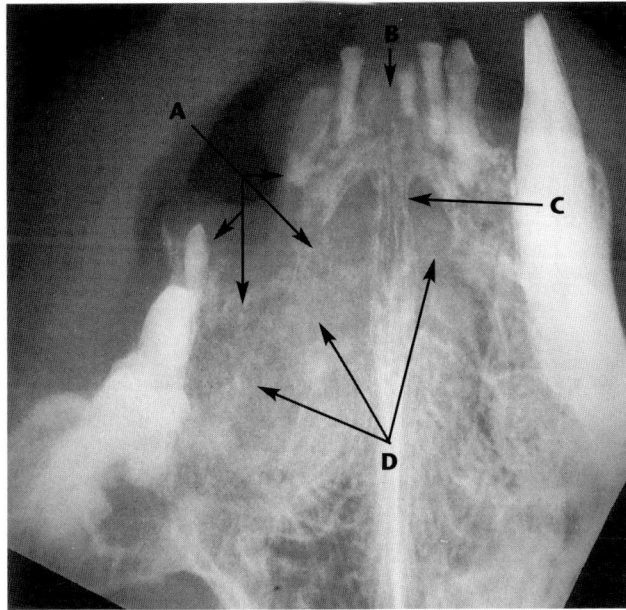

FIGURE 12.6

Contributing Authors:
Anna Fong Revenaugh
and Eva M. Sarkiala-Kessel

Description: Squamous cell carcinoma. A large soft tissue mass with involvement of the right maxilla. Dystrophic calcification can be seen within the mass. There is severe lysis of the maxilla with disruption and loss of teeth. Erosion of the vomer and marked turbinate destruction within the right nasal cavity with evidence of extension into the left side.

Points Identified:

A. Large soft tissue mass involving the right maxilla

B. Dystrophic calcification within the soft tissue mass

C. Severe lysis of the right maxilla

D. Tooth disruption and loss

E. Vomer erosion and turbinate pathology

Diagnostic Keys: Soft tissue mass with dystrophic mineralization. Marked osteolysis of associated bone.

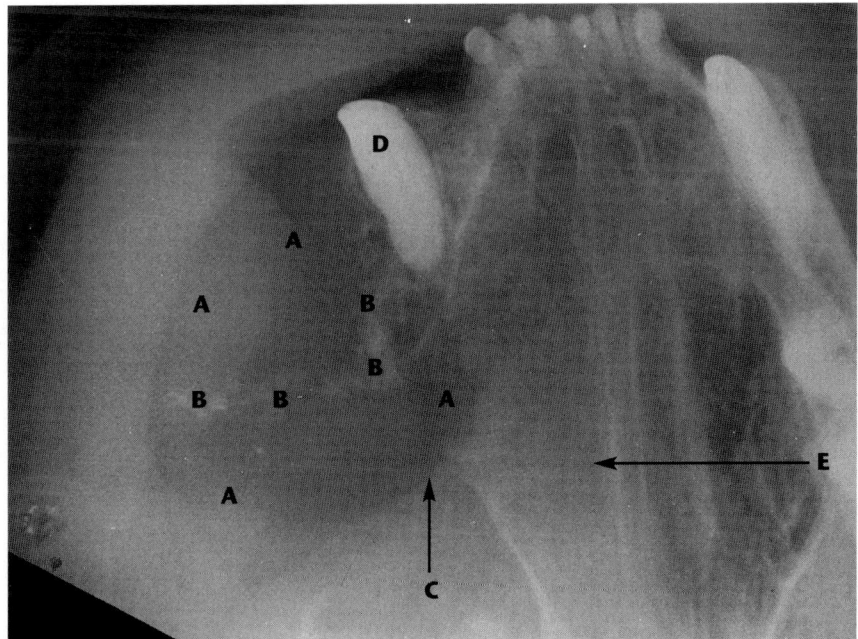

FIGURE 12.7

Contributing Authors:
Anna Fong Revenaugh
and Eva M. Sarkiala-Kessel

Description: Squamous cell carcinoma. A large mass can be seen arising from the soft tissues ventral to and within the intermandibular space. Spiculated periosteal new bone is noted within the mass and along the rostral mandible. The moth-eaten pattern of bone lysis involving the rostral mandible is indicative of the aggressive nature of this tumor.

Points Identified:

A. Spiculated new bone formation within the mass and along the rostral mandible
B. Moth-eaten pattern of bone lysis
C. Tooth and tooth root resorption

Diagnostic Keys: Soft tissue mass with dystrophic mineralization. Marked bone destruction.

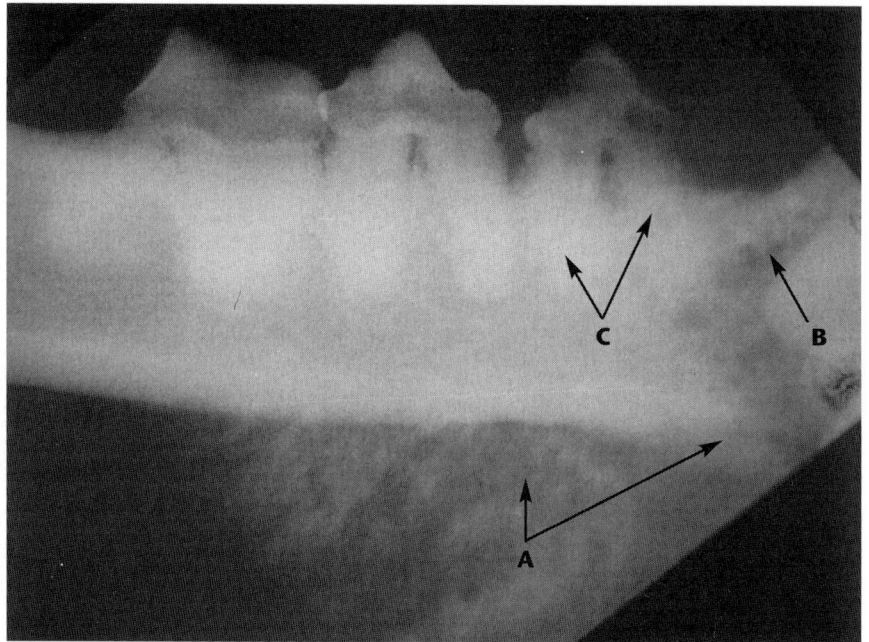

FIGURE 12.8

Contributing Authors:
Anna Fong Revenaugh
and Eva M. Sarkiala-Kessel

Description: Squamous cell carcinoma involving the body of the right hemimandible (post-hemimandibulectomy specimen). The presence of this malignant tumor growing near the cortex caused destruction and rapid elevation of the periosteum, resulting in a proliferation of bony spicules resembling a sunburst. This is an unusual presentation for a squamous cell carcinoma. The differential diagnosis for this radiographic appearance would be osteosarcoma.

Points Identified:

A. Soft tissue mass
B. Spiculated periosteal new bone causing "sunburst" appearance
C. Tooth loss

Diagnostic Keys: Soft tissue mass. Osteoproductive/destructive lesion.

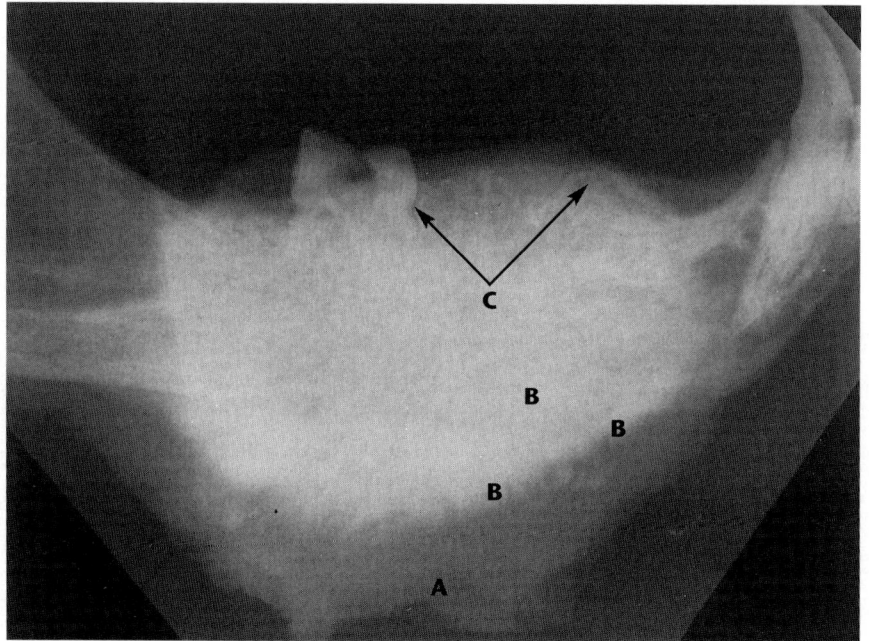

FIGURE 12.9

Contributing Authors:
Anna Fong Revenaugh
and Eva M. Sarkiala-Kessel

Description: Squamous cell carcinoma. This intraoral radiograph reveals severe osteolysis, sclerosis, amorphous periosteal proliferation, and distortion of the rostral mandible. A soft tissue mass is seen associated with the bony lesions. The remaining teeth show evidence of tooth root resorption.

Points Identified:

A. Soft tissue mass around the rostral mandible
B. Severe bony lysis of the rostral mandible
C. Tooth root resorption
D. Bony sclerosis
E. Amorphous periosteal proliferation with distortion of the rostral mandible

Diagnostic Keys: Soft tissue mass. Osteoproductive/destructive lesion.

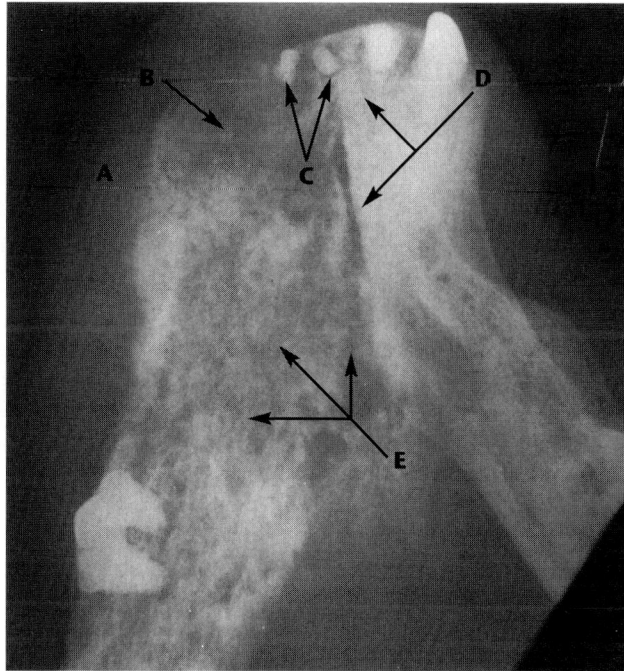

FIGURE 12.10

Contributing Authors:
Eva M. Sarkiala-Kessel
and Anna Fong Revenaugh

Description: Squamous cell carcinoma. An ulcerated lesion at the upper premolar gingiva, extending buccally and palatially. The lesion is packed with food.

Diagnostic Keys: Commonly located on the gingivae. Ulcerated or protuberant. Poorly marginated. Loose teeth may be in the lesion. Food and hair may be packed into the lesion.

Common Errors: The early stages of squamous cell carcinoma in this location may remind the veterinary dentist of severe periodontal disease with mobile teeth.

(See also color plate.)

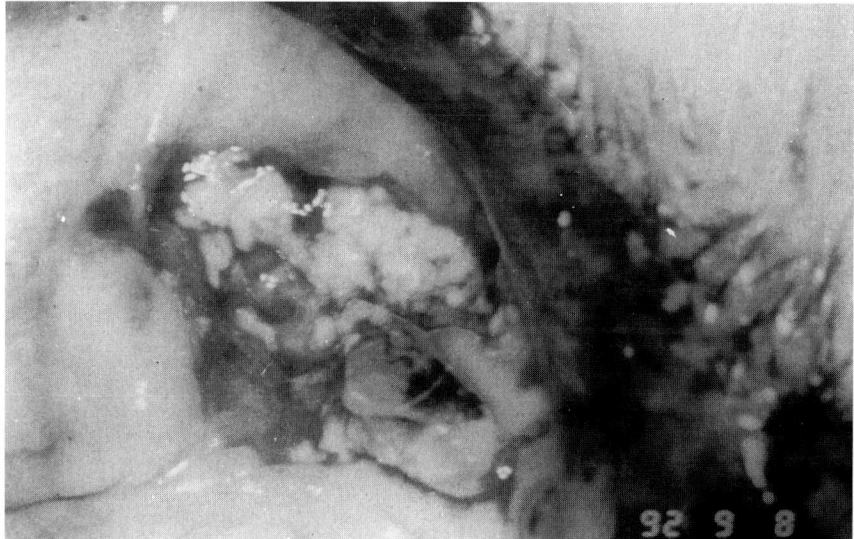

FIGURE 12.11

Contributing Authors:
Eva M. Sarkiala-Kessel
and Anna Fong Revenaugh

Description: Squamous cell carcinoma. A ventral mass at the root of the tongue causing edema of the sublingual frenulum.

Common Errors: Granulation and edema of the frenulum caused by a foreign body trapped beneath the tongue may be reminiscent of sublingual squamous cell carcinoma.

(See also color plate.)

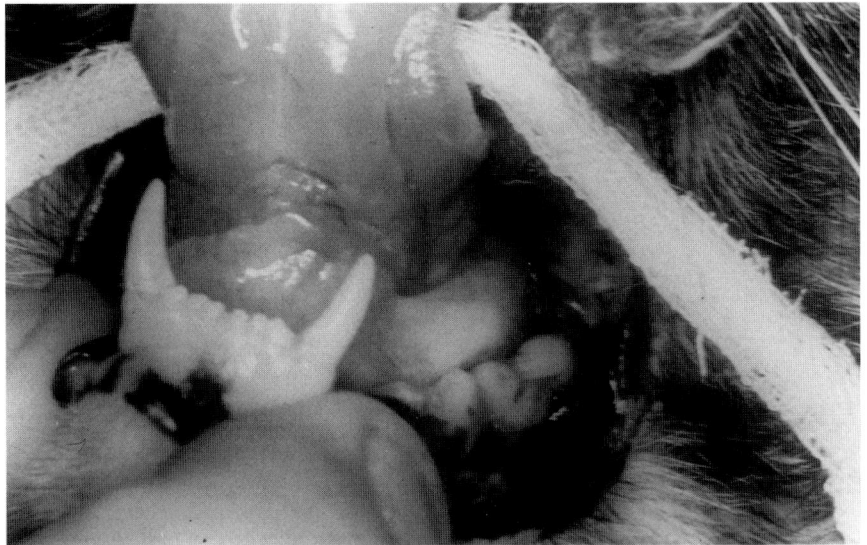

FIGURE 12.12

Contributing Authors:
Eva M. Sarkiala-Kessel
and Anna Fong Revenaugh

Description: Squamous cell carcinoma. A large protuberant lesion on the sides of the caudal tongue and extending into the pharynx.

(See also color plate.)

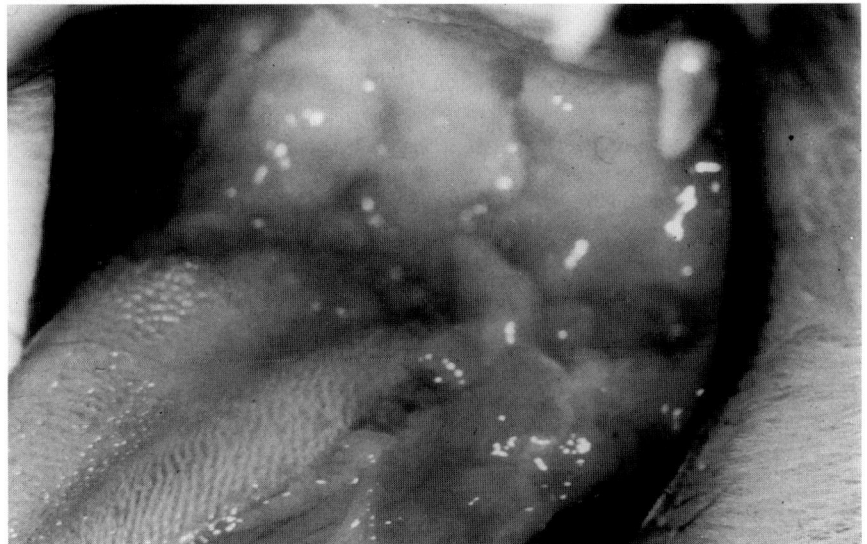

FIGURE 12.13

Contributing Authors:
Eva M. Sarkiala-Kessel
and Anna Fong Revenaugh

Description: Squamous cell carcinoma. An ulcerated lesion of the left upper lip next to the canine tooth.

Common Errors: An electric cord injury may cause necrosis of the lips. Eosinophilic granuloma often occurs on the upper lip of the cat.

(See also color plate.)

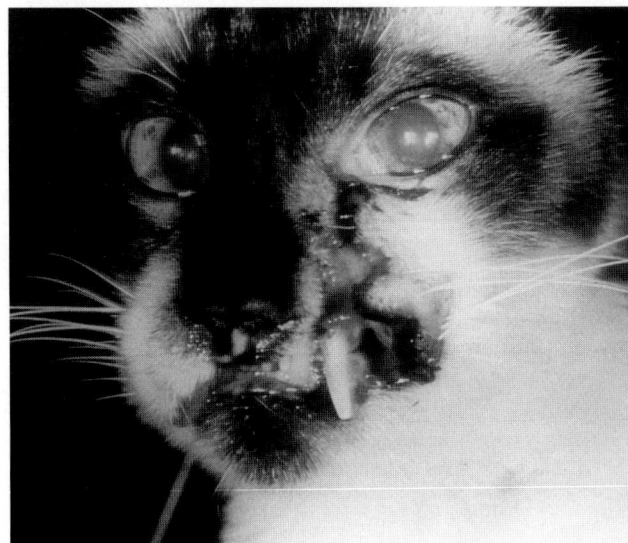

Fibrosarcomas

FIGURE 12.14

Contributing Authors:

Anna Fong Revenaugh
and Eva M. Sarkiala-Kessel

Description: Fibrosarcoma. Soft tissue mass involving the rostral left maxilla. The tumor has caused cortical bone loss. Deviation and erosion of the vomer bone with turbinate destruction is evidence of extension into the nasal cavity. The right rostral maxilla is also involved. There are tooth root lysis and displaced teeth, and several teeth appear to be "floating."

Points Identified:

A. Tooth loss, tooth root lysis
B. Large soft tissue mass—fibrosarcoma
C. Cortical bone destruction
D. Nasal turbinate destruction
E. Vomer bone erosion and deviation

Diagnostic Keys: Locally invasive soft tissue mass. Destruction of adjacent bone and teeth.

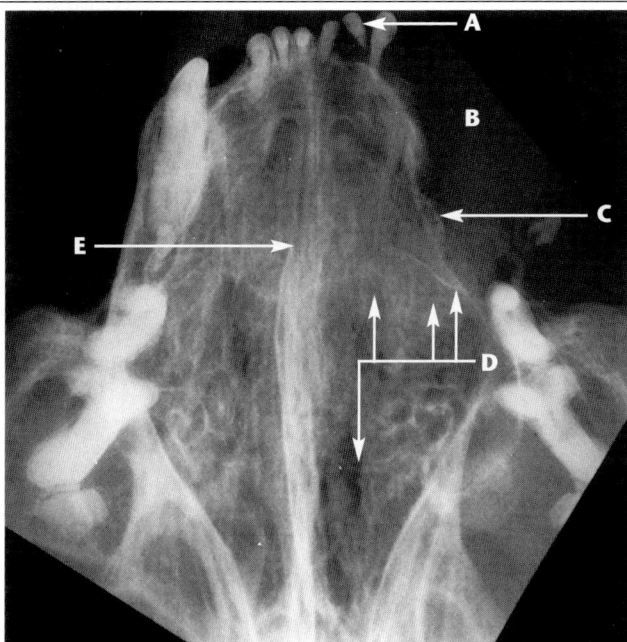

FIGURE 12.15

Contributing Authors:

Anna Fong Revenaugh
and Eva M. Sarkiala-Kessel

Description: Fibrosarcoma. A poorly defined, protuberant mass of the upper gingiva at the premolar-molar area and extending palatially. The upper fourth premolar and first molar can be partially seen.

Diagnostic Keys: Appears frequently on the gingivae. Often firm, smooth, and broad based.

(See also color plate.)

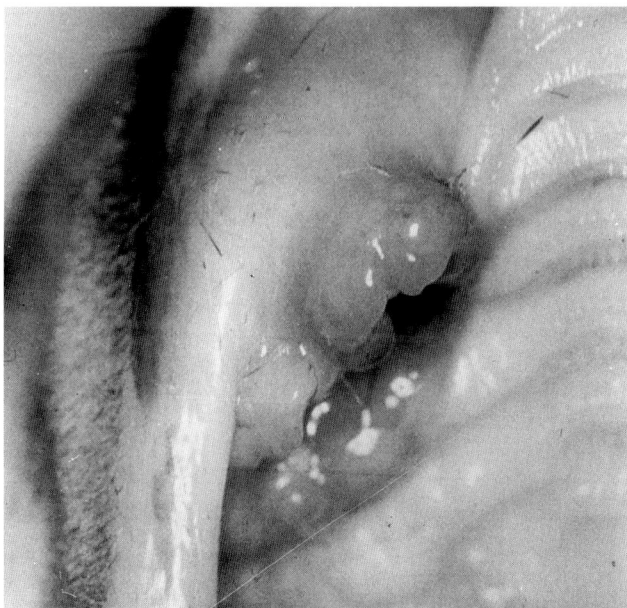

FIGURE 12.16

Contributing Authors:
Anna Fong Revenaugh
and Eva M. Sarkiala-Kessel

Description: Fibrosarcoma. A biopsy specimen after maxillectomy. A poorly defined smooth mass at the premaxilla and maxilla extending from the left side over the midline to the right side of the palate.

(See also color plate.)

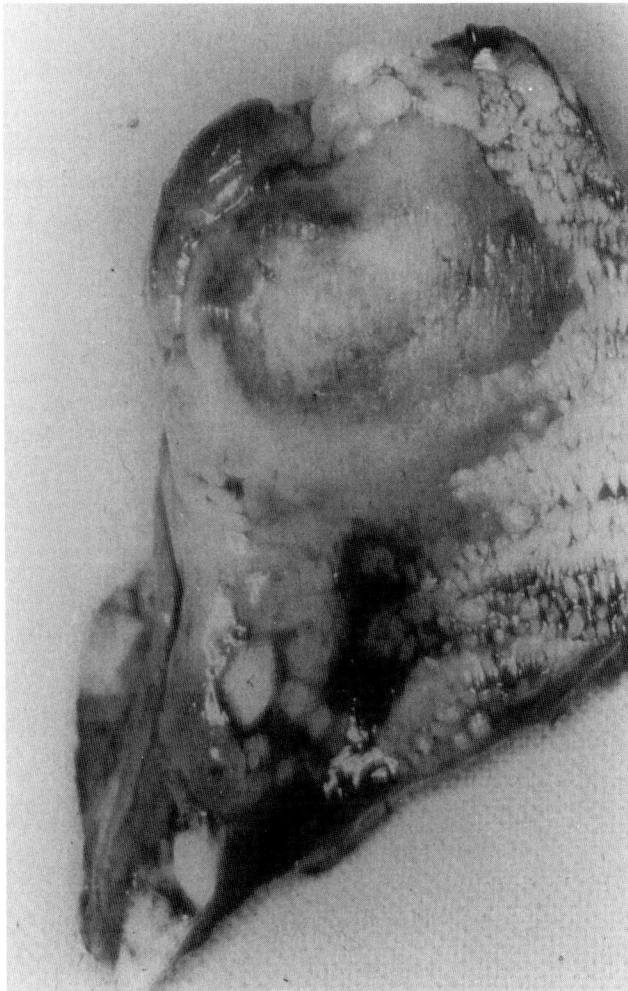

Fibromatous Epulis

FIGURE 12.17

Contributing Authors:
Anna Fong Revenaugh
and Eva M. Sarkiala-Kessel

Description: This radiograph is of a fibromatous epulis. Although epulides are common dental tumors in the canine, they are rarely seen in the cat. As in the canine, this benign tumor is not locally invasive, but can be present radiographically with varying amounts of dystrophic mineralization. A soft tissue mass can be seen around the distal aspect of the lower left first molar. Horizontal bone loss involving the molar and premolars indicates periodontitis.

Points Identified:

A. Soft tissue mass around the distal aspect of the first molar
B. Periodontal disease causing horizontal bone loss

Diagnostic Keys: Soft tissue mass. No local invasion.

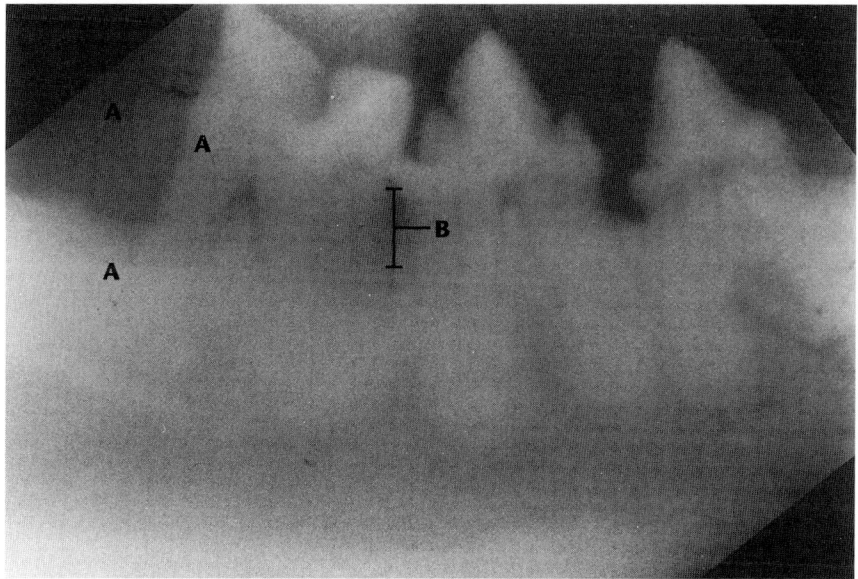

FIGURE 12.18

Contributing Authors:
Anna Fong Revenaugh
and Eva M. Sarkiala-Kessel

Description: Fibromatous epulis in a 6-year-old Persian feline. Although epulides are common dental tumors in the dog, they are rarely seen in the cat. A soft tissue mass can be seen around the distal aspect of the lower left molar (309).

Points Identified: Soft tissue mass around the distal aspect of the first molar.

Common Errors: Failure to biopsy to differentiate from other neoplasms of the oral cavity.

(See also color plate.)

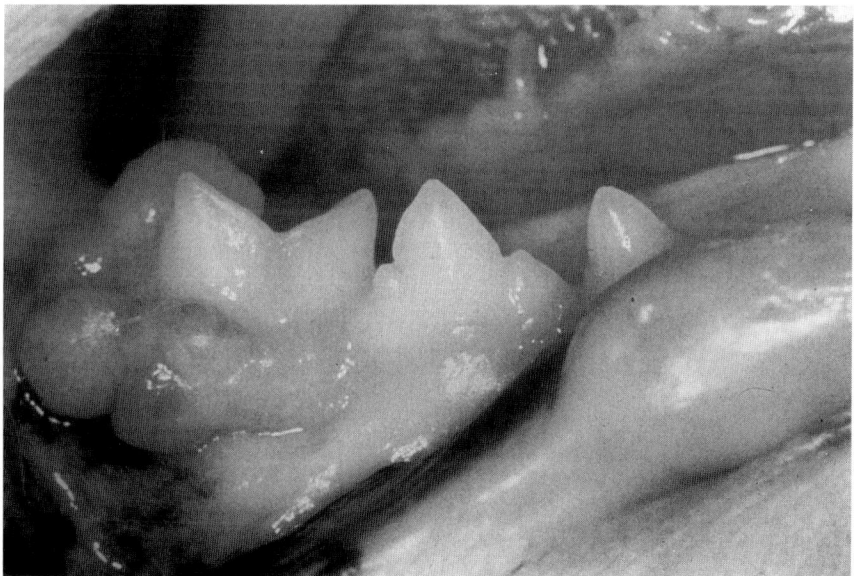

13 Feline Oral Trauma

Dr. Cecilia Gorrel
Dr. Donald H. DeForge

INTRODUCTION

Most jaw fractures are the result of road traffic accidents or falling from high places (i.e., high-rise syndrome) and are frequently compound. Periodontal disease may cause such severe bone loss that spontaneous jaw fractures occur, particularly in the mandible. Rough extraction technique commonly results in fracture of an already weakened mandible. It is therefore advisable to radiograph the jaws before attempting extraction of teeth in an animal with severe periodontal disease.

Mandibular Fractures

Cats commonly suffer mandibular symphyseal fractures, condylar region fractures, and, less commonly, fractures of the body of the mandible.

Upper Jaw Fractures

The upper jaw consists of the premaxilla, maxilla, and nasal bones. All of these are thin plates of bone surrounding an air-filled cavity. They therefore fracture easily at the site of impact.

Biomechanics of Jaw Fracture Repair

The pressures of occlusion tend to push the rostral end of the maxilla dorsally and the rostral end of the mandible ventrally. The caudal areas of these bones, embedded in muscle, are more stable. Hence, the alveolar border of both the maxilla and the mandible is the tension side. The compression side of the maxilla is the nasal chamber and of the mandible is its ventral border.

If a fracture causes malocclusion it is essential to restore and maintain normal or near normal occlusion during the healing process.

Complications

Many of the possible complications of jaw fractures are similar to those elsewhere in the body and are dealt with in the same way. These are soft tissue trama, nonunion, malunion, and infection. The two complications unique to the jaw are malocclusion and endodontic problems.

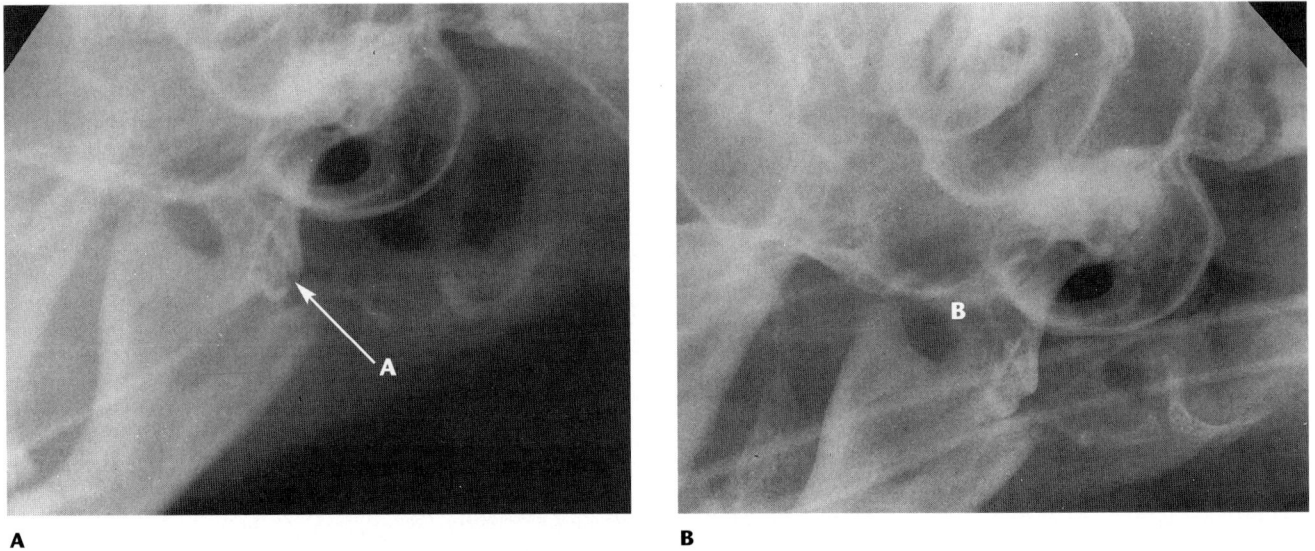

A   B

FIGURE 13.1

Contributing Author:
Mary Suzanne Aller

Description: Radiographs of temporo-mandibular joint (TMJ) of feline hit by car 4 years ago. Clicking noted by owner. Possible TMJ pathology present although clinically normal function, occlusion, eating habits, etc.

Points Identified:

A. Irregular condyloid process
B. Ill-defined articular surface

Diagnostic Keys: This TMJ should be evaluated by C-Scan or MRI before any treatment planning is initiated to verify pathology.

FIGURE 13.2

Contributing Author: Paul Q. Mitchell

Description: Intraoral view of maxilla in an 8-year-old, male, neutered, domestic shorthair presented for oral trauma evaluation.

Points Identified:

A. Rostral extent of maxillary fracture
B. Midportion of maxillary fracture
C. Endodontic files in place

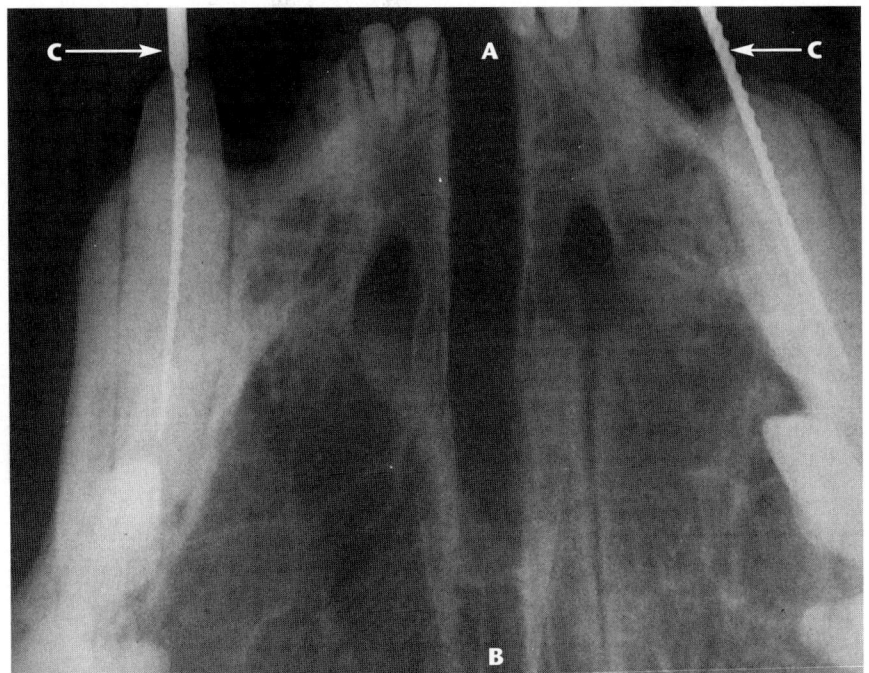

FIGURE 13.3

Contributing Author: Paul Q. Mitchell

Description: Intraoral view of mandible in an 8-year-old, male, neutered, domestic shorthair presented for oral trauma evaluation.

Points Identified:

A. Fracture of mandibular symphysis
B. Full cerclage wire around rostral mandibular fragments
C. Endodontic files in place

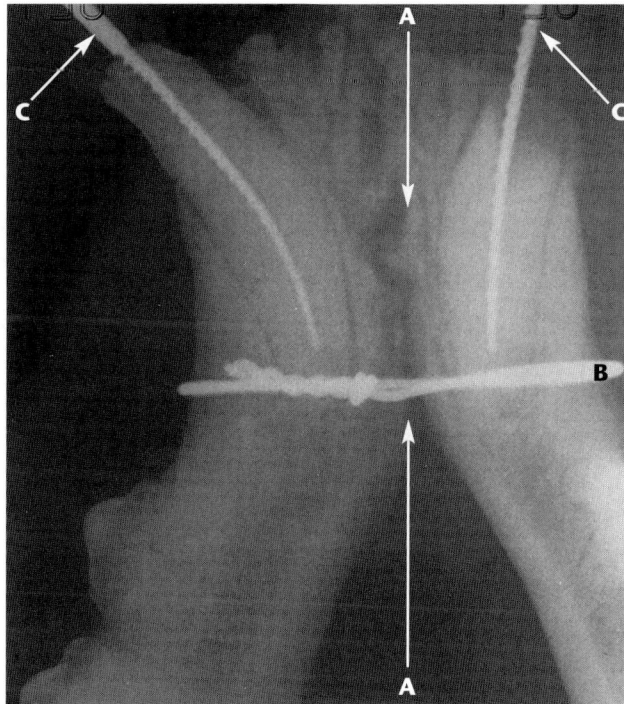

FIGURE 13.4

Contributing Author: Paul Q. Mitchell

Description: Intraoral view of maxilla in a 5-month-old, male, domestic shorthair presented for oral trauma evaluation.

Points Identified:

A. Maxillary fracture
B. Retained fragments of fractured 504
C. Alveolar fracture of 104

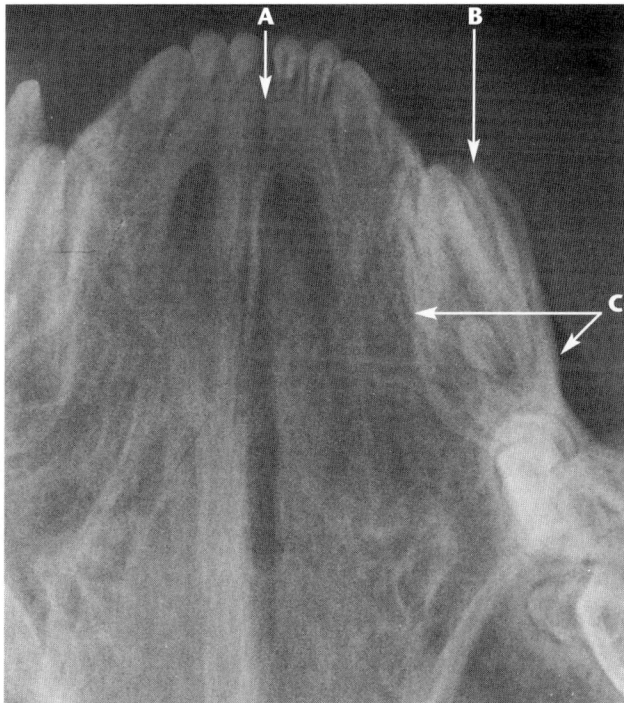

FIGURE 13.5

Contributing Author: Paul Q. Mitchell

Description: Intraoral view of mandible in a 5-month-old, male, domestic shorthair presented for oral trauma evaluation.

Points Identified: Note that the tooth bud of 404 was exposed clinically.

A. 704
B. 804
C. 404 tooth bud
D. Fracture of right hemimandible
E. Fracture of left hemimandible
F. Symphyseal fracture
G. Lingual fracture fragment

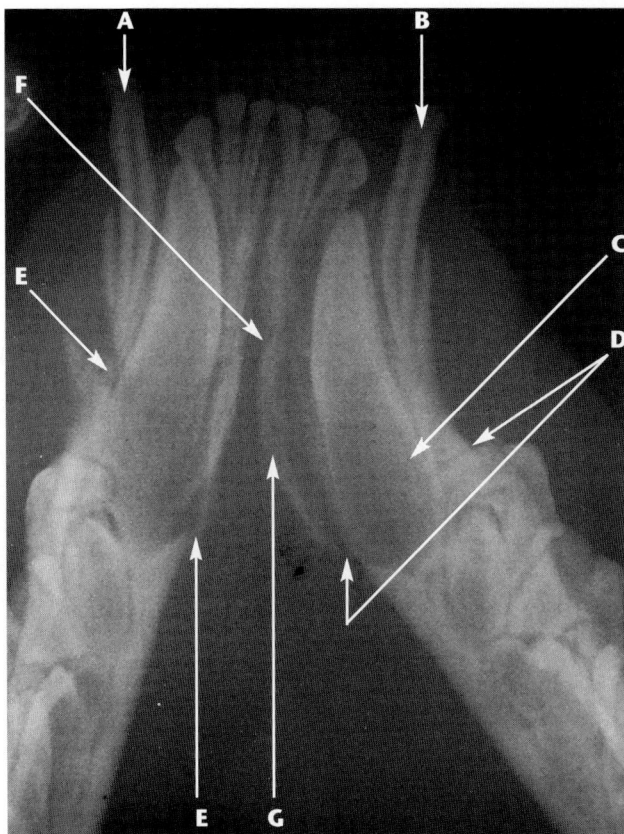

FIGURE 13.6

Contributing Author: Cecilia Gorrel

Description: Mandibular symphysis fracture.

Points Identified: Although mandibular symphysis fractures are common in feline oral trauma, this x-ray allows us to identify the "not so obvious." The central incisors 301/401 have root tip fractures and should be extracted.

A. 301
B. 401
C. Symphyseal fracture

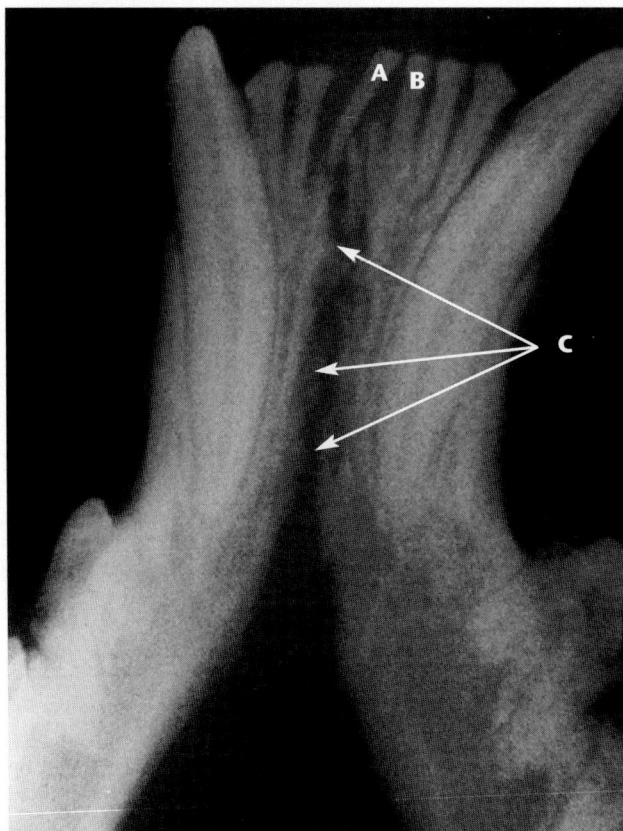

FIGURE 13.7

Contributing Author: Cecilia Gorrel

Description: This displaced mandibular fracture shows a crown fracture in 301 and fibrocartilaginous disjunction in the periodontal attachment apparatus around 304 and 404.

Points Identified:

A. 304
B. 404
C. 301
D. Symphyseal fracture of mandible

Diagnostic Keys: After symphysis repair these teeth, 304 and 404, must be followed up at 3-, 6-, and 12-month intervals to determine whether endodontic treatment is indicated.

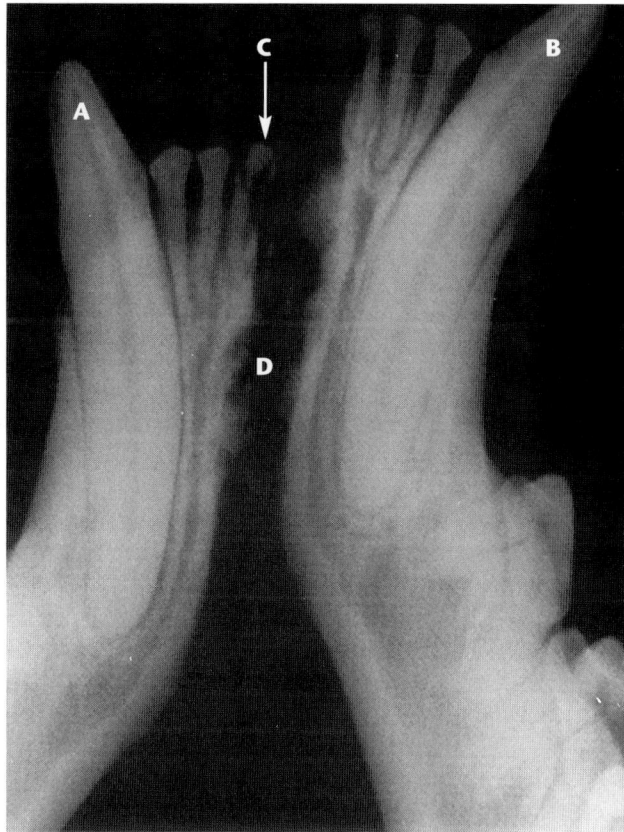

FIGURE 13.8

Contributing Author: Cecilia Gorrel

Description: Maxillary fracture at palatine fissure and parallel fracture between 104 and 103. Both canine teeth had old fractures (Class VI) prior to this recent trauma.

Points Identified:

A. Endodontic lesion with apical root resorption
B. Maxillary fracture
C. Parallel maxillary fracture
D. 103
E. 104
F. 204

Diagnostic Keys: Canine 104 needs conventional and/or surgical endodontic consideration.

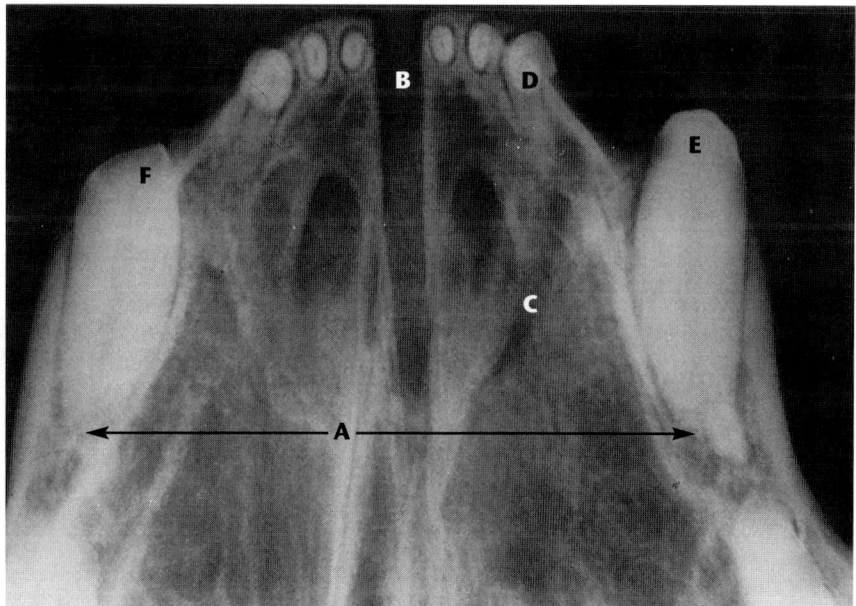

FIGURE 13.9

Contributing Author:
Donald H. DeForge

Description: Multiple maxillary fractures. In the Northeast, in large cities, felines suffer from "high-rise syndrome" (i.e., falling out of windows from multi-story structures). This radiograph shows three fractures and an avulsion.

Points Identified:

A. Triangular incisive bone fracture
B. 104—avulsion
C. 204—Class VI crown fracture and vertical crown-root fracture
D. Fracture of left zygomatic arch

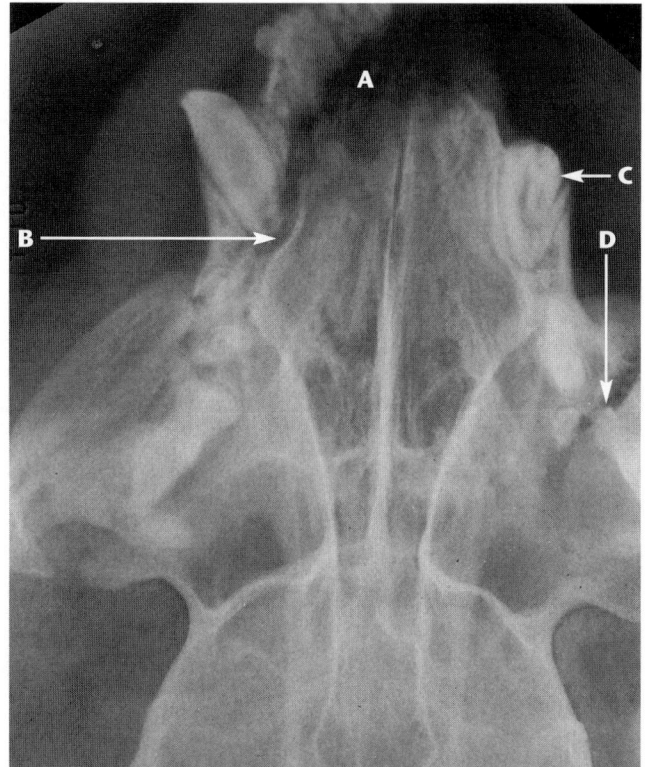

FIGURE 13.10

Contributing Author:
Donald H. DeForge

Description: Maxillary fractures.

Points Identified:

A. Multiple crown-root vertical subcrestal fractures (104)
B. Maxillary fracture at site of mesiobuccal and palatal root 108
C. Zygomatic arch fracture

Diagnostic Keys: All maxillary fractures should be radiographed. Skeletal repair, as well as orodental repair are based on findings.

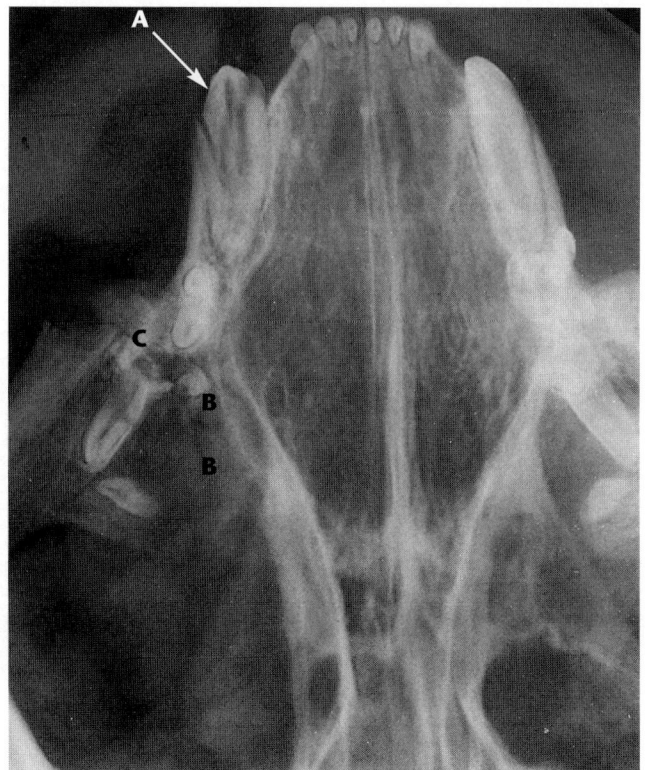

14 Feline Stomatitis Syndrome, Periodontal Disease, and Feline Odontoclastic Resorptive Lesions

Dr. Kenneth F. Lyon
Dr. Chris J. Visser

Dr. Ayako Okuda
Dr. James M.G. Anthony

INTRODUCTION

Periodontitis, which is usually seen in the canine oral cavity, also occurs in the feline oral cavity along with the gingivitis/stomatitis complex (commonly referred to as feline stomatitis) and external and internal odontoclastic resorptive lesions. Although the establishment and progression of nonspecific periodontitis in the feline seems like that in the canine, damage of soft tissue is often more severe and painful in cats than in dogs. It may be postulated that the gingival tissues of cats are not thick enough to protect the oral mucosa, which is thin and sensitive.

We can initially categorize periodontal disease in cats by clinical features:

Grade I: Inflammation is localized only in marginal gingiva. Gingiva is erythematous and edematous due to inflammation without bleeding and abnormal sulcus depth.

Grade II: Moderate inflammation in gingiva and minimal attachment loss can be found with minimal mobility.

Grade III: Established inflammation reveals gingival hyperplasia or recession and attachment loss of 30–50 percent of periodontal ligament with moderate tooth mobility. In this stage gingival sulcus depth starts to appear abnormal (greater than 1 mm).

Grade IV: Severe inflammation of gingiva and 50–75 percent destruction of periodontal ligaments are present with marked tooth mobility and abnormal sulcus depth probings.

Grade V: Tooth should be extracted.

Radiographically in Grades I and II, no significant hard tissue damages can be found on the x-ray images. Periodontitis is established in advanced stages, Grades III, IV, and V, indicating obvious radiographic changes: large periodontal spaces, deep pockets or infrabony pockets, disappearance of alveolar crests, horizontal or vertical bone loss, and ankylosis.

Editors' Comment: This grading system is one of many systems used to define or categorize periodontal disease.

FIGURE 14.1

Contributing Author: Ayako Okuda

Description: Trauma with severe periodontitis, fistulation, and osteomyelitis—chronic case.

Points Identified: The root of the lower left canine is completely ankylosed, judged by no periodontal space. This irregularity of the root surface of the right canine suggests severe root resorption, associated with a fistulation, draining externally just below the lower labial frenulum. The endodontic system of the right canine communicating with the wide periodontal space mesial to the root and the irregular outline of the root canal suggests internal resorption as well as external resorption. The transparency surrounding the right canine indicates the disappearance of all cortical buccal bone and some lingual bone. Irregular aspects of the alveolar bone surrounding both canines, especially on the right, are signs of osteomyelitis.

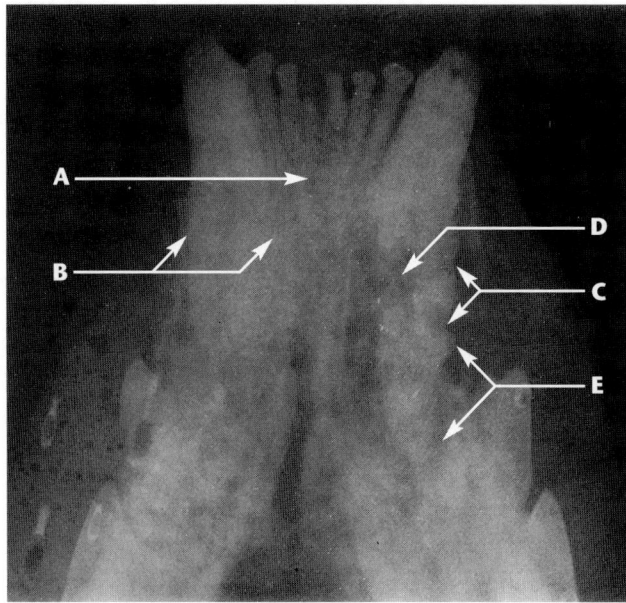

A. Chronic diffuse sclerosing osteomyelitis
B. Unclear periodontal ligament ankylosis
C. External resorption
D. Endodontic involvement (internal resorption)
E. Fistulation from apex to oral mucosa

Diagnostic Keys: Roots of ankylosed teeth have dark outlines, indicating no periodontal space. Irregular radiolucency of alveolar bone is a sign of osteomyelitis.

Common Errors: Malignant tumors.

FIGURE 14.2

Contributing Author: Ayako Okuda

Description: Supererupted canine caused by periodontitis Grade IV with replacement reaction of bone.

Points Identified: Underneath the right supererupted canine a normal radiotransparency can be found within the periodontal space. This supererupted canine was easily displaced. When the length of both canines is compared, the supererupted canine is shorter than the normal canine. This may be possible due to resorption of the apex. The apices of both canines are rounded, presumably due to resorption and/or ankylosis. Irregular appearance of the marginal crestal bone surrounding the affected canine indicates bone resorption and deep pocketing.

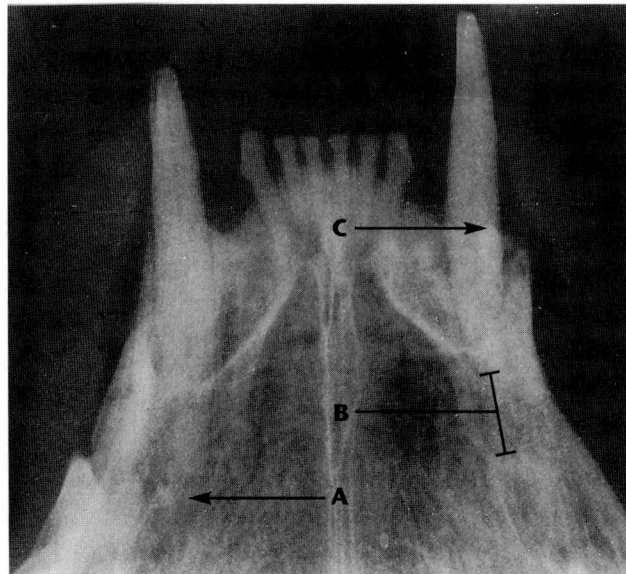

A. Unclear periodontal ligament
B. Supereruption of canine
C. Irregular appearance of marginal crestal bone

FIGURE 14.3

Contributing Author: Ayako Okuda

Description: Grades III–IV periodontitis with root resorption.

Points Identified: Lower third premolar (307) is in an advanced stage of external and internal root resorption; the bulk of the tooth has been mostly resorbed and replaced with bony tissue. Only the crown and the tips of the roots are recognized. The inner wall of the mesial root surfaced against the inter-radicular septa and is ankylosed with alveolar bone, as evidenced by the lack of periodontal space. The apices of the third premolar look bulbous, indicating hypercementosis with ankylosis because of the disappearance of the periodontal ligament. There is an irregular appearance of bone covering both roots of the third premolar, and bone loss is seen between the third and fourth premolars to the mesial root of the fourth premolar (308).

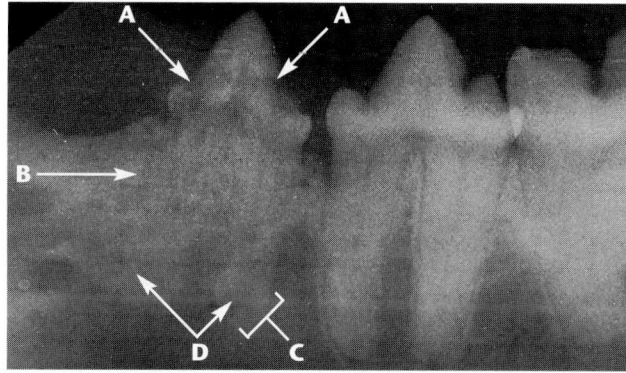

A. Odontoclastic resorptive lesion (ORL) resorption
B. Unclear outline of the roots
C. Hypercementosis
D. Ankylosis

Diagnostic Keys: Deep external resorptive lesions are characterized by replacement with bone or cementum tissue which exhibits a similar radiotransparency.

Common Errors: Osteomyelitis—root resorption and akylosis.

FIGURE 14.4

Contributing Author: Ayako Okuda

Description: Trauma with periodontitis—chronic case.

Points Identified: Both lower canines were broken by an accident. The left canine has a Class I endodontic-periodontic lesion, suggesting infection in the endodontic system extending to apical periodontitis. The small defect on the mesial surface of the root of 204 and wider space on the mesial side of 104 indicate root resorption. The mesial periodontal space of the right canine (104) is wider and more uneven than the distal space, showing a deep pocket. The irregular surface of the root canal suggests a chronic endodontic problem, with internal resorption. The periodontal space surrounding the apex of the right canine is not clear. The rostral part of the mandible shows lucency of the bone, indicating a localized osteomyelitis affecting the symphysis.

A. 104
B. 204
C. Resorption
D. Unclear root apices
E. Fracture

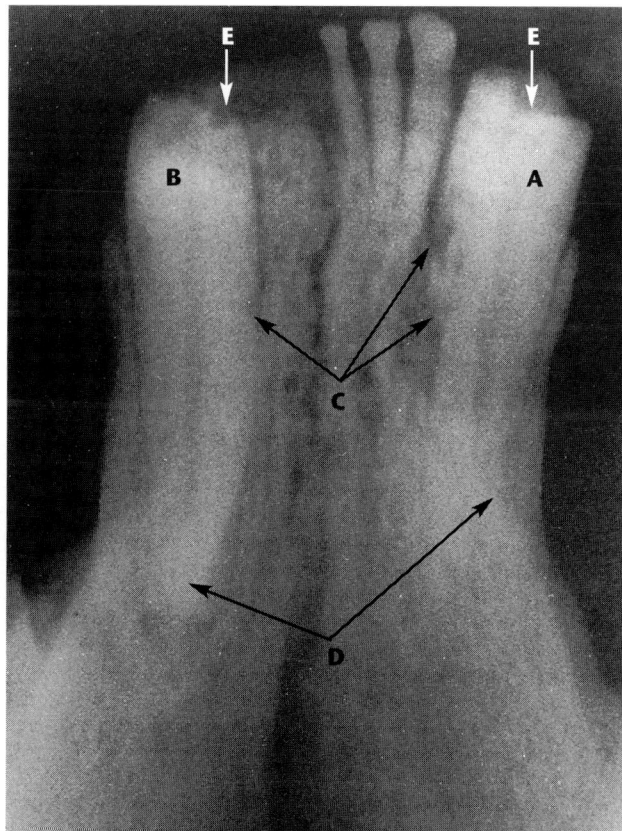

Diagnostic Keys: Chronic trauma with pulp exposure often causes this endo-periodontal problem. The diagnosis for apex lesions of the lower canine should not be confused with the presence of the mental foramen.

FIGURE 14.5

Contributing Author:
James M.G. Anthony

Description: Grade V periodontitis.

Points Identified: Lower fourth premolar (408) is almost displaced because of root resorption and calculus. The chronic inflammation caused resorption of the mesial root of the lower molar. The x-ray shows an irregular surface of the root structure and ankylosis at the apex due to no periodontal space. Loss of crestal bone with deep pockets to the apex is present. The root is covered with calculus deposits making differentiation of the root from calculus uneasy. The crestal bone on the mesial aspect is irregularly lucent.

  A. Difficult recognition of tooth shape
  B. Condensing osteitis
  C. Root resorption, unclear outline
  D. Ankylosis, mesial root 409

Diagnostic Keys: Periodontitis in an advanced stage leads to exfoliation or extraction if identified radiographically.

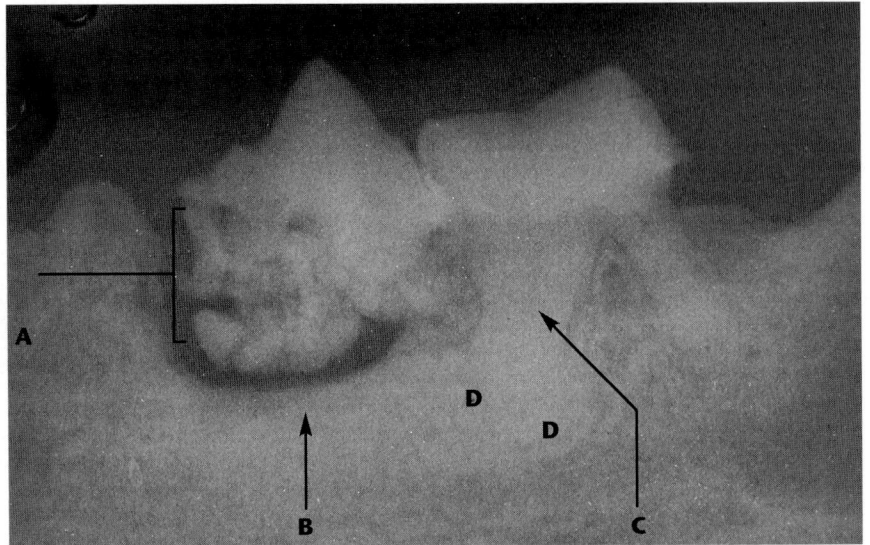

FIGURE 14.6

Contributing Author: Ayako Okuda

Description: Grade IV periodontal disease (see also Figure 14.7).

Points Identified: There is bone loss without external resorption from the distal side of the lower third premolar (307) to the mesial side of the lower molar (309), and both lower third premolars (307/407) have external resorption at the furcation. The cervical area of both the lower canines and the upper left canine was exposed. Hypercementosis can be found on apices of all premolars and molars.

A. Furcation lesion, 407
B. Mental foramen
C. Bone loss
D. Furcation lesion, 308
E. Odontoclastic resorptive lesion (ORL) and furcation lesion, 307

Diagnostic Keys: Severe inflammation of the gingiva and 50–75 percent destruction of the periodontal ligaments is present with marked tooth mobility and sulcus depth.

Common Errors: Acute osteomyelititis, malignant tumors, misdiagnosis.

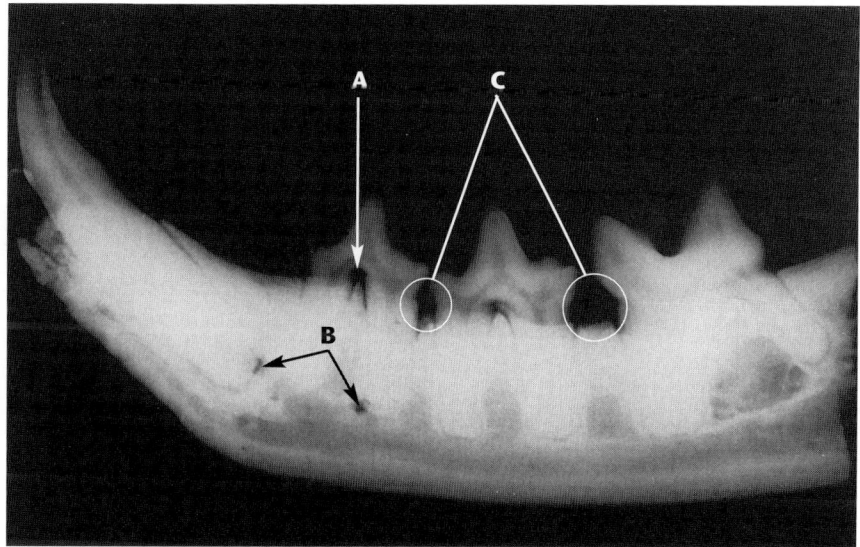

A

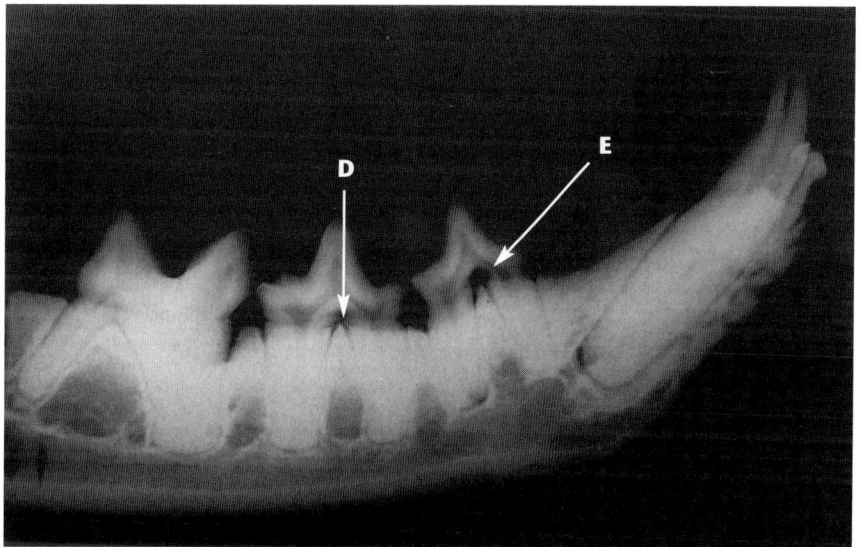

B

FIGURE 14.7

Contributing Author: Ayako Okuda

Description: Grade IV periodontal disease (see also Figure 14.6).

Points Identified: External resorptive lesions can be found at the furcations of the fourth premolar (308) in the left lower jaw and the third premolar (407) in the right lower jaw. They are associated with severe alveolar bone loss.

- A. Crestal bone loss
- B. Odontoclastic resorptive lesion (ORL) and furcation lesion
- C. Horizontal bone loss

Diagnostic Keys: Severe inflammation of the gingiva and 50–75 percent destruction of the periodontal ligaments is present with marked tooth mobility and sulcus depth.

Common Errors: Acute osteomyelitits, malignant tumors, misdiagnosis.

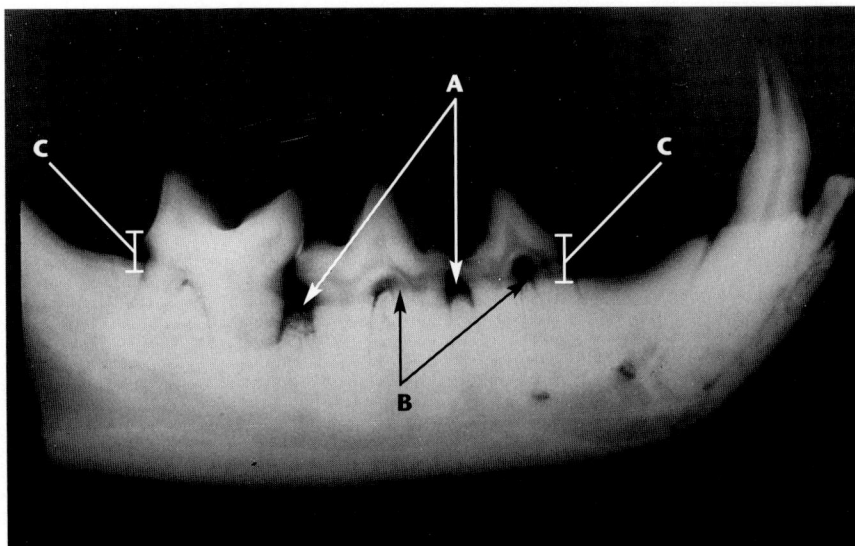

A

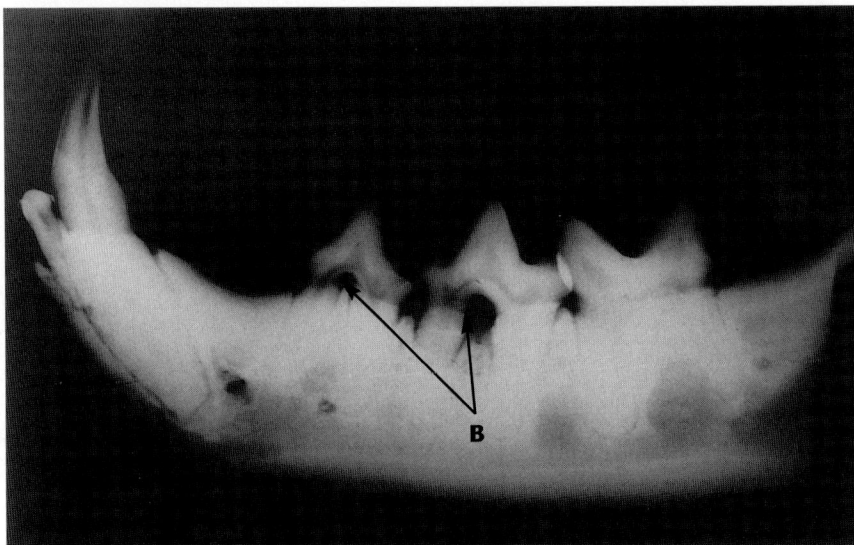

B

FIGURE 14.8

Contributing Author:
James M.G. Anthony

Description: Squamous cell carcinoma with canine fractures.

Points Identified: Radiolucency is extending to alveolar cortical buccal bone.

A. Porous, sponge-like texture of bone
B. Internal resorption
C. Root resorption

Diagnostic Keys: Most malignant tumors, especially squamous cell carcinoma, in the oral cavity furiously invade into alveolar bone because of their enormous migration. However, radiographs cannot indicate the types of tumors. Definite diagnosis should always be made after biopsy and histopathology.

Common Errors: Acute osteomyelitis, severe granuloma or other malignant tumors including odontogenic tumors and severe periodontal disease with gingival hyperplasia can be confused by radiographic interpretation alone.

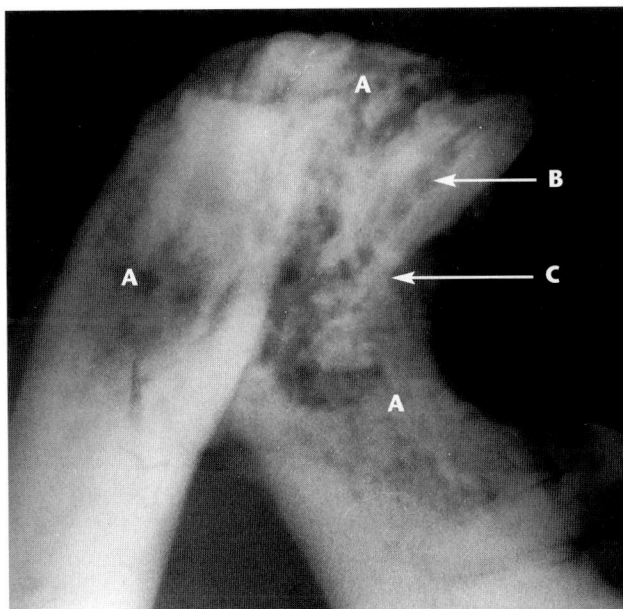

FIGURE 14.9

Contributing Author:
James M.G. Anthony

Description: Early periodontitis.

Points Identified: Gingival recession present on clinical exam, and horizontal bone loss can be seen on x-ray between the lower fourth premolar and the lower molar.

A. Horizontal bone loss

Diagnostic Keys: Immunosuppressive diseases whether bacterial or viral often cause severe gingivitis and/or stomatitis. In advanced stages, periodontal tissue loss and alveolar bone loss can be found, but not always associated with identifiable changes in the x-ray images.

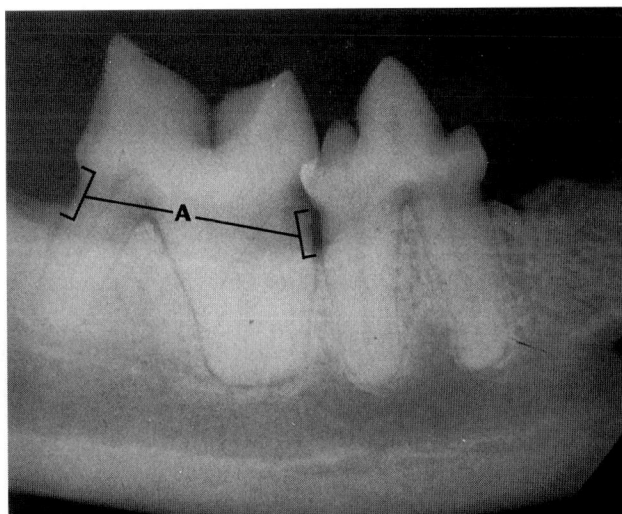

FIGURE 14.10

Contributing Authors:
Ayako Okuda and James M.G. Anthony

Description: Gingivitis/stomatitis.

Points Identified: (View A) Mild horizontal bone loss on the lower molar with hypercementosis of apices of the lower fourth premolar (308) and molar (309).

(View B) Infrabony pocket and root resorption on the lower second and third incisors. Supereruption and calculus on the root of the lower right canine (404). Irregularity on the alveolar bone of lower right canine suggested localization of osteomyelitis.

A. 308
B. 309
C. 404
D. External resorption
E. Horizontal bone loss
F. Early resorption
G. Crestal bone loss
H. Infrabony pocket

Diagnostic Keys: Gingivitis/stomatitis is not a periodontal disease with identifiable changes in the x-ray images. Alveolar bone loss in view A radiograph is not a specific sign of gingivitis/stomatitis. Radiographical changes in view B radiograph are signs of complications of periodontitis.

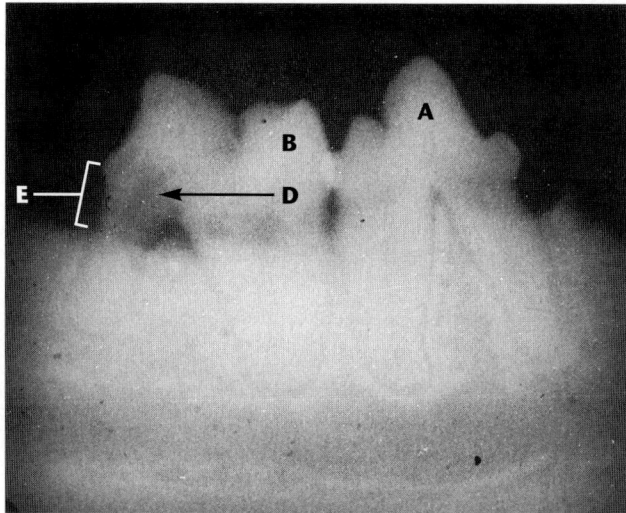

A

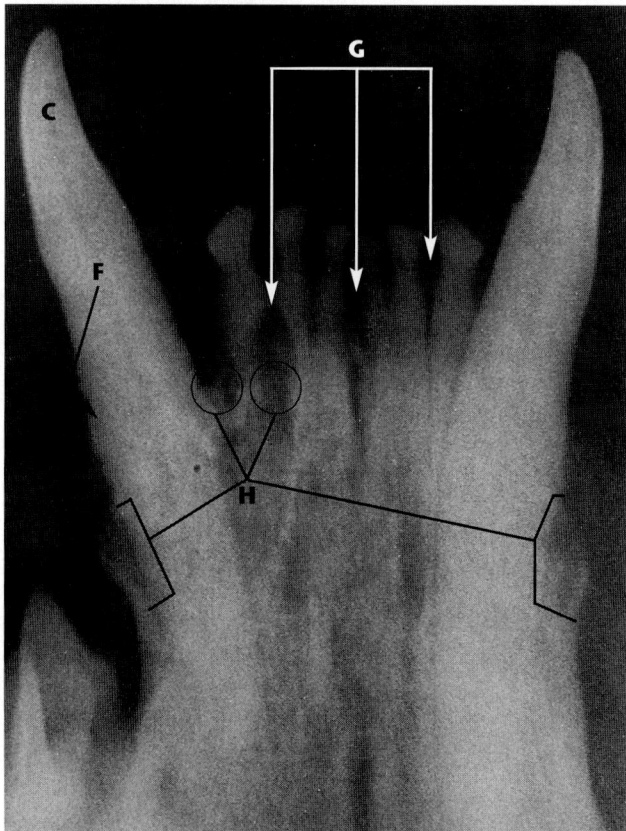

B

FIGURE 14.11

Contributing Author:
James M.G. Anthony

Description: Osteolysis.

Points Identified: Radiolucency is extending into the incisal regions of alveolar bone.

    A. Increased lucency

Diagnostic Keys: Severe periodontal disease, osteomyelitis, malignant tumors, and metabolic disorders can mimic changes seen in this x-ray. Excess parathyroid hormones enhance calcium metabolism, both of bone resorption and bone formation. However, trabecular structures in spongy bone become fragile, and cortical bone turns porous because resorption takes place prior to the formation of bone. Definitive diagnosis should always be made after several tests: serum assay for T_3 and T_4; serum level of calcium; renal profile; parathyroid assay; incisional biopsy; and radiologic exam of the skeletal system. Histopathology is confirmatory if testing is inconclusive.

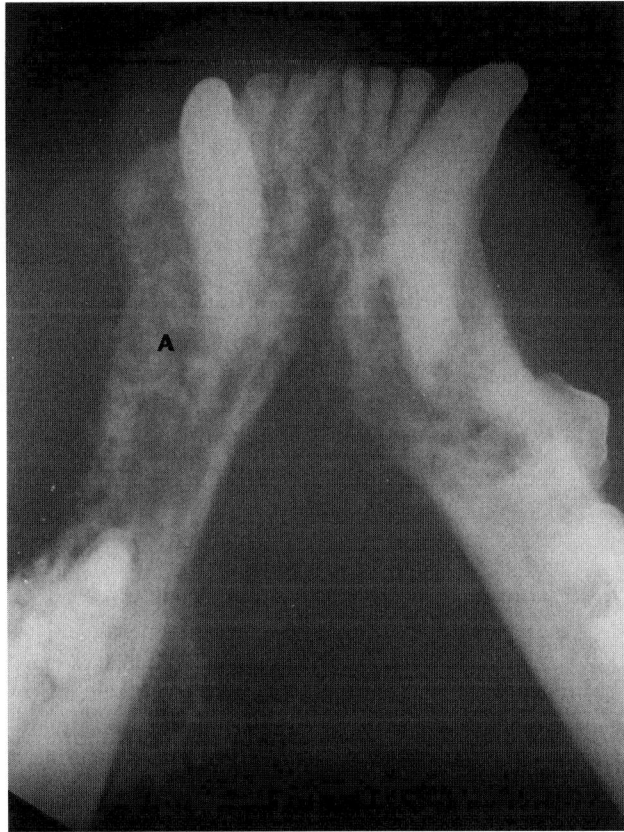

FIGURE 14.12

Contributing Author:

James M.G. Anthony

Description: Grade II periodontal disease.

Points Identified: There are no obvious changes in hard tissue, but attachment loss has been started at the interdental crest of alveolar bone. Besides the slight bone loss of mild periodontal disease, external resorption appears in the cervical area of 309 under the distal and mesial cusps of the lower molar, as indicated by radiolucency.

A. Slight bone loss (horizontal)
B. Horizontal bone loss
C. Odontoclastic resorptive lesion (external resorption), 309

Diagnostic Keys: Non–x-ray soft tissue changes would indicate moderate inflammation in the gingiva and minimal attachment loss. There are no obvious changes in the bone structure on x-ray.

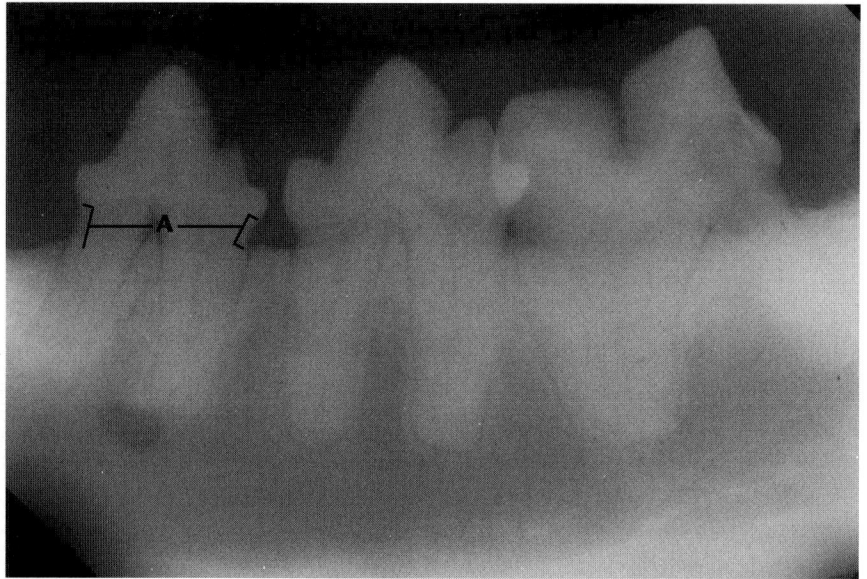

A

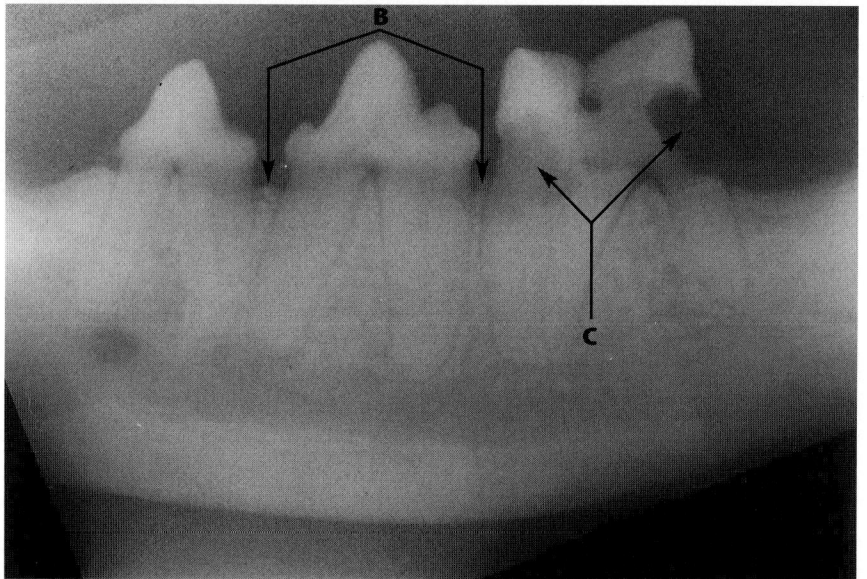

B

FIGURE 14.13

Contributing Author:
James M.G. Anthony

Description: Grades III and IV periodontitis.

Points Identified: Alveolar bone loss in the lower fourth premolar (308), at the interdental alveolar crest between the third premolar (307) and the fourth premolar (308) as well as in the furcation is clear. The cervical region of upper canine (104) is also exposed, indicating early bone loss.

    A. Bony recession, 104
    B. Horizontal bone loss
    C. Furcation lesions

Diagnostic Keys: Established inflammation reveals gingival hyperplasia or recession and attachment loss of 30–50 percent of the periodontal ligament with moderate tooth mobility, which may cause wider periodontal space.

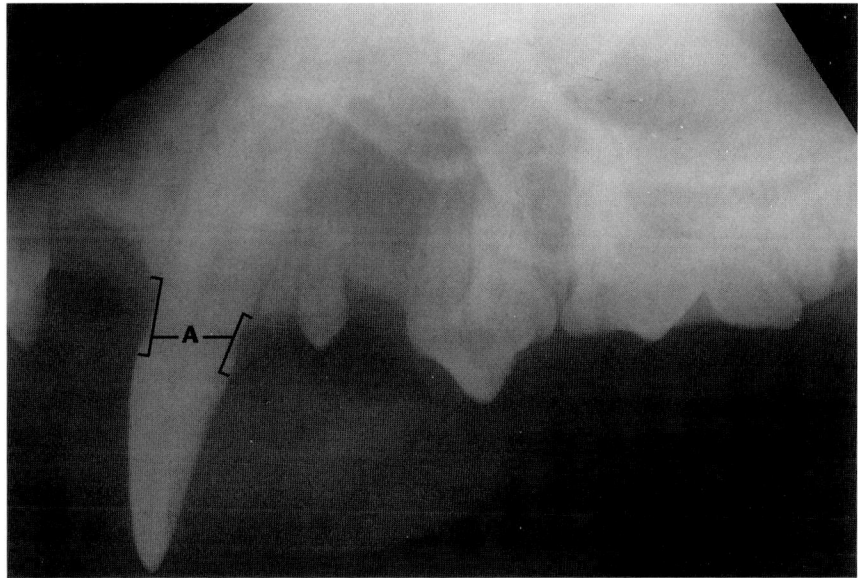

A

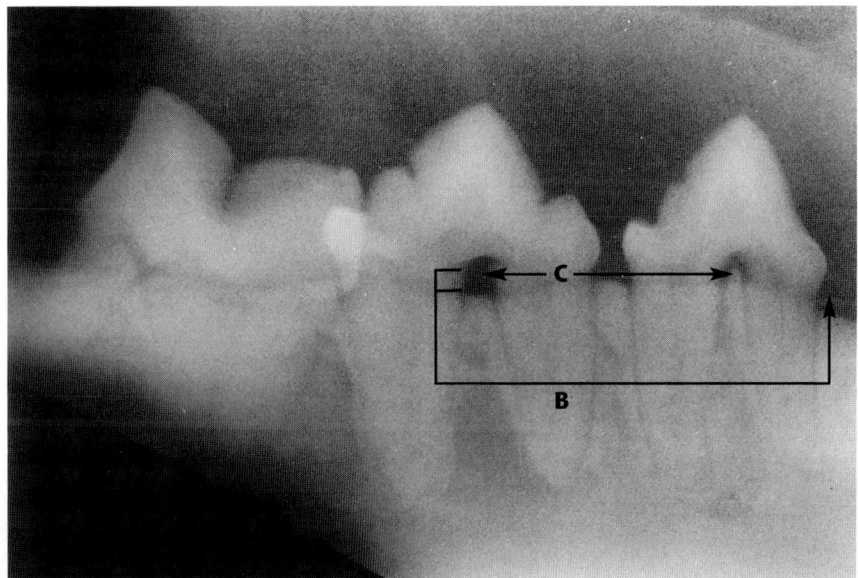

B

FIGURE 14.14

Contributing Author: Ayako Okuda

Description: Grade V periodontitis.

Points Identified: (View A) Root fragments of the fourth premolar (408) and the molar (409) in the mandibular bone remain and are associated with a hypertrophic bone reaction, with exostosis present, around the predisplaced third premolar (407). The root of the lower canine has been partly resorbed and ankylosed.

(View B) Root fragments of the second and third premolars (106, 107) remain in the maxillary bone, and calculus has accumulated heavily on the upper fourth premolar (108). The cementoenamel junction of the upper canine tooth (204) was exposed. This is associated with horizontal bone loss, and the root of the canine (204) has ankylosed, judged by the lack of periodontal ligament space.

A. Exostosis
B. Bony cervical recession, cervical 404
C. Unclear periodontal ligament outline, 404
D. Unfilled bone tissue
E. Root fragments, 408, 409
F. Calculus, 108
G. Unclear periodontal ligament outline
H. Bony cervical recession, cervical 204

Diagnostic Keys: With periodontitis in advanced stages, teeth should be removed. Many foramina in the skull are easily misunderstood as cystic lesions.

Common Errors: Limited radiolucency close to the root apices of the right and the left canine and between the lower fourth premolar and the molar can be found, but not necessarily for identification of periodontal disease.

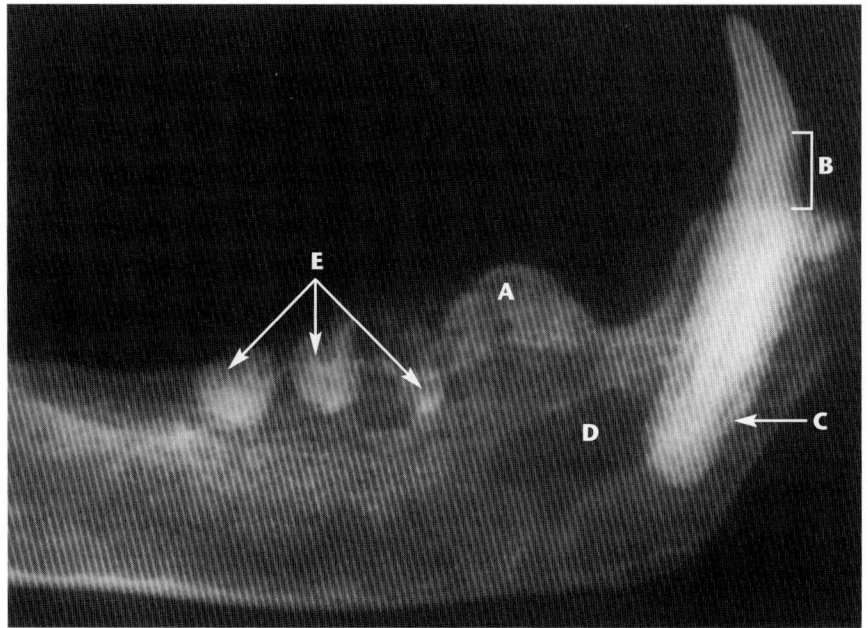

A

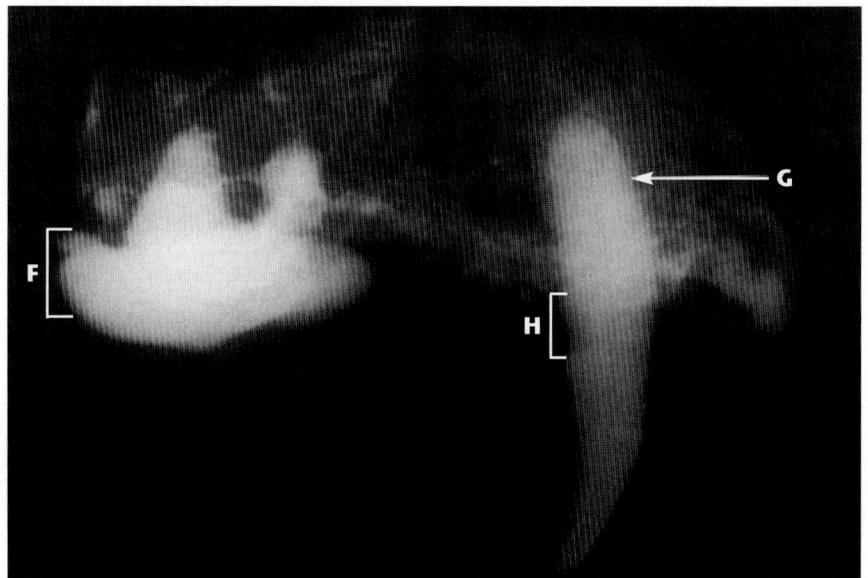

B

FIGURE 14.15

Contributing Authors:
Kenneth F. Lyon and Chris J. Visser

Description: Mandibular molar 309.

Points Identified: Lesion extending through the dentin into the pulp chamber in the area of the cementoenamel junction of the mesial root of 309. Radiopacity in furcation area and at the root apex of the distal root of 309. Loss of periodontal membrance space, 309. Evidence of significant resorption, 307. Note that the soft tissue coronal to the mandible represents the lip margin.

A. Odontoclastic resorptive lesion, mesial root 309
B. Radiopacity, furcation area, 309
C. Radiopacity, apex of distal root, 309
D. Loss of periodontal membrane space, 309
E. 307

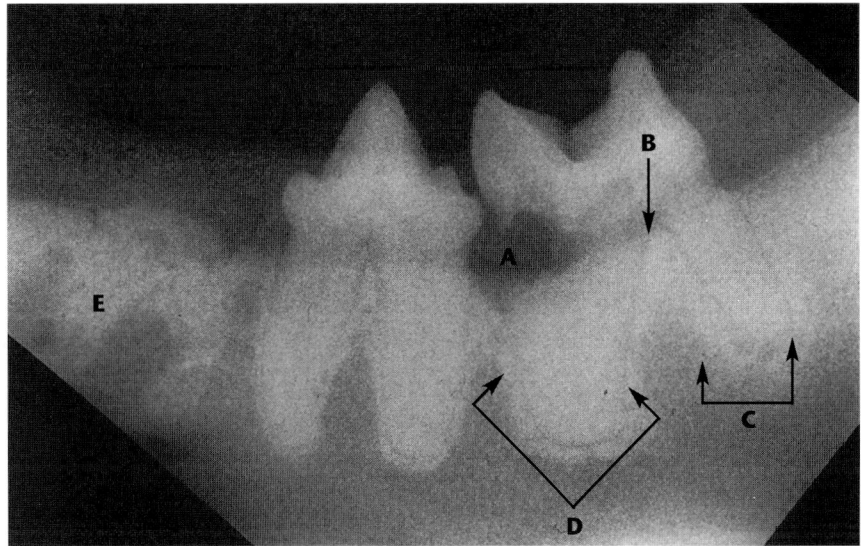

FIGURE 14.16

Contributing Authors:
Kenneth F. Lyon and Chris J. Visser

Description: Mandibular molar 309, mandibular premolar 307.

Points Identified: 309: Resorption of distal root and distal cusp. Loss of periodontal membrane space. Remnant of the apex of the distal root. Sclerotic alveolar crestal bone present. Pulp chamber in the molar not evident (pulp obliteration). Root apex of mesial root has radiopacity.

307: Horizontal bone loss of the alveolar crest with extrusion (supereruption). Resorptive lesions present on the mesial root. Sclerotic alveolar crestal bone present. Periapical lesions present, with obliteration of the periodontal membrane space. The mental foramen evident.

A. Resorption of distal root and distal cusp, 309
B. Remnant of apex of distal root, 309
C. Radiopacity of root apex, mesial root, 309
D. Mental foramen
E. Horizontal bone loss of alveolar crest with extrusion (supereruption), 307

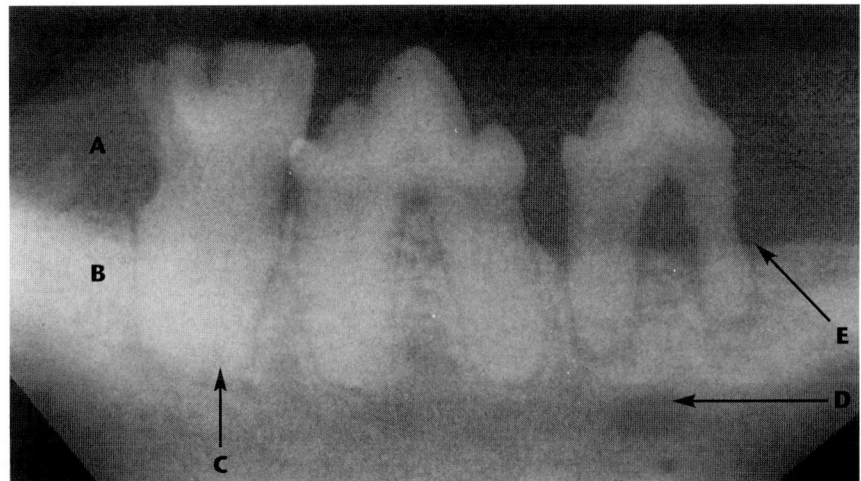

FIGURE 14.17

Contributing Authors:
Kenneth F. Lyon and Chris J. Visser

Description: Maxillary third premolar, 107.

Points Identified: Note loss of distal root structure and focal sclerosing osteomyelitis or osteosclerosis. Resorption is significant, with extension through dentin and the pulp chamber.

A. Resorption extending through dentin and pulp chamber, 107

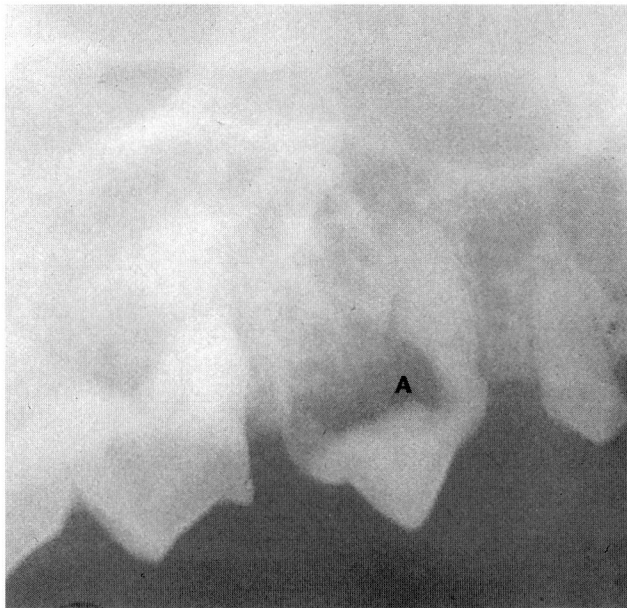

FIGURE 14.18

Contributing Authors:
Kenneth F. Lyon and Chris J. Visser

Description: Mandibular third premolar 407.

Points Identified: Note focal sclerosing osteomyelitis present at the tooth location and normal root structure of the remaining teeth.

A. Tooth structure is not evident
B. Alveolar crestal bone showing exostosis over the tooth site

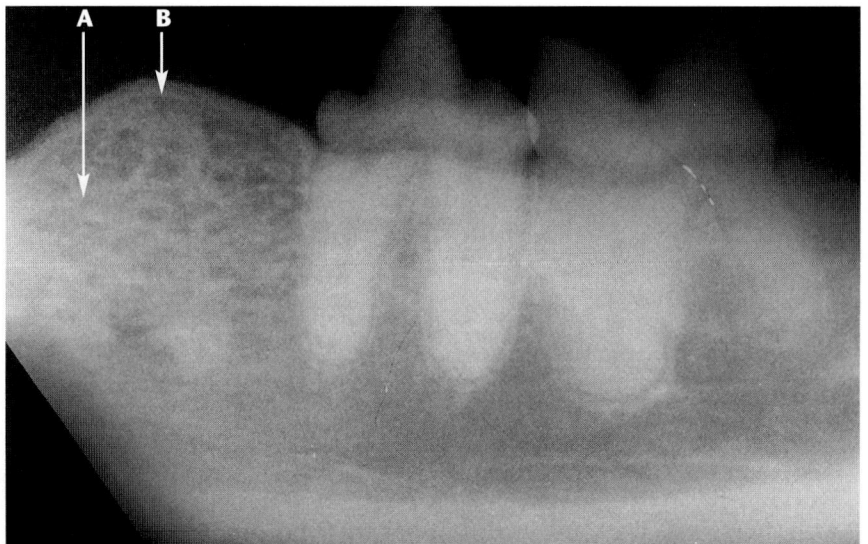

FIGURE 14.19

Contributing Authors:
Kenneth F. Lyon and Chris J. Visser

Description: Mandibular fourth premolar 408.

Points Identified: Note that resorption extends deep into the dentin of the roots.

  A. Mesial crown surface with resorptive lesion (ORL) extending through the dentin into the pulp chamber
  B. Resorption of distal root with ankylosis
  C. Resorption of mesial root with significant focal osteomyelitis
  D. Sclerosing osteomyelitis at site of third premolar (407, lost)

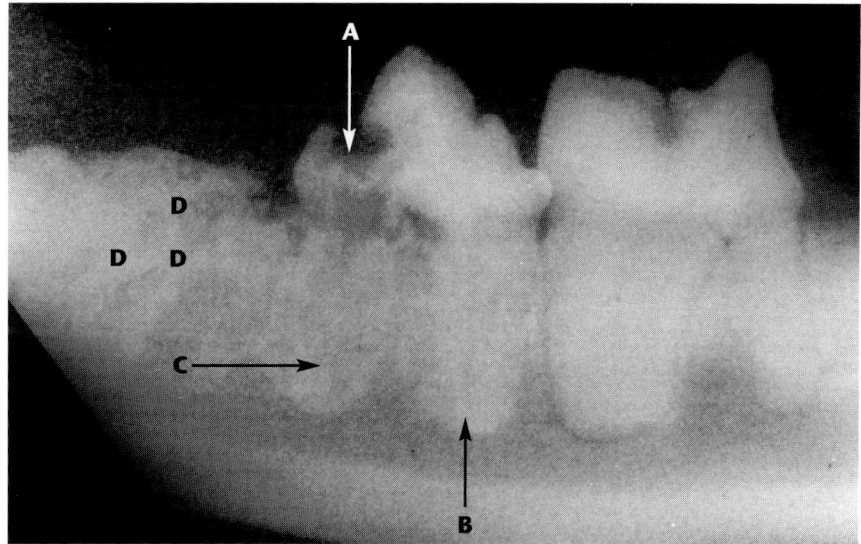

FIGURE 14.20

Contributing Authors:
Kenneth F. Lyon and Chris J. Visser

Description: Maxillary canine 104.

Points Identified: Crown tip has been lost to fracture. No evidence of sclerosing osteomyelitis.

  A. Apical resorption secondary to an endodontically compromised tooth
  B. Note wider pulp canal 104, indicating pulp death at an immature stage of dentinogenesis

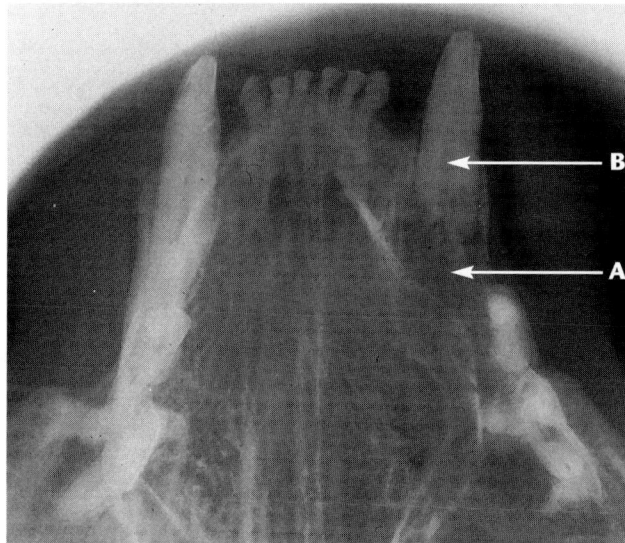

FIGURE 14.21

Contributing Authors:
Kenneth F. Lyon and Chris J. Visser

Description: Mandibular canine 304.

Points Identified: Loss of periodontal membrane space and presence of ankylosis. Subgingival resorptive lesion at the cemento-enamel junction area. Osteomyelitis extends across the rostral mandible.

    A. Lost crown, 304
    B. Resorptive lesion, 304
    C. Ankylosis
    D. Osteomyelitis

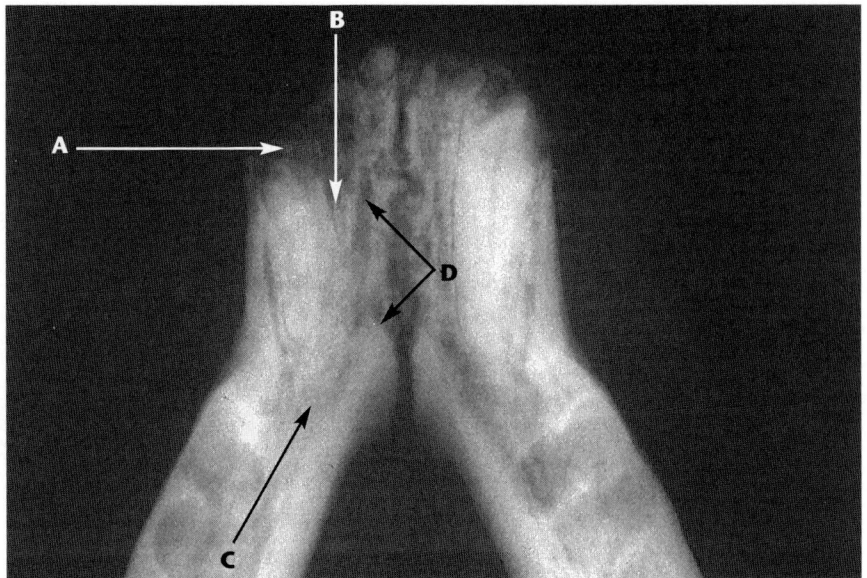

FIGURE 14.22

Contributing Authors:
Kenneth F. Lyon and Chris J. Visser

Description: Mandibular canines and incisors.

Points Identified: Complete resorption of canine and incisor root structures. Extensive osteomyelitis in the symphyseal area. Note that one central incisor is missing.

    A. Complete resorption of the canine root structures
    B. Osteomyelitis
    C. Resorptive lesion extending into the canine crown

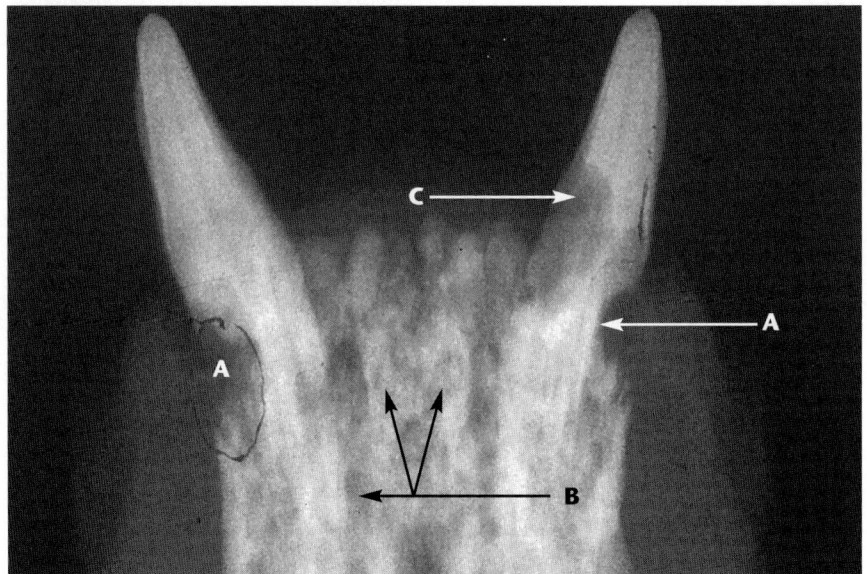

FIGURE 14.23

Contributing Authors:
Kenneth F. Lyon and Chris J. Visser

Description: Mandibular third and fourth premolars (307/308).

Points Identified: Condensing osteomyelitis is present.

A. Resorption of mesial root and furcation area, 307
B. Resorption separating the root apex of the mesial root, 307
C. Resorption of distal root 308, resulting in club-like root apex
D. Vertical alveolar bone loss at distal roots 308 and 309
E. Root resorption, mesial root, 309
F. Condensing osteomyelitis

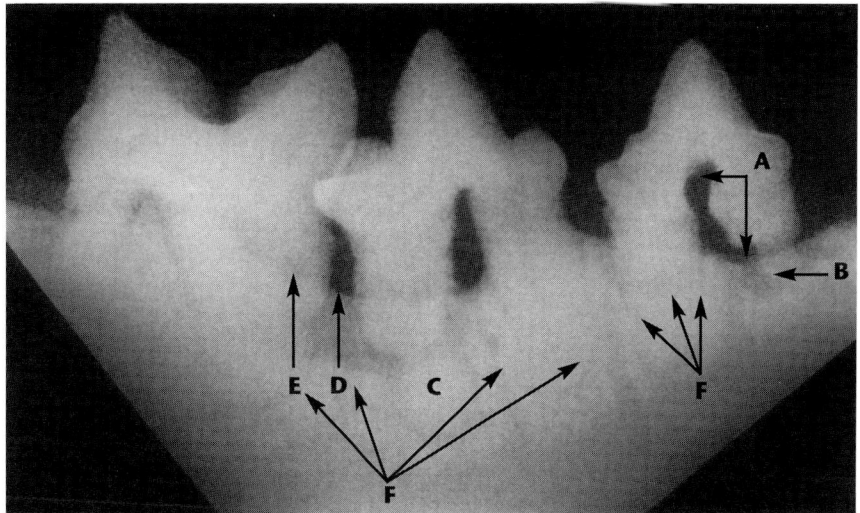

FIGURE 14.24

Contributing Authors:
Kenneth F. Lyon and Chris J. Visser

Description: Mandibular molar 309.

Points Identified: Apical portions of the molar roots. Sharp bur lines showing an attempt to remove tooth structure with a high speed bur. Also note obliteration of periodontal membrane spaces and presence of minimal sclerosis.

A. 309, remaining apical portions of molar
B. 307 (missing)

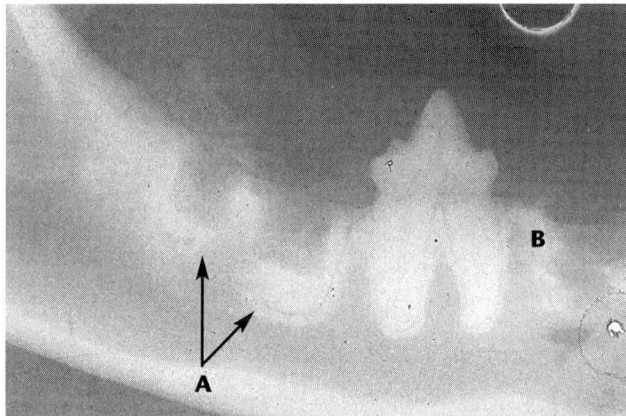

FIGURE 14.25

Contributing Authors:
Kenneth F. Lyon and Chris J. Visser

Description: Maxillary third premolar 207.

Points Identified: On 207 note root resorption at furcation area extending into crown and loss of periodontal ligament space. Also note missing second premolar (206) and resorptive lesion at the furcation of the fourth premolar (208). X-ray tube head for this radiograph was positioned for root elongation to avoid zygomatic arch superimposition over roots.

- A. 206 (missing)
- B. 207
- C. 208
- D. Loss of alveolar bone at fourth premolar (208) with root and furcation exposure
- E. Resorptive lesion at furcation of fourth premolar (208)

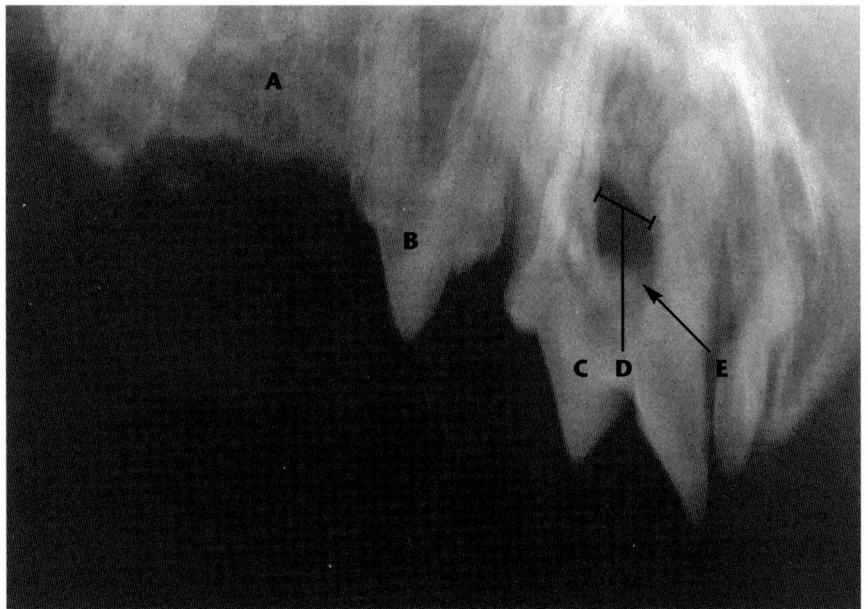

FIGURE 14.26

Contributing Author:
Kenneth F. Lyon and Chris J. Visser

Description: Maxillary molar 109.

Points Identified:

- A. Loss of crown of maxillary molar (109)
- B. Resorption of distal root of fourth premolar (108)
- C. Remnant of root in sclerotic bone of canine (104)
- D. Missing second premolar (106)

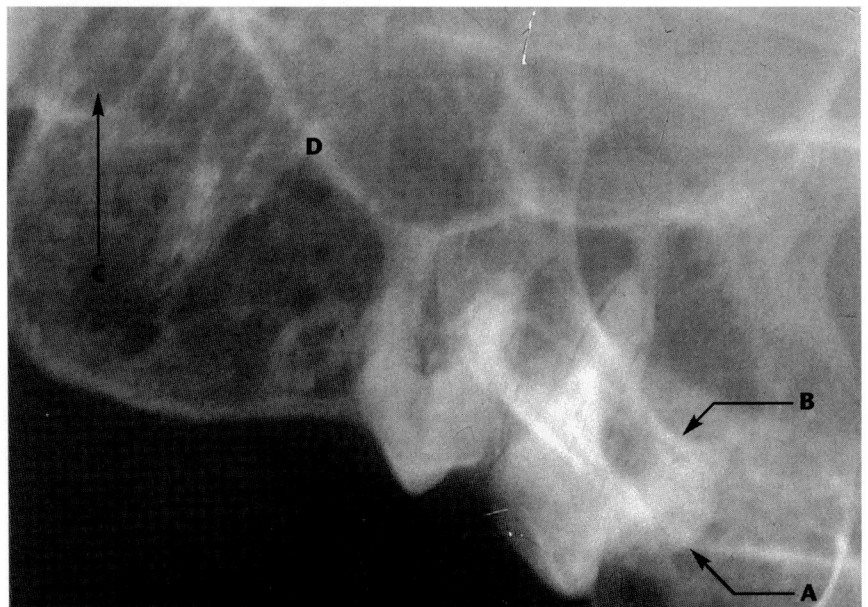

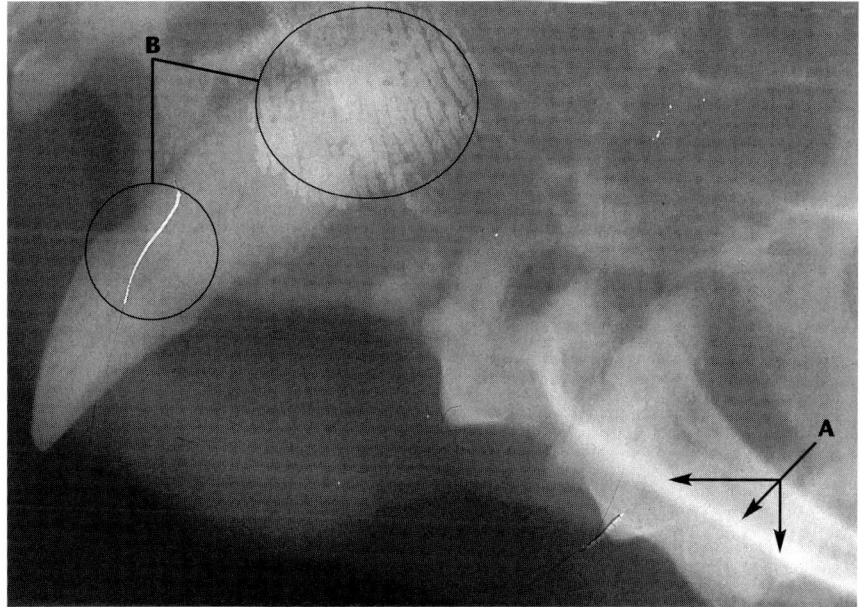

FIGURE 14.27

Contributing Author:
Kenneth F. Lyon and Chris J. Visser

Description: Maxillary fourth premolar 208.

Points Identified: Note loss of periodontal ligament space.

  A. Zygomatic arch overlying roots of third and fourth premolars(207/208)
  B. Artifact over apex of 104 (fingerprint) and scratch mark in body of tooth

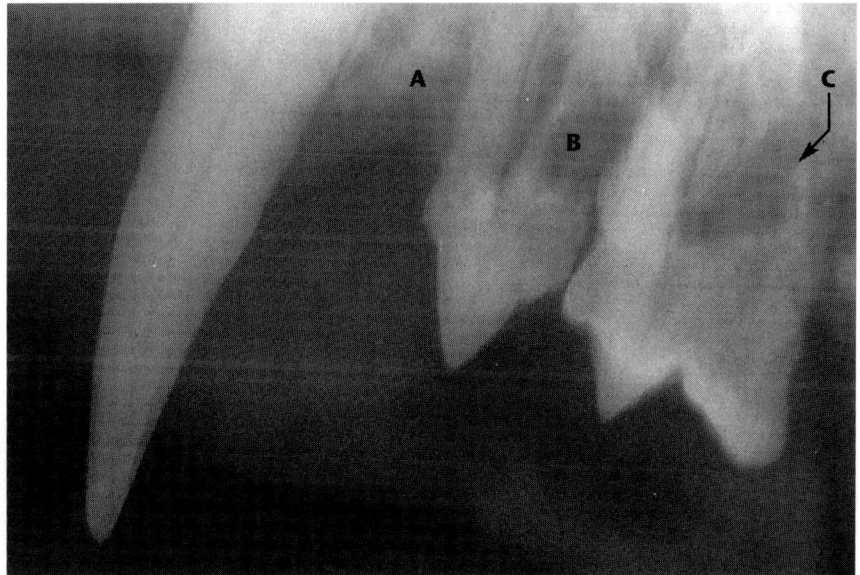

FIGURE 14.28

Contributing Authors:
Kenneth F. Lyon and Chris J. Visser

Description: Maxillary third premolar 207.

Points Identified: Note specific elongation of roots to avoid zygomatic arch superimposition.

  A. 206 (missing)
  B. 207, resorption of distal root
  C. 208, resorption of distal root

FIGURE 14.29

Contributing Authors:
Kenneth F. Lyon and Chris J. Visser

Description: Maxillary canine 104.

Points Identified:

A. Root remnants of both canines with sclerosing osteomyelitis
B. Missing lateral incisor

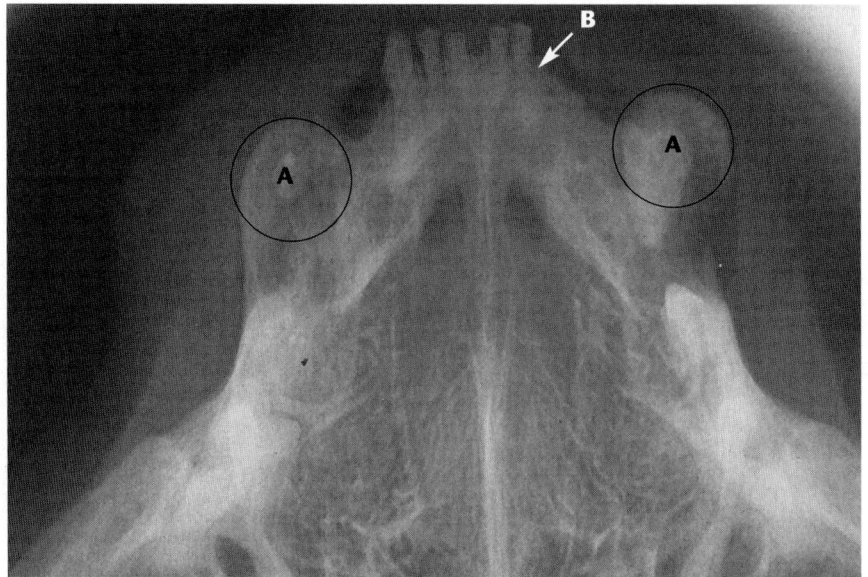

FIGURE 14.30

Contributing Authors:
Kenneth F. Lyon and Chris J. Visser

Description: Maxillary canine.

Points Identified: Note mild root resorption with ankylosis in 104.

A. 204, loss of crown tip
B. 104, deep resorption (ORL) at cementoenamel junction and extending into pulp canal
C. Sclerotic bone in incisor area with resorption of incisors

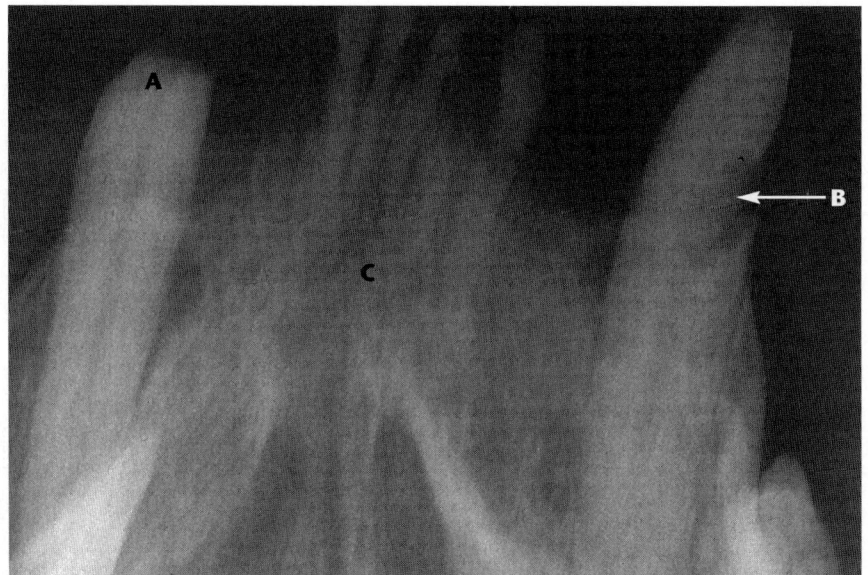

FIGURE 14.31

Contributing Authors:
Kenneth F. Lyon and Chris J. Visser

Description: Maxillary canine 104.

Points Identified:

A. Root remnant of canine tooth (104)

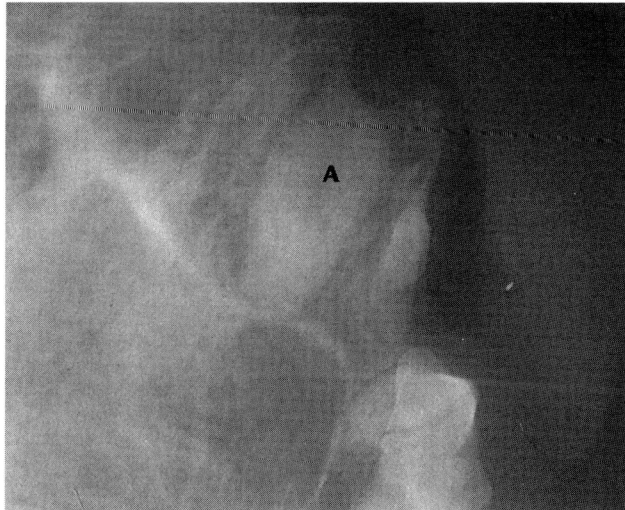

FIGURE 14.32

Contributing Authors:
Kenneth F. Lyon and Chris J. Visser

Description: Mandibular canines.

Points Identified:

A. 304, internal pulp lysis caused by bacterial migration in the pulp canal
B. Periapical radiolucent areas

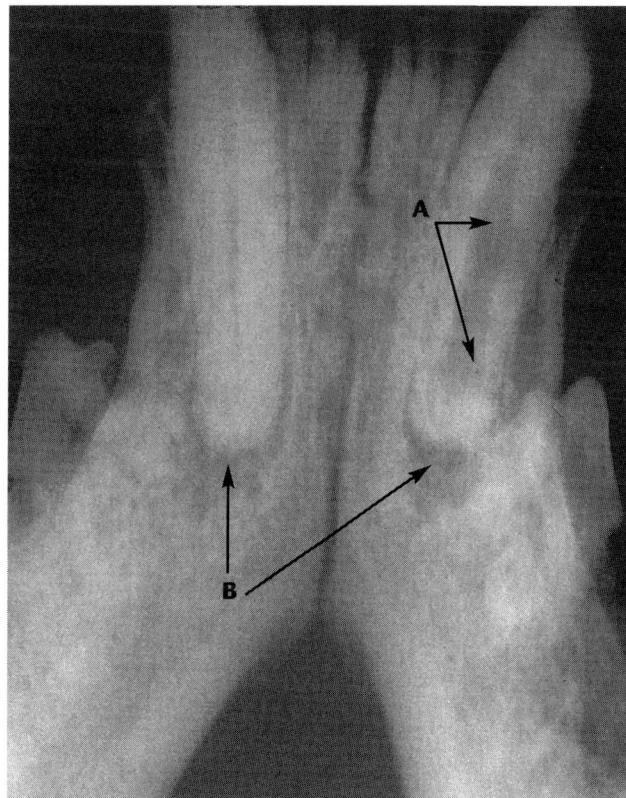

FIGURE 14.33

Contributing Authors:
Kenneth F. Lyon and Chris J. Visser

Description: Mandibular canines.

Points Identified:

A. Advanced internal and external resorption of the canine teeth
B. Sclerotic bone with ankylosis of root remnants
C. Exostosis at third premolar areas where these teeth have been lost to resorption

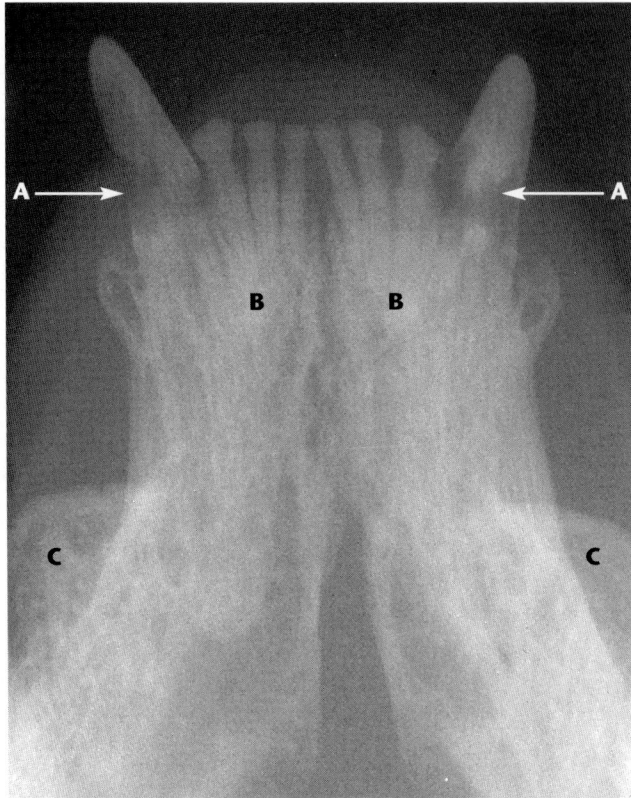

FIGURE 14.34

Contributing Authors:
Kenneth F. Lyon and Chris J. Visser

Description: Mandibular third premolar 307.

Points Identified:

A. Supereruption of third premolar (307)
B. Resorption of distal root of third premolar (307)
C. Periodontal pocket at distal root, 307
D. Resorption 308 and 309 root apices
E. Vertical bone loss, mesial root 309

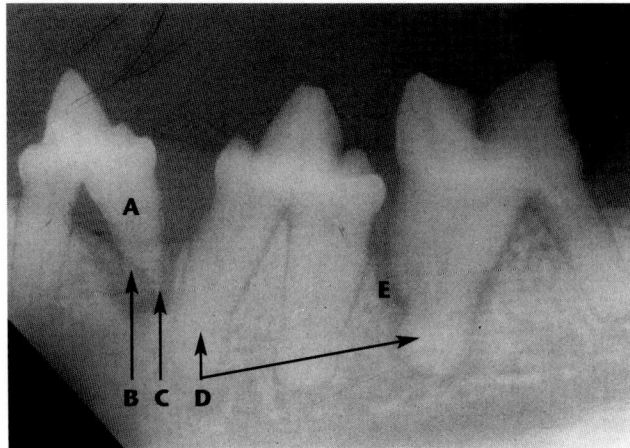

PART THREE

Film Problems

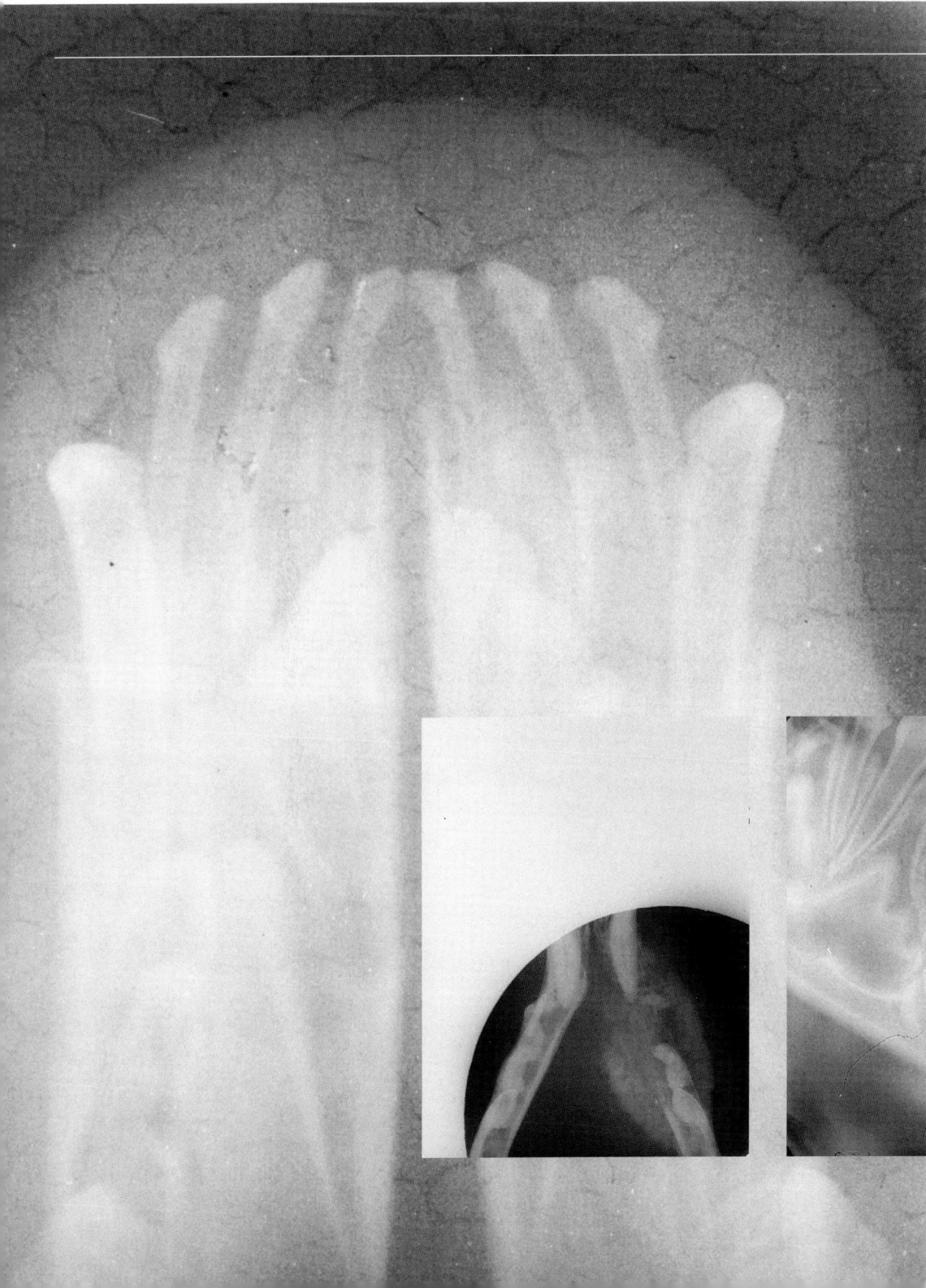

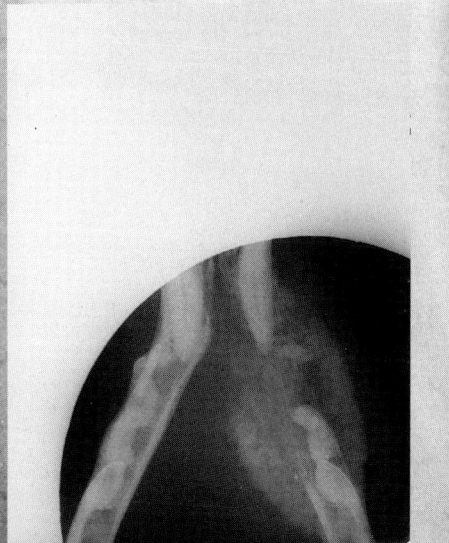

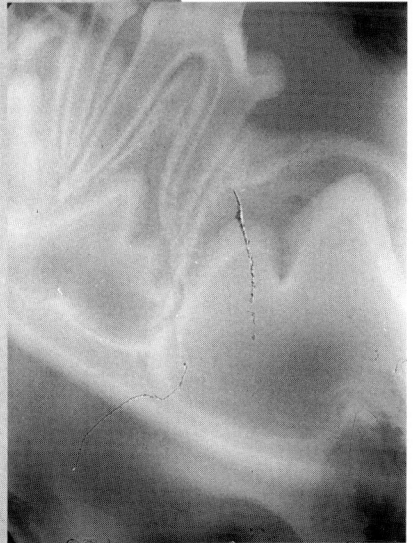

15 Film Artifacts, Visual Illusions, and Technical Errors

Dr. Edward R. Eisner

With contributions by
Linda Klippert, CVT
Katherine A. Jennings, CVT

INTRODUCTION

Radiography is one of the most important diagnostic tools in veterinary dentistry. The astute veterinary dentist can distinguish between artifact and anatomical structure. Faulty technique, foreign matter, and unavoidable technicalities which alter the radiographic image must be identifiable, both so that the clinician can correctly interpret pathology and so that he can improve documentation by correction of the faulty image. Treatment planning depends on accurate interpretation. Gordon J. Christensen, DDS, PhD, Senior Consultant of Clinical Research Associates, Provo, Utah, stated before 2200 dentists at the midwinter meeting in Denver in January 1995 that 25 percent of the intraoral radiographs taken in American dental offices are not legally defensible. It behooves veterinary dentists to hone their radiographic techniques and sharpen their interpretive skills.

A radiographic artifact is a blemish or image in the radiograph that is not present in the roentgen image of the object. In this chapter, examples of unsatisfactory radiographs are collected in four groups: film artifacts and technical errors, visual illusions, materials and foreign objects, and miscellaneous artifacts. Each artifact is identified, and its cause and remedy, if it is not obvious, are briefly explained. With this chapter as a reference, the reader should be able to identify and correct many of the technical radiographic errors which are inherent in the conduct of a busy dental practice.

This chapter shows many unsatisfactory radiographs with the goals of both raising awareness by identification and improving radiographic technique by attention to detail. Notations have been inserted to help prevent as well as evaluate many artifacts and anatomical illusions frequently seen in clinical practice. To practice successful veterinary dentistry, one must possess familiarity with radiographic anatomy, the fundamentals of radiology, and the pathology of dental disease.

X-RAY PLATES

Film Artifacts and Technical Errors

FIGURE 15.1

Contributing Author: Edward R. Eisner

Description: Elongation of the tooth. Positional errors caused by radiographic unit, film, or the patient. In this case elongation is caused by excess positive vertical angulation.

Remedy: Reduce the positive vertical angulation. When the x-ray beam is perpendicular to the tooth axis, this causes the tooth to be elongated. This subject is a 12-year-old standard poodle and shows 107, 108, 109, and 110. It is important to utilize the bisecting angle technique by positioning the primary beam consistently with the same angulation relative to the tooth and the film so that the progress of a condition can be accurately assessed at sequential recall appointments.

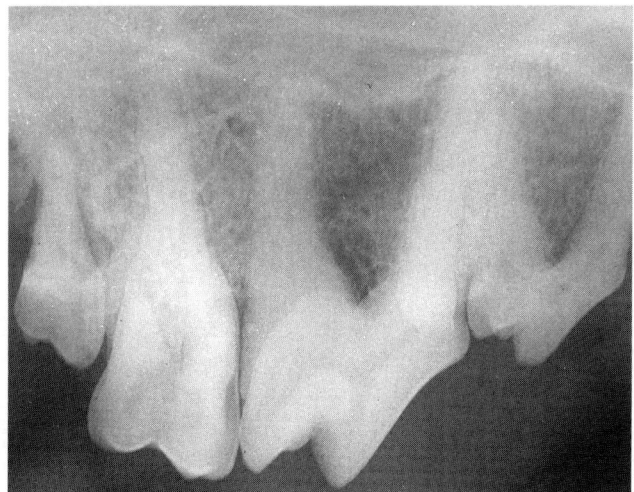

FIGURE 15.2

Contributing Author: Edward R. Eisner

Description: Foreshortening because of inadequate positive vertical angulation.

Remedy: Increase the positive vertical angulation. When the x-ray beam is perpendicular to the film axis, the tooth is foreshortened. Premolar 108 of an 8-year-old Shetland sheepdog is pictured here. The distal root of 108 appears much shorter than it actually is. Molar 109 is seen in occlusal projection.

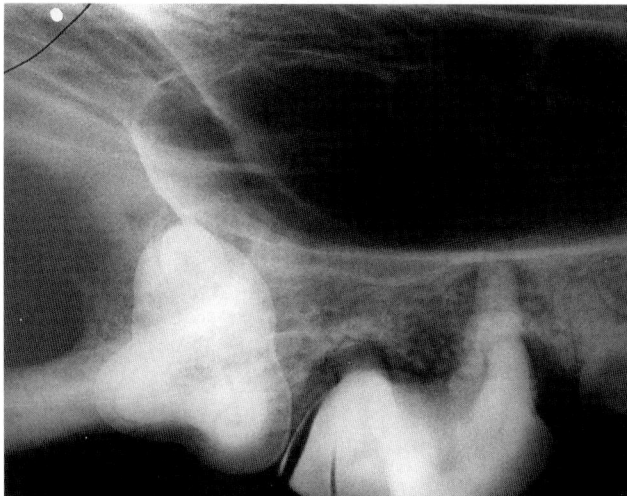

FIGURE 15.3

Contributing Author: Edward R. Eisner

Description: Foreshortening because of inadequate positive vertical angulation.

Remedy: Increase the positive vertical angulation. In this radiograph of a 6-year-old mastiff/Labrador mix, the entire maxillary canine appears much shorter than it actually is in this film of a separated file tip. Poor positioning jeopardizes the effectiveness of treatment planning.

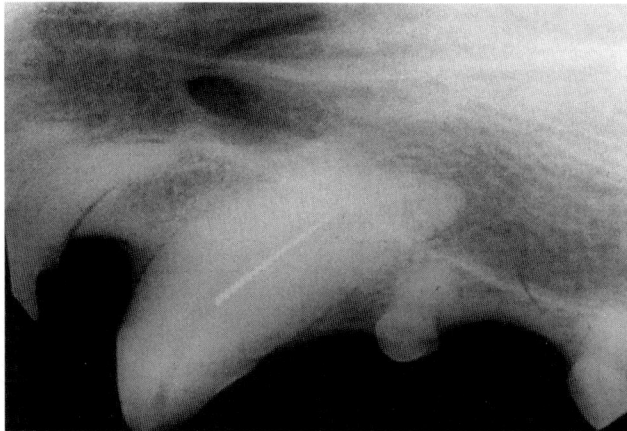

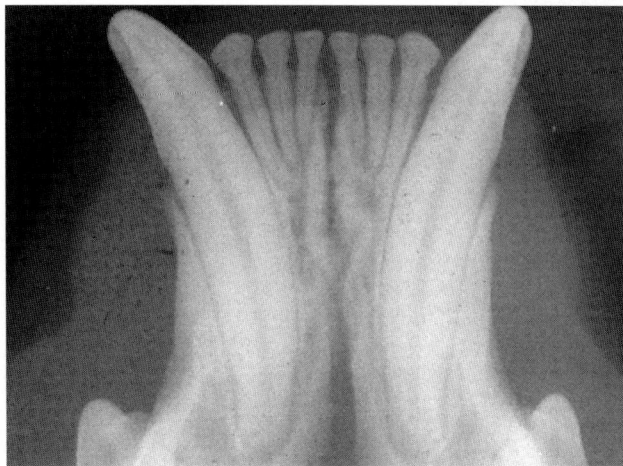

A

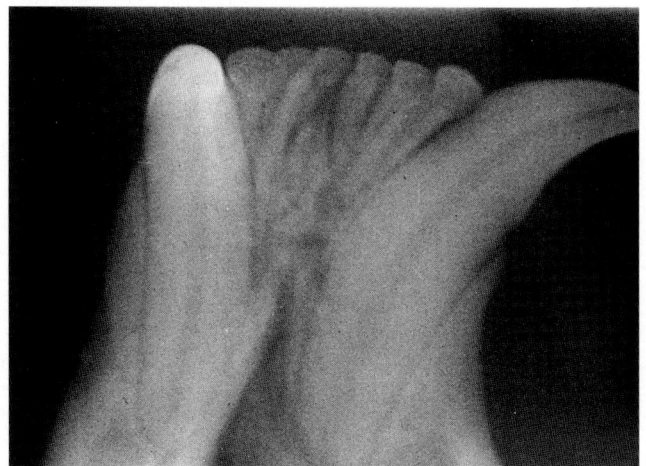

B

FIGURE 15.4

Contributing Author: Edward R. Eisner

Description: View A, good positioning 404; view B, oblique angle 404.

Remedy: Double-check for correct relationship between the primary beam and the tooth. An oblique angle is not always an error. Many times an oblique angle is taken to allow an additional view for a definitive diagnosis.

In this 3-year-old domestic shorthair feline, one can see the difference between good positioning and an oblique angle of the mandibular canine tooth (404).

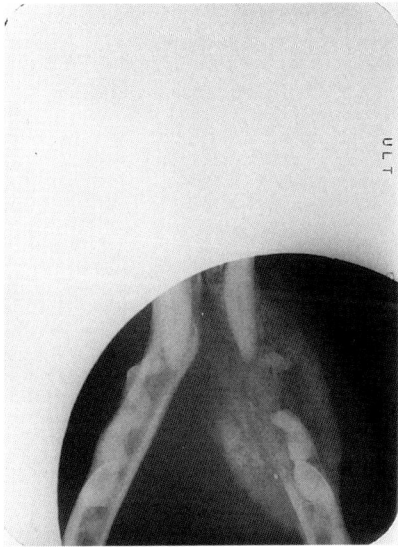

FIGURE 15.5

Contributing Author: Edward R. Eisner

Description: Cone cut. The primary beam may not be centered on the area of interest.

Remedy: Position the cone/collimator so that the x-rays cover the film. This is a good quality dental film of a domestic shorthair feline. The collimator is centered on the area of interest, the osteosarcoma in the mandible, but using a smaller film would have been more efficient.

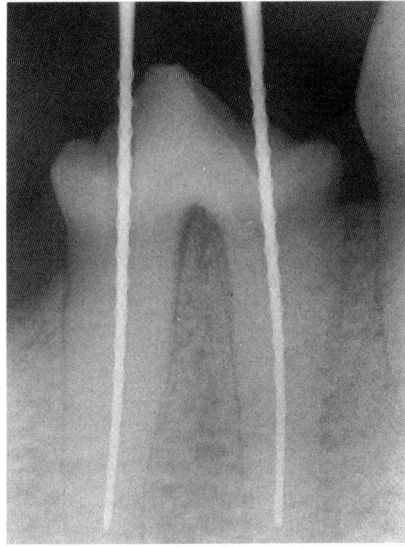

FIGURE 15.6

Contributing Author: Edward R. Eisner

Description: Failure to place the film sufficiently apically has caused inadequate periapical coverage.

Remedy: Move the film farther from the tooth, or reduce the positive vertical angle of the bisecting angle technique. The subject of this film is a 5-year-old golden retriever mix. In this radiograph, root apices cannot be visualized for endodontic evaluation. Often the mandibular vestibule is too shallow to permit parallel radiographic technique, which then necessitates the use of the bisecting angle technique.

FIGURE 15.7

Contributing Author: Edward R. Eisner

Description: Adumbration (poor edge definition of an image on an x-ray film due to crossover x-rays): cervical burn-out, seen as a geometric lack of sharpness of x-ray shadow where the crown meets the root of 104.

Remedy: Correct the horizontal angle to be more perpendicular to the facial surface of the tooth. In this film of an 8-year-old golden retriever, there is reduced sharpness of the image of the cervical region of 104.

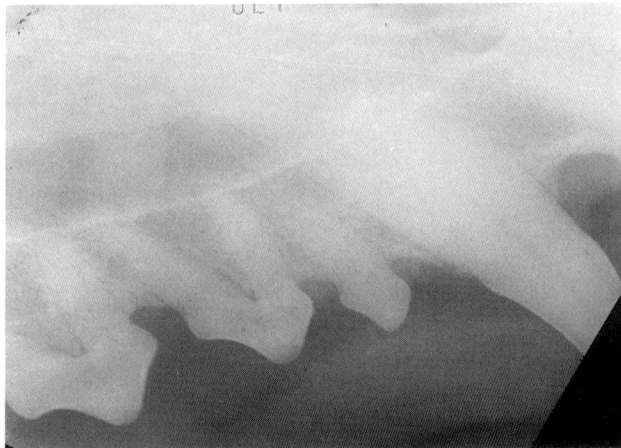

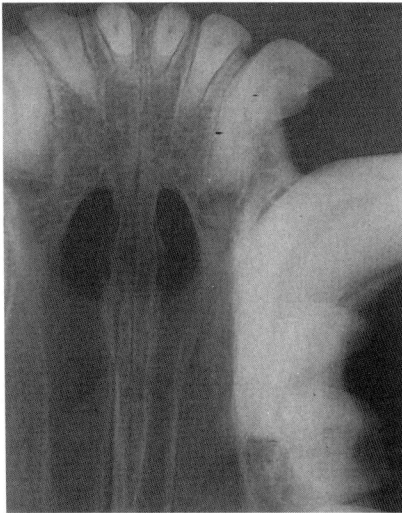

A

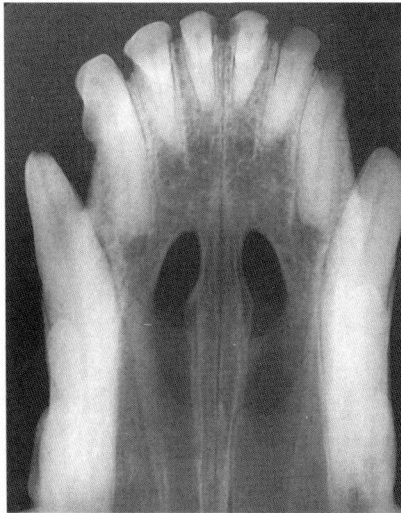

B

FIGURE 15.8

Contributing Author: Edward R. Eisner

Description: View A, a distorted image at one end of the film due to excessive curvature of the film in the patients mouth. View B, proper position of film.

Remedy: Use an appropriately small film packet for the confines of the mouth so that it can be positioned properly without bending.

FIGURE 15.9

Contributing Author: Edward R. Eisner

Description: The black dot superimposed on the tooth is a manufacturer's dimple.

Points Identified:

A. Manufacturer's dimple

Remedy: Place the dimple out of the important field (usually coronally) when radiographing a tooth. In this film of a 3-year-old American Staffordshire terrier, notice the arrow on the film that points to the manufacturer's dimple in the radiograph.

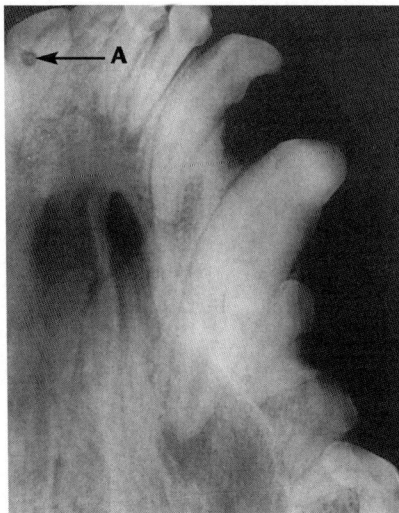

FIGURE 15.10

Contributing Author: Edward R. Eisner

Source: Film for view C provided courtesy of Donald H. DeForge.

Description: Reversed film (film placed wrong side toward tube). When x-rays are partially absorbed by lead backing, "tire track" effect may be seen (when film is placed wrong). Views A and B picture 208 of an 11-year-old Labrador retriever. View C shows pedodontic, canine mandible. View A, correct position (correct side facing tube). View B, inverted position ("tire track,"—film upside down—when lead backing is x-rayed first). View C, "tire track" effect caused by lead backing being on both sides of film (the fault of the manufacturer).

Remedy: Place the film packet so the raised dot faces the tube head.

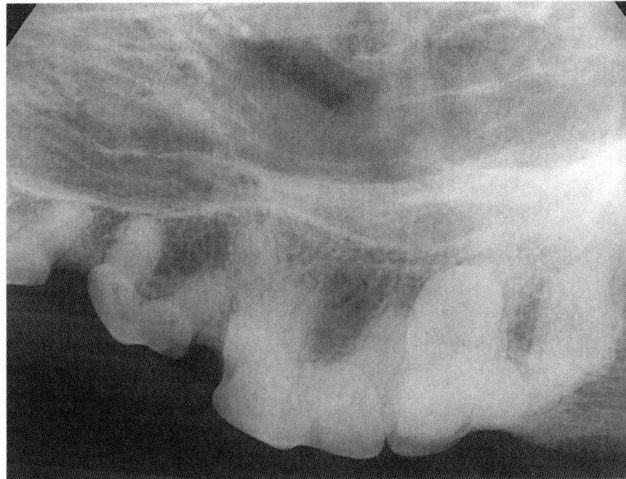

A

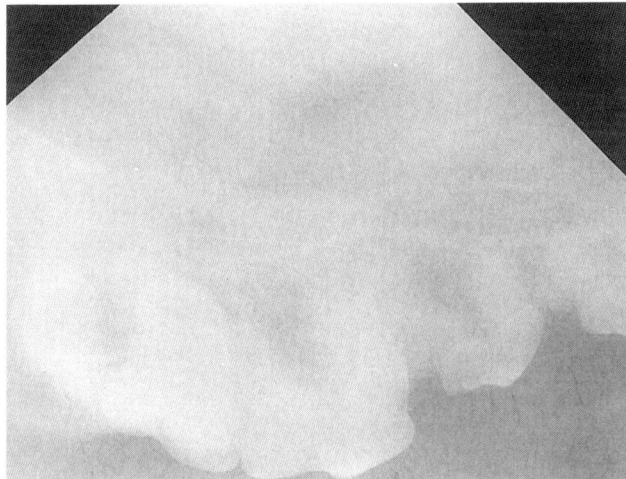

B

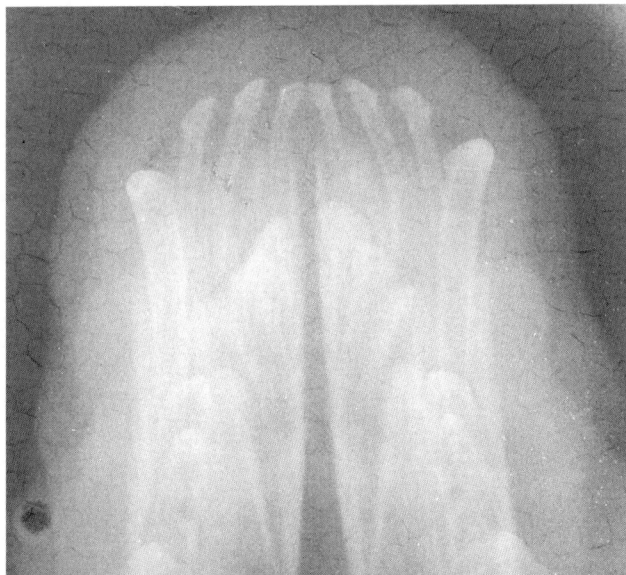

C

FIGURE 15.11

Contributing Author: Edward R. Eisner

Description: Double image (dark film) due to the film being exposed twice to radiation.

Remedy: Place the exposed films by the chairside darkroom in a receptacle immediately after exposure to reduce possibility of using one film packet twice. A second exposure was made on this film of an 11-year-old Labrador retriever.

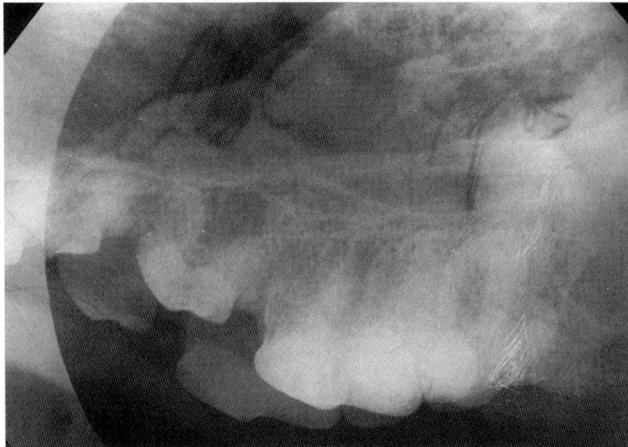

FIGURE 15.12

Contributing Author: Edward R. Eisner

Description: Fogging has occurred due to one of the following: a light leak, the safe light being too close, improper safe filter, scatter (secondary radiation), chemicals, outdated film, film stored in a warm place, or allowing light to penetrate the wrist shields in chairside developer.

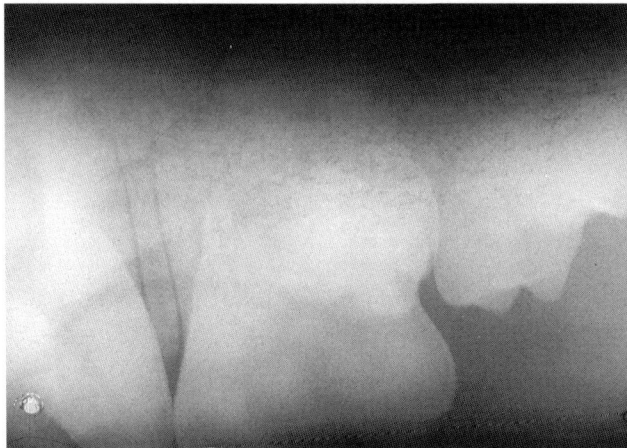

FIGURE 15.13

Contributing Author: Edward R. Eisner

Description: Black marks have formed on the film because of failure to dry the film packet (moisture contamination, from film packet to film or from film packet to hands then to film).

Remedy: Blot the film packet upon removal from the patient's mouth or process it soon after exposure. This film of an 11-year-old Labrador retriever was not dried when removed from the patient's mouth.

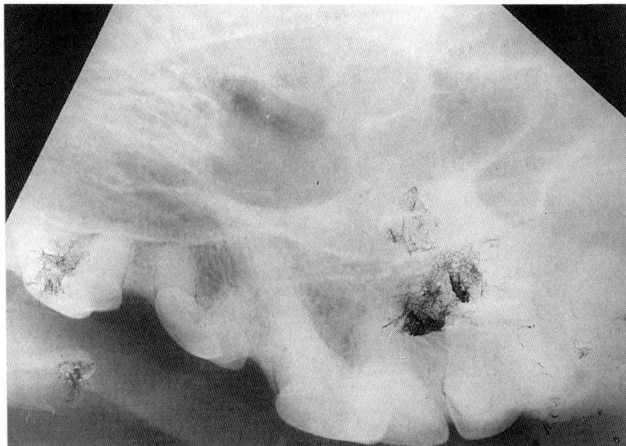

FIGURE 15.14

Contributing Author: Edward R. Eisner

Description: Technical error: There has been a light leak due to a loose lid; note the dark film or dark portion of the film. As one can see in this film of a 9-year-old chow chow, the chairside darkroom lid was loose.

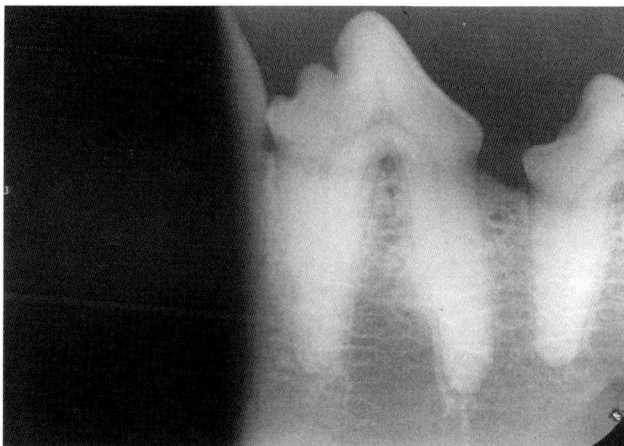

FIGURE 15.15

Contributing Author: Edward R. Eisner

Description: Technical error: In this film of a 4-year-old Yorkshire terrier one can see that a black x-ray has resulted because the packet was opened before being placed inside the chairside darkroom.

FIGURE 15.16

Contributing Author: Edward R. Eisner

Description: In this film of a 6-year-old Maltese, there are clear lines on the film caused by scratched emulsion in the wash.

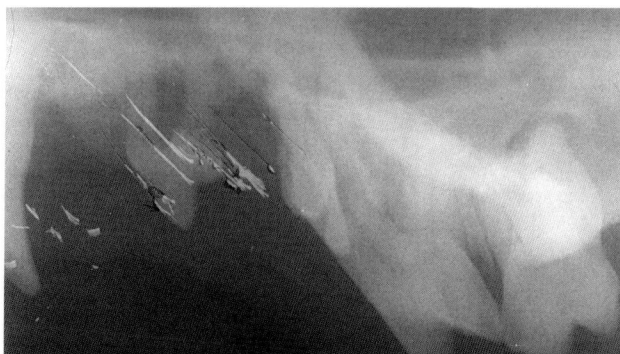

FIGURE 15.17

Contributing Author: Edward R. Eisner

Identification: Plate 17

Description: Dark lines have occurred on this film of a 3½-year-old Maine coon cat because of static electricity. This film was affected out of the packet, but before processing.

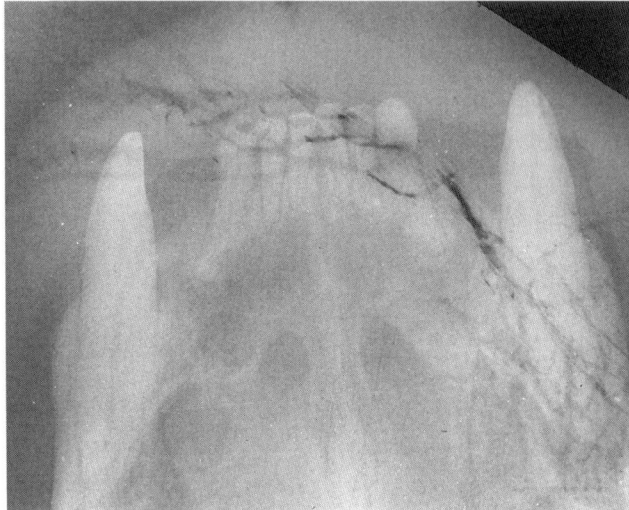

FIGURE 15.18

Contributing Author: Edward R. Eisner

Description: Film was bent, disrupting emulsion as it was removed from the packet causing a light line.

Points Identified:

A. Line caused by disrupted emulsion

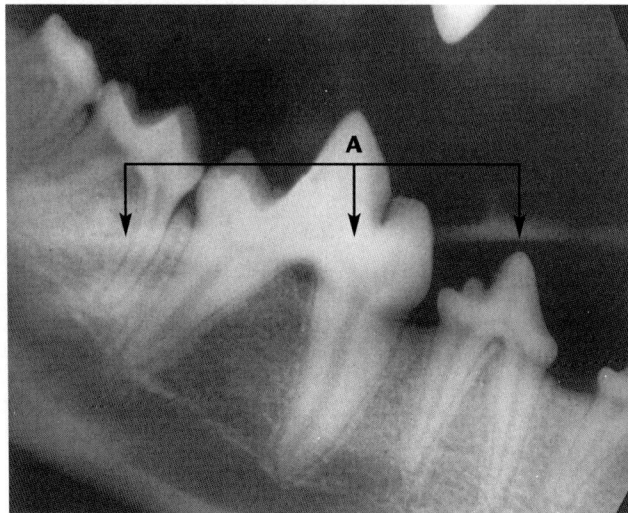

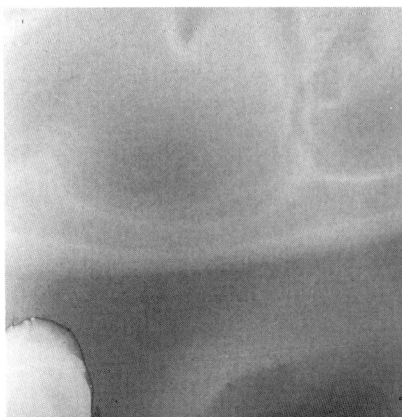

A

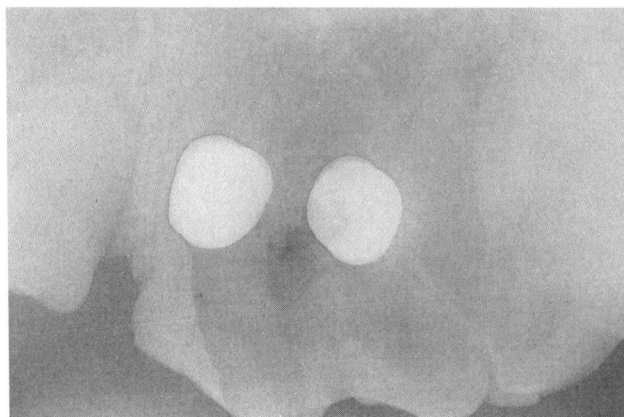

B

FIGURE 15.19

Contributing Author: Edward R. Eisner

Source: Film provided courtesy of Donald H. DeForge.

Description: Drop of fixer contaminated the film prior to processing, causing the white spots, or fixer artifact.

FIGURE 15.20

Contributing Author: Edward R. Eisner

Source: Film provided courtesy of Donald H. DeForge.

Description: Developer artifact: developer splashed onto the film before the film was placed in the developer. Notice the developer artifacts at edges of film and film corners (dark spots on this film).

A. Artifact
B. Scratch

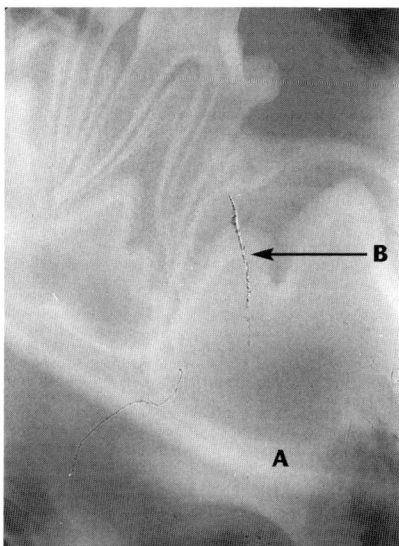

FIGURE 15.21

Contributing Author: Edward R. Eisner

Source: Film provided courtesy of Donald H. DeForge.

Description: Fix contamination after developing process was completed. Grossly, the appearance is similar to the developer contamination, but under radiographic illumination one can notice it is a lighter contamination.

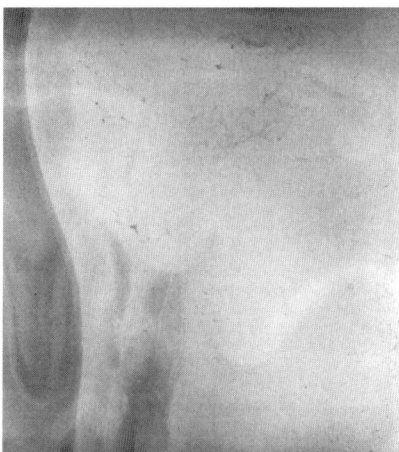

FIGURE 15.22

Contributing Author: Edward R. Eisner

Source: Film for view A provided courtesy of Donald H. DeForge.

Description: View A: Note the darker hues present on the film, caused by developer contamination after the developing process was fully completed.

View B: Note the isolated darkened spots caused by developer spattering. This is the same defect with different presentation.

Points Identified:

A. Dark spots caused by developer spattering

Remedy: Films must be handled carefully after processing.

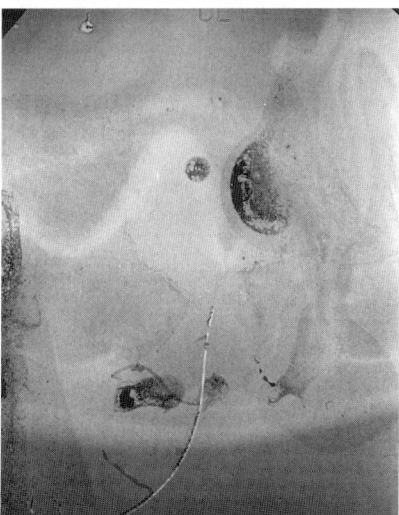

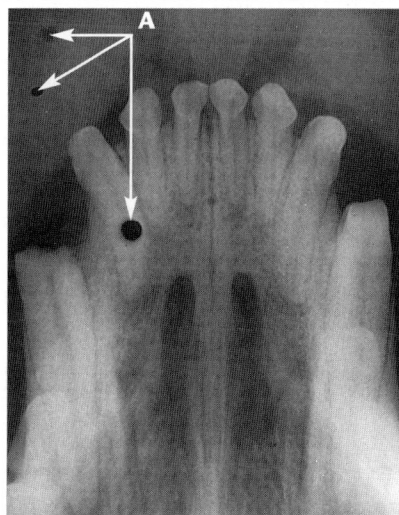

A

B

FIGURE 15.23

Contributing Author: Edward R. Eisner

Source: Film provided courtesy of Donald H. DeForge.

Description: Note the discoloration of the film due to improper rinsing technique.

Remedy: After fixing all dental x-rays should be taken from chairside developer and put in a "running water" rinse for 10 minutes to clear all fixative from the film.

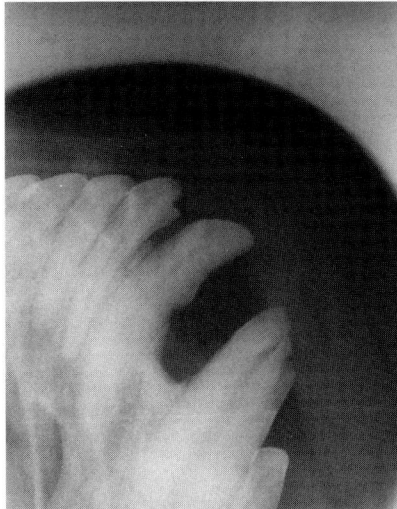

FIGURE 15.24

Contributing Author: Edward R. Eisner

Description: Opaque artifact: Exposed radiograph was developed with black paper, from inside the film packet, still in contact with the film during processing.

Remedy: Use care in removing paper before processing.

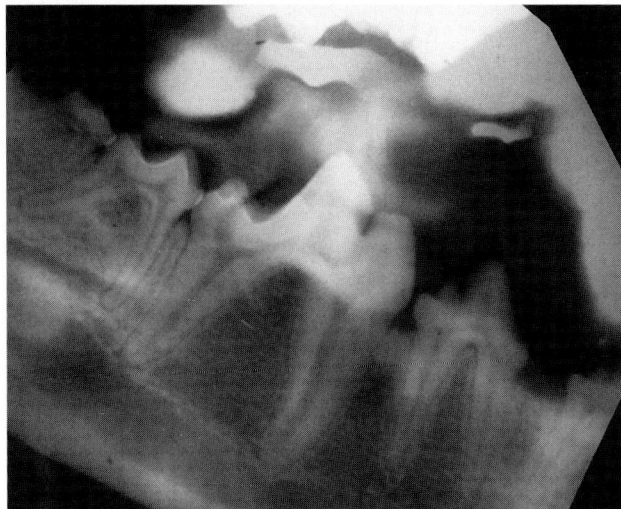

FIGURE 15.25

Contributing Author: Edward R. Eisner

Description: Fluoride-contaminated fingers (white artifacts).

Points Identified:

A. White artifacts

Remedy: Wash hands, or put on clean dry gloves before processing.

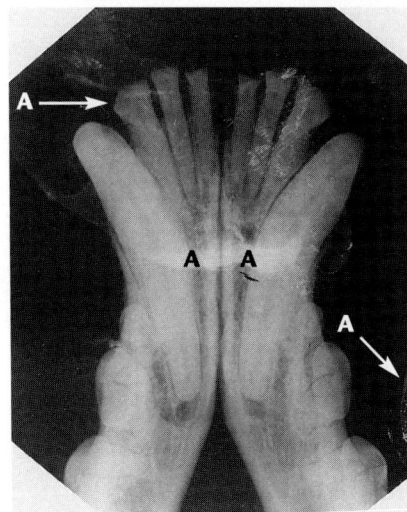

FIGURE 15.26

Contributing Author: Edward R. Eisner

Description: Reticulation or "grainy" film caused by improper temperature of chemicals. [Temperature 80°–90°F or higher causes this problem.]

Remedy: Keep developer, water, and fix at room temperature.

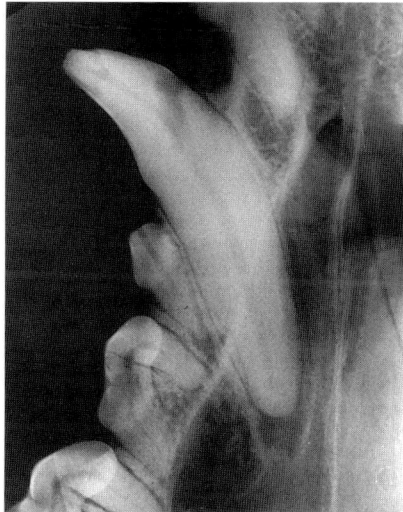

FIGURE 15.27

Contributing Author: Edward R. Eisner

Description: Anatomical superimposition. In this film of a 12-year-old domestic shorthair feline, arrows point to the zygomatic arch superimposed over the root structure of 108.

Points Identified:

A. Superimposed zygomatic arch

Remedy: Correct by making the x-ray beam more perpendicular to the tooth axis, causing elongation of the teeth.

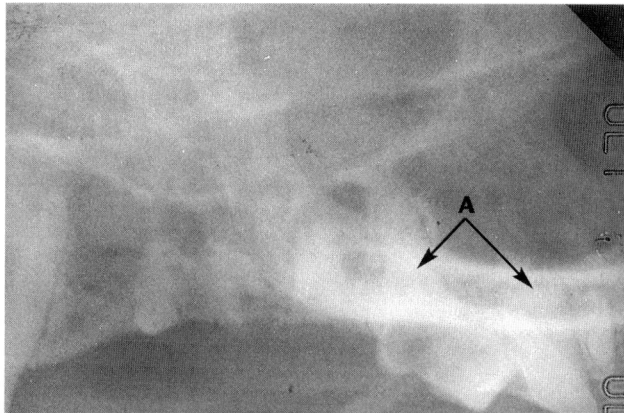

FIGURE 15.28

Contributing Author: Edward R. Eisner

Description: Overlapping contacts caused by improper horizontal angulation. In this film of 208 and 209 in a 12-year-old standard poodle, there is a subtle artifact, but an important one to assess accurately.

Points Identified:

A. Overlapping contacts

Remedy: Correct by taking multiple horizontal (rostral and caudal) angulations.

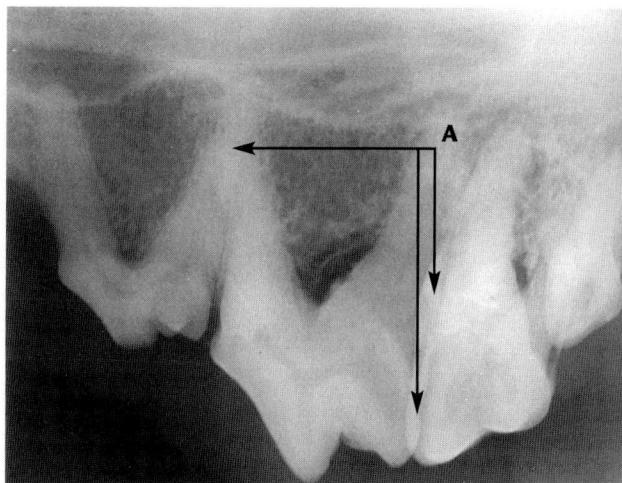

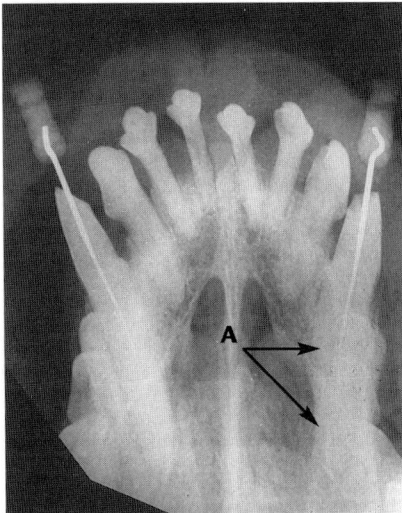

A

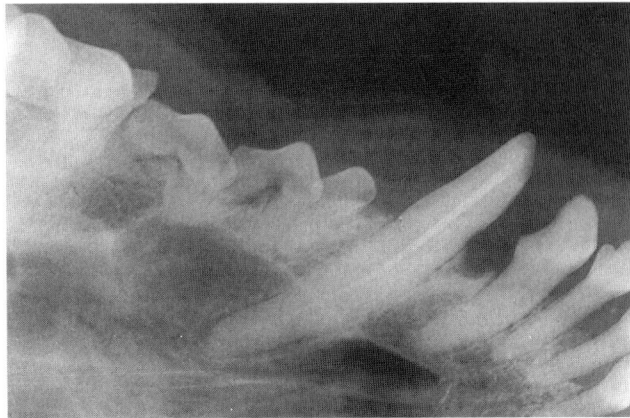

B

FIGURE 15.29

Contributing Author: Edward R. Eisner

Description: Poor visualization caused by superimposed teeth.

Points Identified:

A. 104 superimposed over premolars

Remedy: Take an oblique view. View A, 104 of an 8-year-old cocker spaniel superimposed over the premolars. View B, 104 of the same dog from a maxillary oblique projection.

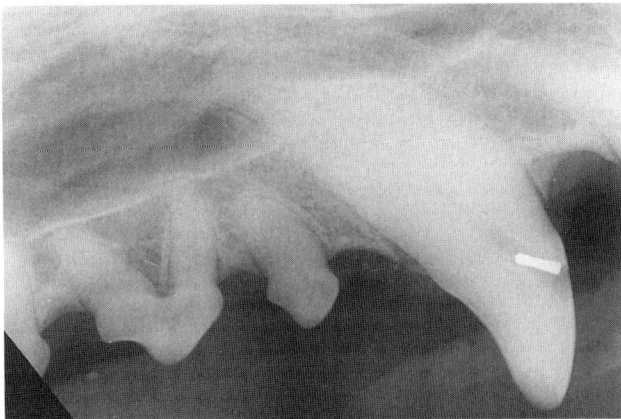

FIGURE 15.30

Contributing Author: Edward R. Eisner

Description: Metal fragments imbedded in the canine tooth. Note the separated bur head in this film of an 8-year-old golden retriever.

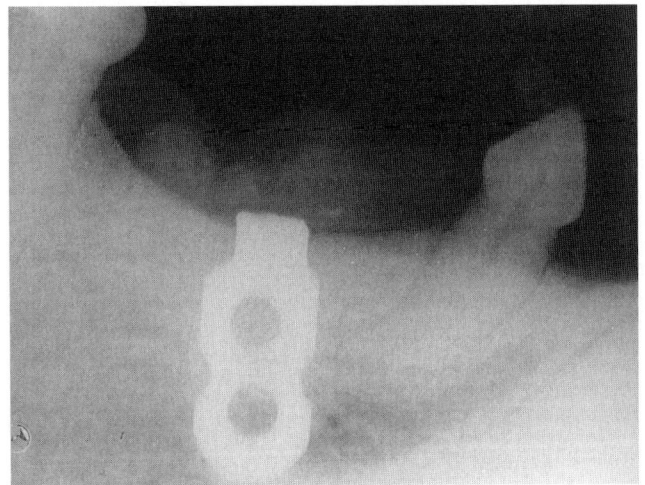

FIGURE 15.31

Contributing Author: Edward R. Eisner

Description: In this film of a 2-year-old German shepherd note the anchor of a prosthesis implant where the crown portion of the prosthesis has been removed.

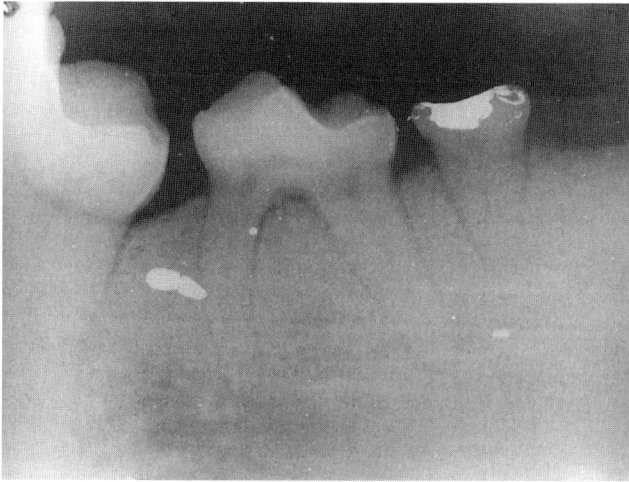

FIGURE 15.32

Contributing Author: Edward R. Eisner

Description: Film of 5-year-old golden retriever mix. Note the Class I amalgam restoration and the amalgam tattoo (contamination) by the mesial root of the second molar.

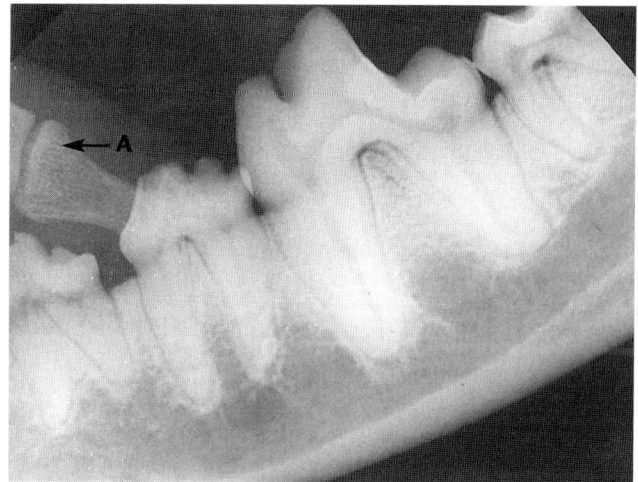

FIGURE 15.33

Contributing Author: Edward R. Eisner

Description: Human finger exposure.

Points Identified:

A. Image of human finger

Remedy: Never stand in the x-ray beam and hold the film. Stand 6 feet from the patient when taking a radiograph. Use film positioning devices to avoid unnecessary radiation exposure.

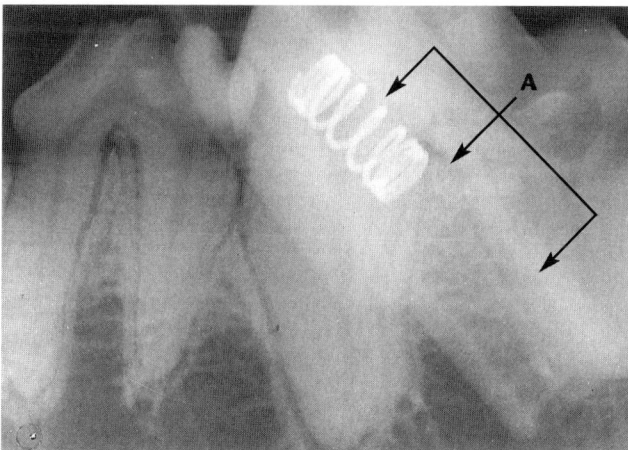

A

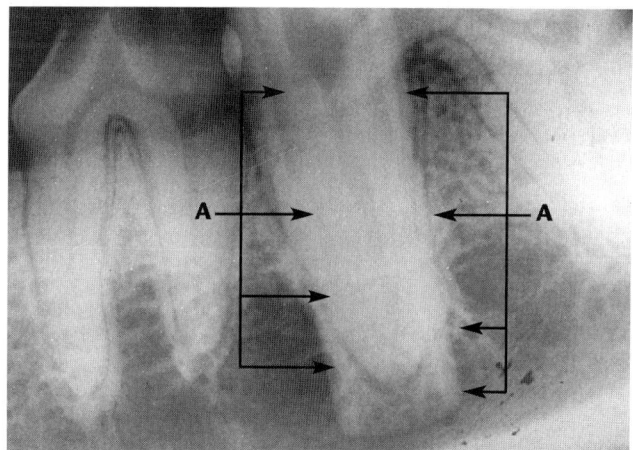

B

FIGURE 15.34

Contributing Author: Edward R. Eisner

Description: Inflation port of the endotracheal tube.

Points Identified:

A. Inflation ports

Remedy: Always be aware of instruments and intraoral mouth props, etc. View A, inflation port with spring in it. View B, inflation port without spring in it.

FIGURE 15.35

Contributing Author: Edward R. Eisner

Description: Endotracheal tube with radiopaque line marker on film of a 6-year-old Samoyed.

Remedy: Always be aware of instruments and intraoral mouth props, etc.

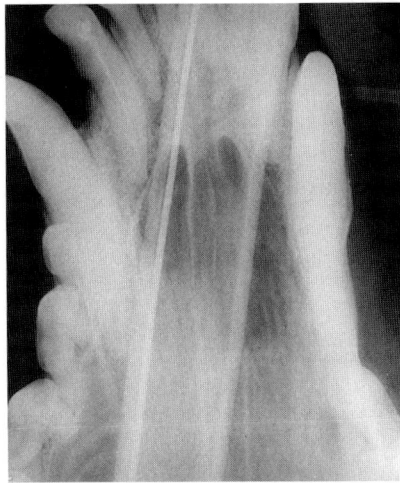

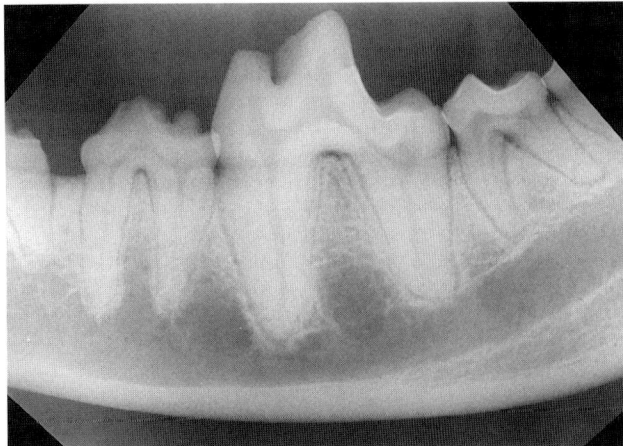

A

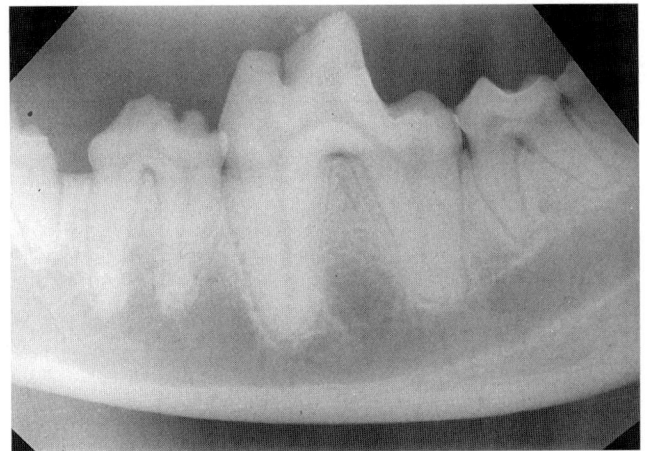

B

FIGURE 15.36

Contributing Author: Edward R. Eisner

Description: A duplicated film will have slightly less detail than the original. View A: Original radiograph. View B: Duplicate film. This film shows slightly less detail than the original.

PART FOUR

Zoo Animals, Rodents, and Rabbits

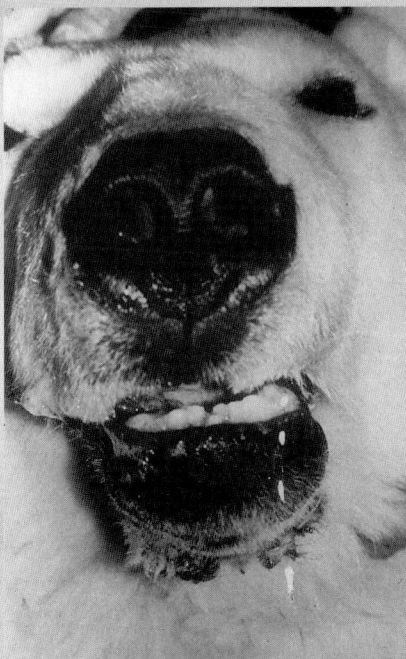

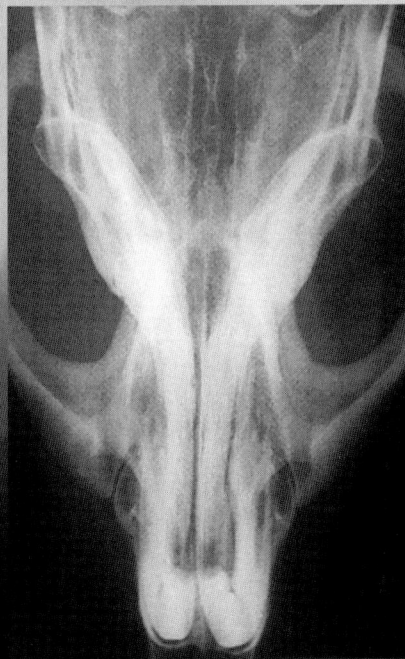

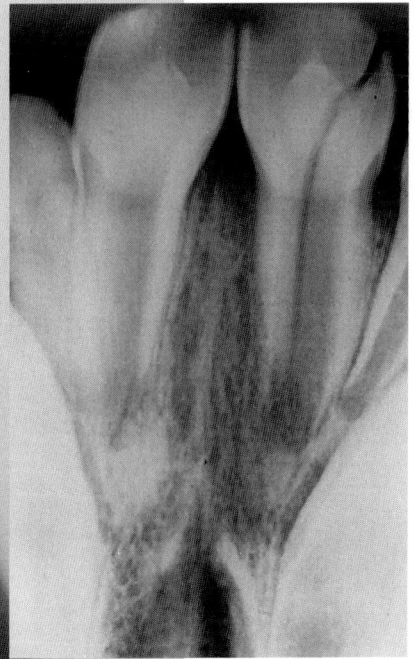

16 Zoo Animal Dentistry

Dr. Laura D. Braswell　　　*Dr. James M.G. Anthony*
Dr. Linda L. Brooks　　　*Dr. Peter Emily*

NONHUMAN PRIMATE ORAL RADIOLOGY DIAGNOSTICS

Dr. Laura D. Braswell
Dr. Linda L. Brooks

Nonhuman primate collections are becoming more numerous in zoos and wild animal parks around the world. As natural habitats are threatened, endangered species are finding protection in these captive environments. Quality medical care is critical for all captive animals, and radiology provides important information for diagnosis and treatment.

This section of the chapter on zoo animals includes examples of radiographs taken on nonhuman primates, housed primarily at Zoo Atlanta Center and Yerkes Regional Primate Research Center at Emory University. Some of these radiographs were taken in general surveys and are diagnostic screening films. Periodontal diseases, caries, endodontic lesions, and examples of normal growth and development are demonstrated.

Radiographic evaluation is an important aspect of dental care in nonhuman primates. The information presented in this section should serve as a basis for comparison for veterinary practitioners involved in the care of nonhuman primates.

Acknowledgments

Special thanks go to Mr. Frank Kiernan for his photographic expertise, to Janet Brewer for her technical assistance, and to Dr. Rita McManamon and Karen Idhe for help in obtaining these primate radiographs.

X-RAY PLATES, NONHUMAN PRIMATES

FIGURE 16.1

Contributing Author: Laura D. Braswell

Description: Intraoral radiograph of a normal arrangement for an incisor in the alveolar bone in an adult rhesus monkey, *Macacca mulatta*.

Points Identified:

A. Nasal septum
B. Apex
C. Pulp
D. Interproximal bone
E. Clinical crown

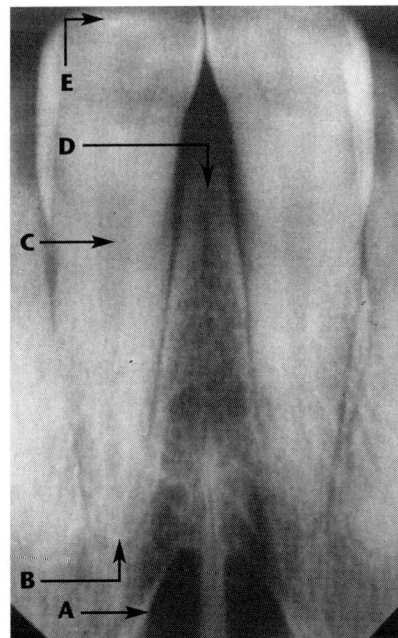

FIGURE 16.2

Contributing Author: Laura D. Braswell

Description: Cephalometric radiograph depicting a lateral skull view of a golden lion tamarin, *Leontopithecus rosalia*, utilizing a 3 occlusal film extraorally.

Points Identified:

A. Incisors
B. Molar

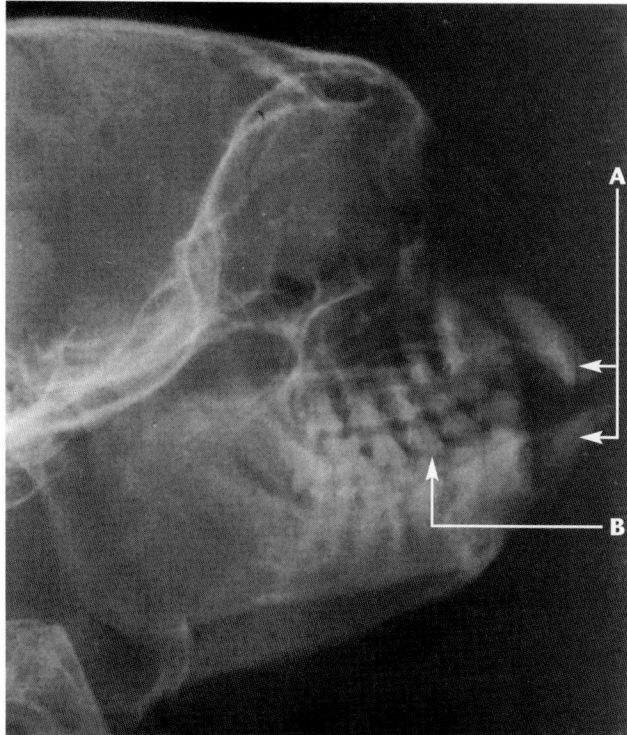

FIGURE 16.3

Contributing Author: Laura D. Braswell

Description: Sialolith (salivary stone) noted during evaluation of an adult female chimpanzee, *Pan troglodytes*.

Source: Used with the permission of Dr. Jack Orkin and the JAVMA.

Points Identified:

A. Incisor
B. Canine
C. Sialolith
D. Body of mandible

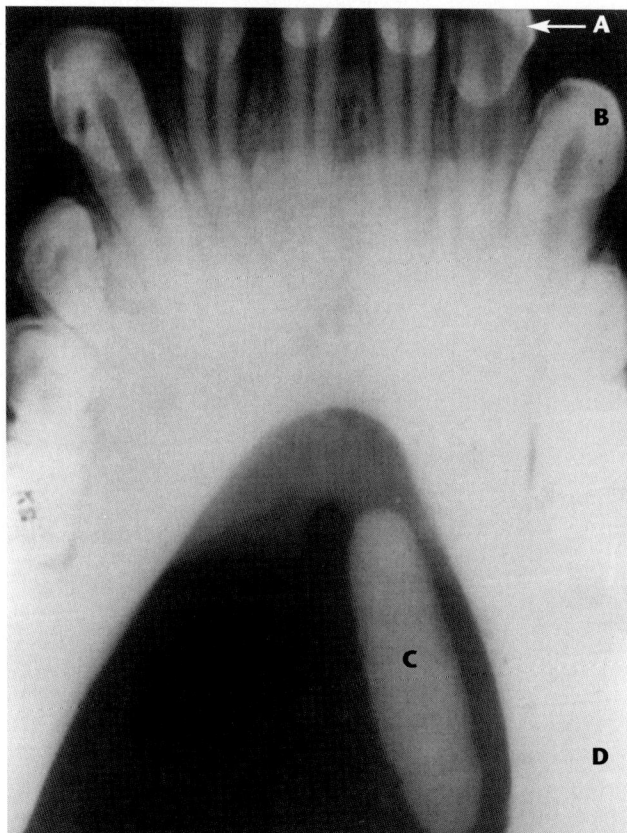

FIGURE 16.4

Contributing Author: Laura D. Braswell

Description: Lateral extraoral view of a dentigerous cyst in an adult female drill, *Papio leucophaeus*.

Points Identified:

A. Cystic enclosure
B. Crown of canine tooth
C. Superior border of rostral bone

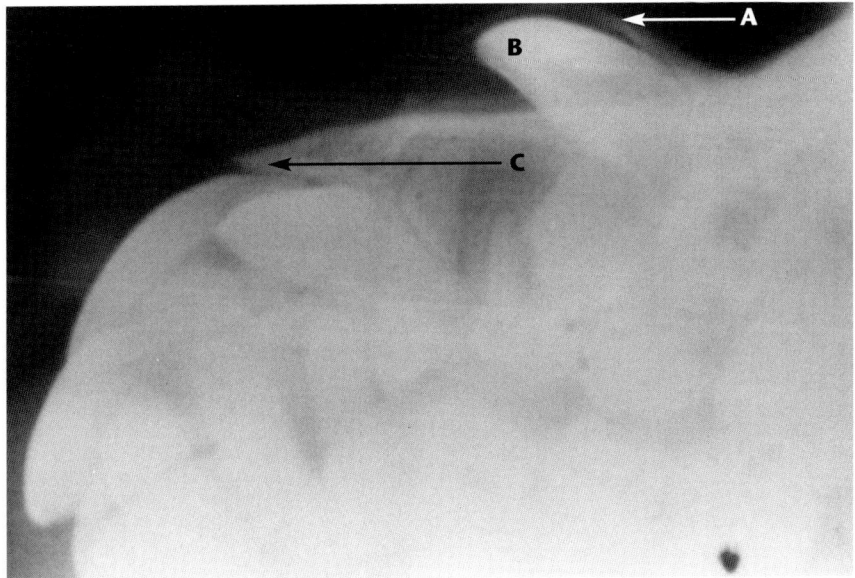

FIGURE 16.5

Contributing Author: Laura D. Braswell

Description: Intraoral occlusal view of the same dentigerous cyst shown in Figure 16.4, demonstrating the circumferential lesion associated with a developing canine tooth crown.

Points Identified:

A. Developed crown of canine
B. Cystic space
C. Lateral incisor
D. Central incisor

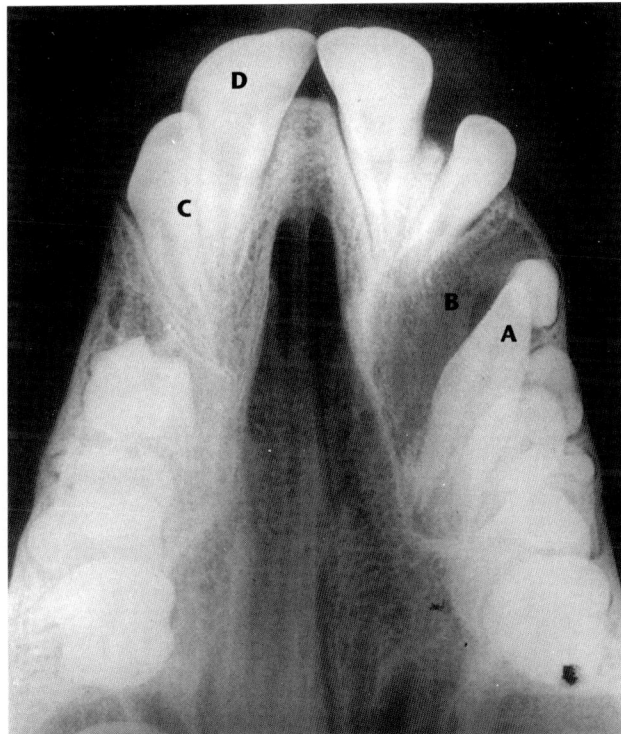

FIGURE 16.6

Contributing Author: Laura D. Braswell

Description: Cephlametric radiographs of an adult female chimpanzee, *Pan troglodytes*, demonstrating benign idiopathic expansion of the anterior maxilla.

Points Identified:

A. Maxillary expansion
B. Maxillary canine
C. Mandibular canine

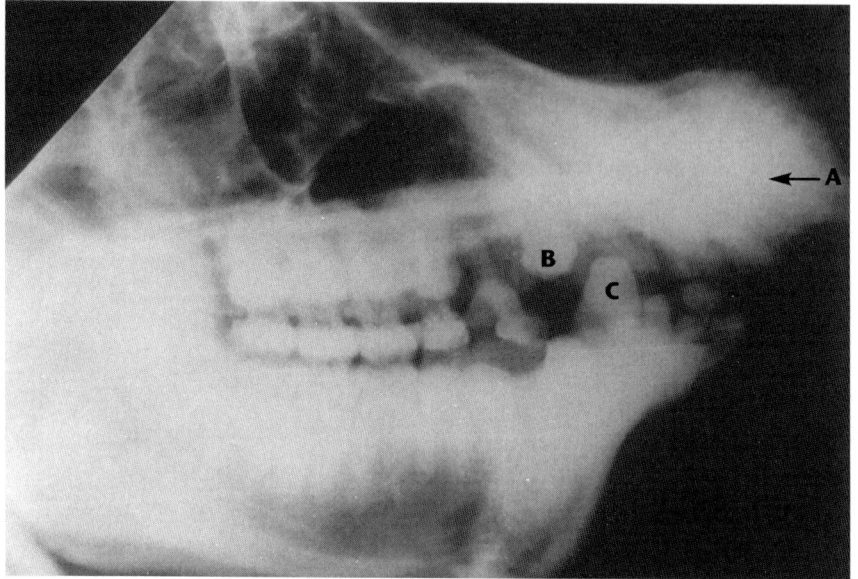

FIGURE 16.7

Contributing Author: Laura D. Braswell

Description: Intraoral occlusal view of the same lesion shown in Figure 16.6, utilizing radiographic cassette and film. Note labial version of anterior dentition.

Points Identified:

A. Canine tooth
B. Lateral incisor
C. Central incisor
D. Maxillary bony expansion

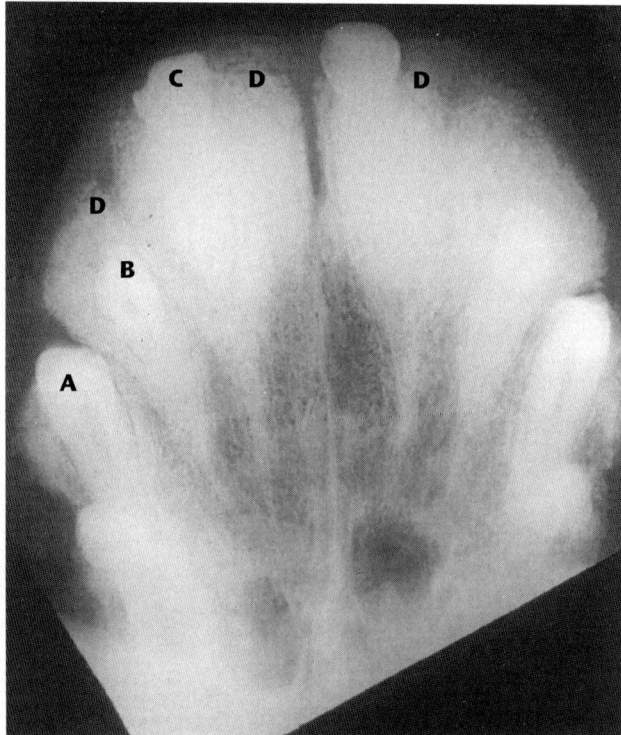

FIGURE 16.8

Contributing Author: Laura D. Braswell

Description: Occlusal decay with carious exposure of distal pulp horn in molars of an adult lowland gorilla, *Gorilla gorilla*. Note the carious lesions in both molars.

Points Identified:

A. Carious lesion
B. Pulpal horn
C. Pulpal chamber
D. Pulpal canal

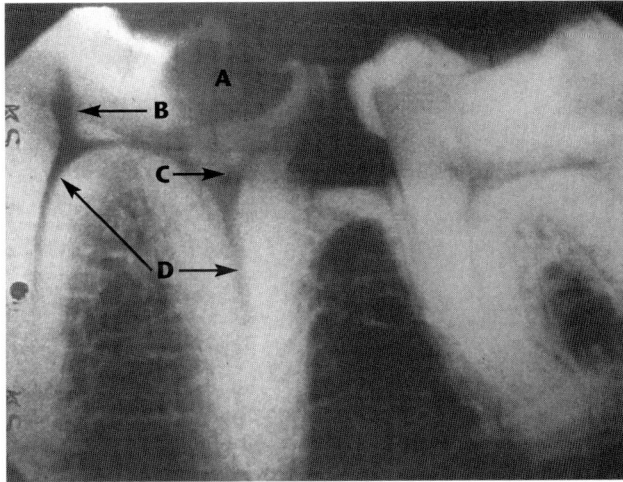

FIGURE 16.9

Contributing Author: Laura D. Braswell

Description: Normal lateral periapical view of adult male lowland gorilla, *Gorilla gorilla*. The roots are elongated moderately due to radiographic technique.

Points Identified:

A. Artifact due to hemostat
B. Buccal trifurcation of root
C. Normal alveolar bone level

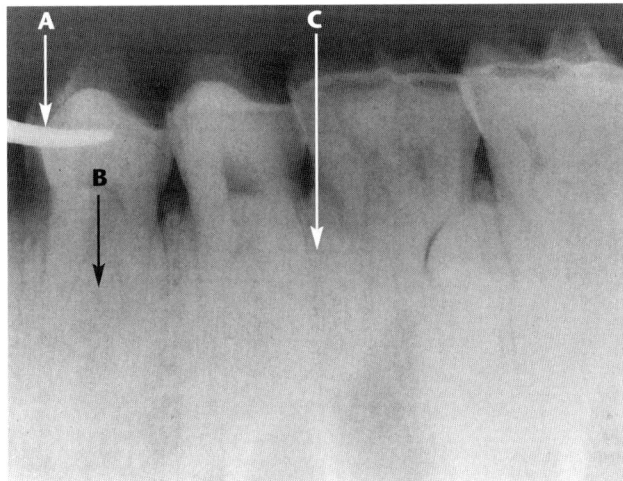

FIGURE 16.10

Contributing Author: Laura D. Braswell

Description: Periapical view of adult male lowland gorilla, *Gorilla gorilla*, revealing a vertical osseous defect on the mesial surface of the maxillary first molar.

Points Identified:

A. Vertical osseous (bony) defect

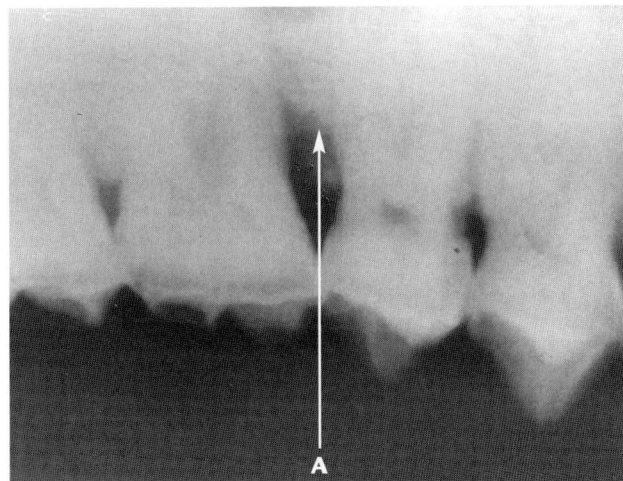

FIGURE 16.11

Contributing Author: Laura D. Braswell

Description: Bitewing radiograph of adult male orangutan, *Pongo pygmaeus*, revealing vertical and horizontal bone loss.

Points Identified:

 A. Vertical bone loss
 B. Horizontal bone loss
 C. Intrafurcal bone loss
 D. Periradicular bone loss

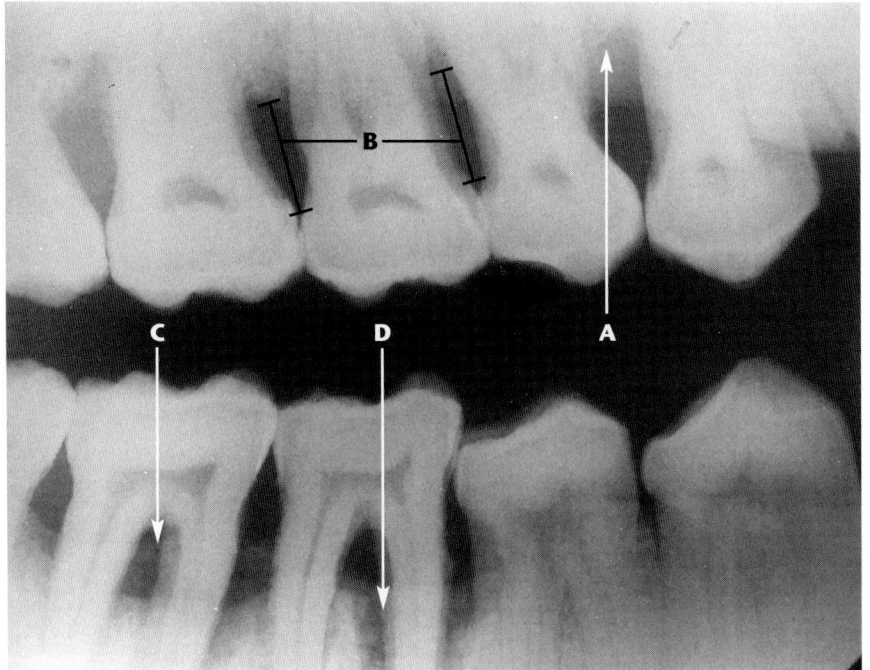

FIGURE 16.12

Contributing Author: Laura D. Braswell

Description: Bitewing radiograph of an adult orangutan, *Pongo pygmaeus*, revealing the presence of pulp stones, calcifications within the pulpal tissue.

Points Identified:

 A. Supernumerary (fourth molar)
 B. Pulpal stones
 C. Cervical "burnout" (radiographic artifact)

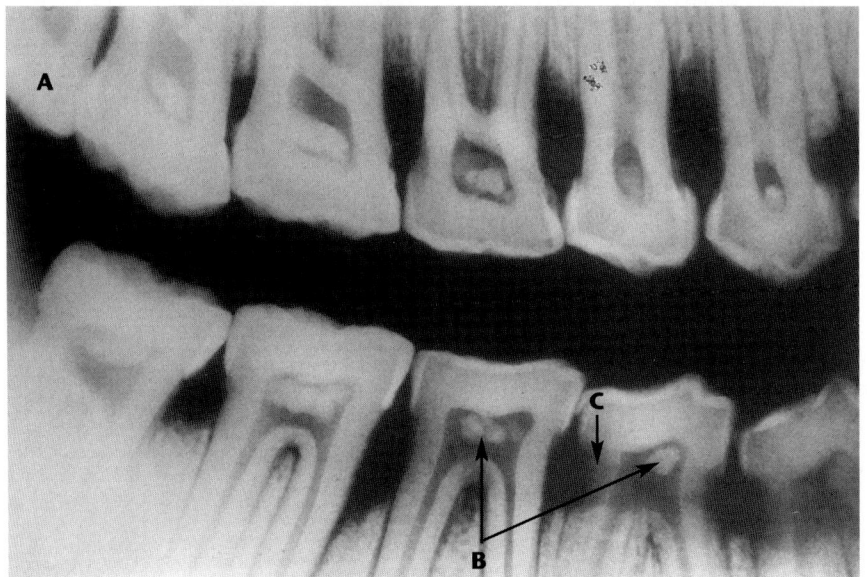

FIGURE 16.13

Contributing Author: Laura D. Braswell

Description: Endodontic lesion associated with a maxillary central incisor in an adult male mandrill baboon, *Papio sphinx*. Note incipent apical pathology on opposite lateral incisor.

Points Identified:

A. Apical lesion
B. Pulp canal
C. Fracture in close proximity to pulp chamber

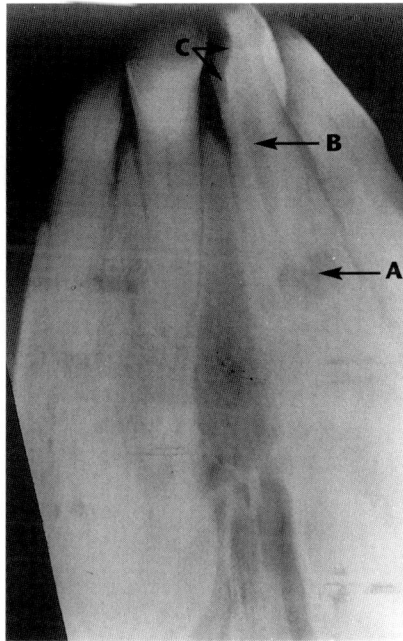

FIGURE 16.14

Contributing Author: Laura D. Braswell

Description: Occlusal view of the maxillary arch on an adult male rhesus monkey, *Macacca mulatta*, demonstrating radiopaque occlusal restorations following a vital pulpotomy procedure. Asymmetry in canal widths indicates cessation of dentinogenesis, which suggests pulpal pathology and possibly pulpal necrosis. This patient must be followed closely and may need conventional endodontics due to failure of the vital pulpotomy procedure. In zoo dentistry, follow-up radiology is advised but not always practical because of need for repeat anesthesia experiences.

Points Identified:

A. Canine tooth pulp (asymmetry in canal width)
B. Radiopaque composite

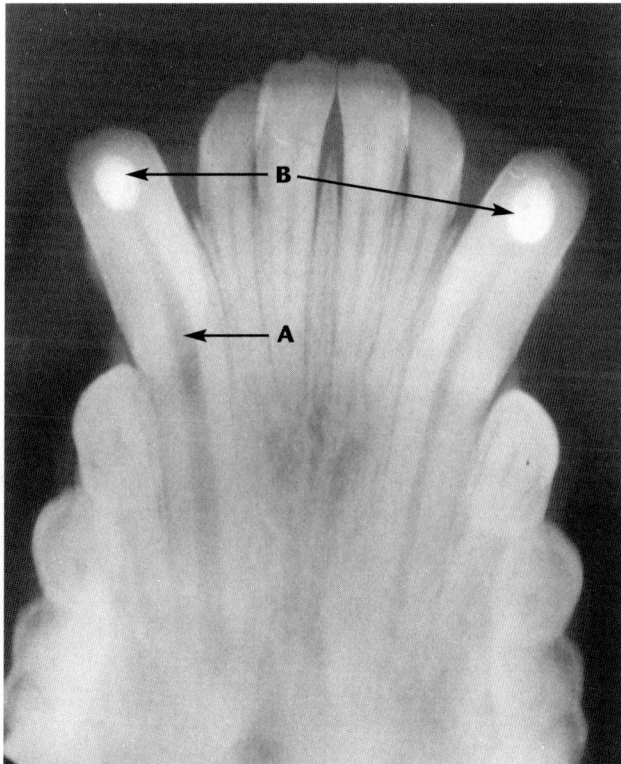

FIGURE 16.15

Contributing Author: Laura D. Braswell

Source: Image provided courtesy of Yerkes Regional Primate Research Center at Emory University, Grant #DEO-8917 of the NIDR of NIH.

Description: Cephlametric film of an adult male rhesus monkey, *Macacca mulatta*, revealing endodontic fill on a maxillary canine tooth as well as a mandibular blade implant and fixed bridge.

Note: Radiolucency in molar peri-implant area in mandibular body. This could mean lack of osseous integration or reactive bone anterior to implant. Also note pathology in periradicular area of mandibular abutment tooth and mandibular canine. Endodontic therapy may be indicated. These teeth must be followed closely radiographically.

Points Identified:

A. Endodontic fill
B. Maxillary canine tooth
C. Gold bridge abutting second premolar
D. Blade implant

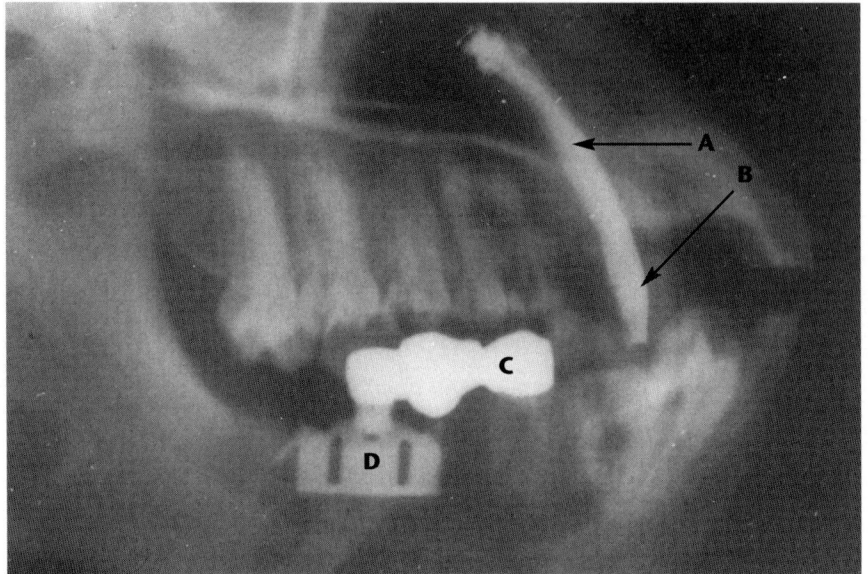

FIGURE 16.16

Contributing Author: Laura D. Braswell

Description: Oblique view of the mandible of a 2-year-old orangutan, *Pongo pygmaeus*, revealing mixed dentition.

Points Identified:

A. Fractured primary canine
B. Primary lateral incisor
C. Primary central incisor
D. Developing lateral incisor
E. Developing permanent canine
F. Developing central incisor

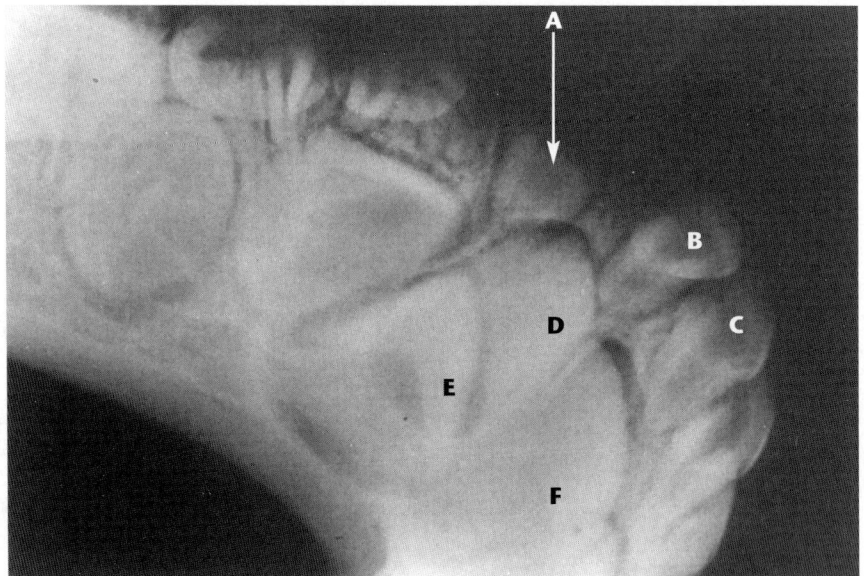

FIGURE 16.17

Contributing Author: Laura D. Braswell

Description: Maxillary occlusal view of a 1-year-old male lowland gorilla, *Gorilla gorilla*, revealing erupted maxillary primary incisors and developing primary and permanent teeth.

Points Identified:

- A. Primary second molar
- B. Developing permanent central incisor
- C. Primary first molar
- D. Primary canine
- E. Primary lateral incisor
- F. Primary central incisor

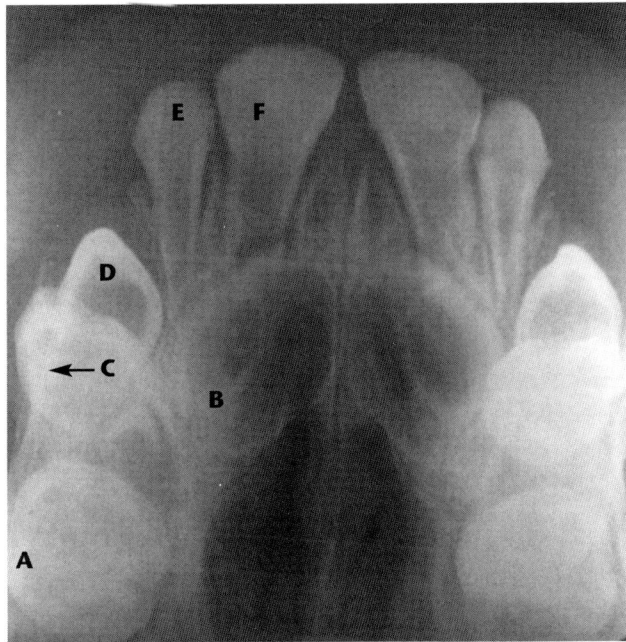

FIGURE 16.18

Contributing Author: Laura D. Braswell

Description: Vertical fracture extending from clinical crown to apex of a maxillary central incisor in an adolescent male orangutan, *Pongo pygmaeus*.

Points Identified:

- A. Developing permanent canine
- B. Apical radiolucency
- C. Vertical root fracture

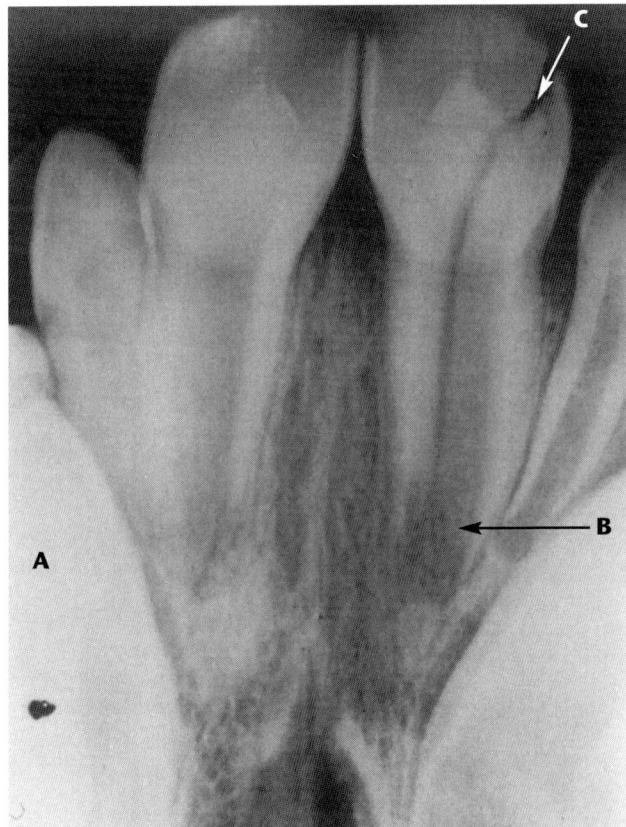

FIGURE 16.19

Contributing Author: Laura D. Braswell

Description: Occlusal view of the maxilla of a female mandrill, *Papio sphinx*, revealing a fractured central incisor with retained root structure.

Points Identified:

A. Fractured central incisor

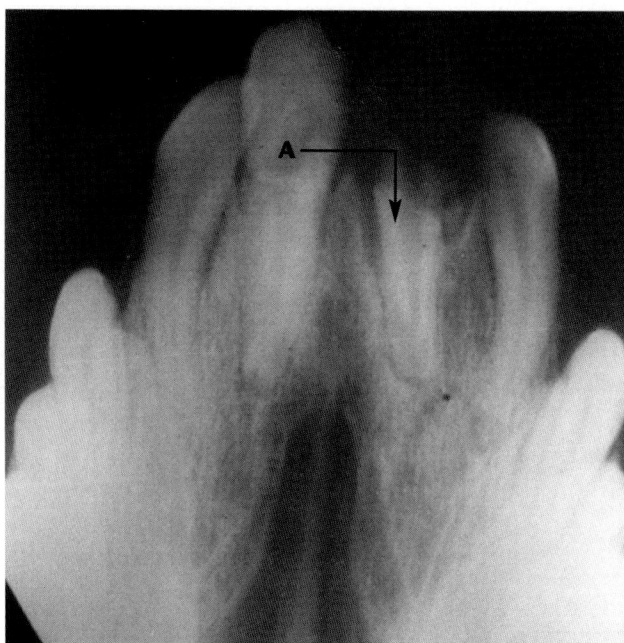

EXOTIC ANIMALS

Dr. James M.G. Anthony
Dr. Peter Emily

The zoo setting is the theater of challenge for the veterinary dentist. The films shown here represent the best field work that can be accomplished under high risk situations.

This area of veterinary radiology demands dedication in the study of the normal regional anatomy of the different species. The oral cavity radiographs taken in the zoo setting are not the same as those commonly taken in a dental operatory. Complete immobilization of these animals is always required and since examination, diagnosis, treatment planning, and treatment are all done at the same time, one must be expeditious in radiography, processing, and interpretation. Difficulties with anesthesia maintenance, on-site development inadequacy (or absence thereof), and species

size and mass variance lead to radiographic challenges; the radiographs shown below are therefore not ideal. They are rather the norm under extenuating circumstances.

At the Metro Toronto Zoo a preventative approach to dental disease and oral examination is followed. All anesthetized animals undergo extra- and intraoral exams with dental radiography if indicated. The following is an amalgamation of different radiographs for interest's sake. Anyone interested in zoo dentistry and oral pathology should allow this information to be the starting point for an educational journey into an exciting field of oral health, diagnosis, and treatment.

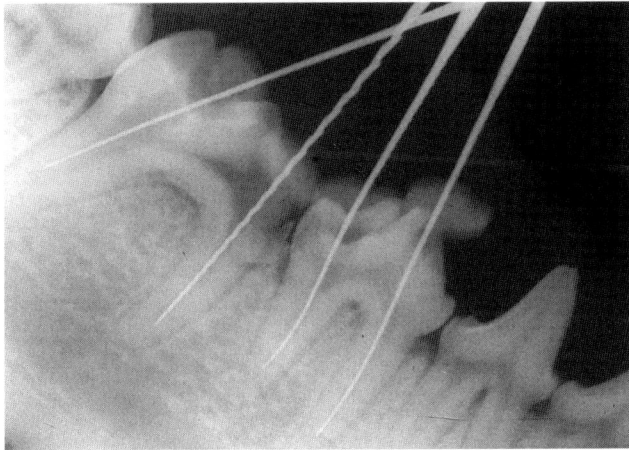

A

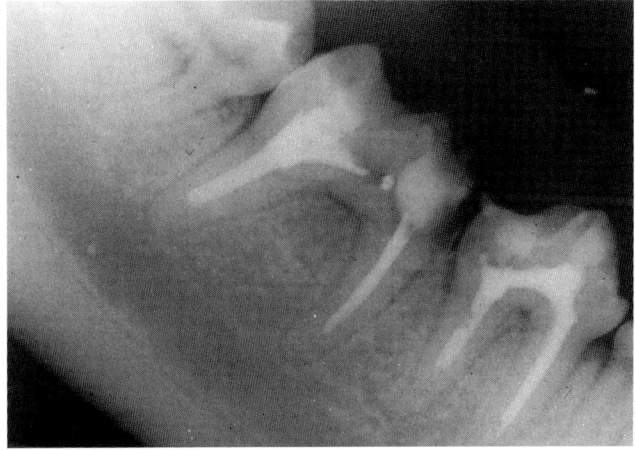

B

FIGURE 16.20

Contributing Author:

James M.G. Anthony

Description: Mandibular premolar and molar pulp exposure (view A) with subsequent endodontic instrumentation and obturation (view B) in a mature red panda (*Ailurus fulgens styani*).

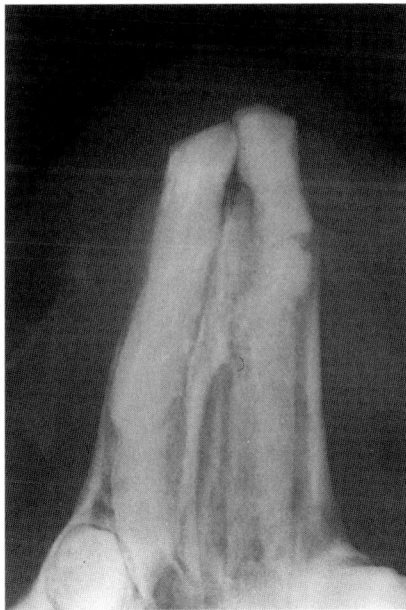

FIGURE 16.21

Contributing Author:

James M.G. Anthony

Description: Bilateral subgingival fracture of the mandibular incisors of a hare (*Lepus capensis*).

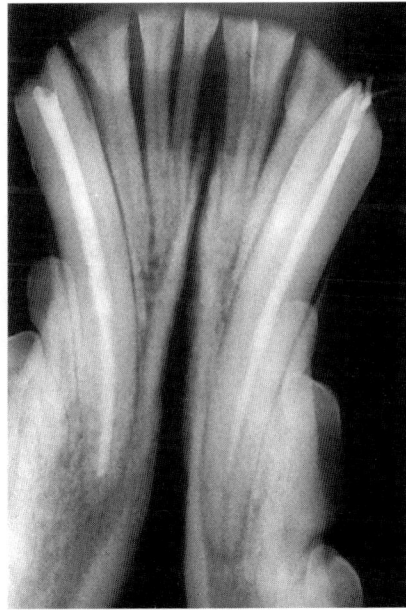

FIGURE 16.22

Contributing Author:

James M.G. Anthony

Description: Fractured mandibular canines after endodontic instrumentation and obturation in a silver fox (*Vulpes vulpes*). Note that there is an apical void in 404.

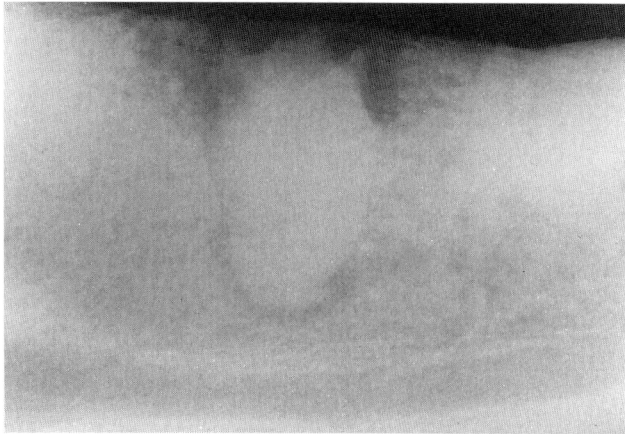

FIGURE 16.23

Contributing Author:
James M.G. Anthony

Description: Retained roots from an old fractured mandibular molar with osteomyelitis in a cougar (*Panthera concolor*).

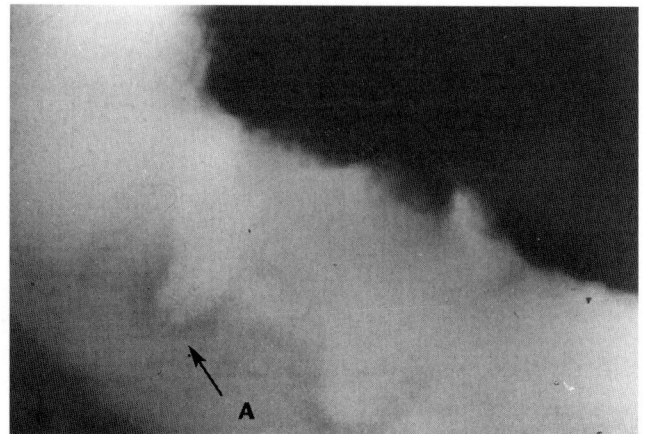

FIGURE 16.24

Contributing Author:
James M.G. Anthony

Description: Retained roots of the last mandibular premolar with apical granuloma (diagnosed by histology) in a lion (*Panthera leo)*. Histology suggested feline odontoclastic resorptive lesions as the cause of crown fracture.

A. Condensing osteitis

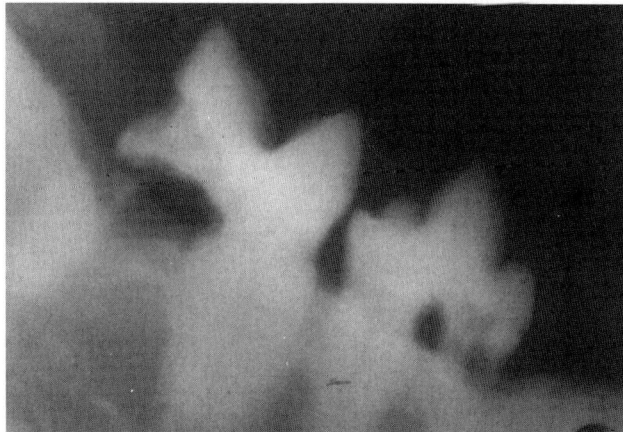

FIGURE 16.25

Contributing Author:
James M.G. Anthony

Description: Mandibular premolar and molar of a Canadian lynx (*Felis lynx canadensis*) with multiple feline odontoclastic resorptive lesions (external resorption).

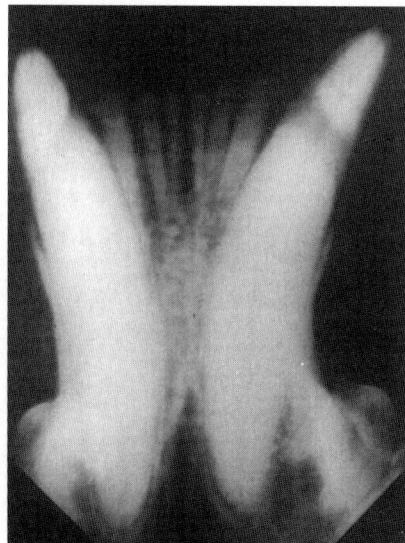

FIGURE 16.26

Contributing Author:
James M.G. Anthony

Description: A Siberian tiger (*Panthera tigris altaica*) with severe bilateral abrasion (cage biter syndrome) of both canines with no pulpal involvement as yet.

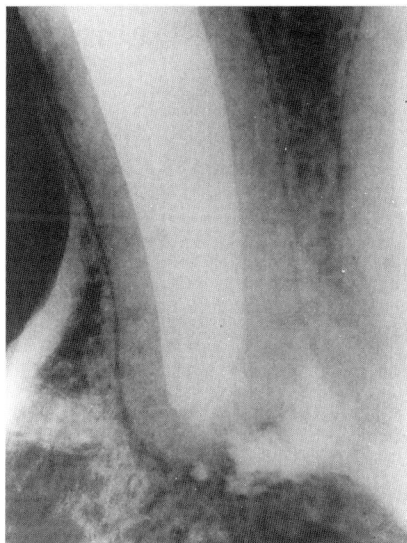

FIGURE 16.27

Contributing Author:
James M.G. Anthony

Description: Endodontic obturation of a Siberian tiger (*Panthera tigris altaica*) mandibular canine showing an apical puff of sealer cement. This canal was 68 mm in length from the gingival margin and 1.8 cm in diameter.

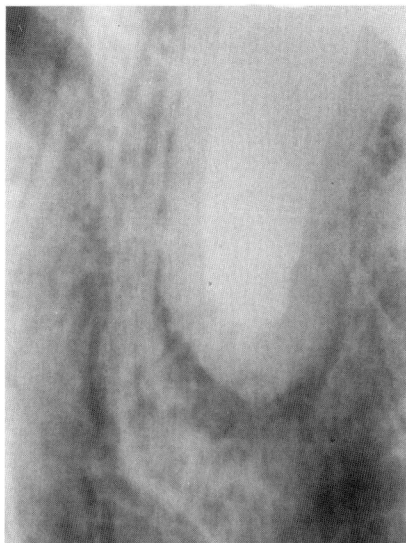

FIGURE 16.28

Contributing Author:
James M.G. Anthony

Description: Endodontic obturation of a Siberian tiger (*Panthera tigris altaica*) maxillary canine with an apical periodontitis. This canal was 79 mm in length from the gingival margin and 2.1 cm in diameter.

FIGURE 16.29

Contributing Author:
James M.G. Anthony

Description: A South African fur seal (*Arctocephalus pusillus pusillus*) with a fractured canine with pulpal exposure and an open apex.

Points Identified:

A. Canine fracture
B. Open apex

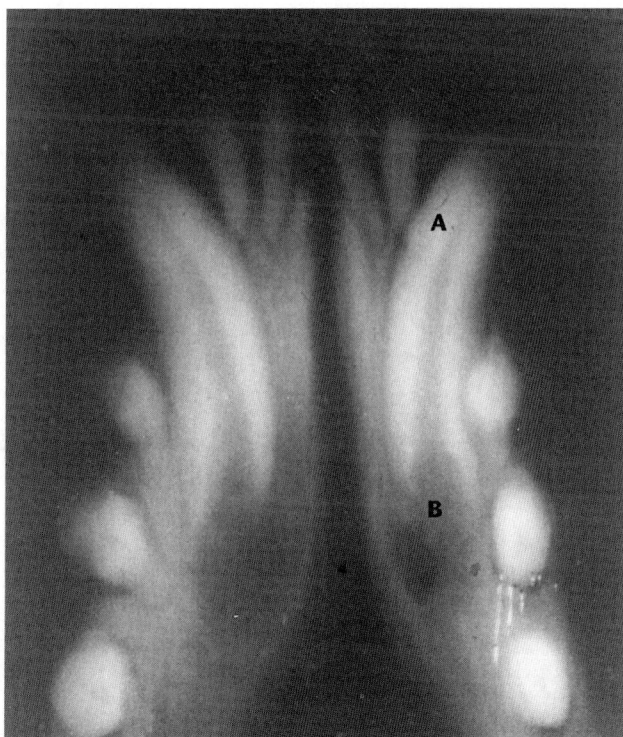

FIGURE 16.30

Contributing Author:

James M.G. Anthony

Description: A common marmoset (*Callithrix jacchus*) with endodontic treatment of both maxillary canines.

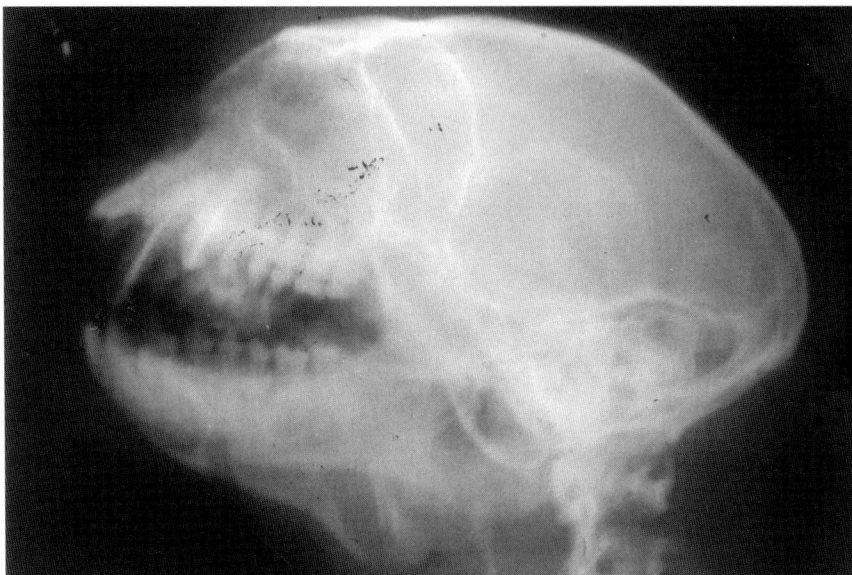

FIGURE 16.31

Contributing Author:

James M.G. Anthony

Description: A gray-headed flying fox (*Pteropus poliocephalus*) with root remnants resulting in a chronic osteomyelitis.

Points Identified:

A. Root remnants and chronic sclerosing osteomyelitis

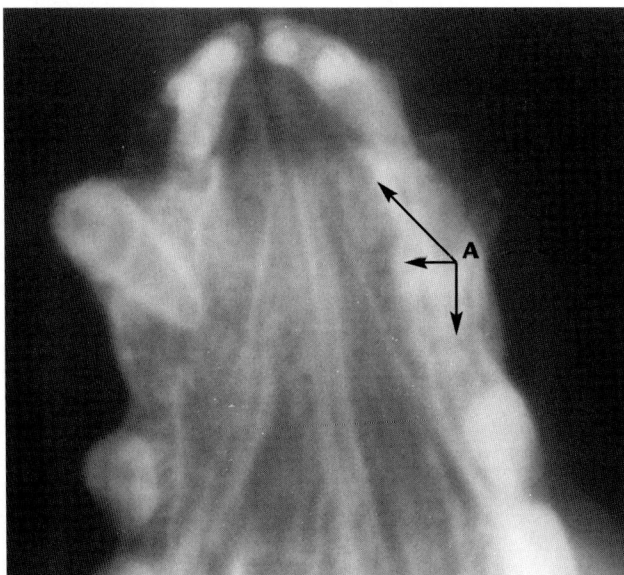

FIGURE 16.32

Contributing Author:

James M.G. Anthony

Description: Tooth root remnant from previous extraction of the maxillary molar in a Grevy's zebra (*Equus grevyi*). Note how the teeth have tipped to fill the diastimal space created by the extraction.

Points Identified:

A. Root remnant from previous extraction

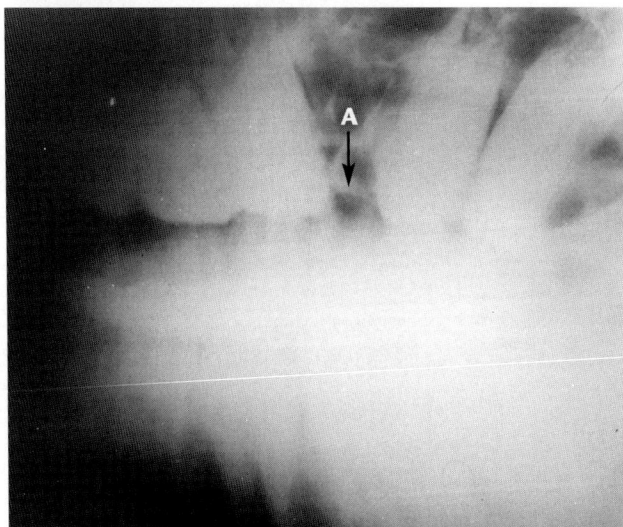

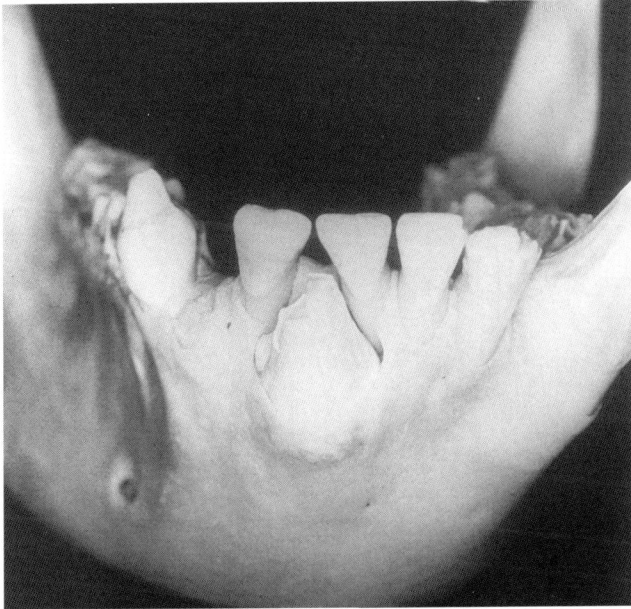

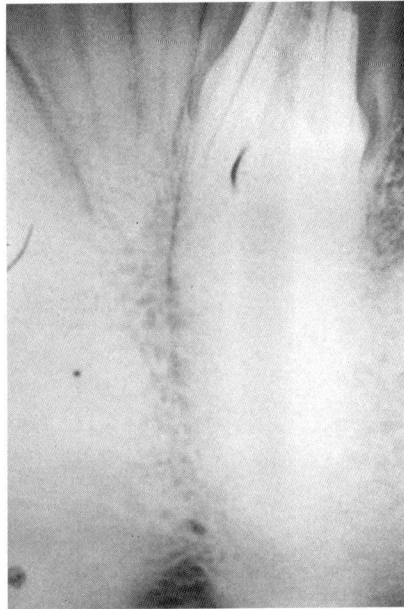

A

B

FIGURE 16.33

Contributing Author: Peter Emily

Description: View A, impacted lower canine in a gorilla. View B, radiograph of the impacted canine.

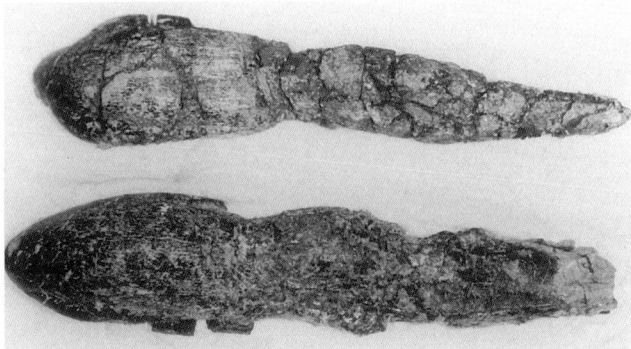

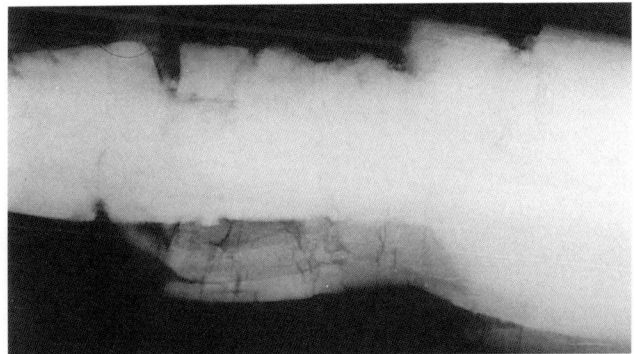

A

B

FIGURE 16.34

Contributing Author: Peter Emily

Description: View A, slide of the tyrannosaur (a homodont). View B, radiograph of premolar and molar area.

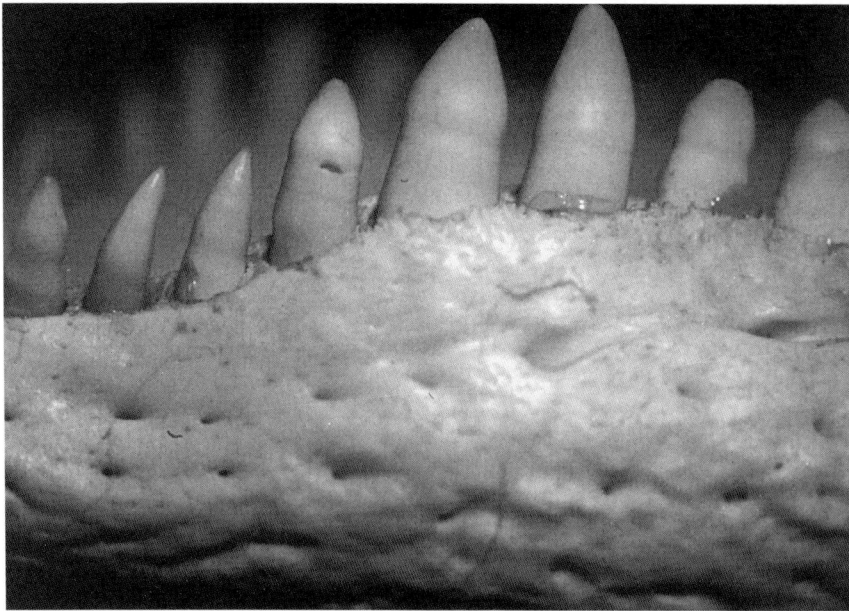
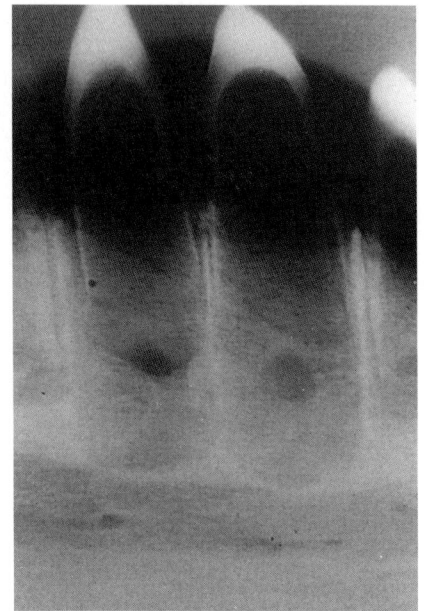

A

B

FIGURE 16.35

Contributing Author: Peter Emily

Description: View A, slide of premolar and molar area, mandible of a crocodile. View B, radiograph of the premolar and molar area.

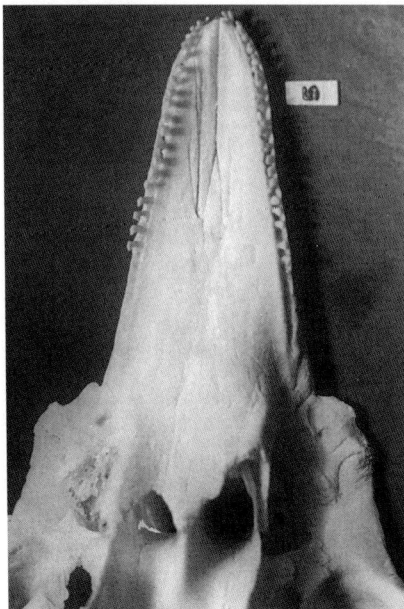
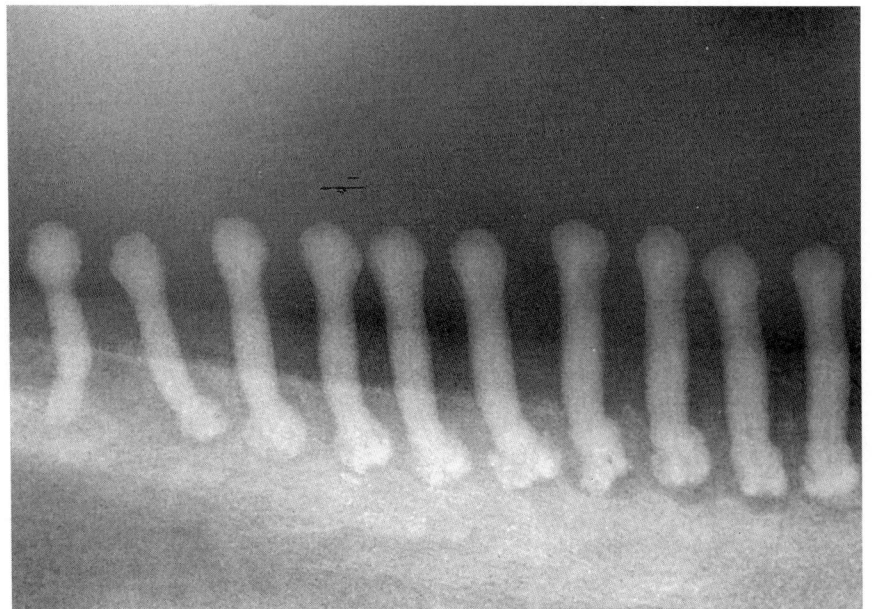

A

B

FIGURE 16.36

Contributing Author: Peter Emily

Description: View A, oral skeletal structure of a river dolphin (homodont). View B, radiograph of the lower premolar and molar area. One should recognize that the river dolphin has 260 teeth.

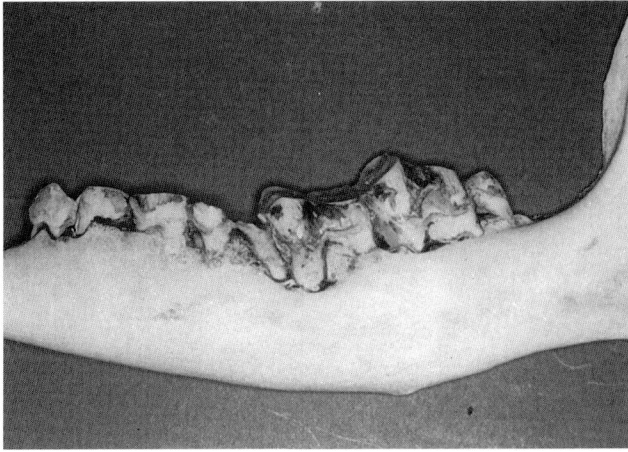

A

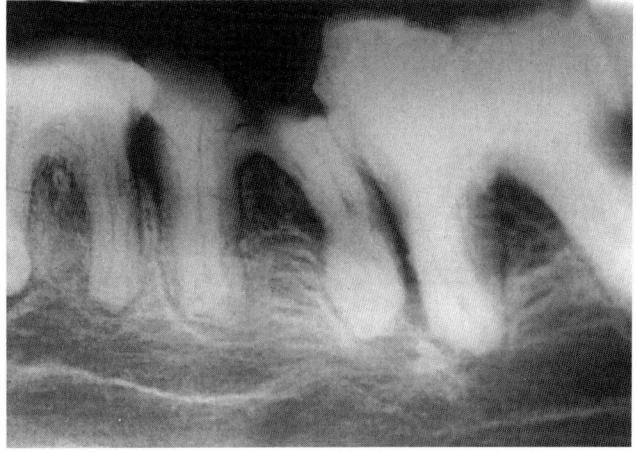

B

FIGURE 16.37

Contributing Author: Peter Emily

Description: View A, mandible axis in a deer; premolar fracture and radicular abscess. View B, radiograph of the premolar fracture and radicular abscess.

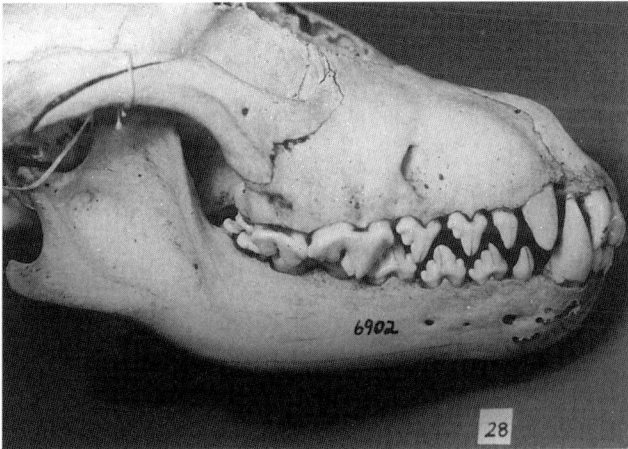

FIGURE 16.38

Contributing Author: Peter Emily

Description: Skull of a wild canine.

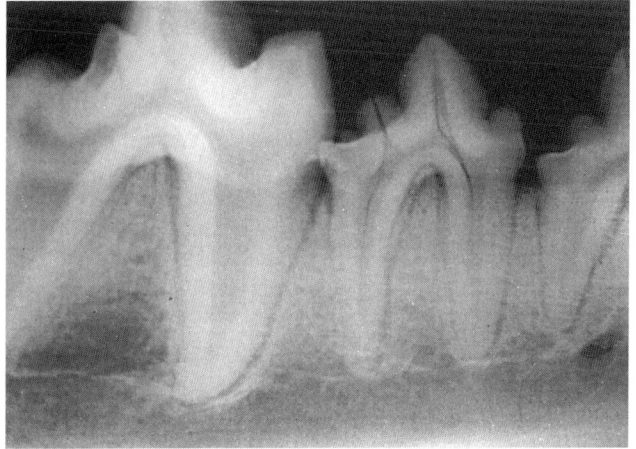

FIGURE 16.39

Contributing Author: Peter Emily

Description: Radiograph of the premolar and molar area of the wild canine seen in Figure 16.38.

FIGURE 16.40

Contributing Author: Peter Emily

Description: White tip shark, occlusal view. Film used is Kodak XRP-5(5×7)-800 speed single.

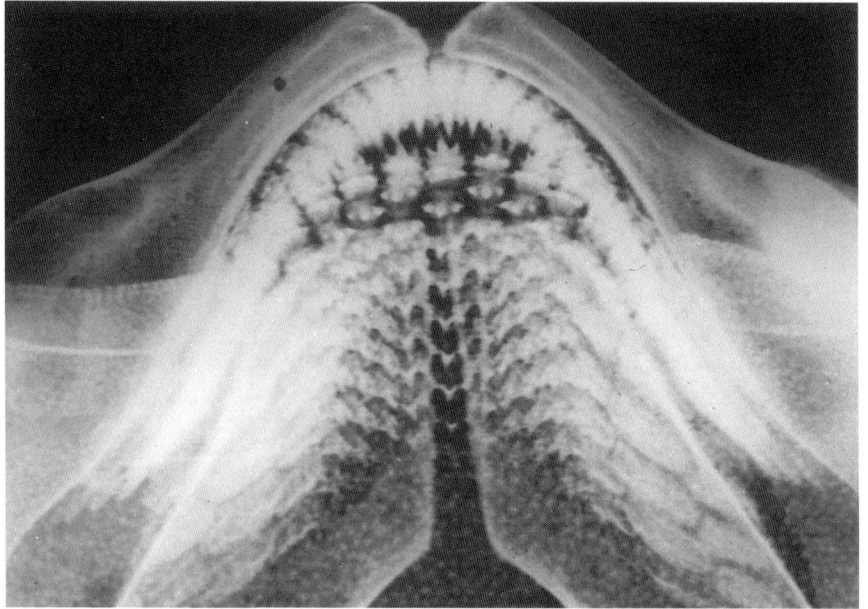

FIGURE 16.41

Contributing Author: Peter Emily

Description: Mandible of a gorilla. Note extensive resorption at lingual gingival surface.

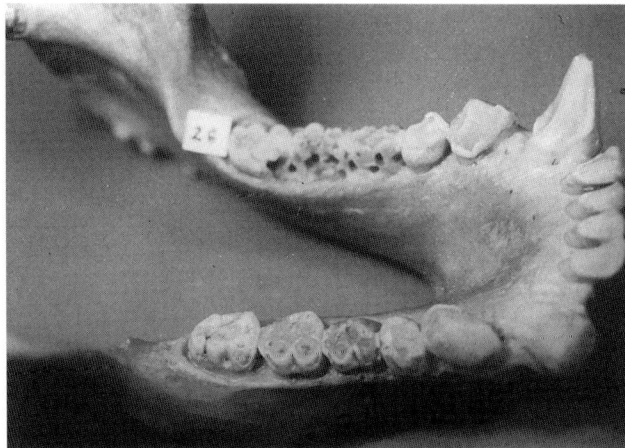

FIGURE 16.42

Contributing Author: Peter Emily

Description: Radiograph of gorilla mandible seen in Figure 16.41, showing odontoclastic resorptive lesions. This is a case worthy of noting.

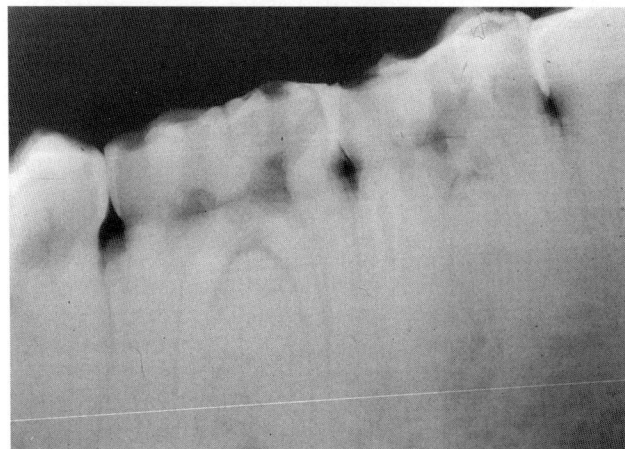

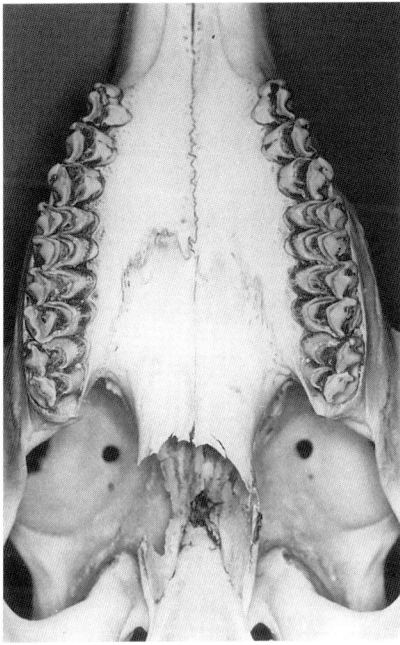

FIGURE 16.43

Contributing Author: Peter Emily

Description: White-tailed deer dentition.

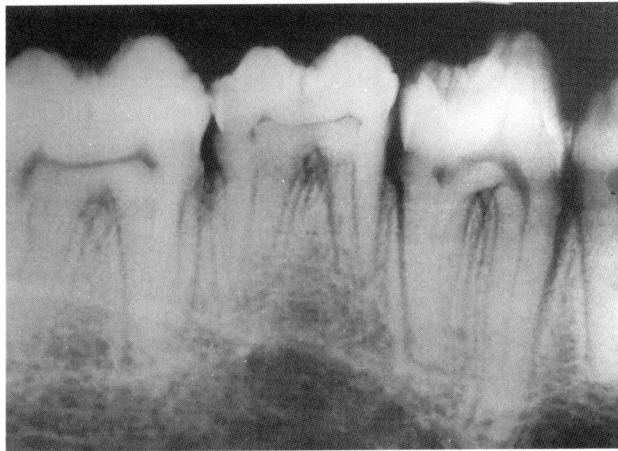

FIGURE 16.44

Contributing Author: Peter Emily

Description: Radiograph of the white-tailed deer dentition shown in Figure 16.43, showing the lower posterior quadrant.

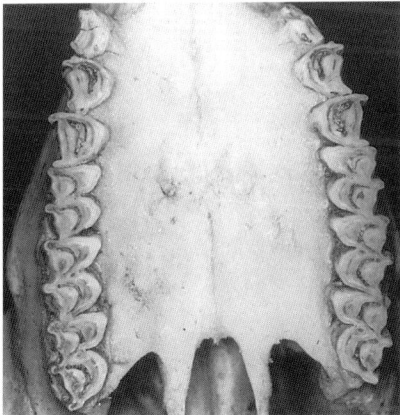

FIGURE 16.45

Contributing Author: Peter Emily

Description: Black buck dentition.

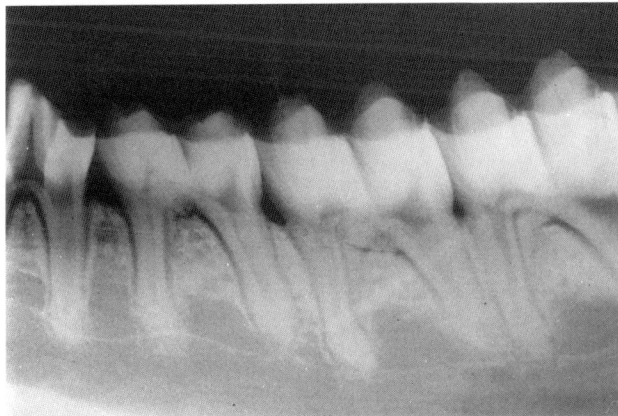

FIGURE 16.46

Contributing Author: Peter Emily

Description: Radiograph of the lower posterior quadrant of a black buck (see Figure 16.45). As a point of interest, note that both the white-tailed deer and the black buck have selenodont brachydont dentition.

FIGURE 16.47

Contributing Author: Peter Emily

Description: Rhinoceros with infra-mandibular abscess.

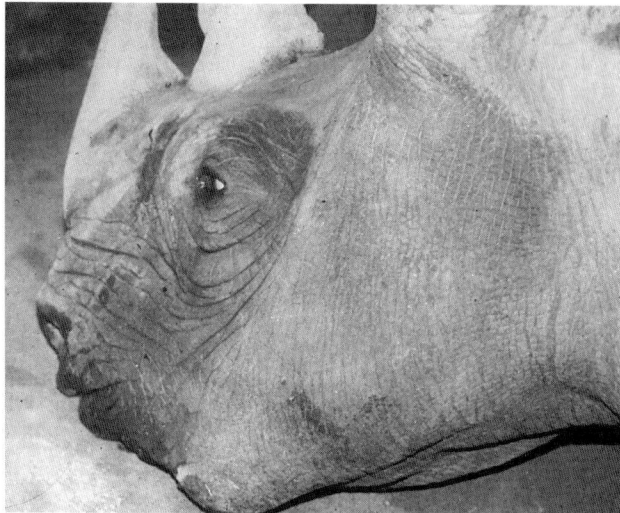

FIGURE 16.48

Contributing Author: Peter Emily

Description: Retrograde access area for endodontics on the rhinoceros seen in Figure 16.47.

(See also color plate.)

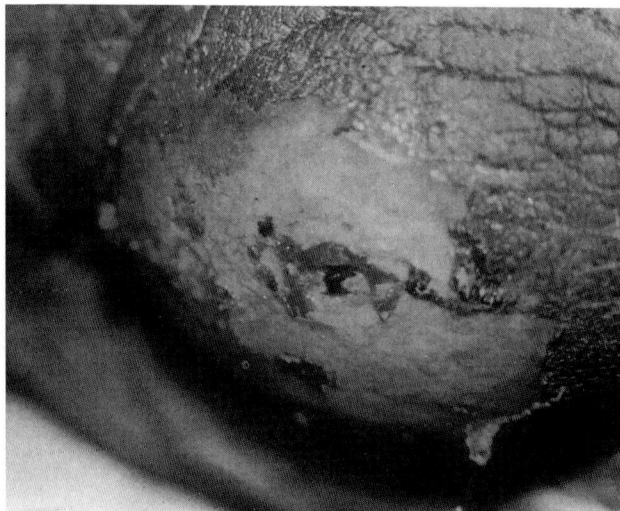

FIGURE 16.49

Contributing Author: Peter Emily

Description: Periapical radiograph of the lower third premolar abscess in the rhinoceros seen in Figures 16.47 and 16.48.

Points Identified:

A. Abscess area

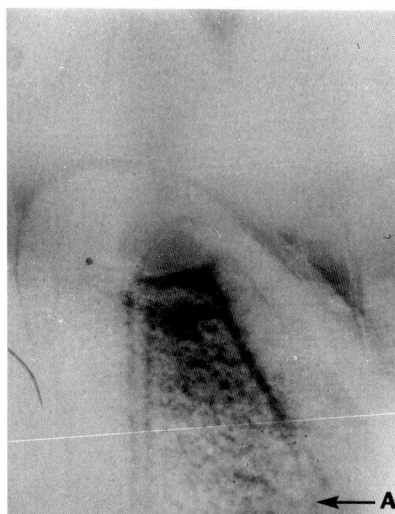

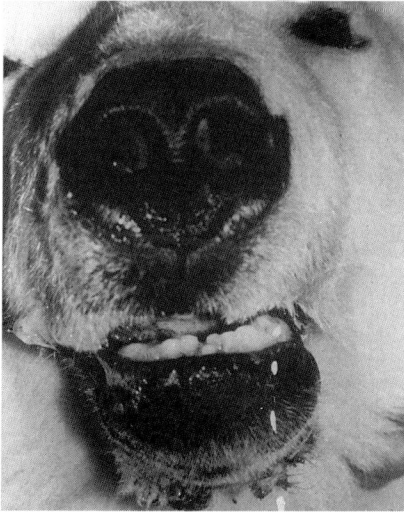

FIGURE 16.50

Contributing Author: Peter Emily

Description: Polar bear, clinical view.

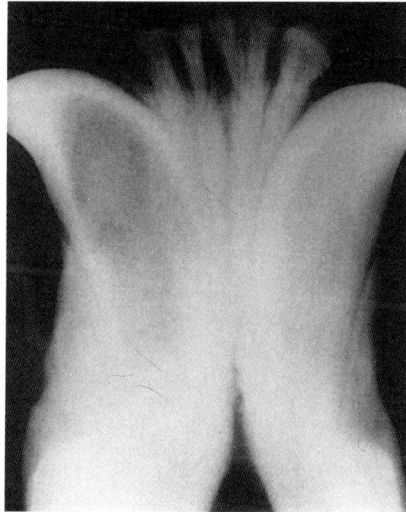

FIGURE 16.51

Contributing Author: Peter Emily

Description: Radiograph showing bilateral difference in pulpal dimensions in the polar bear shown in Figure 16.50.

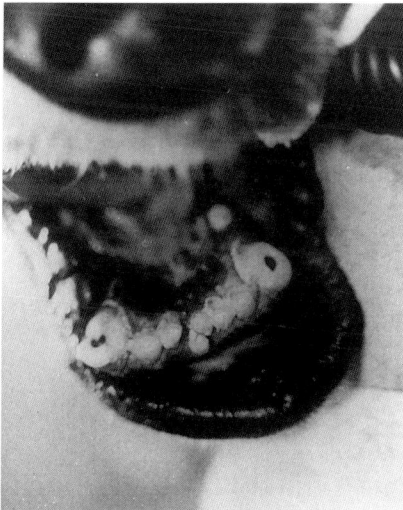

FIGURE 16.52

Contributing Author: Peter Emily

Description: Clinical complications of endodontics in zoo animals. In this polar bear, foreign material found around endodontic openings included small rocks, sticks, straw, and other debris.

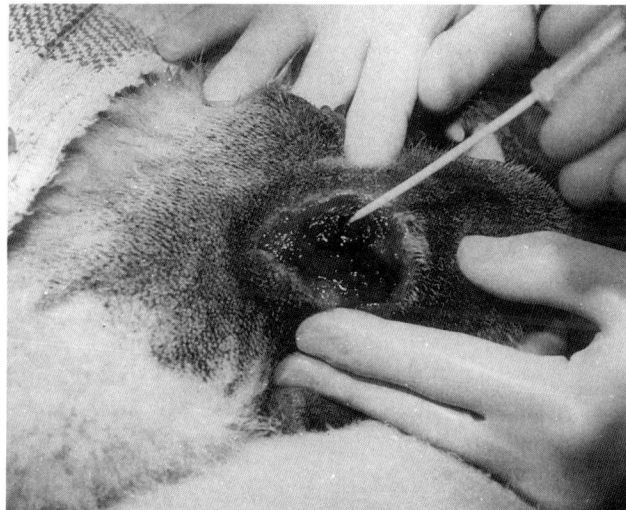

FIGURE 16.53

Contributing Author: Peter Emily

Description: After the conventional endodontic procedure was completed, the root apex was prepared for an additional retrograde apicoectomy. In zoo endodontics, because of the value of the animals and the need for avoidance of repeat anesthesia, it is a good policy to complete orthograde and retrograde endodontics together when a draining tract is present. Follow-up radiography is not possible because of the need for anesthesia. This combination of procedures assures success in most instances. Very few cases are presented without fistulous tracts. The tract is the first sign to the keeper or zoo veterinarian that a problem is present. (See Figures 16.50–16.52.)

*(**See also color plate.**)*

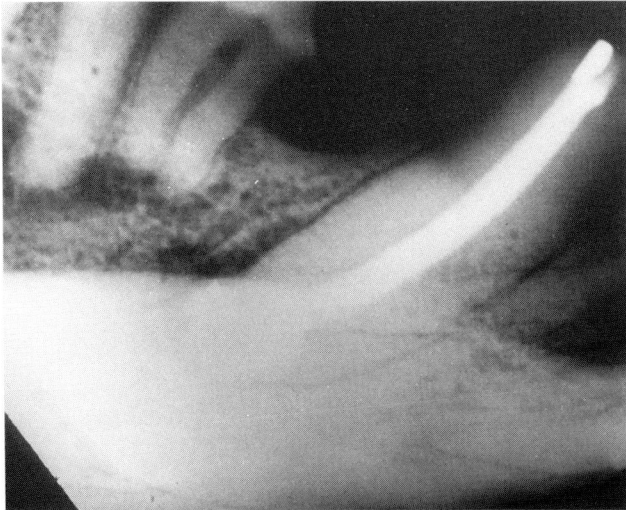

FIGURE 16.54

Contributing Author: Peter Emily

Description: Final radiograph showing conventional and retrograde endodontics; taken with #4-DF50 occlusal film. (Refer to Figure 16.53.)

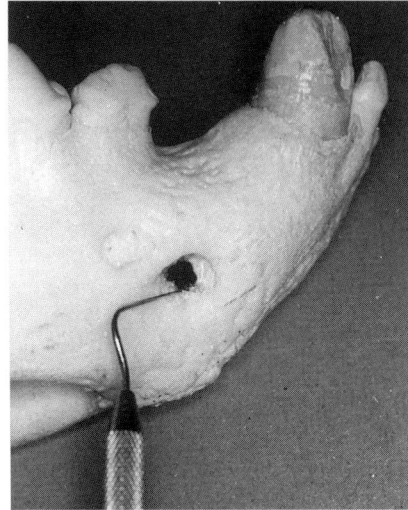

FIGURE 16.55

Contributing Author: Peter Emily

Description: Hyena, postmortem specimen.

(See also color plate.)

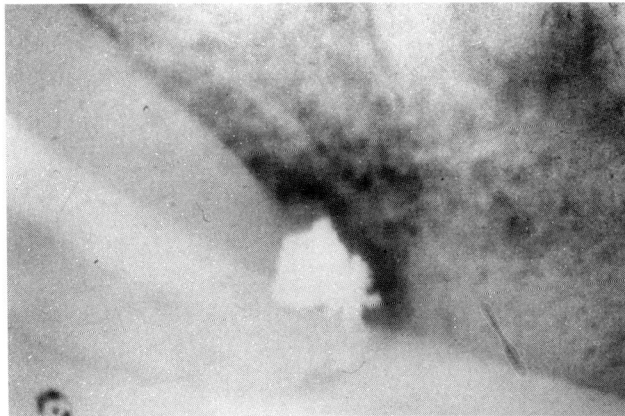

FIGURE 16.56

Contributing Author: Peter Emily

Description: In this hyena, examination and dental radiology show an unsuccessful retrograde endodontic procedure caused by an improper apical seal with amalgam alloy.

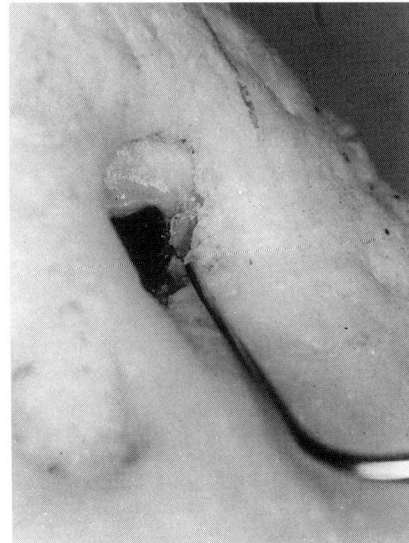

FIGURE 16.57

Contributing Author: Peter Emily

Description: In this view of the hyena (see Figure 16.56) mandible, an explorer points to exposed gutta percha in the endodontic system. An improper apical seal caused microleakage and continued apical pathology. A failed apicoectomy.

(See also color plate.)

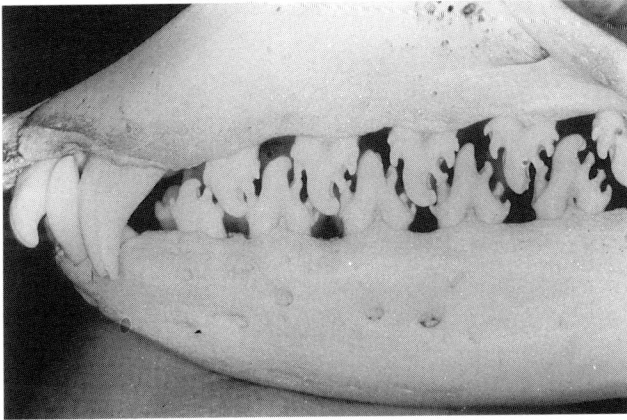

FIGURE 16.58

Contributing Author: Peter Emily

Description: Dentition in a crab seal (skull).

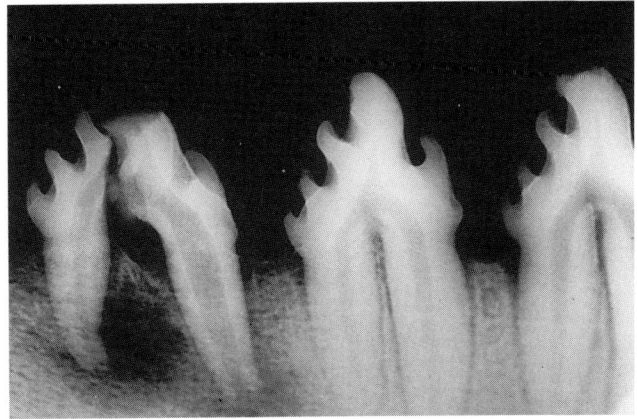

FIGURE 16.59

Contributing Author: Peter Emily

Description: Crab seal. A crown and root fracture with periapical abscessation in the mandible.

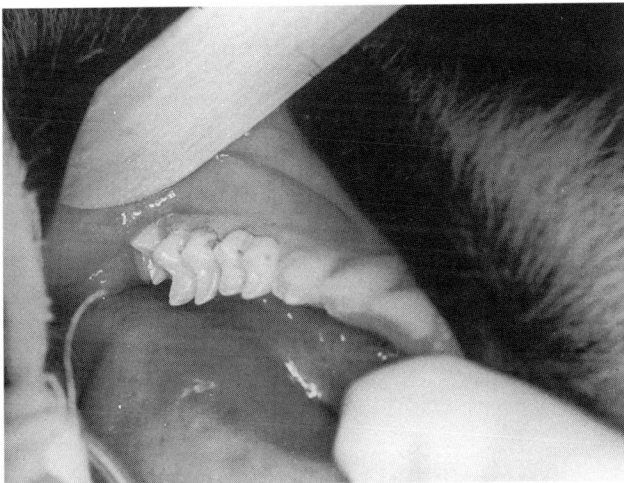

FIGURE 16.60

Contributing Author: Peter Emily

Description: A colobus monkey shown with pericoronitis from a partially erupted lower third molar.

(See also color plate.)

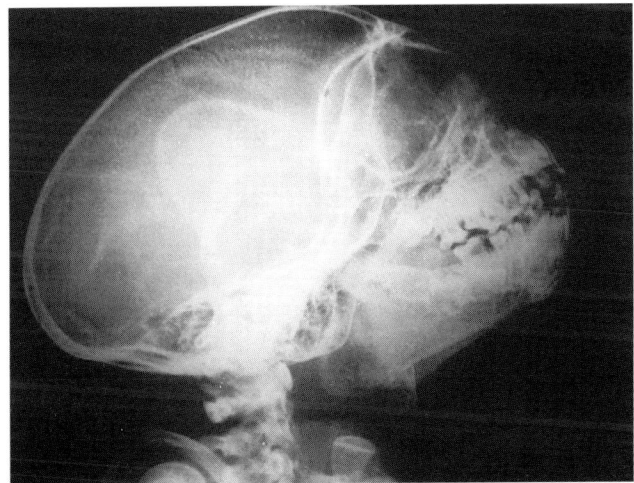

FIGURE 16.61

Contributing Author: Peter Emily

Description: Use of a mammogram x-ray unit to examine dentition in a colobus monkey cranium. In the zoo setting, this unit provides excellent detail for the diagnostics necessary for treatment.

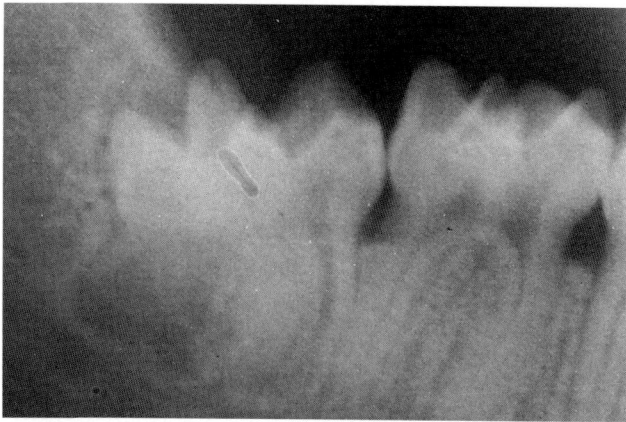

FIGURE 16.62

Contributing Author: Peter Emily

Description: Radiographic examination of patient shown in Figure 16.61. Size 0 intraoral nonscreen film used for examination of third molar.

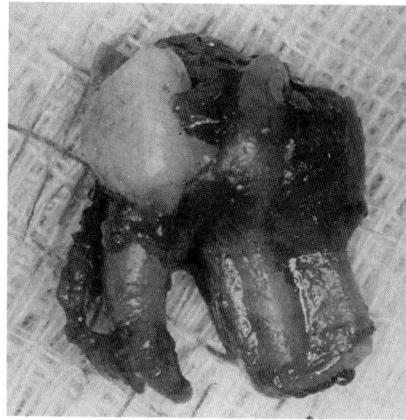

FIGURE 16.63

Contributing Author: Peter Emily

Description: Extracted third molar of colobus monkey (see Figures 16.61 and 16.62).

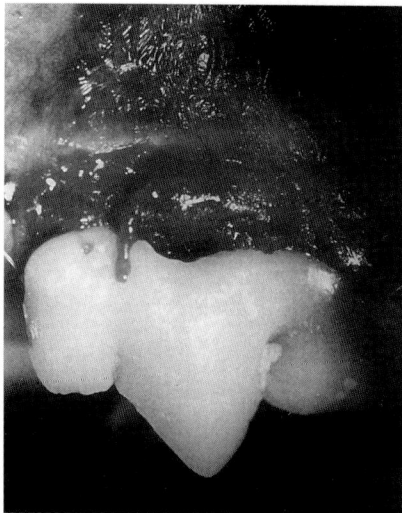

FIGURE 16.64

Contributing Author: Peter Emily

Description: Siberian tiger. This patient exhibited bilateral resorptive lesions of the upper fourth premolars. The lesions did not invade the pulp tissue. There is superimposed caries present.

(*See also color plate.*)

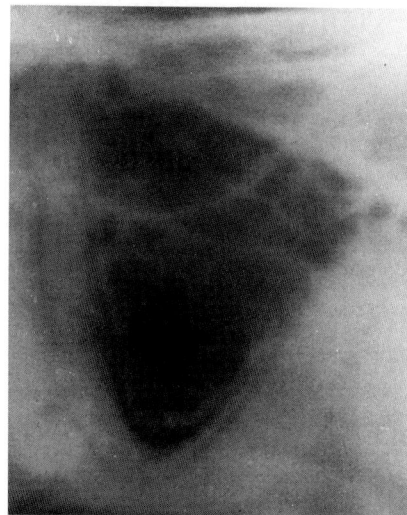

FIGURE 16.65

Contributing Author: Peter Emily

Description: Periapical radiology of Siberian tiger (seen in Figure 16.64) showing no periapical pathology.

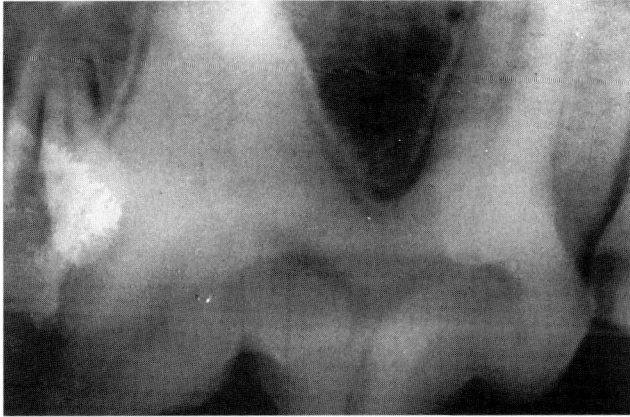

FIGURE 16.66

Contributing Author: Peter Emily

Description: Coronal exposure showing extent of resorption in maxilliary premolars in Siberian tiger shown in Figures 16.64 and 16.65.

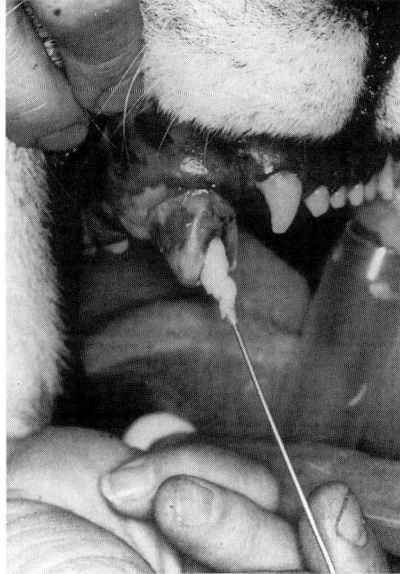

FIGURE 16.67

Contributing Author: Peter Emily

Description: Narrow canal endodontics in a lion. Note occluded apical 3 mm in radiograph of completed endodontic procedure.

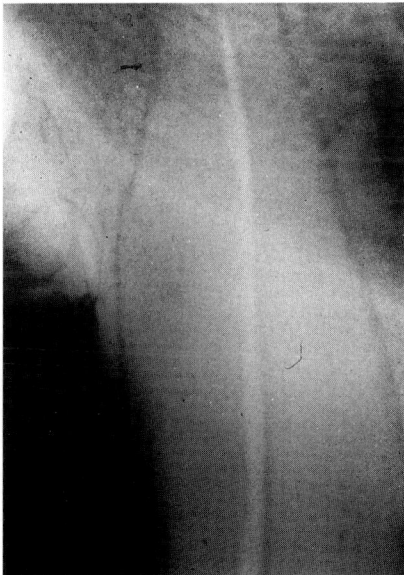

FIGURE 16.68

Contributing Author: Peter Emily

Description: Narrow canal endodontics in a lion. Note occluded apical 3 mm in radiograph of completed endodontic procedure.

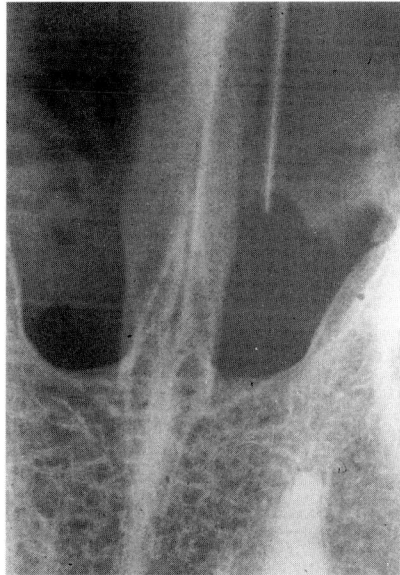

FIGURE 16.69

Contributing Author: Peter Emily

Description: Radiograph taken with XRP-5 Kodak (5×7)-800 single speed film shows the palatal bone destruction caused by fibrosarcoma in a Bengal tiger.

FIGURE 16.70

Contributing Author: Peter Emily

Description: Red kangaroo, mandibular abscess with osteomyelitis.

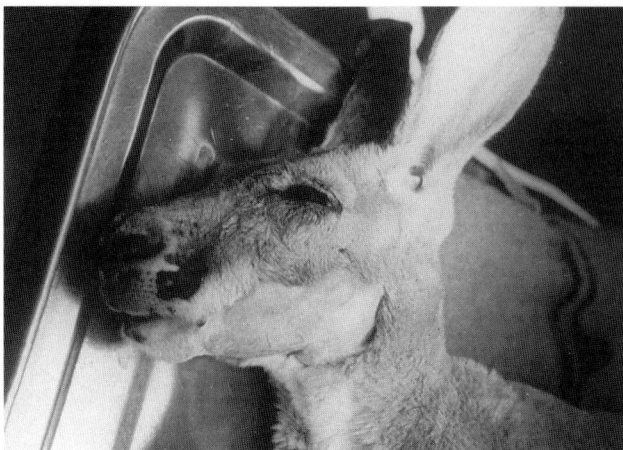

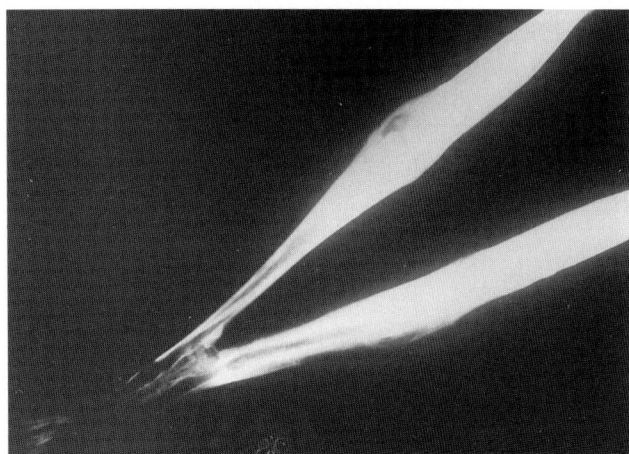

A

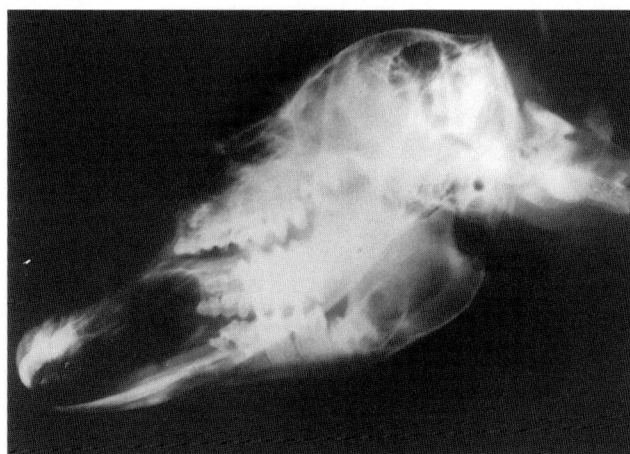

B

FIGURE 16.71

Contributing Author: Peter Emily

Description: Radiographs of mandibular abscess with osteomyelitis in the red kangaroo shown in Figure 16.70.

FIGURE 16.72

Contributing Author: Peter Emily

Description: Wallaby with a mandibular abscess.

(See also color plate.)

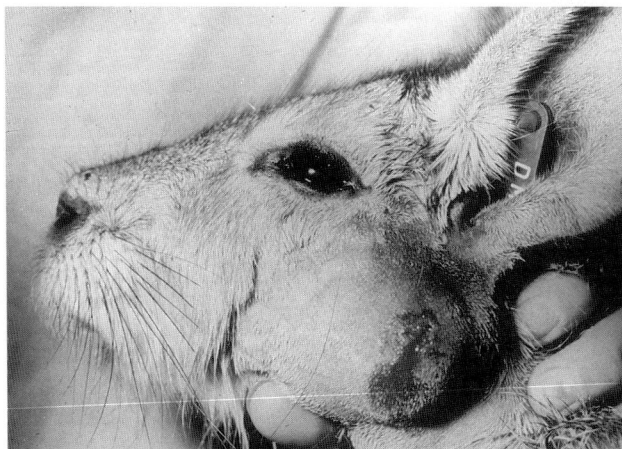

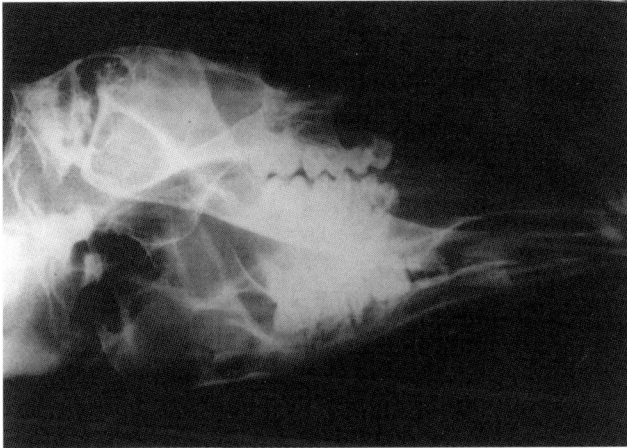

A

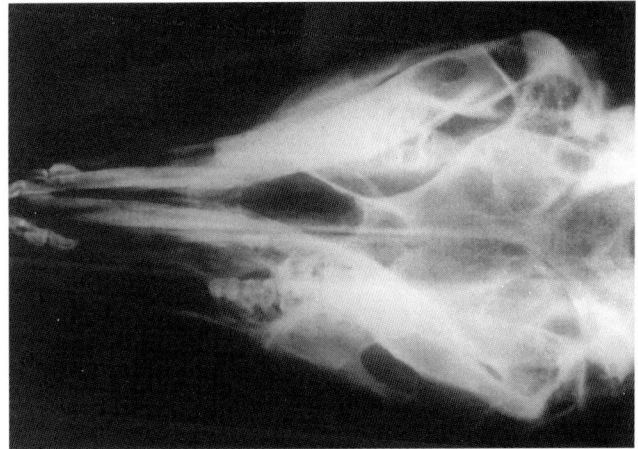

B

FIGURE 16.73

Contributing Author: Peter Emily

Description: Radiographs of abscess noted in Figure 16.72. It should be noted that such abscesses are not the typical "lumpy jaw" seen in domestic cattle. On the other hand, they are usually very aggressive anaerobic infections. The commonly cultured organism is *Fusobacterium necrophorum*. Success rate in therapy is improving, but still poor.

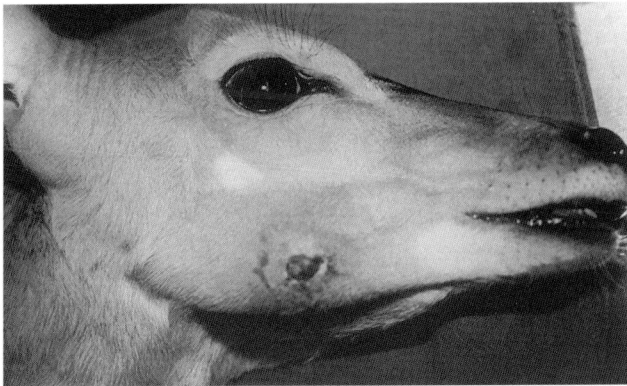

FIGURE 16.74

Contributing Author: Peter Emily

Description: A nyala with a mandibular abscess.

(See also color plate.)

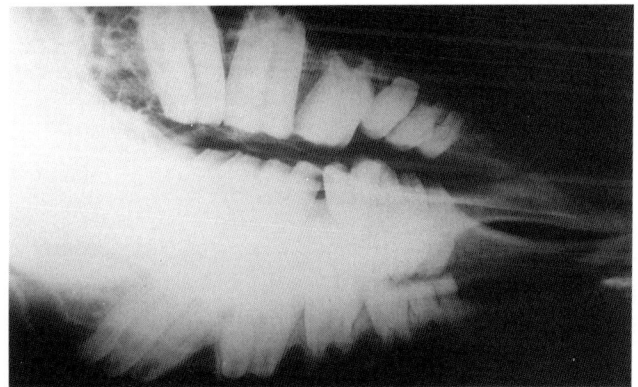

FIGURE 16.75

Contributing Author: Peter Emily

Description: Radiographic examination of an abscessed lower molar. Same species (nyala) as shown in Figure 16.74.

FIGURE 16.76

Contributing Author: Peter Emily

Description: Facial abscess in a Dall sheep (young ram).

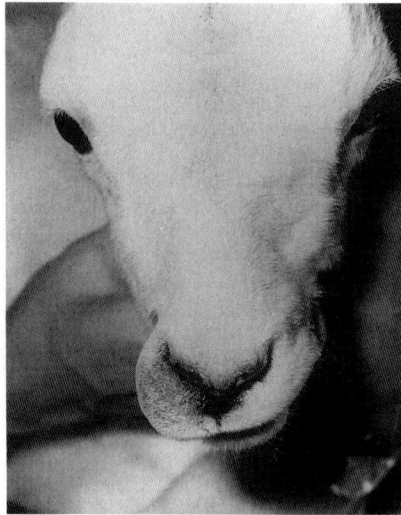

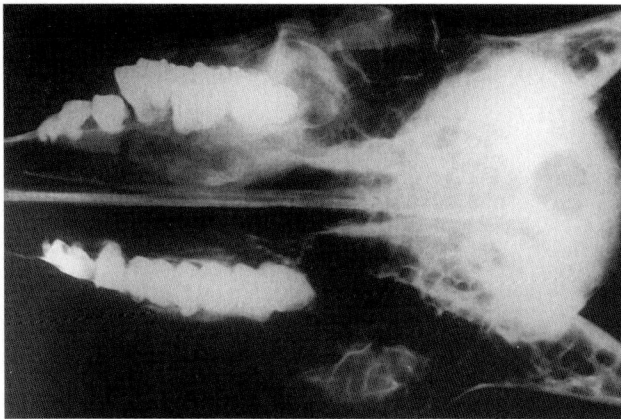

A

FIGURE 16.77

Contributing Author: Peter Emily

Description: Extraoral occlusal and lateral views of mandibular abscessation in the Dall sheep (see Figure 16.76).

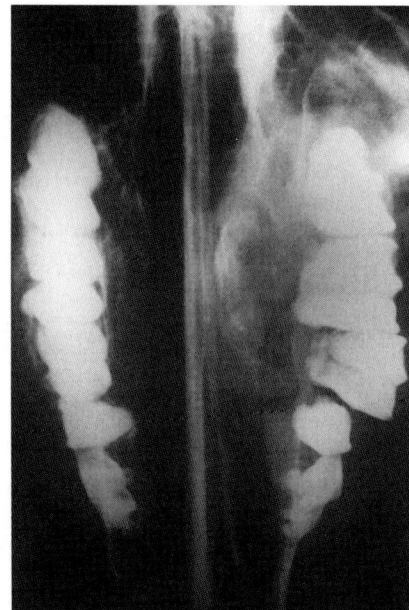

B

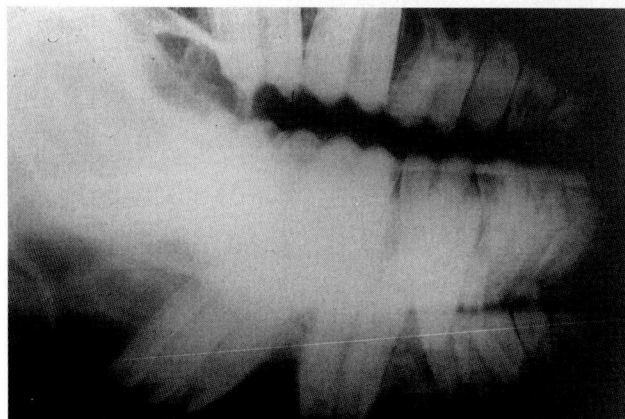

C

FIGURE 16.78

Contributing Author: Peter Emily

Description: A mandibular abscess in a camel with the complicating factor of advanced periodontitis.

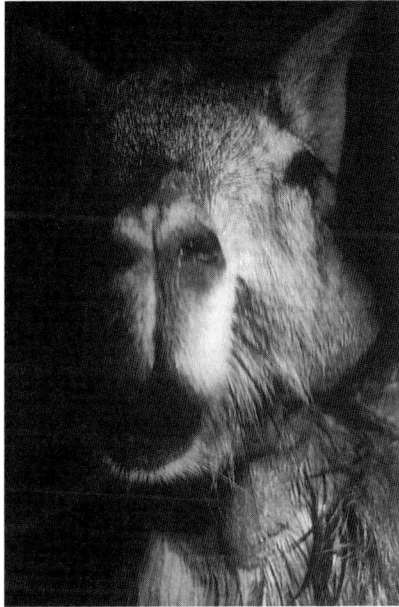

FIGURE 16.79

Contributing Author: Peter Emily

Description: In this radiograph of the camel shown in Figure 16.78 both the advanced bone loss of periodontal disease and an old fracture to the mandible anterior to the first premolar are present.

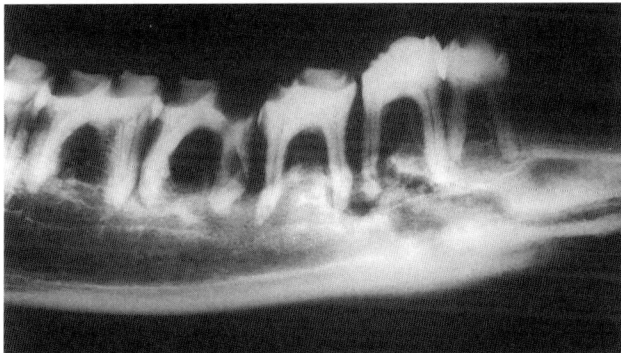

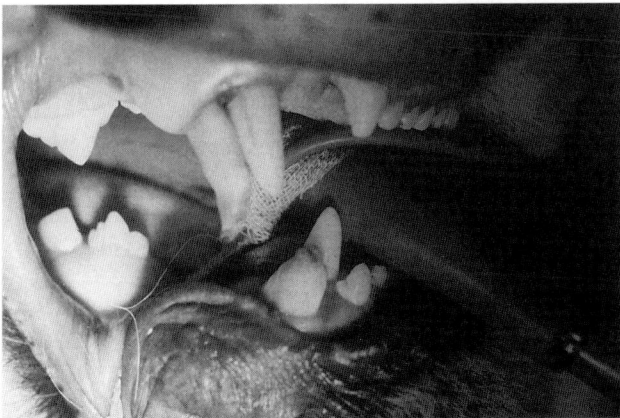

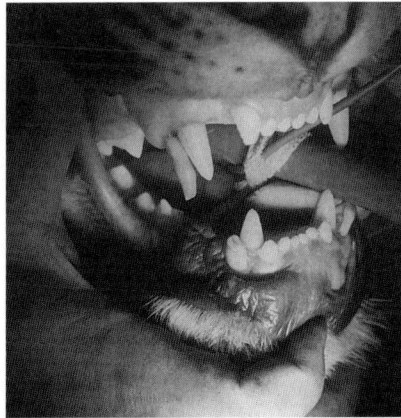

A

B

FIGURE 16.80

Contributing Author: Peter Emily

Description: Retained primary canine in a white Siberian tiger. Also noted in this patient was linguoversion of the mandibular canines.

Not reported commonly, linguoversion may have a genetic linkage to inbreeding in this species to retain the white line.

FIGURE 16.81

Contributing Author: Peter Emily

Description: Radiograph of the retained primary canine shown in Figure 16.80.

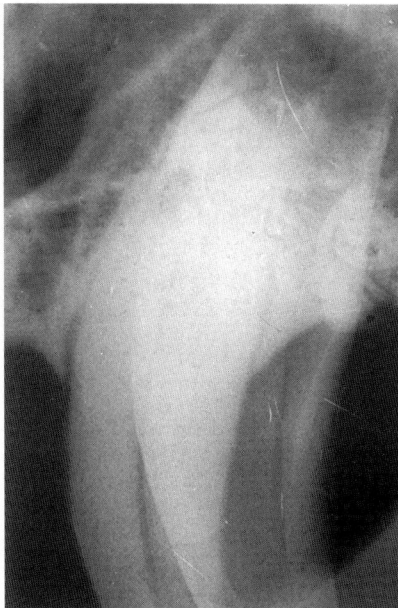

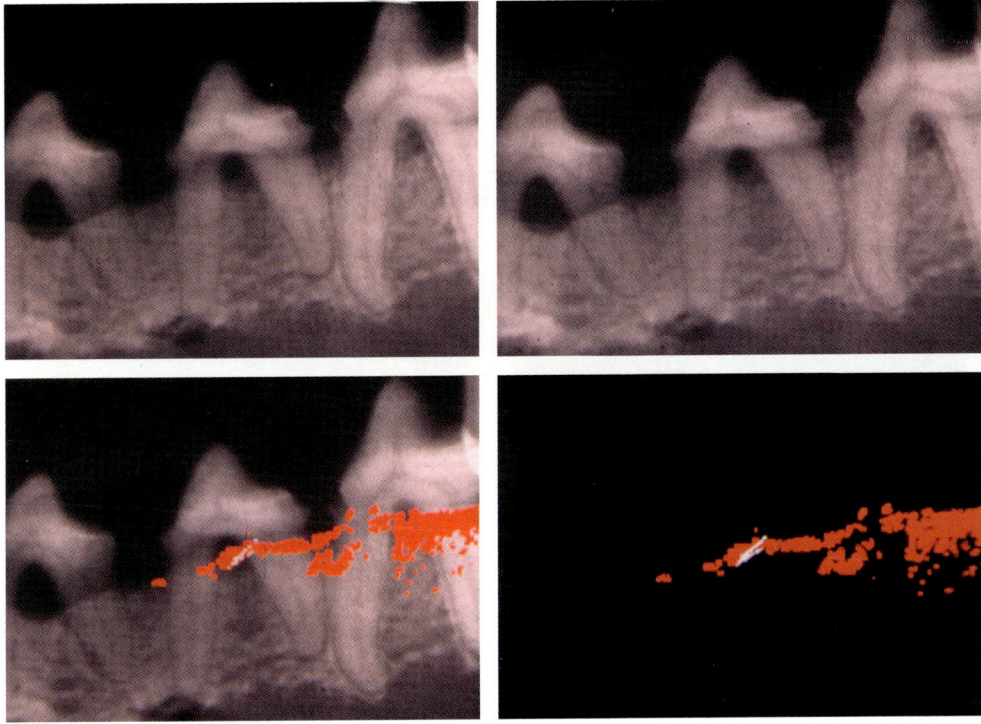

FIGURE 4.20

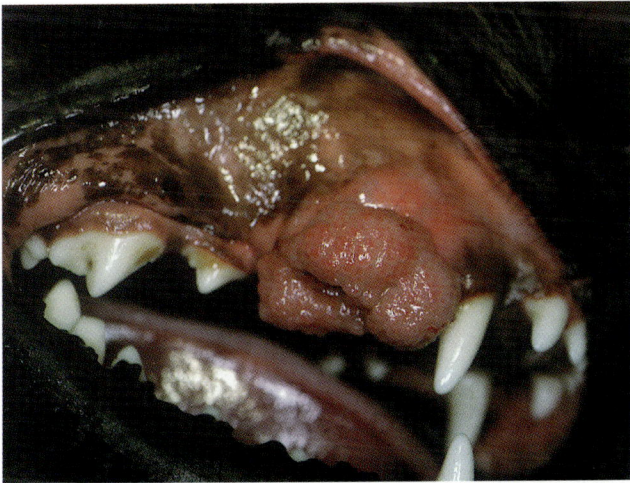

FIGURE 7.9

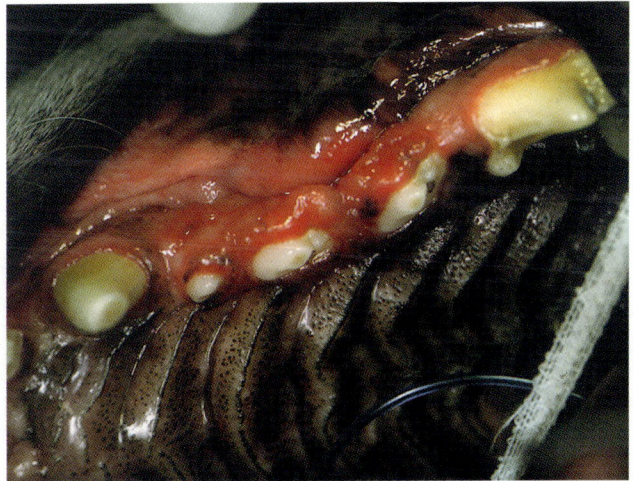

FIGURE 7.14

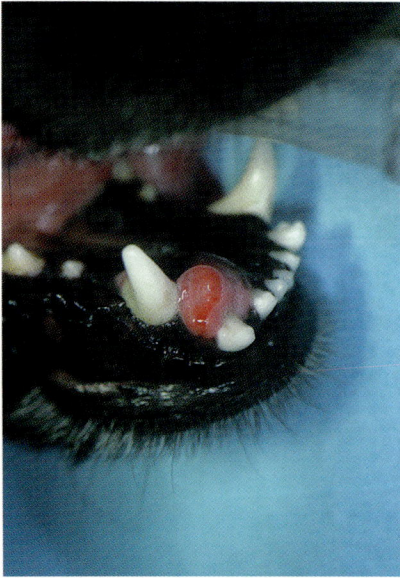

FIGURE 7.17

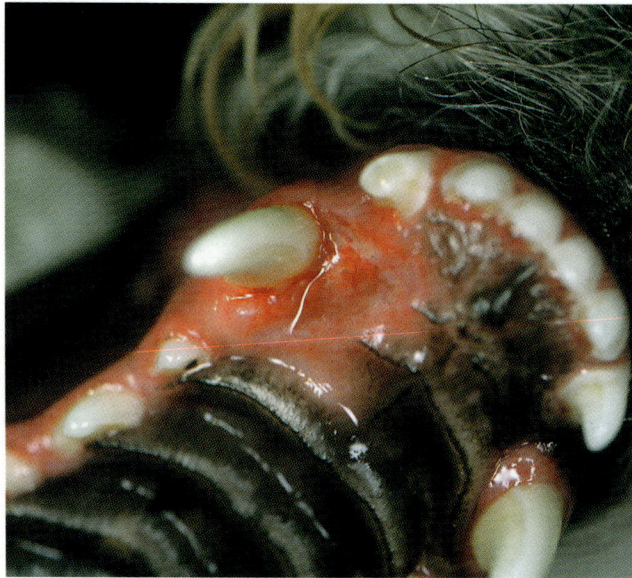

FIGURE 7.24

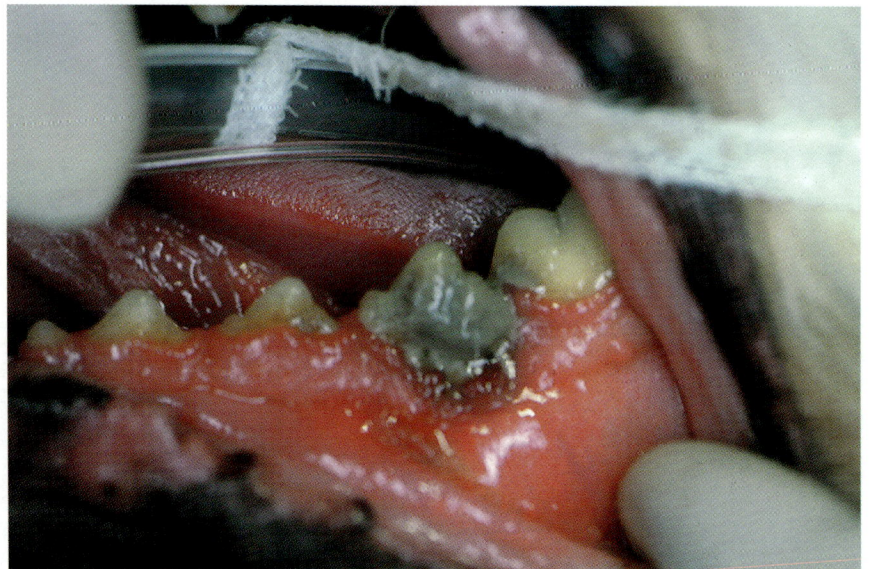

FIGURE 7.26

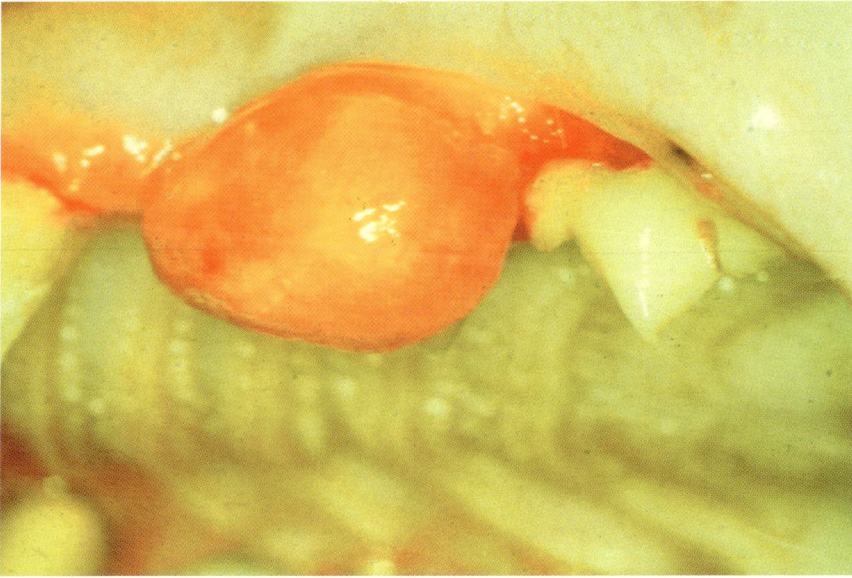

FIGURE 12.2

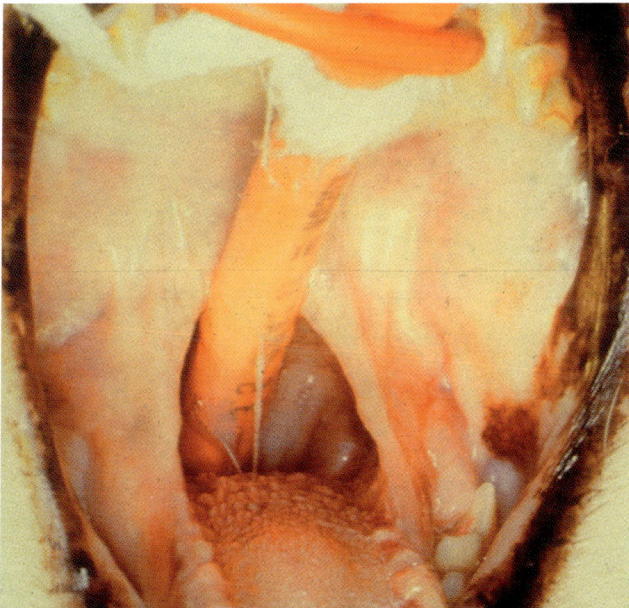

FIGURE 12.3

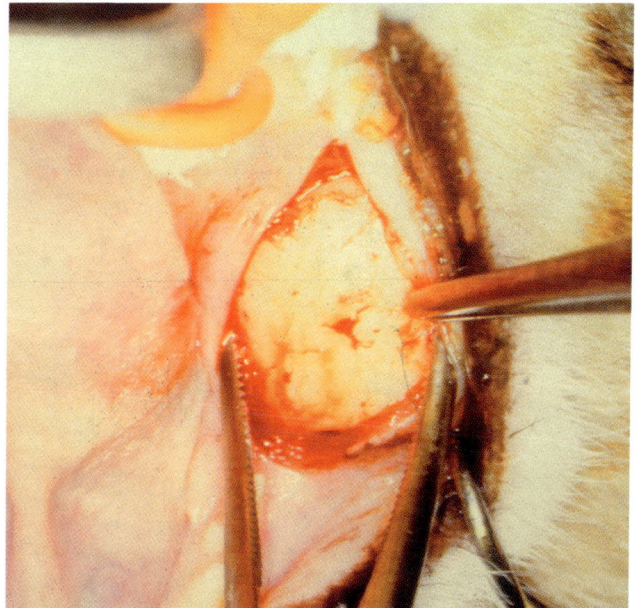

FIGURE 12.4

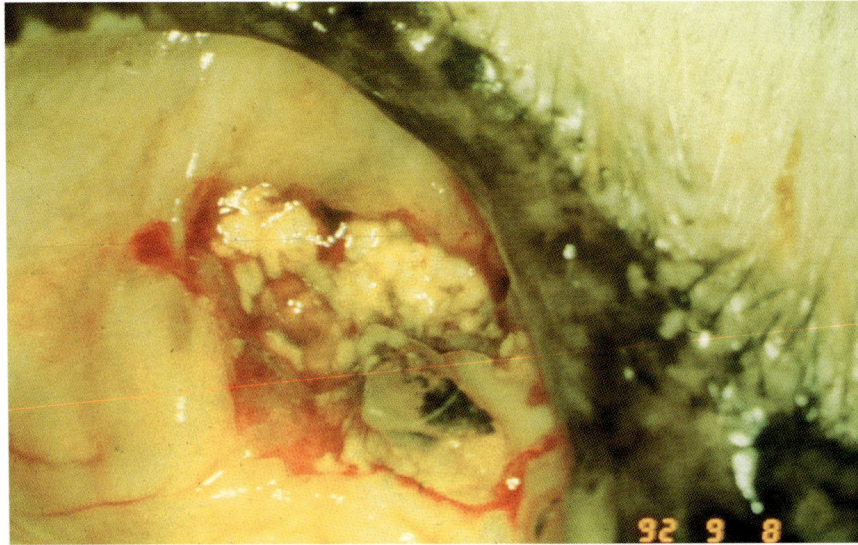

FIGURE 12.10

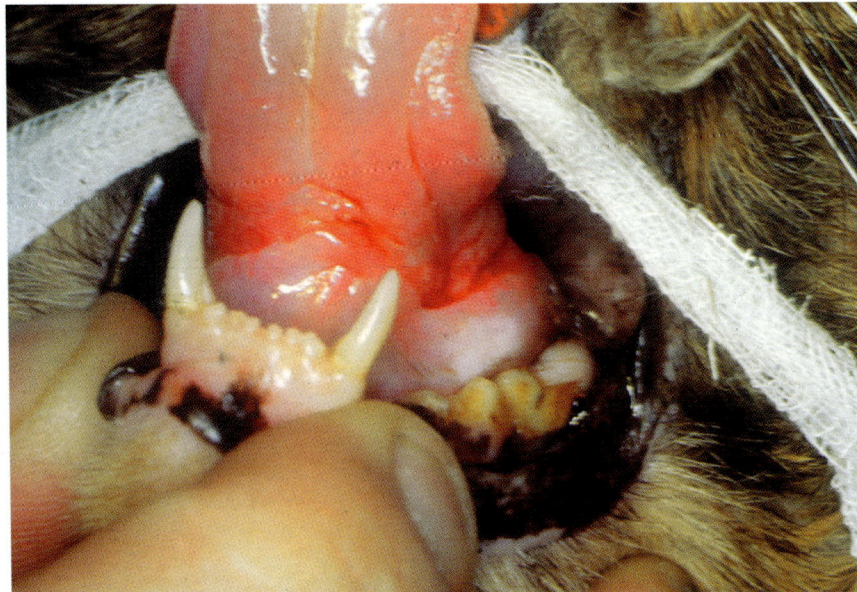

FIGURE 12.11

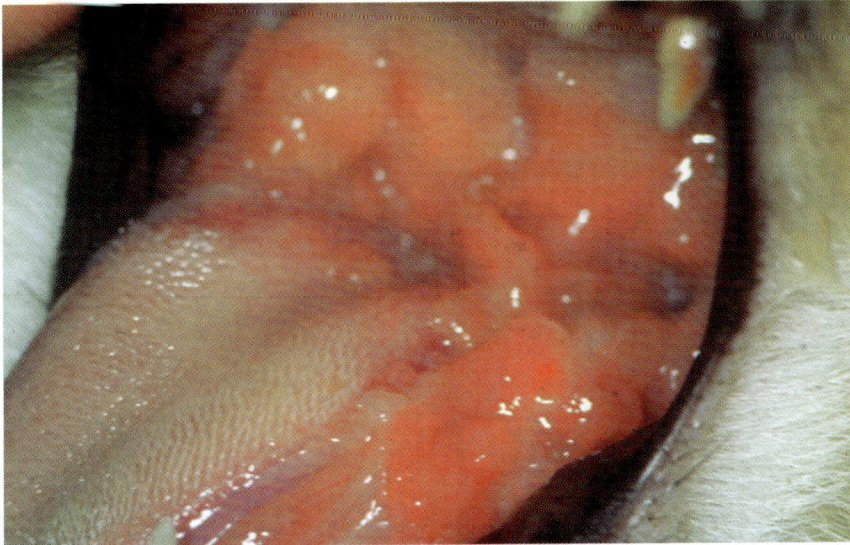

FIGURE 12.12

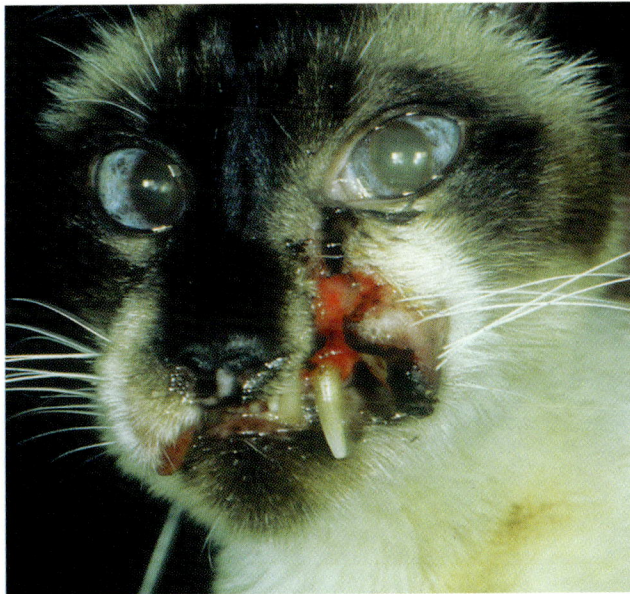

FIGURE 12.13

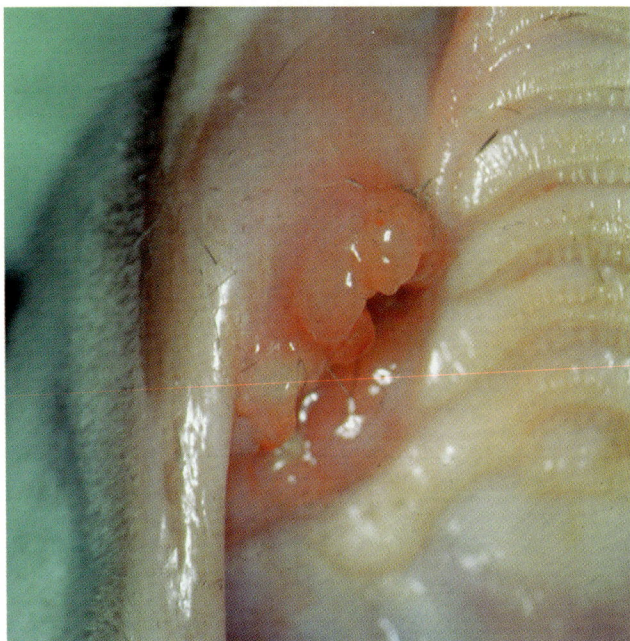

FIGURE 12.15

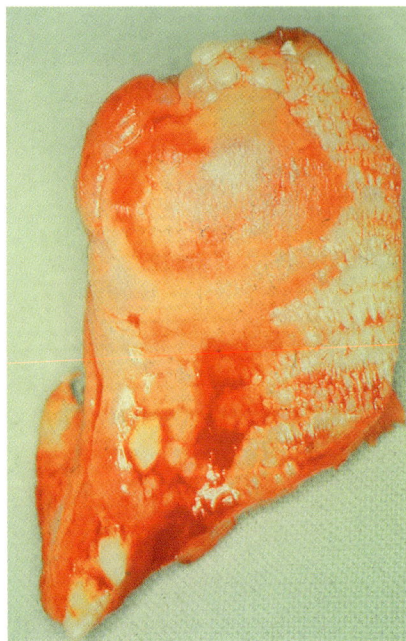

FIGURE 12.16

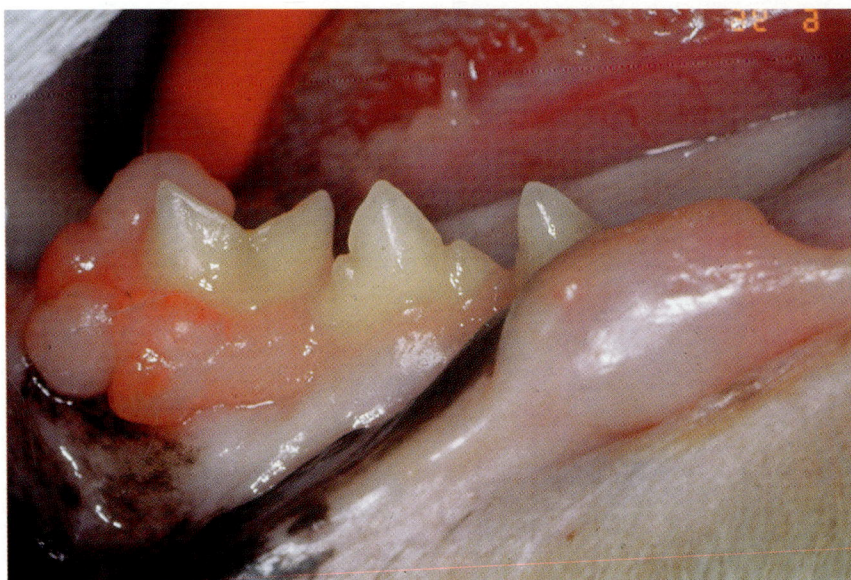

FIGURE 12.18

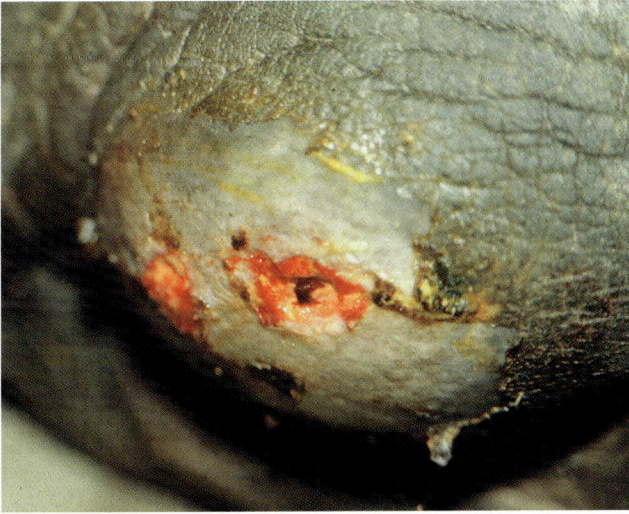

FIGURE 16.48

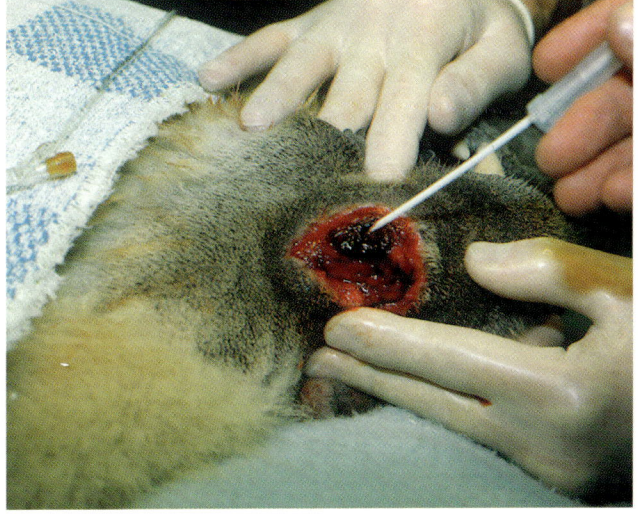

FIGURE 16.53

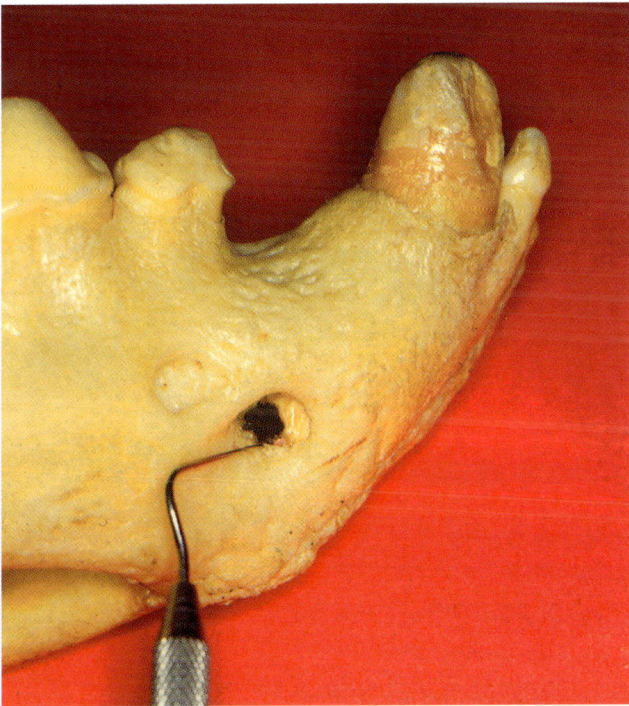

FIGURE 16.55

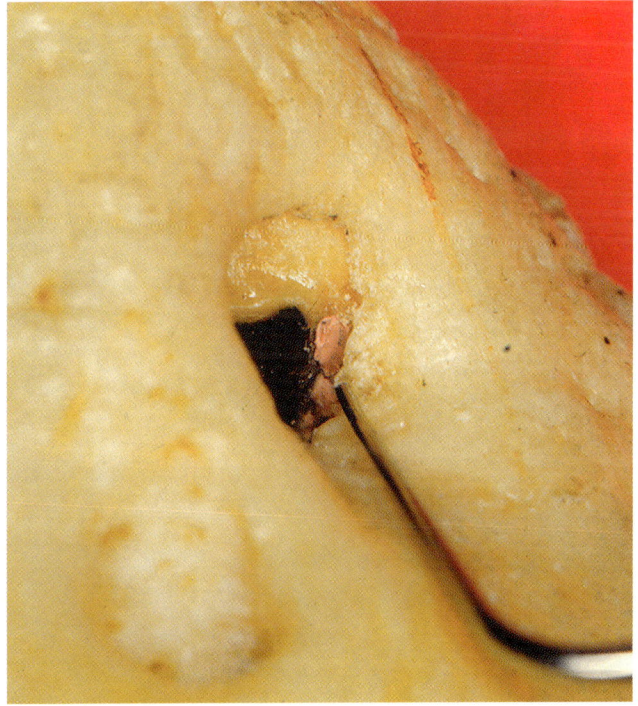

FIGURE 16.57

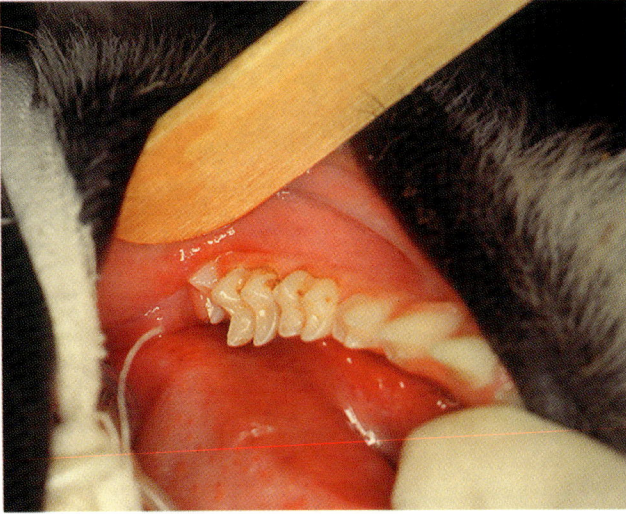

FIGURE 16.60

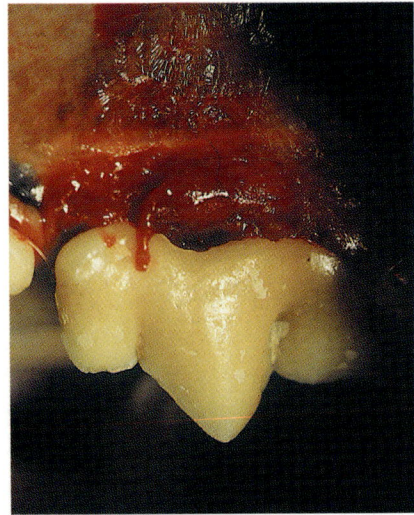

FIGURE 16.64

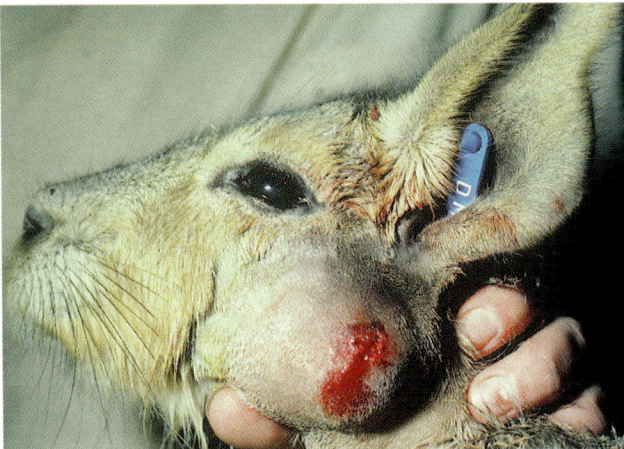

FIGURE 16.72

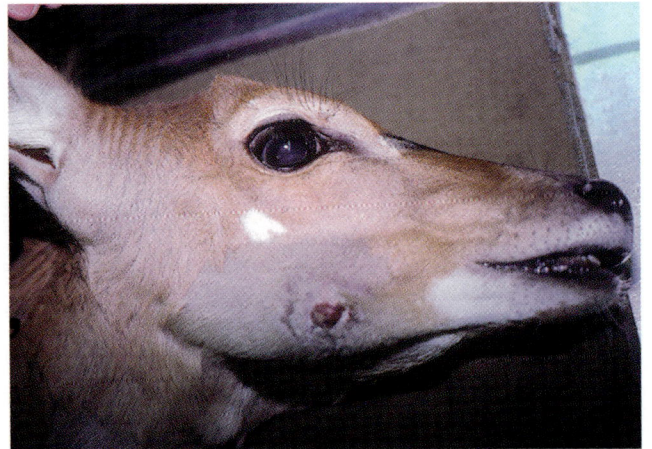

FIGURE 16.74

17 Rodent and Rabbit Radiology

Dr. David A. Crossley

INTRODUCTION: RADIOGRAPHIC DENTAL ANATOMY OF RODENTS AND LAGOMORPHS

Rodents and lagomorphs have a number of oral/dental anatomical features in common. The basic similarity in structure of the incisor dentition with a lack of canine teeth originally led to the classification of lagomorphs within the order Rodentia. Both groups have aradicular hypsodont incisor teeth. These teeth erupt and grow continuously throughout life, never forming anatomical roots. Lagomorphs (rabbits, hares, and cottontails) have a second set of incisor teeth in the maxilla, whereas rodents have one set. Both groups just have a single incisor tooth each side of the mandible. A further difference is that lagomorphs have a deciduous set of teeth, being diphyodont, whereas rodents are mono-phyodont, having a single set of teeth. The lagomorph deciduous teeth, formed in utero, are almost vestigial and usually shed around the time of birth.

There is a basic difference in the relative widths of the maxilla and mandible between rodents and lagomorphs. In rodents the mandibular cheek tooth arcades are generally wider apart than the maxillary arcades (Figure 17.1A). In lagomorphs the situation is reversed (Figure 17.1B), being similar to the situation seen in larger domestic herbivores (cattle and horses), the mandible being narrower than the maxilla.

FIGURE 17.1

Diagrammatic representation of the relative widths of the mandible and maxilla of the chinchilla (view A) and the rabbit (view B). Note the long incisor-to-cheek tooth diastema and the large chewing surfaces of these herbivorous species.

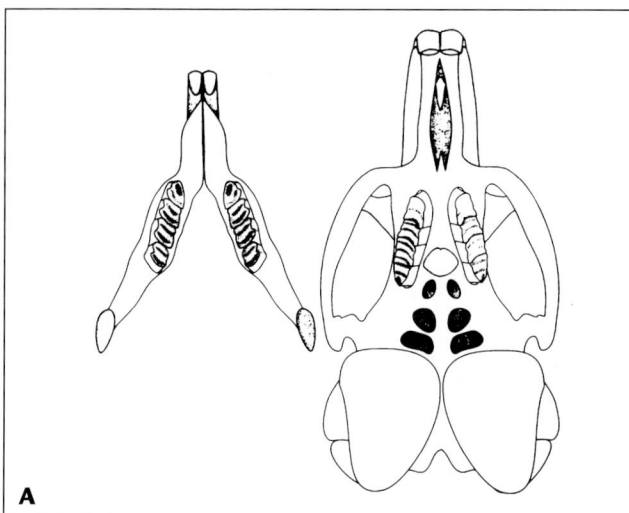

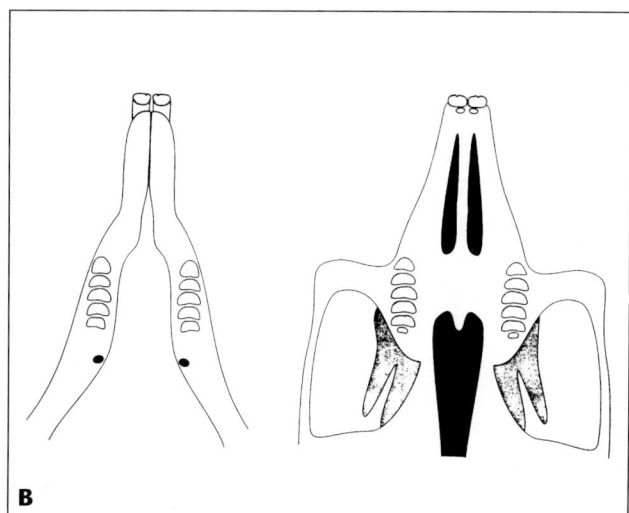

When discussing the molar and, when present, premolar teeth, it is useful to describe them as a functional unit, "the cheek teeth." The function of these teeth is to grind ingested food, as opposed to the incisor teeth which are used for gnawing or slicing the food into manageable pieces. Neither rodents nor lagomorphs have canine teeth, and both have a long gap, the diastema, between the incisors and the cheek teeth.

There are vast numbers of rodent species distributed worldwide, each adapted to a particular environment. In most rodents the enamel of the incisor teeth is a deeply pigmented yellow to orange color, the common exception to this is the guinea pig, which has white incisor teeth. These teeth have thick enamel on the facial/labial surface, which wears more slowly than the labial/palatal tooth surface, leading to the formation of a typical chisel-shaped occlusal surface. The incisors are used for gaining access to, collecting, and cutting up food or bedding. The temporomandibular joints of rodents allow a considerable degree of normal rostrocaudal "gliding" jaw movement so that the incisors can be used for gnawing, a combined rostrocaudal and dorsoventral chewing action.

The cheek teeth have evolved to cope with the foods available in the normal habitat, so with their wide distribution there is considerable variation in rodent cheek tooth dentition. There is a continuous range of cheek tooth dentition extending from species with just two or three small, short crowned molar teeth which have anatomical roots (brachyodont structure) in each quadrant of the jaw, to species with a large chewing surface provided by four or five continuously growing (aradicular hypsodont) cheek teeth, comprising one or two premolars plus three molar teeth in each quadrant. Species with brachyodont molars and a small chewing surface are adapted to cope with nutrient rich food, such as grain, requiring very little chewing. Those species with the largest chewing surfaces on continuously growing cheek teeth have a naturally energy poor diet composed of highly abrasive materials such as tree bark and mountain grasses. Large volumes of such diets must be consumed in order to survive. The teeth are rapidly worn away and grow continuously to replace the lost tooth substance. This growth continues in such animals even if they are fed an unnaturally high energy diet when kept in captivity. The result is overgrowth of the continuously growing cheek teeth. This may show as intraoral (coronal) elongation, root elongation, or a combination of the two. The same problem can affect the incisor teeth when animals are not provided with material to gnaw.

There is much less variation in the dentition of lagomorphs. All lagomorphs feed largely on large volumes of leafy vegetation and have a full set of aradicular hypsodont cheek teeth, like the herbivorous rodents, to compensate for continuous wear. Rabbits, which are the most frequently seen lagomorphs, have two maxillary and one mandibular incisor tooth on each side of the mouth. The structure and the typical wear pattern of the main incisors is similar to that of rodent incisors; however, the second maxillary incisors, which are positioned palatal to the first incisors, may be rudimentary or even absent in domestic rabbits. When present, they are usually worn flat or are beveled the opposite way to the main incisors. Rabbits have six cheek teeth, three premolars plus three molars (the last of which is vestigial in some strains) on each side of the maxilla, and five cheek teeth, two premolars plus three molars, on each side of the mandible.

At rest, the tips of the mandibular incisors rest between the two maxillary incisors (Figure 17.2). The main jaw action in rabbits is a lateral one; however, the incisors are used with a vertical slicing action, cutting their food into short pieces, which can then be ground down by lateral movements of the cheek teeth. The structure of the rabbit temporomandibular joint is different to that of rodents. It does not allow a great deal of rostrocaudal movement so gnawing is not a normal behavior in rabbits. By retracting the mandible a short distance, rabbits raise the mandibular condyle up a "step" in the temporal joint surface, moving the mandibular cheek teeth caudally and dorsally so that they come into occlusion with their maxillary counterparts (Figure 17.3).

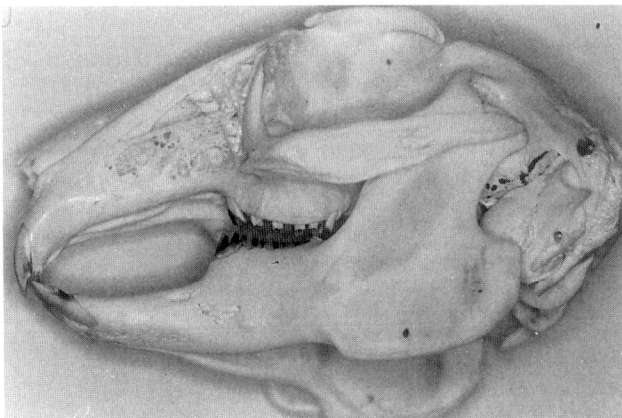

FIGURE 17.2

Photograph of the prepared skull of a mature wild rabbit showing the normal resting jaw position with the incisors in the occlusion and the cheek teeth slightly separated.

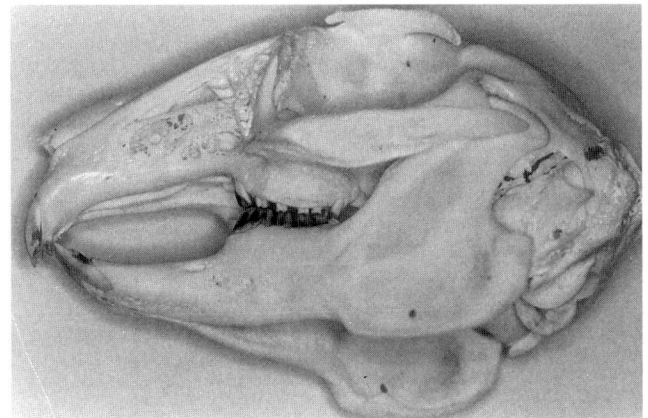

FIGURE 17.3

Photograph of the prepared skull of a mature wild rabbit showing the separation of the incisor teeth with the cheek teeth brought into occlusion.

From a radiological point of view there is a considerable difference in the structure of brachyodont versus aradicular hypsodont teeth. If a radiolucency is detected in the periapical tissues of a tooth with a fully developed anatomical root this is likely to be pathological, whereas radiolucency of the periapical germinal tissues of continuously growing teeth is normal. Once they have erupted, the periodontal ligament of brachyodont teeth is generally very narrow. During eruption the teeth have a wider periodontal ligament space, so this is a normal finding in species with hypsodont teeth. The roots of teeth sit in a bone-lined space, the alveolus. In health, the lining bone appears continuous, but is actually perforated by a large number of very small foramina through which blood vessels reach the periosteum. Loss of this surrounding bone shows radiographically as loss of the lamina dura as seen in man, dogs, and cats. In the continuously growing teeth, the supporting bone around the root apex is frequently affected by pathology. The location of the root apices adjacent to the ventral mandibular border and within the maxillary alveolar bullae often allows accurate radiographic assessment for bone loss in these areas. In small species with brachyodont teeth, periapical assessment is not so easy, particularly for the maxillary teeth. Other possible radiological findings include tooth and jaw fractures, developmental cysts, abscesses, and tumors.

In the author's experience, conscious examination of rabbits and rodents fails to reveal around 70 percent of oral lesions. Examination under anesthesia increases the detection rate to around 50 percent. As many of the lesions affect the tooth roots, only those lesions causing gross pathology are detectable by palpation or visual observation. Radiography alone will not provide a diagnosis and will not show many soft-tissue lesions, but when one has learned interpretation, it allows detection of over 85 percent of the hard-tissue lesions detectable on postmortem examination. This makes it a very important diagnostic tool during investigation of oral and dental disease in lagomorphs and rodents.

Radiographs are two-dimensional representations of three-dimensional structures. In order to obtain an accurate idea of the location of structures and lesions, several views are required. When investigating the head, three standard views are used: dorsoventral, lateral, and rostrocaudal. Additional oblique views are frequently required to separate images from those of overlaying structures. In order to obtain a sufficiently detailed image of the small fine structures associated with the mouth it is necessary to used nonscreen x-ray film. If detail screens are available, screen film can be used, but only gross structures and lesions will be reliably detected. The use of periapical dental x-ray film allows intraoral film placement for certain views, though the narrow oral aperture and long diastema of lagomorphs and rodents makes film placement tricky. Exposure factors of 15 mAs and 75 KVA are a good starting point when using standard nonscreen film or ultraspeed dental film at a 50-cm film-to-subject focal distance for the dorsoventral and lateral views of a rabbit's head. In many cases an increase or decrease in exposure/penetrating power may be indicated in order to improve detail for different structures.

Of the three standard radiographic views, the dorsoventral view is least revealing as regards tooth structure. The maxillary and mandibular teeth are superimposed, making interpretation difficult. It is nevertheless often possible to see root outlines of some of the maxillary teeth as well as the periodontal space of the second incisor and the first and last cheek teeth. A perfect lateral film will provide a great deal more information regarding dentition of rabbits and rodents than the dorsoventral view because teeth and other related structures are more clearly visible. In the rostrocaudal view, the superimposition of the skull over the oral structures necessitates increasing the exposure factors in order to get good results with this view. With careful positioning the rostrocaudal view will reveal any medial or lateral tipping of the cheek teeth.

Rabbits

FIGURE 17.4

Contributing Author: David A. Crossley

Description: Dorsoventral radiographic view of a young adult domestic rabbit.

Points Identified: The periapical lucency of the second maxillary cheek tooth is often visible within the zygomatic process of the maxilla, but it may be obscured by superimposition of the image of the lacrimal process. The zygomatic arch extends caudally beyond the level of the temporomandibular joint [TMJ]. The caudal aspect of the palatine shelf is visible distal to the mandibular symphysis.

A. Periapical lucency of second cheek tooth
B. Lacrimal process
C. Zygomatic process of the maxilla
D. Zygomatic arch
E. Temporomandibular joint
F. Tympanic bulla
G. Palatine shelf, caudal aspect

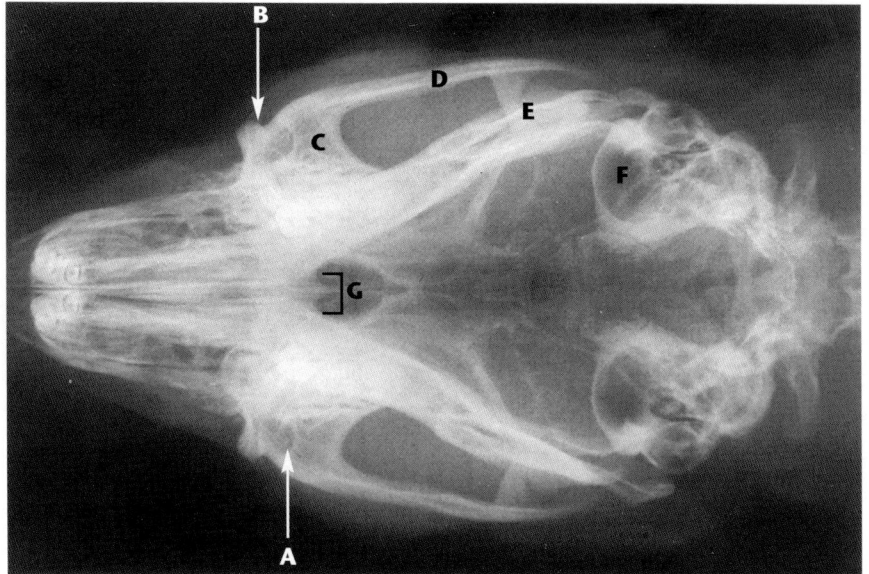

FIGURE 17.5

Contributing Author: David A. Crossley

Description: Lateral radiographic view of a young adult domestic rabbit. Note that the palate and dorsal mandibular borders converge rostrally.

Discussion: This radiograph is not quite a perfect lateral but is well within acceptable limits. This domestic rabbit was with jaw pain following a fall. Careful examination of the film reveals a break in the ventral outline of one side of the mandible. Note that the fracture does not show on the dorsoventral view (Figure 17.4). Note the hyoid apparatus just caudal to the fracture.

Points Identified: The normal radiolucencies of the periapical germinal tissues are clearly seen in this young rabbit.

Note the smooth ventral mandibular border. Also note that both cheek teeth and incisors are in occlusion and that there is a fracture of the mandibular ramus (C).

    A. Tympanic bullae
    B. Soft palate
    C. Break in ventral outline of the mandible due to a fracture
    D. Tongue

    E. Normal apical radiolucencies
    F. Occlusal plane
    G. Hard palate
    H. Nasal bone and turbinate structure
    I. Palatine shelf
    J. Lacrimal bones

Diagnostic Keys: The fact that the cheek teeth are in occlusion at the same time as the incisor teeth indicates that this rabbit has a degree of cheek tooth coronal elongation; however, the palatal and mandibular borders still converge rostrally. This degree of malocclusion is common in domestic rabbits and rarely causes functional problems.

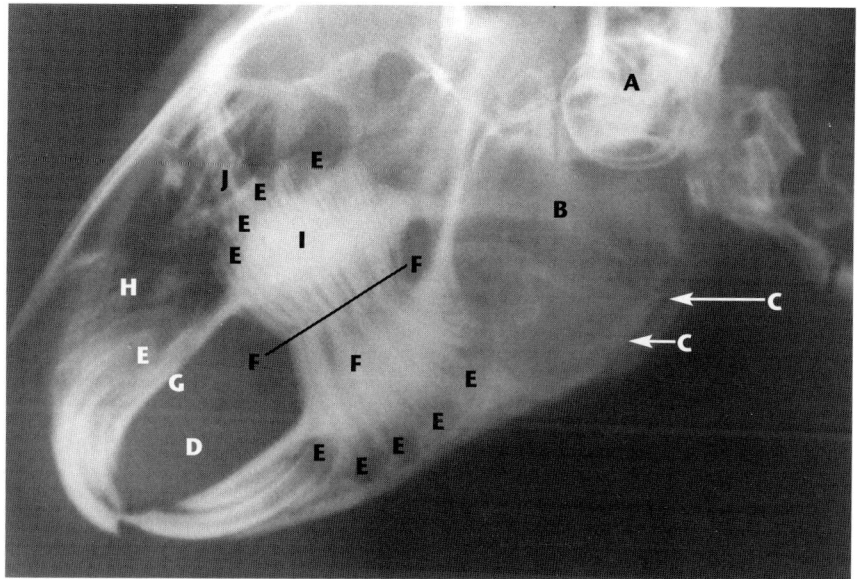

FIGURE 17.6

Contributing Author: David A. Crossley

Description: Rostrocaudal radiographic view of a young adult domestic rabbit. Note clearer view of mandibular fracture than is seen in Figure 17.5.

Points Identified: Note the normal degree of anisognathism (arrows). The temporomandibular joints can be clearly seen as can the fibrous mandibular symphysis. When the head is appropriately angled the occlusal planes of the cheek teeth can be demonstrated.

    A. Mandibular symphysis
    B. Anisognathic dental arcades
    C. Lacrimal process
    D. Temporomandibular joint
    E. Mandibular fracture

Diagnostic Keys: If gross spikes have formed on the teeth, these would be visible. As minute irregularities on the edges of the teeth may cause serious soft-tissue trauma, lack of visible spikes does not rule out this possibility.

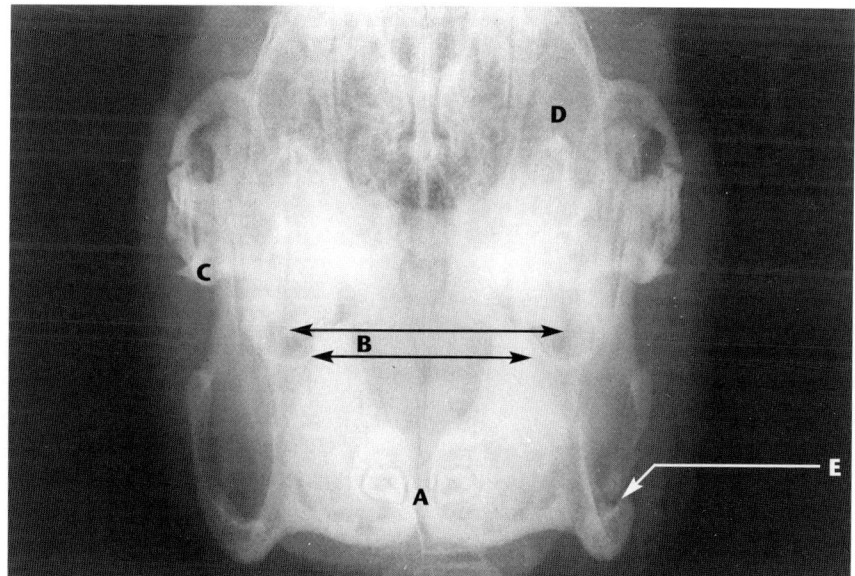

FIGURE 17.7

Contributing Author: David A. Crossley

Description: Rabbit with relative mandibular prognathism. View A, lateral radiographic view of a rabbit less than 1 year old with severe incisor malocclusion due to relative mandibular prognathism. View B, skull of rabbit.

Discussion: Without occlusion and wear, the tight growth curve of the maxillary incisors leads to these teeth curling into the mouth. This causes considerable soft-tissue damage, prevents the mouth closing normally, and leads to secondary overgrowth of the cheek teeth. In most cases, the owner has noticed the overgrown mandibular incisors protruding from the mouth, but does not realize that there is a problem.

Coronal overgrowth of the cheek teeth also forces the mouth open, exacerbating any incisor malocclusion (or causing one if it was not there previously). The jaw is forced open until the palate and dorsal mandibular borders are about parallel. At this stage the resting occlusal forces on the cheek teeth seem to match the eruptive forces. Although eruption stops, root growth continues, leading to root elongation into surrounding tissues.

Points Identified: This rabbit has a marked degree of incisor malocclusion, or really nonocclusion, and there is a radiolucency around the root apices of the mandibular incisor teeth. Note also that the root apices of the maxillary cheek teeth are penetrating the maxillary alveolar bulla within the orbit, and in the mandible there is thinning of the ventral mandibular border adjacent to the periapical tissues.

- A. Apical radiolucency, mandibular incisors
- B. Cheek teeth roots penetrating maxillary alveolar bulla
- C. Thinning of ventral mandibular border due to apical intrusion of cheek tooth roots

Diagnostic Keys: Other factors leading to cheek tooth overgrowth in cases such as this include reduced chewing activity due to reduced food intake due to problems with prehension; reduced chewing activity due to restriction of jaw movement by overgrown incisors; and reduced need for chewing due to inappropriate provision of high-energy foods.

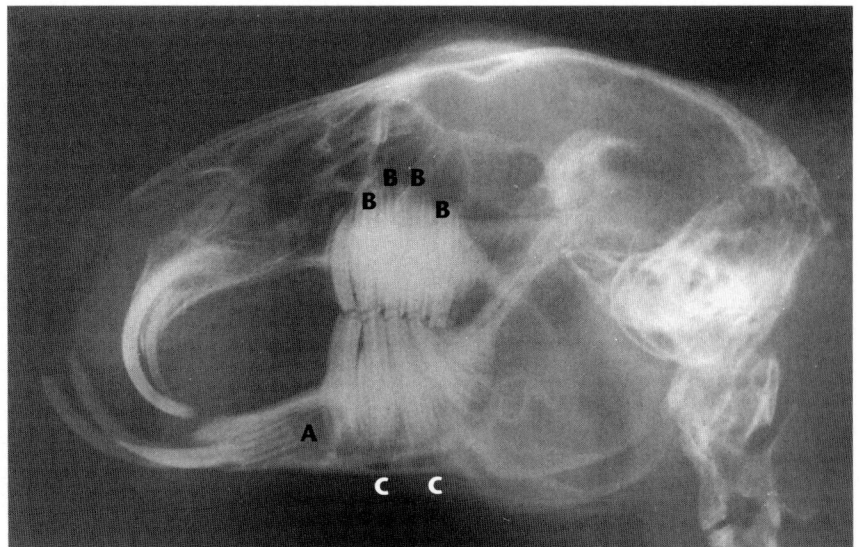

A

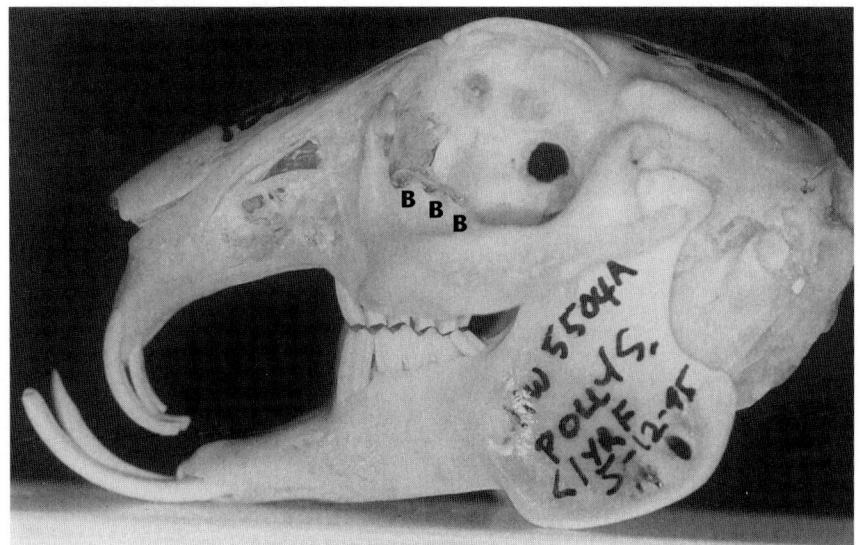

B

FIGURE 17.8

Contributing Author: David A. Crossley

Description: View A, oblique lateral radiograph of a rabbit with early maxillary cheek tooth root elongation. View B, photograph of the prepared skull of the rabbit shown in view A.

Discussion: Oblique positioning separates the images of bilateral structures such as the maxillary alveolar bullae, allowing better interpretation. If a full assessment is required, symmetrical views need to be obtained for both sides. When radiography is used for determining prognosis the localization of lesions to one side or the other is not important.

Points Identified: The root apices of the maxillary first incisors are slightly separated, as are the palatal shadows, occlusal planes and the temporomandibular joints, indicating oblique positioning of the patient.

Note root deformity at the apex of one of the second maxillary premolar teeth and loss of alveolar bulla bone over the apices of the second and third premolars and first two molars on the same side. Compare view A and view B.

Diagnostic Keys: This early root pathology indicates a guarded prognosis. Progression of root pathology is almost inevitable once there is perforation of the supporting periapical bone in species with aradicular hypsodont teeth. Normal chewing leads to discomfort and pain due to tooth movement within the alveolus, causing stretching of the exposed periosteum at the root apex.

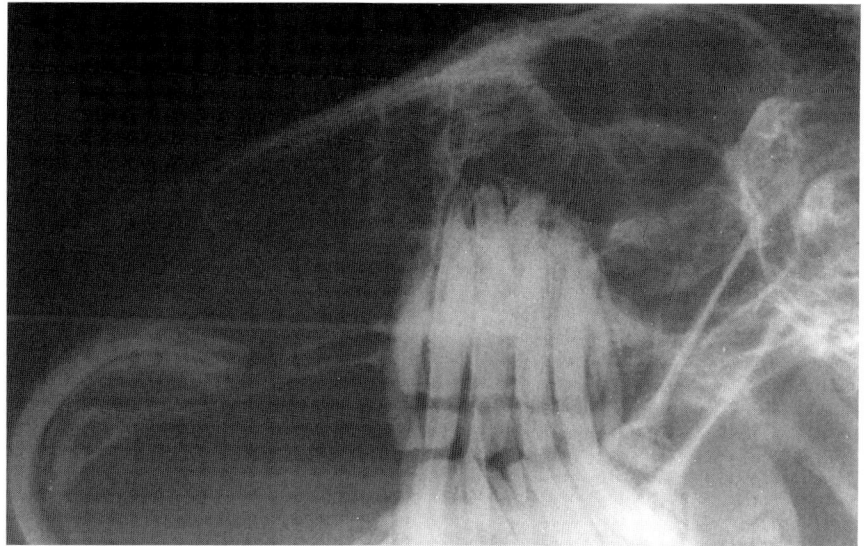

A

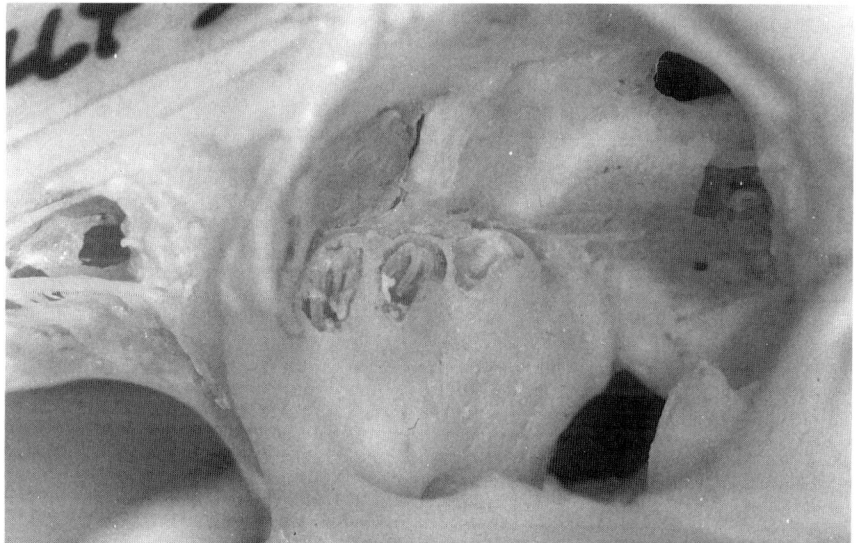

B

FIGURE 17.9

Contributing Author: David A. Crossley

Description: Lateral radiographic view of a dwarf rabbit with severe cheek tooth pathology.

Normal Anatomy: Rabbit cheek teeth should be arranged in neat rows with clearly defined structure, the opposing arcades meeting perpendicular to an almost horizontal occlusal plane.

Points Identified: This rabbit has a grossly abnormal cheek tooth occlusion with severe coronal overgrowth of several maxillary teeth and excessively short mandibular teeth. The root structure of both maxillary and mandibular teeth is also abnormal. The ventral mandibular borders had grossly palpable hard swellings which are associated with tooth root elongation and pathology seen in the radiograph. The root apex of one of the mandibular first molar teeth can be seen penetrating the cortical bone plate.

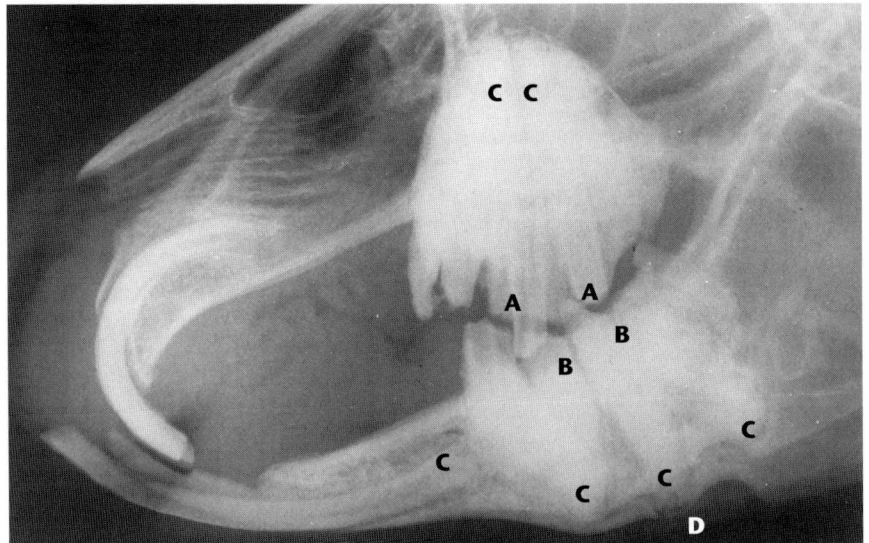

A. Coronal overgrowth of maxillary teeth
B. Excessively short mandibular teeth
C. Tooth root elongation
D. Root apex penetrating cortical bone plate

Diagnostic Keys: Incisor malocclusions are very common in dwarf and lop breeds of rabbit. In this case the incisor problem is the least significant factor. The prognosis is for this animal is grave. Treating the incisor malocclusion will just prolong this rabbit's suffering.

FIGURE 17.10

Contributing Author: David A. Crossley

Description: Radiograph (lateral view) of a lop breed rabbit with incisor and cheek tooth malocclusion and a large mandibular abscess. Although it is not possible to differentiate between structures on the left and right on a lateral view, many diagnostic and prognostic features are visible.

Points Identified: Note malocclusion associated with relative mandibular prognathism (not possible to assess jaw length accurately as the temporomandibular junction is not shown). The dotted line in the radiograph approximates the normal ventral mandibular border.

A. Coronal overgrowth of maxillary first incisor teeth, curling into mouth and forcing it open
B. Widening periodontal ligament, palatal surface of the maxillary first incisor teeth and adjacent side of second incisors ("pig teeth")
C. Maxillary first incisor apices, root elongation and deformity
D. Very irregular occlusal planes
E. Gross distortion of the bony ventral mandibular border with evidence of periosteal reaction and new bone deposition

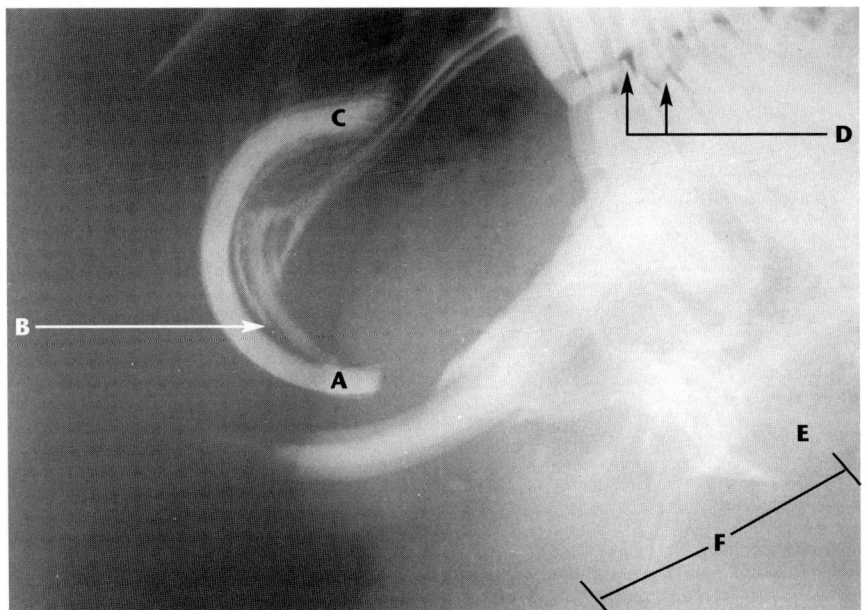

F. Single, large soft-tissue mass (the abscess) centered around the location of the mandibular premolar root apices

Diagnostic Keys: This is a lop breed rabbit, so it is likely that there is a significant degree of brachycephalism rather than true mandibular prognathism in this animal. Grossly deformed mandibular cheek tooth root structure is commonly seen in such cases. Note that dorsal border of rostral mandible is parallel to the ventral border of incisive bones.

In healthy wild rabbits the normal pattern is for the palate and dorsal mandibular borders to converge toward the incisor teeth as seen in 0-normal rabbit occlusion. The root apices are adjacent to the "palatal" bone plates, but there is no evidence of bone perforation. The vaguely locular appearance over the mandibles is caused by multiple root abscesses developing within the opposite mandible. These additional abscesses could be recognized clinically as palpable bony swellings.

FIGURE 17.11

Contributing Author: David A. Crossley

Description: Mandibular lesion. Lateral (view A) and dorsoventral (view B) radiographs of a rabbit with chronic incisor malocclusion which had been managed for several years by coronal reduction using a bur in a high-speed dental handpiece. The rabbit was admitted for investigation of a unilateral ventral mandibular swelling which had developed over an 8-week period.

Points Identified:

A. Incisor teeth trimmed using a dental bur prior to radiography

B. Root elongation of the larger maxillary incisor teeth. The root apices are adjacent to and beginning to penetrate the palatal surface of the incisive bones

C. Obvious root elongation of the maxillary cheek teeth

D. Palate and dorsal mandibular border parallel, indicating cheek tooth coronal overgrowth

E. Indistinct and somewhat uneven cheek tooth occlusal planes

F. Distortion of ventral mandibular border

G. Tipped mandibular cheek teeth. (Note also displacement and deformation of the roots.)

H. Increased, diffuse radiodensity in the mandibular body

I. It is not possible to determine whether radiodensity and tipped mandibular cheek teeth are unilateral or bilateral features from the lateral view (A), but the dorsoventral view (B) clearly shows a unilateral mandibular deformity

Diagnostic Keys: Unilateral mandibular abscessation is quite a common finding in rabbits which have had their incisor teeth fractured (or shortened by clipping). Apart from the immediate severe pain and the trauma to the periodontal structures caused by tooth fracture or clipping, pulp infection is common.

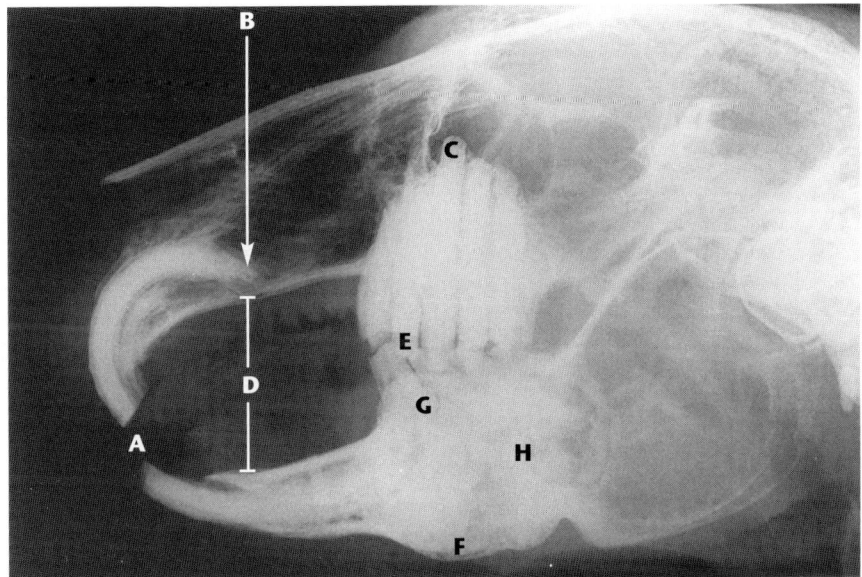

A

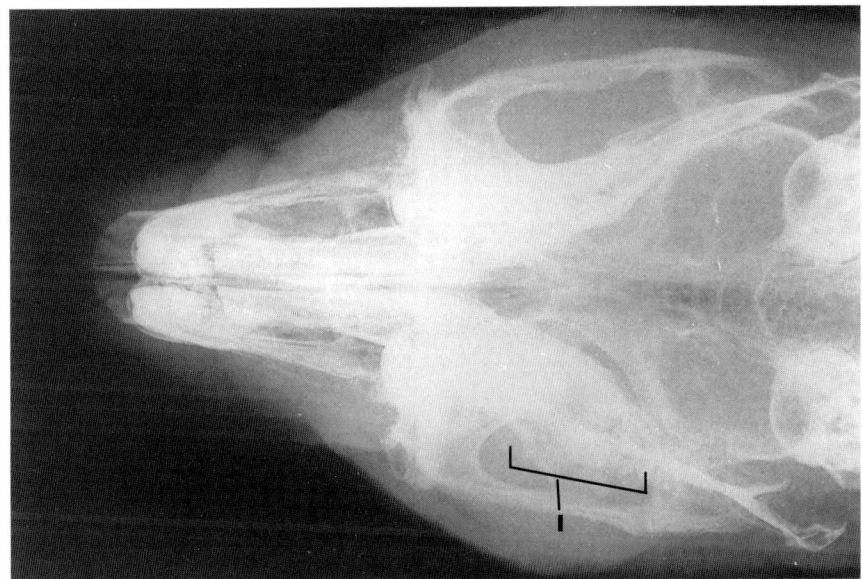

B

If not treated adequately, endodontic abscessation follows. As the mandibular incisor root apices are level with the premolar teeth, it can be difficult to distinguish the origin of the abscess even using radiography.

The changes shown in the case illustrated here are not typical of jaw abscessation. The mandibular lesion was a malignant melanoma unassociated with the incisor malocclusion.

FIGURE 17.12

Contributing Author:
Dr. Mary Suzanne Aller

Description: Rabbit with maloccluded cheek teeth (mandible) resulting from increased occlusal pressure. View A, lateral extraoral view; view B, lateral intraoral view; view C, maxilla, occlusal intraoral view.

Points Identified: Severe coronal elongation in cheek teeth and upper incisors. Severe root elongation in upper and lower cheek teeth. Root elongation in upper large central incisors (Is) and root deformity in upper small accessory incisors (IIs). Defect in mandibular premolar, crown and root. Note the irregular occlusal surface of the cheek teeth, characteristic of "wave mouth." Lower incisors: One or both lower incisors show short roots and deformed or missing crown (one incisor could be missing altogether), and there are marked bone changes, mainly lytic changes rostrally and sclerotic changes toward the apical region.

- A. Maxillary incisor I
- B. Maxillary incisor II
- C. Sclerotic apical region
- D. Wave mouth
- E. Resorptive lesion
- F. Root apices penetrating supporting bone

Diagnostic Keys: This rabbit had primary cheek tooth malocclusion, which caused secondary incisor malocclusion. Root penetration of the ventral mandibular cortex causes rapid development of a problem with minimal remodeling. This is common for rapid progression due to feeding of a "supportive" diet when animals exhibit inappetence: There is not tooth wear from the soft/liquid food, but the tooth is still growing. Defect in mandibular premolar may be a resorptive lesion, defective tooth formation, or a combination; secondary caries may also be present.

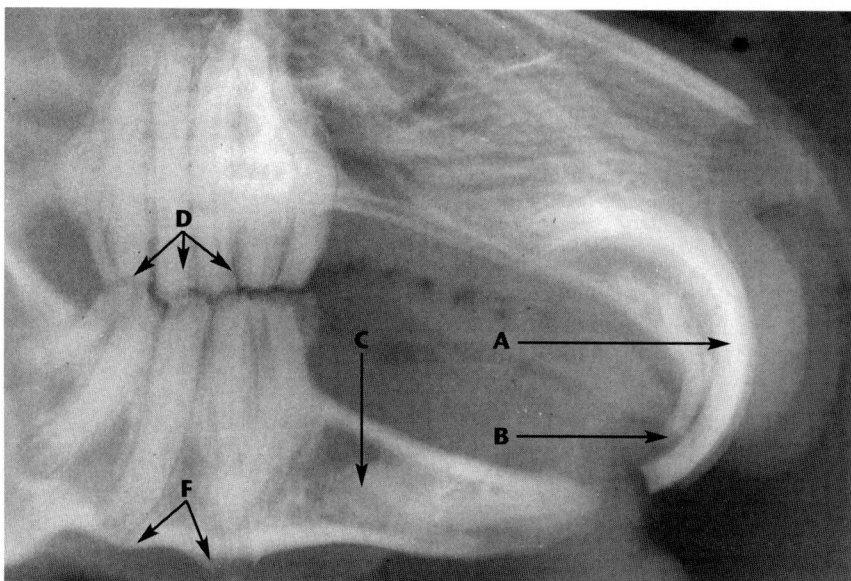

A

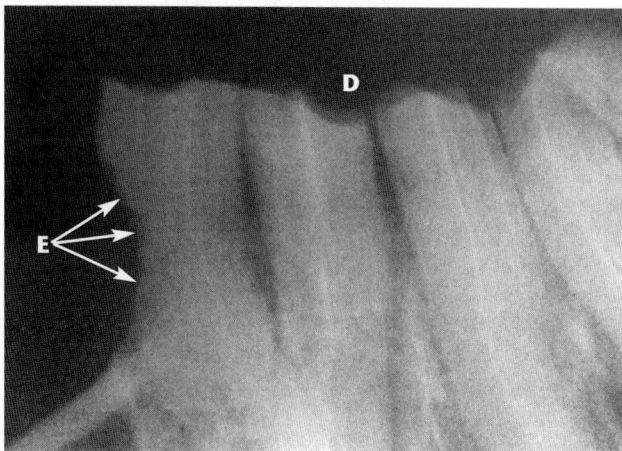

B

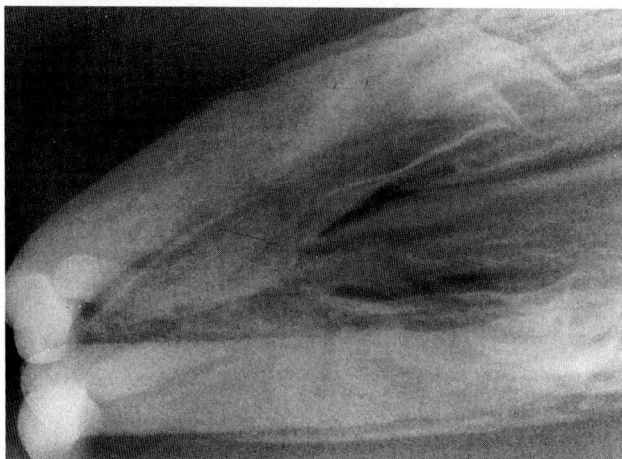

C

Rodents

The three standard anatomical views of the head are applicable to rodents as well as rabbits. In most cases the dorsoventral view is least informative due to the superimposition of the maxilla and mandible.

The rostrocaudal view clearly demonstrates the temporomandibular joints. This view is only really helpful for demonstrating dental problems in species with continuously growing cheek teeth and a horizontal occlusal plane such as the chinchilla. In the guinea pig the steep angulation of the occlusal planes and the divergent cheek tooth arcades make interpretation difficult.

When screening for dental problems in rodents, the lateral radiographic view is usually most useful. When a unilateral problem is suspected, and in species with steeply angled occlusal planes, two oblique views are necessary in order to assess the situation more accurately. In larger rodents it may be possible to use intraoral film placement to improve the accuracy of interpretation.

FIGURE 17.13

Contributing Author: David A. Crossley

Description: Dorsoventral radiograph of a rat's head.

Points Identified: Superimposition of the maxillary and mandibular molar teeth masks all detail of this area. Note the narrow maxilla, wide zygomatic arches, and small tympanic bullae.

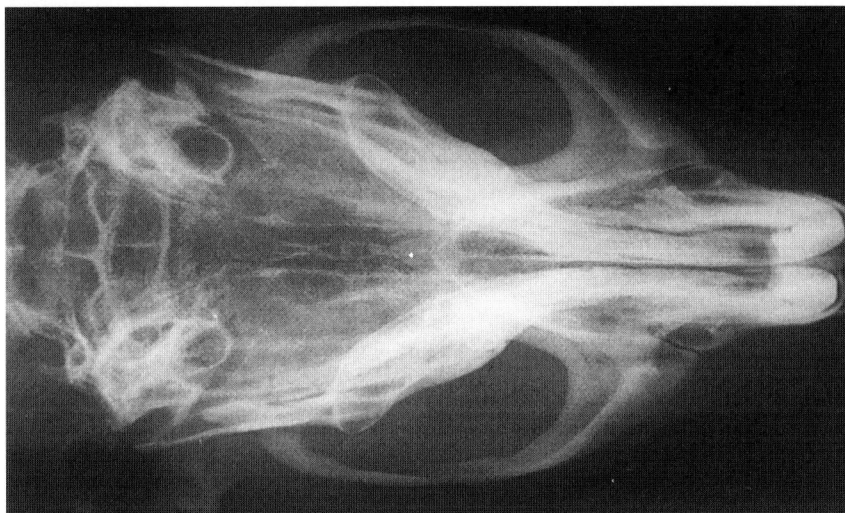

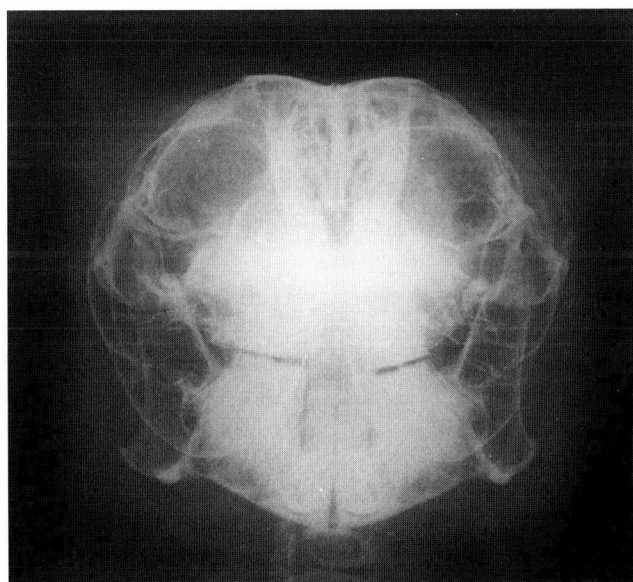

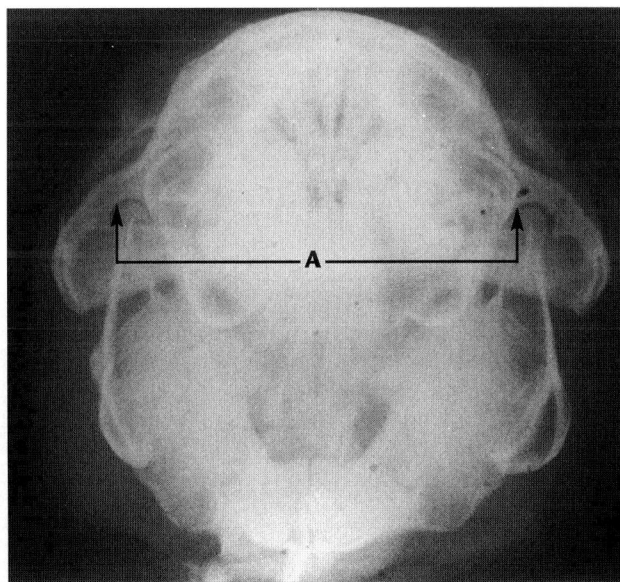

A

B

FIGURE 17.14

Contributing Author: David A. Crossley

Description: Rostrocaudal radiograph of a healthy chinchilla (view A) and a guinea pig with tooth overgrowth (view B).

Points Identified: View A, note how smooth the occlusal planes are and that the cheek teeth are very short. View B, note that the guinea pig's temporomandibular joint (TMJ) has a long temporal groove which is easily demonstrated radiographically.

A. Temporomandibular joints

FIGURE 17.15

Contributing Author: David A. Crossley

Source: Radiograph courtesy of Robert B. Wiggs.

Description: Lateral view of a healthy rat's dentition.

Points Identified: Incisor tooth morphology clearly seen. Note curvatures of the maxillary and mandibular incisor teeth and the location of the root apices. Cheek teeth can be clearly seen to have short crowns and fully developed anatomical roots.

Diagnostic Keys: At rest, the cheek teeth are normally held in occlusion with the incisors separated, giving a retrognathic appearance to the mandible.

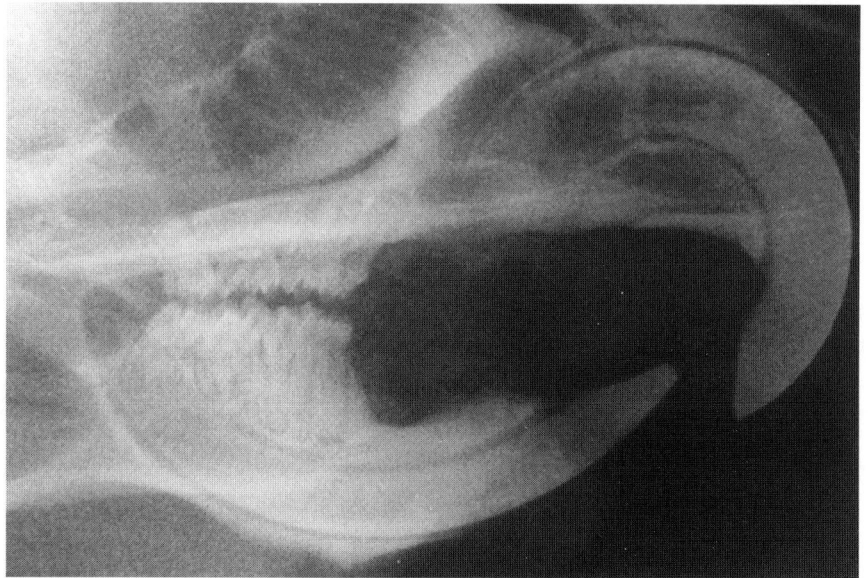

Chinchillas

Chinchillas seem particularly prone to cheek tooth overgrowth and malocclusion problems. The cheek teeth continue growing at a normal rate even when wear is inadequate. There is initially continued eruption into the mouth. This leads to increased resting pressure on the teeth. As chinchillas normally have short and fairly straight cheek tooth roots the eruption pressure is very low. The occlusal pressure soon matches the eruption pressure, and eruption ceases. Continued root growth leads to root elongation, and the apices penetrate through the supporting alveolar bone. Once this has happened the condition is irreversible.

Various degrees of cheek tooth overgrowth can be recognized clinically. Unfortunately animals are rarely presented in the early stages of disease when correction is possible. Routine radiography of chinchillas presented for inappetence, weight loss, nasal, orofacial, and ocular signs improves the detection rate considerably. It is important to remember that in many cases there is no visible intraoral lesion; however, root elongation can be readily detected radiographically.

The tooth root elongation and penetration of the supporting bone is demonstrated best by use of computed tomography (CT). This technique provides cross-sectional radiographic images. While CT scanning provides the best method of detecting tooth root elongation in the living animal and would be a useful screening technique, it cannot generally be justified due to both lack of general availability of CT facilities and expense.

FIGURE 17.16

Contributing Author: David A. Crossley

Description: Lateral view of a healthy chinchilla.

Points Identified: Cheek teeth with short crowns and roots. Periapical germinal tissues showing as areas of radiolucency. Note the large tympanic bullae and the smooth occlusal plane. Note clear incisor tooth morphology.

Diagnostic Keys: At rest the cheek teeth are normally held in occlusion, with the incisors separated, giving a retrognathic appearance to the mandible.

Points Identified:

   A. Periapical germinal tissues
   B. Tympanic bullae
   C. Occlusal plane

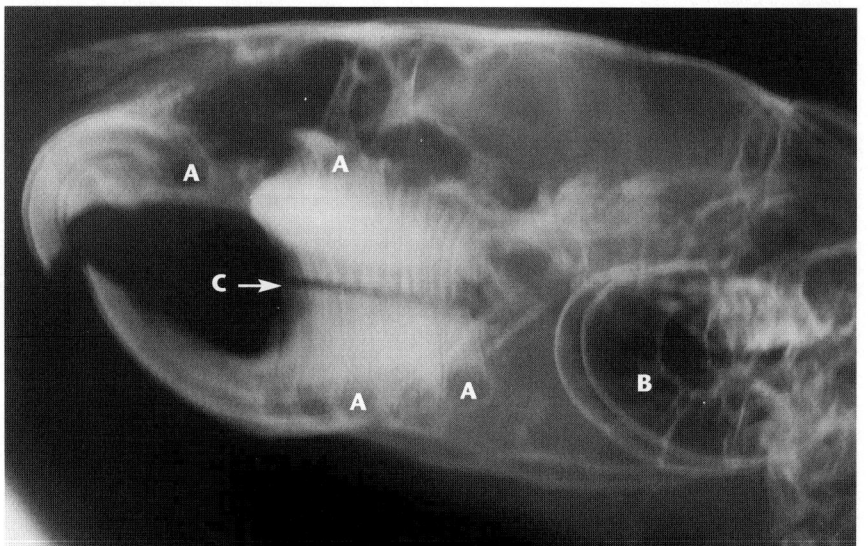

FIGURE 17.17

Contributing Author: David A. Crossley

Description: Lateral view of a chinchilla with advanced cheek tooth overgrowth.

Points Identified:

A. Note elongated cheek tooth roots penetrating the supporting bone on the ventral mandible. Intraoral overgrowth of cheek teeth, forcing the mouth open and causing secondary incisor malocclusion.

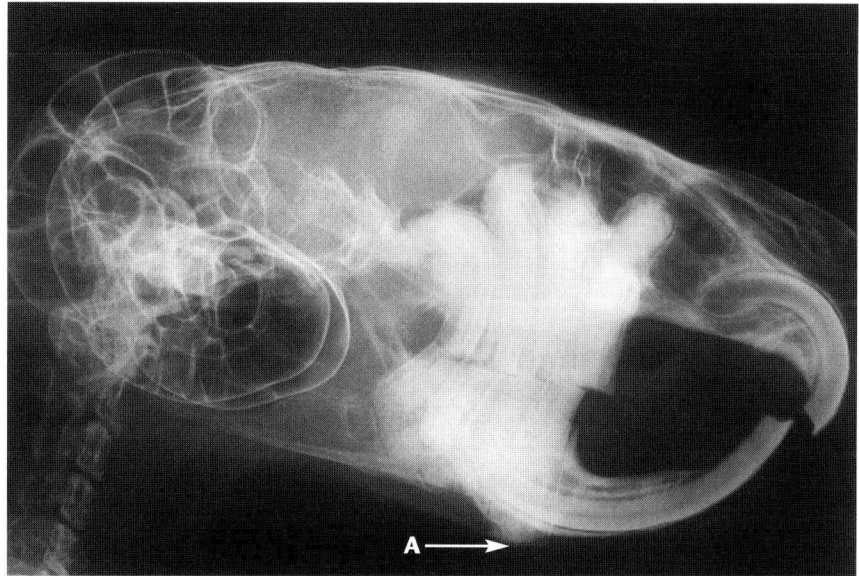

FIGURE 17.18

Contributing Author: David A. Crossley

Description: Two cross-sectional CT images of the chinchilla shown in Figure 17.16. Left image shows situation at the level of the second molar teeth. Right image shows situation at the level of the first molar teeth.

Points Identified:

A. Maxillary tooth roots penetrating into the orbit. Penetration of mandibular roots into the ventral border of the mandible.
B. Gross "spike" formation on lateral occlusal edges of the maxillary teeth
C. Chinchilla's eyes

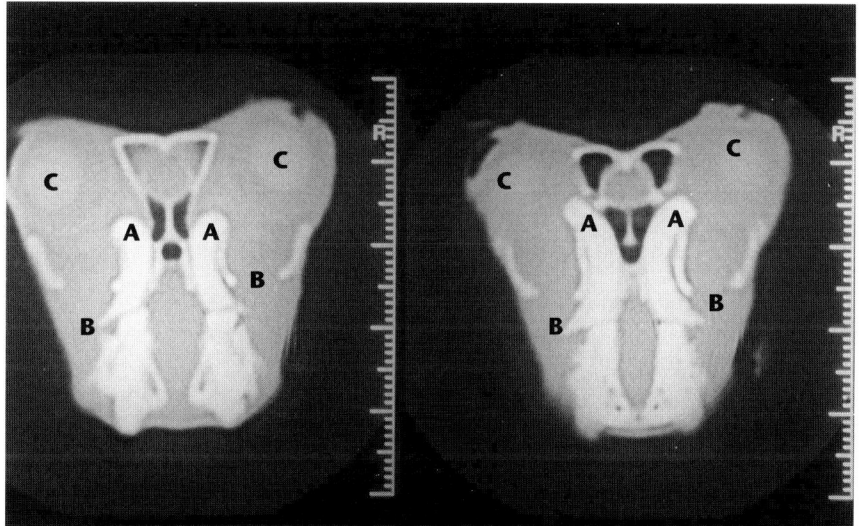

APPENDIX 1

COMPUTED TOMOGRAPHY AND MAGNETIC RESONANCE IMAGING IN VETERINARY DENTISTRY AND ORAL SURGERY DIAGNOSTICS

Dr. Anna Fong Revenaugh

Until recently, the radiograph was the most effective diagnostic tool for evaluating oral/dental disease. Successful interpretation of radiographs is affected by many variables including image quality, knowledge of anatomy, and experience.[1] Errors such as overlooking the involvement of nearby structures, underestimating the extent of the disease process, or coning out the lesion can occur. Radiographs suffer other drawbacks. Detection of bone lysis is not seen on radiographs until there is 30–50 percent bone loss.[2] The complex anatomy of the skull will cause superimposition of some structures and distortion in the shape and size of others.[3] The new technologies of computed tomography (CT) and magnetic resonance imaging (MRI) offer solutions to those problems. CT and MRI furnish highly detailed images without the problems of distortion and superimposition. The entire skull is imaged in a short amount of time.[4-7] These alternate imaging modalities are being performed at university veterinary medical teaching hospitals, large veterinary referral centers, and associated human hospitals.

Computed tomography takes multiple x-ray projections of an object, computer processes the numerical data, and reconstructs the object's internal structure.[8] CT scanners come in various types or "generations." A third generation CT scanner consists of an x-ray tube and detectors that rotate around the patient.[9] A projection is made by passing the x-ray beam through a very thin "slice" of the patient and measuring the transmitted radiation. A single image is produced from the thousands of projections that are obtained. The image on the screen is made up of many pixels that represent blocks of tissue ("voxels"). The shades of gray that are assigned to each pixel in the image matrix are dependent upon what tissues are being examined. The image can be manipulated to highlight only tissues of a certain density such as bone or brain or teeth.[8] The data can also be used to obtain an image of the object in another plane or to reconstruct a three-dimensional model of the subject.[41] CT is considered to be superior in resolving bone detail when compared to radiographs and MRI.[10,11]

MRI, like CT, examines very thin "slices" of the patient's body. Instead of radiation, MRI uses a magnetic field thousands of times more powerful than that of the earth.[12] This strong magnetic field causes the protons of the hydrogen atoms within the body to act like spinning bar magnets and line up along the lines of force. A radio signal is then pulsed perpendicular to the main magnetic field. This excites some of the aligned protons into a higher energy state. At the end of the pulsed radio signal the hydrogen protons realign with the main magnetic field.[7,13,14] The energy released and the time it takes for realignment ("relaxation time") is read, measured, and translated into an image. The physical and chemical nature of the environment surrounding the excited hydrogen nuclei determines the relaxation times.[7,15] The radio-frequency pulse sequences can be varied in duration and strength in order to highlight the characteristics of certain tissues ("T1-weighted," "T2-weighted," or "proton density" type images).[7,12] Intravenously injected paramagnetic contrast agents will cross the blood-brain barrier, enter abnormal tissues, and enhance lesions that may not have been evident on the survey scan.[7] Overall image quality is vastly superior with MRI; cortical bone, however, is not well imaged due to its lack of hydrogen content.[16] Implications of bone and teeth involvement on MRI can be made because cancellous bone yields a strong signal from the marrow fat while cortical bone and dental enamel is dark.[17]

CT and MRI are used extensively in human medicine to assess all areas of the body. Maxillofacial surgeons use these multiplanar modalities to preoperatively assess tumor extension, to assess temporomandibular joint disorders, and to localize injuries to the facial skeleton.[18,19] Dental applications include precise imaging of orofacial soft tissues and air spaces, developmental defects, suitability for dental implant treatment, and caries detection.[17,20,21] Comparisons of the accuracy of dental radiographs with CT for assessing infra-alveolar bone loss and interradicular furcation involvement have been done. CT proved to be very sensitive in detecting defects and was more precise in estimating the extent of the lesion than radiographs.[22,23] Computed tomography is being used to determine the external and internal morphology of the tooth for endodontic research.[24] The different signal intensities seen in various locations within the tooth on an MRI scan accurately portray the pulp chamber, periodontal membrane, and dental pulp tissue.[25]

The use of CT and MRI in veterinary medicine is growing. Atlases have mapped out various parts of the canine and equine body as they appear on CT and MRI examination.[8, 26–35] Articles describe the detection and differentiation of infectious diseases from neoplastic diseases of the nasal cavity, intraorbital and periorbital lesions, various types of brain tumors, and localization of spinal cord disease.[4,5,16,36–38,40] Few articles specific to CT/MRI and veterinary dentistry have been done. Kirkland, et al. have documented the age-related changes in the cheek teeth of horses using radiographs, CT, and histology.[39] As accessibility to these diagnostic techniques improves, the shortage of information should improve.

Veterinary schools are turning out practitioners who understand the use of these new technologies and radiologists who are skilled in CT/MRI interpretation. At this time the major obstacles to their use in veterinary dentistry are cost and accessibility. The benefits of having such highly sensitive and accurate imaging techniques should overcome these limitations in the near future.

References

1. Thrall, DE. Introduction to radiographic interpretation. In *Textbook of Veterinary Diagnostic Radiology*, 2nd Edition. Philadelphia:WB Saunders, 1994.

2. Kealy, JK. *Diagnostic Radiology of the Dog and Cat*. Philadelphia:WB Saunders, 1987.

3. Morgan, JP and Silverman, S. *Techniques of Veterinary Radiography*, 4th Edition. Ames:Iowa State University Press, 1992.

4. Codner, EC, Lurus, AG, Miller, JB, Gavin, PR, Gallina, A, Barbee, DD. Comparison of computed tomography with radiography as a noninvasive diagnostic technique for chronic nasal disease in dogs. *J Am Vet Med Assoc* 202(7):1106–10 (April 1993).

5. Park, RD, Beck, ER, LeCouteur, RA. Comparison of computed tomography and radiography for detecting changes induced by malignant nasal neoplasia in dogs. *J Am Vet Med Assoc* 201 (11):1720–24 (December 1992).

6. Beuf, O, Briguet, A, Lissac, M. In vitro magnetic resonance imaging of rodent teeth. *Oral Surg Oral Med Oral Pathol Oral Radiol Endod* 84(5):582–85 (November 1997).

7. Thomson, CF, Konegay, JN, Burn, RA, Drayer, BP, Hadley, DM, Levesque, DC, Gainsburg, LA, Lane, SB, Sharp, NJH, Wheeler, SJ. Magnetic resonance imaging–a general overview of principles and examples in veterinary neurodiagnosis. *Vet Rad & Ultrasound* 34(1):2–17.

8. Feeney, DA, Fletcher, TF, Hardy, RM. Atlas of Correlative Imaging Anatomy of the Normal Dog. Philadelphia:WB Saunders Company, 1991.

9. Coulam, CM, Erickson, JJ. Equipment considerations in computed tomography. In *The Physical Basis of Medical Imaging*. New York:Appleton-Century-Crofts, 1981.

10. Hogeboom, WR, Hoekstra, HJ, Mooyaart, EL, Freling, NJ, Veth, RP, Postma, A. MRI or CT in the preoperative diagnosis of bone tumours. *Eur J Surg Oncol* 18(1):67–72 (1992).

11. Virapongse, C, Mancuso, A, Fitzsimmons, J. Value of magnetic resonance imaging in assessing bone destruction in head and neck lesions. *Laryngoscope* 96(3):284–291 (1986).

12. Dennis, R. Magnetic resonance imaging and its application to veterinary medicine. *Vet Int* 6(2):3–10 (1993).

13. Clark, JA. The MRI signal and its generation. In *Magnetic Resonance Imaging for Technologists*. Seminar at the University of California School of Medicine, Department of Radiology, 1986.

14. Hendrick, RE. The AAPM/RSNA physics tutorial for residents. Basic physics of MR imaging: an introduction. *Radiographics* 14(4):829–46 (July 1994).

15. Bradley, WG, Shelden, CH. Nuclear magnetic resonance imaging: Review of early clinical experience. *Am J Surg* 146(1):85–87 (1983).

16. Adams, WH, Daniel, GB, Pardo, AD, Selcer, RR. Magnetic resonance imaging of the caudal lumbar and lumbosacral spine in 13 dogs (1990–1993). *Vet Rad & Ultrasound* 36(1):3–13 (1995).

17. Gray, CF, Redpath, TW, Smith, FW. Pre-surgical dental implant assessment by magnetic resonance imaging. *J Oral Implantol* 22(2):147–153 (1996).

18. Caldemeyer, KS, Mathews, VP, Righi, PD, Smith, RR. Imaging features and clinical significance of perineural spread or extension of head and neck tumors. *Radiographics* 18(1):97–110 (1998).

19. Harms, SE, Wilk, RM. Magnetic resonance imaging of the temporomandibular joint. *Radiographics* 7(3):521–542 (1987).

20. Bodner, L, Sarnat, H, Bar-Ziv, J, Kaffe, I. Computed tomography in pediatric oral and maxillofacial surgery. *ASDC J Dent Child* 63(1):32–38 (1996).

21. Matteson, SR, Deahl, ST, Alder, ME, Nummikoski, PV. Advanced imaging methods. *Crit Rev Oral Biol Med* 7(4):346–395 (1996).

22. Fuhrmann, RA, Bucker, A, Diedrich, PR. Assessment of alveolar bone loss with high resolution computed tomography. *J Periodontal Res* 30(4):258–263 (1995).

23. Fuhrmann, RA, Bucker, A, Diedrich, PR. Furcation involvement: Comparison of dental radiographs and HR-CT-slices in human specimens. *J Periodontal Res* 32(5):409–418 (1997).

24. Nielsen, RB, Alyassin, AM, Peters, DD, Carnes, DL, Lancaster, J. Microcomputed tomography: An advanced system for detailed endodontic research. *J Endod* 21(11):561–568 (1995).

25. Lockhart, PB, Kim, S, Lund, NL. Magnetic resonance imaging of human teeth. *J. Endod* 18(5):237–244 (1992).

26. Burk, RL. Computed tomographic anatomy of the canine nasal passages. *Vet Rad & US* 33(3):170–176 (1992).

27. Fike, JR, LeCouteur, RA, Cann, CE. Anatomy of the canine orbital region: Multiplanar imaging by CT. *Vet Rad* 25(1):32–35 (1984).

28. Fike, JR, LeCouteur, RA, Cann, CE. Anatomy of the canine brain using high resolution CT. *Vet Rad* 22(6):236–243 (1981).

29. Smallwood, JE, George, TF. Anatomic atlas for computed tomography in the mesaticephalic dog: Thorax and cranial abdomen. *Vet Rad & US* 34(2):65–84 (1993).

30. Smallwood, JE, George, TF. Anatomic atlas for CT in the mesaticephalic dog: Caudal abdomen and pelvis. *Vet Rad & US* 33(6):143–146 (1992).

31. George, TF, Smallwood, JE. Anatomic atlas for computed tomography in the mesaticephalic dog: Head and neck. *Vet Rad & US* 33(4):217–240 (1992).

32. Kraft, SL, Gavin, PR, Wendling, LR, Reddy, VK. Canine brain anatomy on MRI. *Vet Rad* 30(1):147–158 (1989).

33. Morgan, R, Daniel, GB, Donnell, RL. Magnetic resonance imaging of the normal eye and orbit of the dog and cat. *Vet Rad & US* 35(2):102–108 (1994).

34. Denoix, J-M, Crevier, N, Roger, B, Lebas, J-F. Magnetic resonance

imaging of the equine foot. *Vet Rad & US* 34(6):405–411 (1993).

35. Kaser-Hotz, B, Sartoretti-Schefer, S, Weiss, R. CT and MRI of the normal equine carpus. *Vet Rad & US* 35(6):457–461 (1994).

36. Turrel, JM, Fike, JR, LeCouteur, RA, Higgins, RJ. Computed tomographic characteristics of primary brain tumors in 50 dogs. *J Am Vet Med Assoc* 188(8):851–856 (1986).

37. LeCouteur, RA, Fike, JR, Scagliotti, RH, Cann, CE. Computed tomography of orbital tumors in the dog. *J Am Vet Med Assoc* 180(8):910–913 (1982).

38. Karkkainen, M, Punto, LU, Tulamo, R-M. Magnetic resonance imaging of canine degenerative lumbar spine disease. *Vet Rad & US* 34(6):399–404 (1993).

39. Kirkland, KD, Baker, GJ, Manfra, MS, Eurell, JA, Losonsky, JM. Effects of aging on the endodontic system, reserve crown, and roots of equine mandibular cheek teeth. *Am J Vet Res* 57(1):31–38 (1996).

40. Burk, RL. Computed tomographic imaging of nasal disease in 100 dogs. *Vet Rad & US* 33(3):177–180 (1992).

41. Kraus, MS, Mahaffey, MB, Girard, E, Chambers, JN, Brown, CA, Coates, JR. Diagnosis of C5-C6 spinal luxation using three-dimensional computed tomographic reconstruction. *Vet Rad & US* 38(1):39–41 (1997).

APPENDIX 2

THE MODIFIED TRIADAN SYSTEM: NOMENCLATURE FOR VETERINARY DENTISTRY

Dr. Michael R. Floyd

The goal of any dental nomenclature system should be to provide a logical, exact, nonconfusing, easy-to-learn-and-use method of describing teeth. An effective system should function equally well when spoken, handwritten, typed, printed, stored, or retrieved. For veterinary dentists, the ideal system would identify the same tooth in different species with the same designation.

Animal Nomenclature from Human Nomenclature

In January 1972, the International Dental Federation adopted a new, two digit, "user friendly" nomenclature system for use in the human dental patient. This New System eliminated the plus and minus signs of the Haderup System and the brackets of the Winkel System.[1] The New System has many advantages, not the least of which is its compatibility with computer technology. It is, however, more commonly used in Europe than in the United States.

In the New System, the first of the two digits represents the *quadrant* in primary or secondary dentition, beginning with 1 for the upper right and proceeding clockwise around the mouth to 4 for the lower right quadrant. In primary dentition, the numbers start with 5 in the upper right and proceed to 8 in the lower right quadrant. The second digit refers to the *location and anatomical description* of the tooth. The teeth are numbered consecutively from 1 to 8, starting at the midline and proceeding distal. Since the teeth in each quadrant are homologous, each tooth with the same second digit is the same type of tooth. For example, 14, 24, 34, and 44 are all first premolars (bicuspids).

Following the acceptance of the New System for human dental nomenclature, Professor Dr. Med. Dent. H. Triadan, a dentist at the University of Bern, Switzerland, introduced a similar system for animals.[2] Due to the fact that many animals, including [Triadan's] canine model, have more than nine teeth in an arcade, the Triadan System for animals utilizes three digits instead of two digits.

Just as [in] the New System, the first digit of the Triadan Sys-

tem identifies the quadrant starting with 1 in the upper right and ending with 4 in the lower right. The teeth are numbered consecutively beginning with 01 at the midline and proceed distal. For example, the dog's upper right fourth premolar is 108, and [its] lower right fourth premolar is 408 (Figure A2.1). However, Triadan failed to address the problem of numbering teeth in species, such as the feline, which are missing teeth compared to the canine. In 1990, West-Hyde established the anatomic description of feline dentition which accounted for the anatomic numbering sequence of teeth in this species.

The Modified Triadan System

A veterinary dentist may have patients of several different species with varying dental formulas. In order for a dental numbering system to be user-friendly, the tooth numbers should be consistent from species to species. A tooth with the same anatomical designation should have the same identifying number regardless of species.

In introducing a modification of the Triadan System, gaps are left in the numbering sequence where there are missing teeth. For example, the first premolar encountered in the feline left maxilla (ULP2) is numbered 206, not 205.[2,3] The two lower right premolars are 407 and 408, not 405 and 406 (Figure A2.2).

With the Modified Triadan System, all canine teeth end in 4, and all first molars end in 9 ("The Rule of 4 and 9"). This system applies equally well to all domestic species. In addition to being an easy system to learn, it also reinforces the relationship between teeth of the upper and lower arcades. Furthermore, the use of this system provides the veterinary dentist with a method to understand the comparative anatomic relationship between teeth of various species by referring to their common identifying numbers.

Conclusions

The Modified Triadan System has [a] distinct advantage over anatomical notation in that it is equally easy to write, type, speak, print, store, and retrieve. It leaves no room for confusion about left and right, upper and lower, or comparative evaluations between species even when one species has a reduced den-

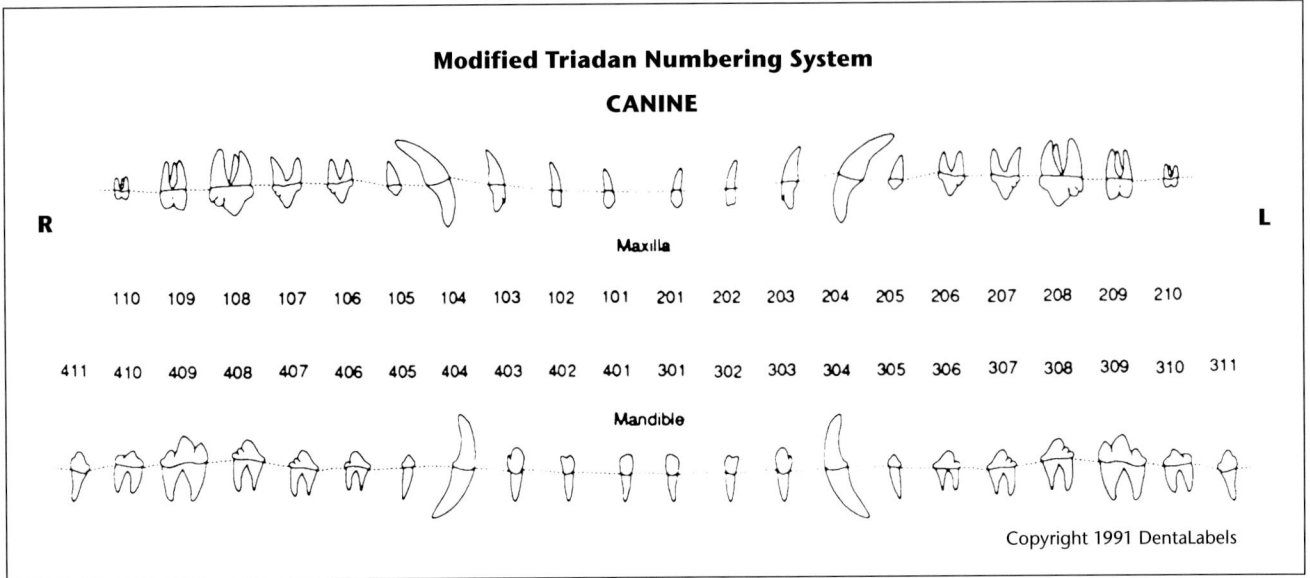

Modified Triadan Numbering System

CANINE

FIGURE A2.1

Canine chart for the Modified Triadan System.

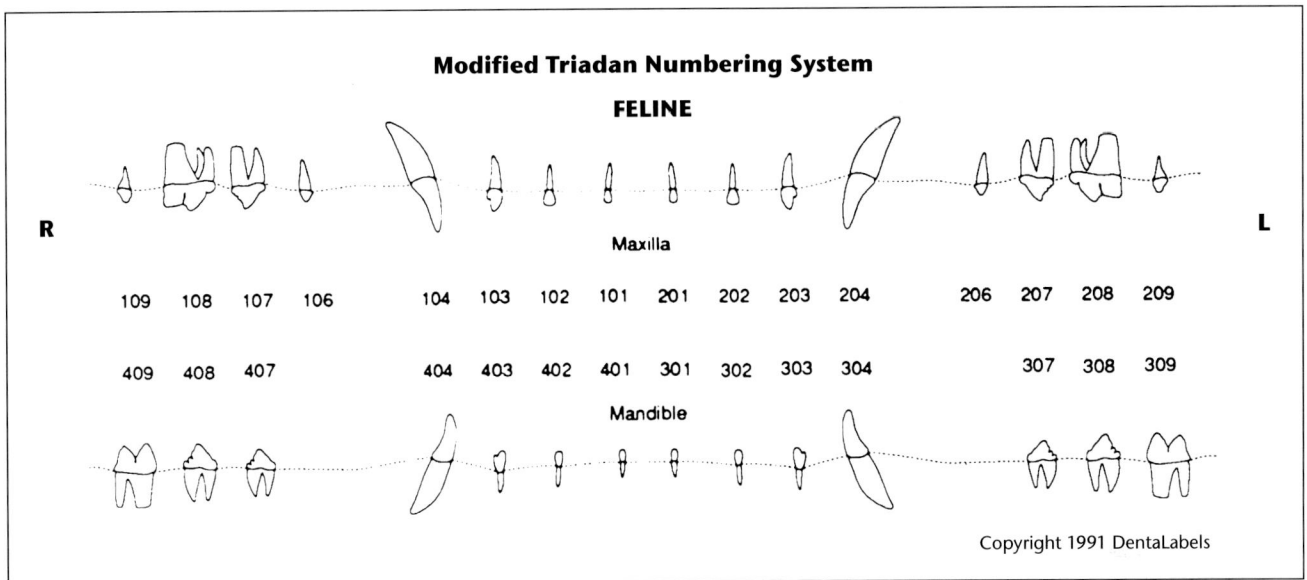

Modified Triadan Numbering System

FELINE

FIGURE A2.2

Feline chart for the Modified Triadan System.

tition. It allows exact communication when charting or otherwise speaking about teeth. Regular users of the Modified Triadan System quickly learn the numbers and appreciate the accuracy and simplicity of this system.

Reprinted with permission of Michael R. Floyd, DVM, FAVD, from the *Journal of Veterinary Dentistry*. The Modified Triadan System: Nomenclature for veterinary dentistry. *J Vet Dent* 8(4) (1991).

References

1. Triadan H. Tierzahnheilkunde: Zahnerhaltung (Fullungstherapie mit "Composite Materials" und Endodontie) bei Affen und Raubtieren. *Schweiz Arch Tierheilkd* 114:292 (1972).

2. West-Hyde L. The enigma of feline dentition. *J Vet Dent* 7(3):16–17 (1990).

3. Eisenmenger E, Zetner K. Tooth and jaw. In *Veterinary Dentistry*. Philadelphia: Lea and Febiger, 1985, 9–10, 16.

GLOSSARY OF Veterinary Dental Terminology

INTRODUCTION AND SPECIAL ACKNOWLEDGMENT

It is impossible to communicate in veterinary dentistry without a consistent vocabulary. Over the years, terms and definitions have been used which do not completely apply to veterinary dentistry because of incorrect application or inappropriate adaptation from human to veterinary usage. In this Glossary of Veterinary Dental Terminology, we have attempted to select only those definitions which apply to veterinary dentistry specifically. There will be those that question our choices and definitions. To those we welcome open dialogue as veterinary dentistry continues to grow into the twenty-first century. This glossary is a starting point. As the companion to the radiology atlas, it will open doors and become a valuable resource as our field expands.

Two sources must be gratefully acknowledged. The American Academy of Periodontology has allowed complete access to defin-

itions from their *Glossary of Periodontal Terms*—1992—Third Edition. A second thank you goes to the publishing house of Butterworth-Heinemann for usage of terms from the *Concise Illustrated Dental Dictionary* by F. J. Harty—Second Edition.

Both of these sources in human dentistry have allowed us to begin a glossary in veterinary dental terms that is complete and accurate. This freedom of exchange of medical/scientific knowledge lends credence to its composition. As veterinary dentistry continues to grow, cooperation of this type with human dentistry will allow both fields to mutually benefit. The authors again deeply thank those mentioned above for their help.

Ben H. Colmery III, DVM
Donald H. DeForge, VMD

A

Aberrant—varying or deviating from the usual or normal course, form, or location.[1]

Abscess—localized collection of pus in a cavity formed by the disintegration of tissues.[1]

> **Acute a.**—abscess that runs a relatively short course, producing pain and local inflammation.[1]

> **Apical a.**—inflammatory condition characterized by pus formation involving the tissues surrounding the apex of a tooth.

> **Chronic a.**— Abscess of comparatively slow development with little evidence of inflammation. There may be an intermittent discharge of purulent matter. 2. Long-standing collection of pus. It may follow an acute abscess.[1]

> **Periodontal a. (parietal a.)**—localized purulent inflammation in the periodontal tissues; also called lateral periodontal abscess.[1]

> **Pulpal a.**—inflammation of the dental pulp characterized by the formation of pus.[1]

Abutment—tooth, root, or implant used to support and/or anchor a fixed or removable prosthesis.[1]

Accretion—accumulation on the teeth of foreign materials such as plaque, material alba, and calculus.[1]

Acid etching—partial demineralization of a selected area of tooth substance by the use of dilute acid in order to provide a clean and mechanically retentive surface for the retention of selected types of restorative materials such as composite and glass ionomer cements.[2]

Actinobacillus actinomycetecomitans—small, Gram-negative, nonmotile, facultatively anaerobic, rod-shaped bacteria found in subgingival and marginal plaque. Implicated as a major pathogen in localized juvenile periodontitis in man.[1]

Adenocarcinoma—malignant epithelial tumor arising from glandular structures. Also applies to tumors with a glandular growth pattern.[2]

Adenoma—benign epithelial tumor derived from glandular tissue.[2]

Adumbration—poor edge definition of an image of an x-ray film due to cross over of x-rays (also see penumbra).[2]

Aerobe—a microorganism that can live and grow in the presence of molecular oxygen.[1]

Alginate—salt of alginic acid (obtained from seaweed) which, when mixed with water in the recommended proportions, forms an irreversible hydrocolloid gel used for dental impressions.[2]

Allograft—a bone grafting material from one individual donor placed in another individual donor.

Alloplast—synthetic bone grafting material which is chemically deriven.

Alveolar bone—compact bone that composes the alveolus (tooth socket). The fibers of the periodontal ligament insert into it.[1]

Alveolar crest—the most coronal portion of the alveolar process.[1]

Alveolitis—inflammation or infection of the empty socket after extraction.

Alveolus—the socket in the bone into which a tooth is attached by means of the periodontal ligament.[1]

Alveoplasty—a general term used to describe the surgical reshaping of the alveolar ridges.[2]

Ameloblast—ectodermally derived cell primarily responsible for the formation of enamel (amelogenesis).[2]

Ameloblastic fibroma (fibroameloblastoma)—a locally invasive, destructive, odontogenic neoplasm consisting of proliferating odontogenic epithelium in a fibrous stroma.

Amelogenesis imperfecta—an imperfection in which enamel formation and/either calcification is defective.

Amputation, root—removal of a root from a tooth.[1]

Amyloid producing odontogenic tumor (calcifying epithelial odontogenic tumor)—an odontogenic tumor that develops in tissues that produce teeth. Amyloid is a starch-like protein-carbohydrate complex that is deposited abnormally in some tissues during certain chronic disease states, such as amyloidosis.

Anachoresis—blood-borne infection in which micro-organisms are attracted toward certain local lesions while the rest of the body appears to remain immune from these organisms.[2]

Anaerobe—a microorganism that can live in partial or complete absence of molecular oxygen.[1]

Anisocephalic—Asymmetrical maxilla lengths.

Anisognathic—Asymmetrical jaw lengths (mandible).

Ankylosis—solid fixation of a tooth resulting from fusion of the cementum and alveolar bone, with obliteration of the periodontal membrane.

Anodontia—congenital absence of the teeth.[1]

Anomaly—deviation from the norm.

Antagonist—in dentistry, a tooth in one jaw which occludes with a tooth in the other jaw.[2]

Anterior cross bite—an orthodontic malocclusion in which canine, premolar and molar occlusion is normal, but one or more mandibular incisors are anterior to the maxillary incisors.

Antrum—a cavity or chamber, especially in a bone.[1]

Apex—the root tip end of a tooth.

Apex of root—the terminal portion of the tooth root.

Apexification—more correctly termed *root end closure induction*. Process whereby an immature permanent tooth apex is induced to continue root formation or to produce a calcific barrier across the root canal. This is generally achieved by the use of calcium hydroxide paste dressing to the canal.[2]

Apical—referring to the tip or apex of the tooth root and its immediate surroundings.[2]

> **A. delta**—numerous small perforations into the apex that allow passage of vessels and nerves into the root canal of the tooth (found in the canine and feline).

> **A. foramen**—a single opening at the apex that allows passage of vessels and nerves into the root canal of a tooth (found in humans).

Apicoectomy (apicectomy, apicotomy, apectomy, root resection, root amputation)— the surgical removal of the apex of a tooth root.[1]

Archwire—in orthodontics, a length of fine stainless steel wire contoured to the dental arch and fitting into brackets or other orthodontic attachments on the buccal or labial aspects of the teeth.[2]

Articulation—1. The contact relationships of mandibular teeth with maxillary teeth in excursive movements of the mandible. 2. A junction or union between two or more bones. 3. A skeletal joint.[1]

Articulator—a mechanical device representing the temporomandibular joint and jaw members to which maxillary and mandibular casts may be attached.[1]

Astringent—in dentistry, agent used to contract gingival tissue away from a crown preparation in order to facilitate impression taking.[2]

Attachment apparatus—a term commonly used to designate the cementum, periodontal ligament, and alveolar bone.[1]

Attachment, new—the union of connective tissue or epithelium with a root surface that has been deprived of its original attachment apparatus. This new attachment may be epithelial adhesion and/or connective adaptation or attachment and may include new cementum.[1]

Attenuation—in radiology, the process by which a beam of radiation is reduced in energy when it passes through matter.[2]

Attrition—loss of tooth substance or of a restoration as a result of mastication or of occlusal or approximal contact between the teeth.

Autograft—a bone grafting material from one individual donor to that same individual.

Avascular—lacking in blood supply (e.g., tooth enamel).

Avulsion—traumatic removal of a tooth from its socket.[2]

Axis—1. A real or imaginary straight line passing through the center of a body. 2. "Long axis of a tooth," the central lengthwise line through the crown and the root.[1]

B

Basal bone—the bone of the mandible and maxilla exclusive of the alveolar process.[1]

Base narrow canines—linguoversion of the canine teeth usually concomitant with a narrow mandible.

Bed—the surgically-prepared recipient site for a graft.

Benign—describes a tumor that is not malignant (e.g., papilloma). It does not destroy the tissues from which it originates, nor does it spread to other parts of the body. Generally recurrence is unlikely following excision.[2]

Beta-lactam antibiotics—antibiotics containing a beta-lactam ring; the penicillins, cephalosporins, monobactams (aztreonam), and carbapenums (imipenem-cilastatin).[1]

Beta-lactamase—a bacterial enzyme that accounts for the major resistance mechanism to beta-lactam antibiotics by opening the beta-lactam ring of penicillins and cephalosporins.[1]

Bifurcation—the anatomic area where roots of a two-rooted tooth divide.[1]

Bifurcation invasion—the extension of pulpitis or periodontitis into a bifurcation.[1]

Biological width—a physiologic space controlled by the body's defense and immune system to maintain a normal equilibrium in restorative dentistry. Most often described in relationship to a full jacket crown restoration and the base of the gingival sulcus with it epithelial attachment. If the biological width is invaded upon an inflammatory response with crestal bone resorption and apical migration of the periodontal tissues can occur. The normal biological width for the canine is 2-3mm. (Fifty percent being supracrestal connective tissue and 50 percent being junctional epithelial tissue.)

Biopsy—the removal and examination, usually microscopic, of tissue for the purpose of establishing a histopathological diagnosis. May also refer to the tissue specimen obtained by this procedure.[1]

> **Excisional b.**—the removal of an entire lesion, including a significant margin or contiguous, normal-appearing tissue for microscopic examination and diagnosis.[1]

> **Incisional b.**—the removal of a selected portion of a lesion and, if possible, adjacent normal-appearing tissue for microscopic examination and diagnosis.[1]

Bisecting angle—in radiology, technique in which the beam of radiation is directed perpendicularly toward an imaginary line which bisects the angle formed by the plane of the film and long axis of the tooth.[2]

bis-GMA (Bowen's resin)—the resin system most commonly associated with dental restorative materials.[2]

Bite—the act of incising and crushing between the teeth.[1]

Bone fill—the clinical restoration of bone tissue in a treated periodontal defect. Does not address the presence or absence of histologic evidence of new connective tissue attachment or the formation of a new periodontal ligament.[1]

Bowen's resin—*See* bis-GMA.[2]

Boxing—(of an impression) Provision of a wall, usually of wax, to form a box around an impression to reduce time and effort in subsequently trimming and shaping plaster models. It is attached to the perimeter of the impression to contain the cast material until it has set.[2]

Brachygnathia—a lower jaw of inadequate length.

Brachyodonts—species with teeth with anatomic roots that stop growing once erupted. These are closed rooted teeth with a short anatomical crown in relation to the anatomical root (i.e., canines, felines, most carnivores, molars of rats, mice, and hamsters).

Bridge—prosthesis which replaces one or more clinical crowns of missing natural teeth.[2]

B. retainer—restoration cemented to an abutment tooth which provides retention for a bridge.[2]

Broach—hand instrument attached to a broach holder and used in endodontic treatment to demonstrate pulpal exposures and root canals, and to remove debris and necrotic tissues.[2]

Barbed b.—broach made in assorted sizes, similar to smooth broach but with barbs pointing toward the handle. Used mainly for extirpation of vital pulps, and the removal of necrotic tissue and dressing from the root canal.[2]

Bruxism (tooth grinding)—a habit of grinding, clenching, or clamping teeth. The force so generated may damage both tooth and attachment apparatus (common in humans, but also found in animals).[1]

Buccal—term denoting the surfaces of premolars and molars facing toward the cheeks. Pertaining to or adjacent to the cheeks.[2]

Buccoversion—the deviation of a tooth from the normal line of the dental arch toward the cheek.[1]

Bundle bone—a type of alveolar bone, so called because of the "bundle" pattern caused by the continuation of the principal (Sharpey's) fibers into it.[1]

Bur—rotary milling tool with sharp blades or various shapes, designed to fit into a handle. Term also used for small rotary diamond instruments. Consists of a cutting portion (the head), the shaft which attaches the bur to the handle, and a generally tapering shank which joins the head to the shaft.[2]

Burnisher—hand instrument with rounded edges, used to polish or burnish the surface of metallic restorations by rubbing.[2]

Butt joint—joint in which two flat surfaces are brought together without overlapping.[2]

C

Calcified epithelial odontogenic tumor—slowly growing locally invasive neoplasm that is diagnosed histologically by the appearance of cords of epithelial cells, amyloid spherules, and foci of calcification.

Calcium hydroxide—salt of calcium used to encourage the formation of reparative dentine. The powder may be mixed with water to form a paste, or it may be obtained ready mixed in tubes. It is placed in deep cavities as a seal and a protective lining, or in direct contact with the pulp in endodontic procedures.[2]

Calculus, dental (tartar)—a hard concretion that forms on teeth or dental prostheses through calcification of bacterial plaque.[1]

Subgingival (seruminal) c.—calculus formed apical to the gingival margin; often brown or black, hard, and tenacious.[1]

Supragingival (salivary) c.—calculus formed coronal to the gingival margin; usually formed more recently than subgingival calculus.[1]

Canal, root—the portion of the dental pulp cavity in the root of a tooth.[1]

Accessory (lateral) root c.—a lateral branch of the main root canal most often found in the apical half of the roots and in furcation areas.[1]

Cancellous bone—bone having a reticular, spongy, or lattice-like structure.[1]

Canine—the long pointed tooth, just distal to the incisors in each quadrant, used for tearing, also commonly referred to as fangs.

Carat—the carat of an alloy refers to the parts of gold in an alloy in 24 parts. For example, 22 carat gold has 22 parts of gold and 2 parts of other metals, 24 carat being pure gold.[2]

Carcinoma—a malignant growth of epithelial cells tending to infiltrate the surrounding tissues giving rise to metastases.[1]

Caries—a localized and progressive disintegration of a tooth usually beginning with the dissolution of the enamel and followed by bacteria invasion of the dentinal tubules.[1]

Carnassial—referring to the maxillary fourth premolar and the mandibular first molar.

Carver—hand instrument with a blade or nib used to contour the surface of filling materials in their plastic state, waxes, models, and patterns (e.g., Ward's, Frahm's, LeCron's).[2]

Cast, study or diagnostic—a positive replica of the teeth and adjacent tissues usually formed by pouring plaster into a matrix or impression.[1]

Caudal—toward the tail.

Cavity—in dentistry, a condition caused by caries, trauma, abrasion, erosion or attrition, resulting in the loss of hard tissue. Refers to such cavities only and should not be applied to a tooth preparation.[2]

Cavity, pulp—the internal space within a tooth, which normally houses the dental pulp.[1]

Cement—in dentistry, term covering materials used for luting, lining, and as a permanent (e.g., silicate, glass-ionomer) or temporary (e.g., zinc phosphate, zinc oxide, etc.) filling. The components are mixed in their correct proportions to provide a plastic mass which sets in due course.[2]

Cementation—process of cementing a restoration in place by the use of a luting agent or cement.[2]

Cementicle—a calcified, spherical body composed of cementum, lying free within the periodontal ligament, and attached to the cementum or imbedded within it.[1]

Cementoblast—cell concerned with the formation of cementum.[2]

Cementoclasia—disintegration of the cementum of a tooth.

Cementocyte—cell found in the cellular layer of cementum. Some-what stellate-shaped cell with radiating thin processes. A product of cementoblast cells which have remained in the newly formed cementum.[2]

Cementoenamel junction (CEJ)—imaginary line formed between the cementum and enamel at the anatomical neck of the tooth where amelogenesis takes place.[2]

Cementogenesis—the development or formation of cementum.[1]

Cementoma—generally benign proliferation of odontogenic connective tissue in the mandible or maxilla which produces cementum or cementum-like tissue. Often associated with the apices of teeth.[2]

Cementosis—a condition characterized by proliferation of cementum, also called dental exostosis.

Cementum—This substance covers the root and contains the collagenous fibers of the periodontal ligament that anchor the teeth to alveolar bone. Cementum resorption and deposition continue throughout life. Cementum is thickest toward the tooth apex and thinnest at the CEJ.

> **Acellular c.**—that portion of the cementum that does not incorporate cells.[1]

> **Cellular c.**—that portion of the cementum that contains cementocytes. It is found primarily in the apical third of the root.[1]

Cephalosporins—broad spectrum beta-lactam antibiotics chemically related to and having the same mechanism of action as the penicillins.[1]

Ceramics—general term for dental porcelain work.[2]

Cervical—in dentistry, the area where the tooth crown joins the root.[2]

> **C. line**—line around a tooth marking the junction of the enamel of the crown and the cementum of the root.[2]

> **C. burnout or c. radiolucency**—the radiolucency seen at the margin of a tooth and sometimes mistaken for caries.[2]

Cervix—a neck or constricted portion; specifically, the narrowed region at the junction of the crown with the root of a tooth.[1]

Chamber, pulp—that portion of the pulp cavity within the anatomic crown of the tooth.[1]

Cheek teeth—collective term for molars and premolars.[2]

Chlorhexidine—a bis-biguanide antiseptic agent used to prevent colonization and kill or inhibit microorganisms on surfaces of skin, mucous membranes, and teeth.[1]

Chronic diffuse sclerosing osteomyelitis—an extensive or widespread radiopaque lesion. Because of the diffuse pattern the border between the sclerosis and the normal bone is not always clear.

Chronic ulcerative paradental stomatitis (CUPS)—an exaggerated ulceration of the buccal, labial, or lingual mucosa in advanced periodontitis. Also, referred to as a "kissing" lesion.

Cingulum—bulge or ridge found on the palatal or lingual aspects of incisor and canine teeth, near to their cervical margins.[2]

Cleft—fissure or elongated opening which occurs due to failure of parts to unite during development.[2]

> **C. lip (harelip)**—congenital condition (sometimes involving the maxillary bone) in which there is a developmental defect along the normal lines of fusion of the lip tissues, causing a cleft or fissure.[2]

> **C. palate**—lack of fusion along the normal developmental lines of the palate.[2]

Clindamycin—a lincosamide antibiotic with a broad spectrum of bacteriostatic activity particularly against anaerobes.[1]

Clinical root—that portion of the anatomical root attached to the alveolar bone by the periodontal ligament.[2]

Collimator—diaphragm or tube lined with an x-ray absorbing material designed to restrict the size of the x-ray beam.[2]

Commissure—the union of the upper and lower lips at the angles of the mouth.[1]

Compact bone—bone substance that is dense and hard.[1]

Computerized tomography (CAT scan)—the technique by which multidirectional x-ray transmission data through a body are mathematically reconstructed by a computer to form an electrical cross section (slice) of a patient's anatomy.[1]

Concrescence—fusion of two normally separate parts.[2]

Concretion—an inorganic mass in a natural cavity or in a tissue of an organism.[1]

Condenser—in dentistry, a hand instrument designed to pack restorative materials into a prepared tooth cavity.[2]

Condensing osteitis—chronic focal sclerosing osteomyelitis also known as condensing osteitis is a circumscribed radiopaque mass of sclerotic bone surrounding the periapical area of the tooth root. The radiopacity stands out in distinct contrast to the trabecular pattern of the normal bone. It is a reaction of the bone to a low grade infection.

Cone—in radiography, that part of the x-ray apparatus which determines the minimum anode-to-film distance and indicates the direction of the central axis of the x-ray beam.[2]

Contact—the touching of surfaces of two adjoining or occluding teeth.

Contra-angle—instrument having two or more off-setting angles along its shank in order to bring the working end closer to the long axis of the handle.[2]

Contralateral—situated on, pertaining to, or affecting the opposite side, as opposed to ipsilateral.[1]

Contrast, radiographic image—the visible differences in photographic or film density produced on a radiograph by the structural composition of the object or objects radiographed. Radiographs made with higher kilovoltage (90 kV) have a longer scale contrast and appear dull by comparison with those made at lower voltages, but they have improved image character for interpretation.[1]

Copal—resin obtained from tropical trees and used in a solvent as varnish.[2]

Coping—thin, cast-metal cap, without external undercuts, that is fitted over a preparation.[2]

> **Transfer c.**—base metal or resin cap used to obtain precise relative locations during the taking of impressions of multiple preparations.[2]

Core—correctly shaped and well-retained substructure to a partial or full veneer crown. May be a part of a post and core system and may be cast or prefabricated. A core may also be constructed of amalgam or composite resin and retained by pin fixation.[2]

Cornu—synonym for pulp horn.[2]

Coronal—in the direction of the tip of the crown.

Coronal pulp—the part of the dental pulp contained in the crown portion of the pulp cavity.

Coronitis—soft tissue inflammation around an erupting tooth crown.[2]

Cortical bone—the compact bone at the surface of any given bone.[1]

Cortical plate—hard bone covering the inner and outer surface of the alveolar process.[2]

Cranial—toward the head.

Crazing—pattern of minute hair-like cracks on the surface of porcelain and acrylic polymers.[2]

Creep—to slowly change shape, as do heated metals and ceramics under load. Amalgam restorations may flow or creep under heavy masticatory forces.[2]

Crest—a projection or ridge. In periodontics, usually refers to the most coronal portion of the alveolar process.[1]

Crestal bone—referring to the most coronal extent of the alveolar bone.

Cribriform plate, dental—the alveolar bone proper.[1]

Cross bite—an abnormal relation of a tooth or teeth of one arch to its/their antagonists in the other arch due to lateral deviation of tooth position or abnormal jaw position.[1]

Crowding—discrepancy between tooth sizes and arch length resulting in malalignment and abnormal contact relationships between teeth.[1]

Crown—the part of the tooth that is covered with enamel or a dental restoration and normally projects beyond the gingival margin.[1]

> **Anatomic c.**—the portion of a natural tooth that extends from its cementoenamel junction to the occlusal surface or incisal edge.[1]

> **Cast c.**—metal veneer crown, full or partial, and constructed by the casting process.[2]

> **Clinical c.**—the portion of a tooth that extends occlusally or incisally from the margin of the investing soft tissue, usually gingiva.[1]

> **Jacket c.**—full veneer crown completely covering the prepared stump of a tooth and having a cervical shoulder. Constructed of porcelain or acrylic resin and cemented into place.[2]

Crown, lengthening of clinical—a surgical procedure designed to increase the extent of supragingival tooth structure for restorative or esthetic purposes by apically positioning the gingival margin, removing supporting bone, or both. May be accompanied by orthodontic tooth movement.[1]

Crown-root ratio—the relationship between the extra-alveolar arm of the tooth and the intra-alveolar arm of the tooth as determined radiographically.[1]

CT—computed tomography. *See* Appendix 1.

Curettage—scraping or cleaning the walls of a cavity or surface by means of a curette.[1]

> **Apical (periapical) c.**—Surgical removal of tissue or foreign material surrounding the apex of a tooth.[1]

> **Closed c.**—performed via the gingival crevice without flap reflection.[1]

> **Gingival c.**—the process of debriding the soft tissue wall of a periodontal pocket.[1]

> **Open c.**—facilitated by reflection of a soft tissue flap.[1]

> **Root c.**—scraping or cleaning the walls of a cavity or surface by means of a curette.[1]

Cusp—referring to the crown.

Cyclosporine—an immunosuppressant and antifungal agent used to prevent rejection in organ transplant recipients. It can be associated with gingival overgrowth.[1]

Cyst—a pathologic cavity lined by epithelium and usually containing fluid or semisolid material.[1]

> **Apical periodontal c.**—the most common odontogenic cyst; involving the apex of a root and resulting from the inflammatory reaction to a nonvital pulp.[1]
>
> **Dentigerous c.**—forms around the crown of an unerupted tooth or odontoma.[1]
>
> **Developmental c.**—results from a formative aberration.[1]
>
> **Gingival c.**—found within the gingiva, most commonly in the mandibular canine-premolar region. Believed to be derived from epithelial rests of the dental lamina.[1]
>
> **Odontogenic c.**—a class of cysts derived from odontogenic epithelium. Primordial, dentigerous, and lateral periodontal cysts fall into this classification.[1]
>
> **Primordial c.**—an odontogenic cyst resulting from degeneration of the enamel organ of a developing tooth bud.[1]
>
> **Radicular c.**—a cyst along the root of a tooth. Previously the term was used synonymously with what is now more correctly referred to as an apical periodontal cyst.[1]
>
> **Residual c.**—a cyst in the maxilla or mandible that remains after the associated tooth as been removed.[1]

Cytokines—a broad family of humoral factors that mediate important roles in growth, differentiation, and tissue damage by cellular receptors.[1]

D

Dappen pot—small glass or plastic receptacle for drugs and liquids used in dentistry.[2]

Debridement—the removal of inflamed, devitalized, or contaminated tissue or foreign material from or adjacent to a lesion.[1]

Decortication—removal of cortical bone. Often used to describe multiple penetrations of the cortical surface of an intrabony defect.[1]

Dehiscence—in dentistry, a vertical defect of the alveolar margin.[2]

Demineralization—decalcification; loss of mineral salts.[1]

Dens in dente—"tooth within a tooth." A developmental tooth anomaly in which there is an invagination within the primary tooth wholly or partially lined with enamel.

Dens invaginatus—developmental tooth anomaly in which there is deep invagination lined with enamel on the lingual or palatal surface of the primary tooth (used interchangeably with dens in dente).

Dental alveoli—the bony cavities or sockets in the mandible or maxilla in which the roots of teeth are attached.

Denticle (pulp stone)—a calcified mass of dentin, which may be free within the pulp, attached to the pulpal wall, or embedded in the dentin.[1]

Dentigerous cyst—a subgingival cyst containing or producing teeth or rudimentary teeth.

Dentin—The main component of the tooth and consists of many tubules containing sensory nerve fibers. Harder than bone it is covered by enamel on the crown and cementum on the root.

Diastema—a space between two adjacent teeth in a dental arch.[1]

Die—the positive reproduction of a prepared tooth or teeth in a suitable hard material such as amalgam, stone or plaster.[2]

Dilaceration—1. A tearing apart. 2. A distortion of the root or crown of a tooth resulting from an injury during tooth development. Through common usage, the term now includes teeth with sharply angulated and deformed roots.[1]

Diphyodonts—species with both a primary dentition and secondary or permanent dentition that replaces the primary (i.e., primates, canines, felines, and domestic herbivores).

Disclosant—a dye (tablet or solution) used to stain dental plaque. Used primarily as an aid in oral hygiene instruction.[1]

Distal—that aspect of the tooth facing toward the caudal direction of the arch. For incisors, the distal aspect is lateral toward the midline of the arch.

Distocclusion—the abnormal posterior or distal relationship of the mandibular to the maxillary teeth as in an Class II malocclusion.[1]

Distomesial lateral oblique view—referring to a view of the teeth in which the horizontal angulation of the x-ray beam is toward the distobuccal aspect of the teeth and passes through to the palatal or lingual aspect mesially. Most often used for maxillary premolars.

Ditching—characteristic effect seen at the periphery of an amalgam restoration and its junction with the enamel of the tooth.[2]

Dorsoventral view—referring to the passage of the x-ray beam from the dorsal aspect through to the ventral aspect of the animal.

Dysplasia, periapical cemental (cementoma)—a process of unknown origin in which the periapical bone of vital teeth is replaced first by a fibrous type of connective tissue, and then by an osseocementoid tissue. During its early stages this abnormality appears radiolucent and with time the center becomes opaque. It is classified as an odontogenic tumor.[1]

E

EBA cement—reinforced zinc oxide-eugenol cement.[2]

Eburnation—the change in carious dentine from a soft decalcified mass to a hard, polished, black-to-brown state.[2]

Ectopic—referring to an abnormal position of a tooth.

Edentulous—toothless. Without natural teeth in the mouth, as when born or following total tooth removal.

Edge-to-edge bite—malocclusion in which the mandibular and maxillary incisors occlude along their incisal edges and do not overlap. Also referred to as an "even bite."

Embedded tooth—if the eruption process has ended and the tooth is below the mucosa it is embedded.

Enamel—Crown formation is completely and entirely within the bones of the jaw. Enamel is formed by ameloblasts and is generally thickest at the apex of the crown. Its hydroxyapatite crystalline components are laid down in flattened hexagonal rods which are generally perpendicular to the surface of the tooth. Enamel is incapable of healing after eruption because it lacks viable connective tissue or epithelial covering.

> **E. pearl**—a small, focal mass of enamel formed apical to the cementoenamel junction.[1]

> **E. projection**—an apical extension of enamel, usually toward a furcation.[1]

Endodontia—the branch of dental science concerned with the dental pulp and related tissues.[2]

Endodontics—procedures used to preserve the health of the dental pulp and periapical tissues, and the treatment of the diseased pulp to enable the tooth (or part of the tooth) to be retained in function.[2]

Endodontic stops—device to fix the depth to which an instrument has been introduced into a root canal and to prevent it from being advanced farther.[2]

Enostosis—a bony growth located within a bony cavity or extending centrally from the cortical plate.[1]

Eosinophilic granuloma—Eosinophilic granuloma complex appears in the oral cavity in two different forms: 1. Eosinophilic ulcer is a well-circumscribed, ulcerated lesion most commonly found on the upper lip of the cat. It is usually nonpainful and nonpuritic. 2. Eosinophilic granuloma is found in a nodular pattern in the oral cavity often on the palate. The etiology is unknown.

Epithelialization (epithelization)—healing by growth of epithelium over connective tissue.[1]

Epithelium, oral—the tissue serving as the lining of the intraoral surfaces. It extends into the gingival crevice and adheres to the tooth at the base of the crevice.[1]

> **Crevicular e.**—the nonkeratinized epithelium of the gingival crevice.[1]

> **Junctional e.**—a single or multiple layer of nonkeratinizing cells adhering to the tooth surface at the base of the gingival crevice. Formerly called epithelial attachment.[1]

Epulis—a nonspecific term for any tumor of the gingiva.[1]

Eruption, active—normal movement of a tooth into or toward the oral cavity from its developmental position in the alveolar bone.[2]

Erythromycin—a bacteriostatic macrolide group of antibiotics that has both Gram-positive and Gram-negative antibacterial spectra and acts by inhibiting ribosomal protein synthesis.[1]

Eschar—a slough caused by cauterization or by application on some corrosive substance.[1]

Even bite—occlusal contact of upper and lower teeth (incisors) at the cusps.

Exfoliation—natural loss of a deciduous tooth prior to its replacement by its permanent successor. Also used to describe loss of teeth in advanced periodontitis due to disruption in support of periodontal apparatus.

Exodontics (exodontia)—the subject of and the techniques used in the extraction of teeth or parts of them.[2]

Exostosis—a benign bony growth projecting outward from the surface of a bone.[1] May be due to a chronic inflammation, constant pressure on the bone, or tumor formation. It may influence the positioning of a prosthesis.[2]

Expansion devices, spring loaded—a fixed orthodontic device producing predetermined finitely measured pressure meant to move teeth by tipping them or other movements.

External resorption—begins on the root surface and extends into the dentin.

Extirpation—complete removal or eradication of tissue. In endodontics, commonly used to describe the complete removal of vital dental pulp.[2]

Extraoral—outside of the oral cavity.

Extrusion—1. Condition of being forced or thrust out of a normal position. 2. In dentistry, the movement of a tooth to a new position beyond its normal alignment.[2]

F

Facet—a flattened or worn spot on the surface of a hard body, as on a bone or a tooth.[1]

Facially—toward the face or labially.

Facioverted—teeth or a tooth abnormally situated toward the face or lips.

Fenestration—a window-like aperture or opening, such as may be found in the alveolar bone over the root of a tooth.[1]

FFD—the distance from the focal spot on the x-ray tube's target to the film.

Fibroma—a benign neoplasm consisting largely of fibrous or fully developed connective tissue.

Fibromatosis, gingival—a diffuse, fibrous overgrowth of the gingiva; can be idiopathic, hereditary, or associated with drug administration.[1]

Fibropapilloma (fibroepithelial papilloma)—the common wart, which is composed of epithelial and connective tissue.

Fibrosarcoma—a sarcoma that arises from collagen-producing fibroblasts. Fibrosarcoma tends to invade local tissues rapidly, causing bony destruction. Local recurrence is common, but metastasis occurs late in the course of the disease.

Filled resin (composite resin; composite filling material)—resin-based filling material consisting of an organic polymer matrix such as methylmethacrylate or polymer precursors such as bis-GMA, to which has been added an inert inorganic material such as quartz, aluminum silicate or glass in the form of rods or beads. Polymerization of the matrix may be initiated by chemical catalysts or by ultraviolet or visible light.[2]

Filling, retrograde—an amalgam or other restoration placed in the apical portion of a tooth to seal the root canal following surgical removal of a periapical lesion and/or the end of the root.[1]

Fistula—an abnormal canal joining the cavities of two hollow organs or the cavity of an organ and the surface of the body.[1]

> **Oroantral f.**—an abnormal opening between the maxillary sinus and the mouth.[1]
>
> **Orofacial f.**—an abnormal opening between the cutaneous surface of the face and mouth.[1]
>
> **Oronasal f.**—an abnormal opening between the nasal cavity and the mouth.[1]

Flap—a loosened section of tissue separated from the surrounding tissues except at its base.[1]

> **Envelope f.**—a flap retracted from a horizontal linear incision, as along the free gingival margin, with no vertical incision.[1]
>
> **Gingival f.**—a flap that does not extend apical to the mucogingival junction.[1]
>
> **Modified Widman f.**—a scalloped, replaced, mucoperiosteal flap, accomplished with an internal bevel incision, that provides access to root for root planing.[1]
>
> **Mucogingival f.**—a flap that includes both gingiva and alveolar mucosa.[1]
>
> **Mucoperiosteal (full thickness) f.**—a mucosal flap (usually gingiva and alveolar mucosa) that includes the periosteum.[1]
>
> **Partial thickness (split thickness) f.**—a surgical flap of mucosa and connective tissue that does not include the periosteum.[1]
>
> **Pedicle f.**—a surgical flap with lateral releasing incisions.[1]
>
> **Positioned f.**—a surgical flap that is moved laterally, coronally, or apically to a new position.[1]
>
> **Sliding f.**—a pedicle flap (partial thickness) moved to a new position (also called rotating).[1]

Foramen—a natural opening or passage, particularly into or through a bone.[1]

Foreshortening—in radiography, the decrease in length of the radiographic image of the tooth due to incorrect technique.[2]

Freeway space—the space between the opposing maxillary and mandibular teeth when the mandible is suspended in the nonopened position.

Frenulum—a restraining portion or structure. On the ventral surface of the tongue, the lingual mucosa forms an unpaired, median mucosal fold, the lingual frenulum, which primarily connects the body of the tongue to the floor of the mouth. The lower lip is attached to the mandible at the level of the first premolar tooth by a frenulum.

Furcation—anatomical area where the root of a multirooted tooth divides.[1]

Fusion teeth—a condition in which two crowns, two pulp chambers, and two distinct root canals exist. With fusion teeth there will be one less tooth noted in the arcade as fusion with the sister tooth occurs.

G

Gemination teeth—condition in which twin tooth forms develop from a single bud or follicle. They have two crowns, two separate pulp chambers, and a common root canal system.

Giant cell tumor—a neoplasm containing abnormally large tissue cells that often have more than one nucleus and may appear as mergers of several normal cells: 1. A rare bone tumor of dogs and cats with benign and malignant variants. 2. Carcinoma of the thyroid. 3. Peripheral giant cell reparative granuloma: Uncommon, pedunculated or sessile lesion of the gingivae or alveolar ridge which is usually due to trauma.

Gingiva—this tissue overlies the bony alveolar processes of the maxilla and mandible and surrounds the tooth. The gingiva is the first line of defense against periodontal disease, protecting the bone and supporting tooth structures.

> **Attached g.**—the portion of the gingiva that is firm, dense, stippled, and tightly bound to the underlying periosteum, tooth, and bone.[1]
>
> **Free g.**—that part of the gingiva that surrounds the tooth and is not directly attached to the tooth surface.[1]
>
> **Marginal g.**—the most coronal portion of the gingiva. Often used to refer to the free gingiva that forms the wall of the gingival crevice in health.[1]

Gingival—referring to the gingiva.

G. crevice (g. sulcus)—the shallow fissure between the marginal gingiva and the enamel or cementum.[1]

G. enlargement—an overgrowth or increase in size of the gingiva.[1]

G. hyperplasia—an enlargement of the gingiva due to an increase in the number of cells.[1]

G. hypertrophy—an enlargement of the gingiva due to an increase in the size of cells.[1]

G. papilla—that portion of the gingiva that occupies the interproximal spaces. The interdental extension of the gingiva.[1]

G. pocket—a pathologically-deepened gingival crevice that does not involve loss of connective tissue attachment. Frequently observed when there is gingival enlargement.[1]

Gingivoplasty—a surgical reshaping of the gingiva.[1]

Glossalgia—pain in the tongue.[1]

Granuloma—a reactive nodule consisting of modified macrophages resembling epithelial cells surrounded by a rim of mononuclear cells, usually lymphocytes, and often containing giant cells.[1]

Apical g.—circumscribed granulomatous tissue adjacent to the apex of a tooth.[1]

Guided tissue regeneration (GTR)—a technique used in periodontology in which various materials are used to guide the path of epithelial cell regeneration.[2]

H

Halitosis—bad breath.

Harelip—a congenital anomaly affecting the lips in which the two sides of the primary palate fail to fuse normally.

Hedstrom file—tapered, flexible, hand-held file consisting of a series of sharp, conical-shaped blades. Used in endodontic treatment to smooth, clean, and enlarge root canals.[2]

Hemangiosarcoma—a malignant tumor characterized by rapidly proliferating, extensively infiltrating, anaplastic cells derived from blood vessels and lining irregular, blood-filled, or lumpy spaces.

Hemimandibulectomy—surgical excision of the mandible on one side.

Hemisection—the surgical separation of a multirooted tooth, especially a mandibular molar, through the furcation in such a way that a root and the associated portion of the crown may be removed.[1]

Hertwig's epithelial root sheath—an extension of the enamel organ (cervical loop). Determines the shape of the roots and initiates dentin formation during tooth development. Its remnants persist as epithelial rests of Malassez in the periodontal ligament.[1]

Heterodont—possessing teeth of several shapes, such as incisors, canines, premolars, and molars.[2]

Horizontal bone loss (HBL)—a full thickness loss of crestal bone secondary to periodontal disease, parallel to the cementoenamel junction, involving multiple teeth within a dental arch. Suprabony pockets can be noted in HBL in which the level of the receding epithelial attachment remains coronal to the alveolar crestal bone.

Hydroxyapatite (HA)—an inorganic compound, $Ca_{10}PO_46$ (OH_2), found in the matrices of bone and teeth which gives rigidity to these structures. Synthetic forms are used in ridge augmentation and intrabony defects and for coating dental implants.[1]

Hypercementosis—excessive development of secondary cementum on the surfaces of tooth roots. Often leads to loss of apical lamina dura.

Hyperthermia for oral tumors—use of supranormal temperatures to produce tumor regression. Studies suggest heat sensitivity is determined by tumor physiology. Hypoxia, low pH, reduced blood flow, and cells in the "S" phase of mitosis are factors that contribute to the lethal effects of heat on tumor cells.

Hypodontia (oligiodontia)—developmental absence of a number of teeth.[2]

Hypsodonts—species with roots that erupt and grow continually and never form full anatomical roots. These teeth have long anatomical crowns in relation to the anatomical root (i.e., rodent and lagomorph incisors, lagomorph, chinchilla, and Guinea pig cheek teeth, and domestic herbivores—including horses, cows and sheep).

Aradicular h.—continually growing teeth; those without roots (i.e., lagomorphs and rodents).

Radicular h.—continually erupting teeth that eventually close their roots (i.e., horses).

I

Iatrogenic—an abnormal mental or physical condition induced in a patient by the effects of treatment.[1]

Idiopathic—of unknown causation.[1]

Immobilization, tooth—any procedure that renders a tooth fixed or nonmobile. In periodontics, it refers to splinting of teeth.[1]

Impacted—a tooth prevented from normal eruption, occlusion, or extraction due to overlying bone, adjoining teeth, or other pathology.

Impaction—state of being firmly lodged or wedged.[2]

> **I., tooth**—situation in which a tooth is so placed that it is unable to erupt normally. May be due to a wedging against another tooth or teeth or to the abnormal development or sitting of the tooth.[2]

Implant, oral—1. An alloplastic material or device that is surgically placed into the oral tissue beneath the mucosal or periosteal layer or within the bone for functional, therapeutic, or esthetic purposes. 2. To insert a graft or alloplastic device into the oral hard or soft tissues for replacement of missing or damaged anatomical parts, or for stabilization of a periodontally compromised tooth or group of teeth.[1]

> **Endosseous i.**—an implant placed into the alveolar process and/or basal bone which, via an abutment or a connector, will protrude through the mucoperiosteum for support and attachment of a prosthesis or other device.[1]

> **Osseointegrated i.**—a direct structural and functional connection between ordered, living bone and the surface of an immobile, load-bearing implant.[1]

Implant abutment—that part of an implant system that connects the implant with a prosthesis or other device.[1]

Implant fixture—a synonym for an implant, especially an endosseous implant.[1]

Impression—a reproduction in a negative form of areas of the oral cavity.[1]

Incision—a cut or surgical wound made by a knife, electrosurgical scalpel, laser, or other such instrument.[1]

> **External bevel i.**—reduces the thickness of the mucogingival complex from the outside surface, as in gingivectomy.[1]

> **Internal (inverse, reverse, or inverted) bevel i.**—reduces the thickness of the mucogingival complex from the sulcar side.[1]

> **Releasing i.**—made to enhance the mobility of a periodontal flap.[1]

Incisors—one of six anterior teeth in the jaw used for cutting, grooming, and prehension.

Inclined plane, telescoping metallic—a dental laboratory produced noncorrosive metal inclined plane device cemented in place and designed to allow natural growth of the palate and maxilla in growing animals while a desired orthodontic tipping of teeth occurs.

Induction—the act or process of causing to occur as induction of bone formation.[1]

Interalveolar—located between the alveoli.[1]

> **I. septum**—alveolar and trabecular bone between contiguous teeth.[1]

> **I. crest**—the coronal edge of the interdental bony septum.[1]

Interdental—situated between the proximal surfaces of teeth in the same dental arch.[1]

> **I. space**—the space between adjacent teeth in the same arch.[1]

Interdigitation—the interlocking or fitting of opposing parts, as the cusps of the maxillary and mandibular posterior teeth.[1]

Interference—a tooth contact that interferes with harmonious mandibular movement.[1]

Interfurcation—the area between and at the base of the roots of a multirooted tooth.[1]

Internal resorption—begins adjacent to the pulp and extends into the dentin.

Interocclusal clearance (freeway space)—the space between the maxillary and mandibular opposing teeth when the mandible is suspended in postural (rest) position.[1]

Interproximally—between two adjoining teeth.

Interradicular—between the roots of teeth.[1]

Intrabony or Infrabony—within a bone.[1]

> **I. pocket**—periodontal pocket, the base of which lies below the margin of the surrounding alveolar bone. It is described according to whether it has one, two, or three bony walls.[2]

Intraoral—inside the oral cavity.

Invasive resorption—also called cervical resorption; originates in the cervical region of the tooth just below the epithelial attachment. The resorption invades into the dentin and can extend coronally or apically.

Irreversible pulpitis—an inflammatory condition of the pulpal tissues that cannot be resolved leading to pulp necrosis and death. Usually associated with bacterial pulpitis, this condition is only treatable with root canal therapy or apicoectomy.

J

Junction—a place of meeting or coming together, as of two different tissues.[1]

> **Cementodentinal j.**—the area of union of the dentin and cementum.[1]

> **Cementoenamel j.**—the area where enamel and cementum meet at the cervical region of the tooth.[1]

> **Dentinocemental j.**—the junction of dentin and cementum.[1]

> **Dentinoenamel j.**—the junction of dentin and enamel.[1]

> **Mucogingival j.**—the junction of gingiva and alveolar mucosa.[1]

Junctional epithelium (dentinogingival junction, epithelial cuff)—epithelium at the base of the gingival sulcus which attaches the gingiva to the enamel or cementum.[2]

K

kVp—kilovolt peak.

L

Labioversion—any deviation from the normal line of the dental arch toward the lip.[1]

Lamella—a thin layer, plate, or scale, as of bone.[1]

Lamina dura—the layer of compact bone forming the wall of a tooth alveolus. The alveolar bone.[1]

> **Crestal l. d.**—the layer of compact bone at the alveolar crest.[1]

Laser—light amplification by stimulated emission of radiation. A device that transforms light of various frequencies into an extremely intense, small, and nearly nondivergent beam of monochromatic radiation in the visible region with all the waves in phase. Capable of mobilizing immense heat and power when focused at close range, it is used as a tool in surgical procedures, diagnosis, and physiologic studies.[1]

Lateral—away from the midline.

Lingual—facing toward the tongue.

> **L. hemangioma**—a benign tumor consisting of a mass of blood vessels and located on the tongue.

Linguoocclusion—an occlusion in which a tooth or group of teeth is located lingually to its normal position.[1]

Linguoversion—a tooth or teeth abnormally situated toward the tongue.

Luxation—1. Dislocation or displacement. 2. Partial or complete dislocation of a tooth from its alveolus.[1]

Lymphocyte—a spherical cell of the lymphoid series, 7–20 μm in diameter with a large, round nucleus and scant cytoplasm. It is the principal cell involved in the immune response. There are two major populations, T(thymus-dependent)-lymphocytes and B(bursa-equivalent)-lymphocytes. B-lymphocytes may differentiate and become antibody-producing plasma cells, while T-lymphocytes are involved in a variety of cell-mediated immune reactions.[1]

Lymphohistiocytic sarcoma—a sarcoma involving lymphocytes and histiocytes.

Lymphokine—soluble factors released from lymphocytes that transmit signals for growth and differentiations of various cell types.[1]

Lymphoma (lymphosarcoma)—lymphoid neoplasm primarily affecting lymph nodes or other solid visceral organs such as the spleen or the liver. Lymphoma is classified based on anatomic site, e.g., multicentric, alimentary, mediastinal, and cutaneous lymphoma, and extranodal forms.

M

mA—milliampere.

Macula, macule—a small spot, perceptibly different in color from the surrounding tissue. It is neither elevated nor depressed from the surface.[1]

Malalignment, dental—the displacement of a tooth from its normal position in the dental arch.[1]

Malignant—in the case of neoplasm, having the properties of anaplasia, invasion, and metastasis.[1]

> **M. melanoma**—melanomas are neoplasms arising from melanocytes, dendritic cells of neuroectodermal origin, or melanoblasts. Typical for malignant melanoma is rapid local infiltration, frequent recurrence rate, and high likelihood of metastasis to regional lymph nodes and the lungs.

Malocclusion—lack of proper relations of opposing teeth when the jaws are closed.

> **Class II (distocclusion)**—the dental relationship wherein the mandibular dental arch is posterior to the maxillary arch.

> **Class III (mesiocclusion)**—the dental relationship wherein the mandibular dental arch is anterior to the maxillary arch.

Mandibular—referring to the lower jaw.

> **M. quadrant**—referring to the half of the lower jaw as divided by the median sagittal plane.

Mast cell tumor—a connective tissue tumor composed of mast cells that contain large basophilic granules. Mast cell tumors are malignant in approximately 50 percent of dogs and in the majority of cats.

Mastication—the process of chewing food in preparation for swallowing and digestion.[1]

Masticatory system—the organs and structures functioning in mastication, including the jaws, teeth with their supporting structures, temporomandibular articulation, mandibular musculature, tongue, lips, cheeks, oral mucosa, and associated nervous system.[1]

Maxillary—referring to the upper jaw.

Maxillary quadrant—referring to the half of the upper jaw as divided by the median sagittal plane.

Melanoma—a neoplasm made up of melanin-pigmented cells. When used alone, the term refers to malignant melanoma.[1]

Melanoplakia—pigmented patches on the oral mucosa.[1]

Mental foramen—openings on the lateral part of the mandible, opposite the second premolar, for passage of the mental nerve and vessels.

Mesial—that aspect of the tooth facing toward the rostral direction of the arch. For incisors, the mesial aspect is medial toward the midline of the arch.

Mesiobuccal—that aspect of the tooth that is both mesial and buccal. Also referring to the mesial root of the maxillary fourth premolar that is lateral to the mesiopalantine root.

Mesiodens—supernumerary tooth usually malformed and lying in the midline of the anterior maxilla between the central incisors.[2]

Mesiodistal lateral oblique view—referring to a view of the teeth in which the horizontal angulation of the x-ray beam is towards the mesiobuccal aspect of the teeth and passes through to the palatal or lingual aspect distally. Most often used for maxillary premolars.

Mesiopalatal/mesiopalantine—that aspect of the tooth that is both mesial and palatal. Also referring to the mesial root of the maxillary fourth premolar that is medial to the mesiobuccal root.

Mesioversion—the location of a tooth nearer than normal to the median line of the face along the dental arch.[1]

Metaplasia—a change from one adult cell type to another form which is not normal to that tissue.[1]

Metastasis—transfer of disease from one body part or organ to another not directly connected to it. Classically, the transfer of cells, as in malignant tumors, or the transfer of pathogenic microorganisms.[1]

Metronidazole—an antibiotic with a spectrum confined to obligate anaerobes, some microaerophilic organisms, and some anaerobic protozoa that acts to damage or inhibit DNA synthesis; may include a disulfiram-like reaction.[1]

Microdontia—condition in which the teeth are abnormally small.[2]

Microglossia—condition in which the tongue is abnormally small.[2]

Micrognathia—underdevelopment of the mandible and/or the maxilla.[2]

Mineralize (calcify)—the precipitation of calcium and other salts into an organic matrix to form a hard deposit, such as dental calculus.[1]

Minimum bactericidal concentration (MBC)—the minimum concentration of an antimicrobial agent required to kill a pure population of bacteria in vitro.[1]

Minimum inhibitory concentration (MIC)—the minimum concentration of an antimicrobial agent required to inhibit the growth and/or reproduction of a pure population of bacteria in vitro.[1]

Mobility, tooth—the degree of looseness of a tooth beyond physiologic movement.[1]

Modified Triadan System—a nomenclature numbering system in which the quadrants are designated by the 100, 200, 300, and 400s and the tooth is assigned a position number within its quadrant. *See* Appendix 2.

Molars—the posterior teeth with an occlusal surface for grinding, except for the mandibular molar in cats.

Monophyodont—species with a single set of teeth without precursors or successors (i.e., rodents and lagomorphs, or rabbits).

Morbidity—the condition of being diseased.[1]

MRI—magnetic resonance imaging. *See* Appendix 1.

Mucobuccal fold—the cul-de-sac formed where the mucous membrane is reflected from the mandible or maxilla to the cheek.[1]

Mucocele (mucus retention cyst)—collection of mucus within the tissue arising from a salivary gland. May be due to blockage of a salivary duct.[2]

Mucogingival—a generic term used to describe the mucogingival junction and its relationship to the gingiva, alveolar mucosa, frenula, muscle attachments, vestibular fornices, and floor of the mouth.[1]

Mucogingival junction—the junction of the gingiva and the alveolar mucosa.[1]

Mucolabial fold—the line of flexure of the oral mucosa membrane as it passes from the mandible or maxilla to the lip.[1]

Mucoperiosteum, oral—the complex of mucous membrane and periosteum that surrounds and invests the maxilla, mandible, and teeth.[1]

Mucosa—a mucous membrane.

> **Alveolar m.**—mucosa covering the basal part of the alveolar process and continuing without demarcation into the vestibular fornix and the floor of the mouth. It is loosely attached to the periosteum and is movable.[1]

> **Masticatory m.**—the gingiva and the mucosal covering of the hard palate.[1]

> **Oral m.**—the tissue lining the oral cavity.[1]

Mucositis—inflammation of a mucous membrane.[1]

Myxosarcoma—fibrosarcoma-like tumor that contains myxomatous (mucus-like) tissue. Myxosarcoma is infiltrative but metastasis are uncommon.

N

Nasopharyngeal polyp—a small tumor-like growth in the nasopharynx that projects from a mucous membrane surface. In cats inflammatory polyps arise from the nasal cavity and auditory canal.

Neck—that region of the tooth where the crown joins the root, also called the cementoenamel junction.

Neoplasm—a new, abnormal, uncontrolled growth arising from a given tissue.[1]

Neurofibrosarcoma—a fibrosarcoma of nerve tissue that results from the abnormal proliferation of Schwann cells.

Neutrophil—the predominant polymorphonuclear leukocyte comprising up to 70 percent of the peripheral white blood cells that is important in infection and injury repair. May have impaired function in some forms of early onset periodontitis.[1]

Nonworking side (balancing or contralateral side)—the side opposite the working side.[2]

O

Obtundent—an agent or remedy that lessens or relieves sensibility or pain. Soothing, deadening, dulling.[1]

Occlude—1. To bring together; to shut. 2. To bring or close the mandibular teeth into contact with the maxillary teeth.[1]

Occlusal—refers to the tooth surface that occludes with the opposing tooth.

Odontalgia—toothache; pain in a tooth.[1]

Odontoblast—a connective tissue cell found in the odontoblastic layer of the dental pulp that is responsible for deposition of dentin.[1]

Odontoclast—a multinucleated giant cell found associated with resorption of dentin.

Odontogenic—1. Tooth-forming. 2. Arising in tissues that give origin to the teeth.[1]

Odontogeny—origin and formative development of the teeth.[2]

Odontoma—a developmental anomaly consisting of a calcified mass of enamel, dentin, and cementum that may or may not resemble a tooth.[1]

Odontoplasty—the reshaping of a portion of a tooth.[1]

OFD—the distance from the object being x-rayed to the film.

Oligodontia—formation of less than a full complement of teeth. Those teeth that are present are usually smaller than normal.[1]

Open bite—a condition in which certain teeth cannot be brought into the proper occlusal contact with their antagonists.[1]

Operculum—the flap of mucosa over a partially erupted tooth.[1]

Oroantral fistula—abnormal opening between the oral cavity and the maxillary sinus.[2]

Orthodontics—that branch of dental science concerned with the study of the growth, development, and infinite variations of the face, jaws, and teeth, and with dentofacial abnormalities and their corrective treatment.[2]

Orthograde root filling—root filling normally carried out in a root canal through the coronal access cavity.[2]

Orthopantograph—a panoramic radiograph that includes images of the maxilla and mandible on a single extraoral film.[1]

Osseoconductive—a product that will aid in the regeneration of bone in an osseous site.

Osseoinductive—a product that will aid in the generation of new bone in any site; if you put this grafting material into any tissue it could cause bone to grow. From a practical standpoint, only autogeneous bone grafts and bone can do this currently. New materials are being developed that are osseoinductive. Freeze dried bone and irradiated bone are *not* osseoinductive, because the cells that make it osseoinductive are killed in treatment.

Osseointegration—is defined as the direct bone anchorage to an implant body, which will provide a foundation to support a prosthesis.[2]

Osseoproductive—is currently considered an improper and ill defined term. It has been used incorrectly as a substitute for osseopromotive.

Osseopromotive—a product that stimulates the growth of new bone, either osseoconductively or osseoinductively.

Osseous—bony; pertaining to bone.[1]

Ossification—1. The natural process of bone formation. 2. The hardening (as of muscular tissue) into a bony substance.

Ostectomy—the excision of bone or portion of a bone. In periodontics, ostectomy is done to correct or reduce deformities caused by periodontitis in the marginal and interalveolar bone and includes the removal of supporting bone.[1]

Osteitis—inflammation of bone involving the Haversian spaces and canals and their branches.[1]

> **Condensing (formative, sclerosing) o.**—osteitis associated with increased bone density.[1]

Osteoblast—a cell which arises from mesenchymal tissue and is associated with the formation of bone.[1]

Osteoclast—a large, multinuclear cell associated with the resorption of bone.[1]

Osteocyte—an osteoblast that has become embedded within the bone matrix.[1]

Osteogenesis—development of bone; formation of bone.[1]

Osteogenic—any tissue or substance with the potential to induce growth or repair of bone.[1]

Osteoid—the organic matrix of bone; developing bone that has not undergone calcification.[1]

Osteoma—a benign tumor composed of bone tissue.

Osteomyelitis—local or generalized infection of bone and bone marrow, usually caused by bacteria introduced by trauma or surgery, by direct extension from a nearby infection, or via the bloodstream.

Osteoperiosteal—pertaining to bone and its periosteum.[1]

Osteoplasty—reshaping of the alveolar process to achieve a more physiologic form without removal of supporting bone.[1]

Osteoporosis—abnormal rarefaction of bone.[1]

Osteosarcoma—a malignant tumor of the bone, composed of anaplastic cells derived from mesenchyme.

Osteosclerosis—*See* Osteitis, condensing.

Overgrowth—excessive enlargement of a part due to an increase in size of the constituent cells (hypertrophy) or an increase in their number (hyperplasia).[1]

Overhang—excess of dental filling material extending beyond cavity margin.[1]

Overjet—the horizontal projection of the maxillary incisors beyond the mandibular incisors when the jaws are in habitual occlusion.[1]

P

Pachyglossia—abnormal thickness of the tongue.[2]

Palatal—facing toward the palate.

Papilla—any small, nipple-shaped elevation.[1]

> **Incisive p.**—the elevation of soft tissue covering the foramen of the incisive or nasopalatine canal.[1]

Papilloma—a benign, pedunculated, cauliflower-like neoplasm of epithelium. May have a viral etiology.[1]

Paralleling technique—periapical radiographic technique in which a film holder is used to align the film parallel to the long axis of the tooth and also to allow the central ray to pass perpendicular to the plane of the film.[2]

Pathognomonic—characteristic or symptomatic of a disease. A sign or symptom on which a diagnosis can be made.[1]

Pathosis—a disease entity; a morbid condition.[1]

Pedicle—a stem-like or narrow base part, such as the stalk by which a nonsessile tumor is attached.[1]

Penicillin—a generic name for a related group of antibiotics differing in antibacterial spectrum, oral absorption, and resistance to beta-lactamase enzymes. Classified as penicillin G and congeners (penicillin V), antistaphylococcal penicillins (methicillin, dicloxacillin), extended-spectrum penicillins (ampicillin and amoxicillin), and extended-spectrum penicillins with beta-lactamase inhibitors (amoxicillin and clavulanate, ampicillin and sublactam).[1]

Penumbra—partial or imperfect shadowing of an object. In radiology it is influenced by the object-to-film or focus-to-subject distance.[2]

Periapical—relating to tissues surrounding the apex of a tooth, including the periodontal ligament and alveolar bone.[1]

Pericoronitis—acute inflammation of the gingiva and/or mucosa surrounding a partially erupted tooth.[1]

Periodontal—situated or occurring around a tooth; pertaining to the periodontium.[1]

> **P. bony defects:**

>> **Crater**—a cup- or bowl-shaped defect in the interalveolar bone with bone loss nearly equal on the contiguous roots. The facial and lingual/palatal walls may be of unequal height. A type of intrabony/infrabony defect.[1]

>> **Funnel-shaped d.**—an intrabony/infrabony resorptive lesion involving one or more surfaces of supporting bone; may appear moat-like.[1]

>> **Furcation invasion**—pathologic resorption of bone within a furcation.[1]

>>> **Class I f. i.**—a minimal, but notable, loss of bone in a furcation.[1]

>>> **Class II f. i.**—a variable degree of bone destruction in a furcation but not extending completely through the furcation.[1]

>>> **Class III f. i.**—bone resorption extending completely through the furcation.[1]

>> **Infrabony/Intrabony d.**—a periodontal defect surrounded by two or three bony walls or a combination of these.[1]

Periodontal disease—those pathologic processes affecting the peridontium; most often gingivitis and periodontitis.[1]

Periodontal dressing (pack)—a protective material applied over the wound created by periodontal surgical procedures.[1]

Periodontal ligament—This is a network of connective tissue structures that attaches and supports the tooth in the alveolus. They cushion the tooth and bone from occlusal forces. The periodontal ligament is in a constant state of repair and remodeling in response to multiple stimulations. On x-ray, the periodontal ligament is a radiolucent space seen between the lamina dura of the alveolus and the cementum of the tooth.

Periodontal pocket—a pathologic fissure between a tooth and the crevicular epithelium, limited at its apex by the junctional epithelium. It is an abnormal apical extension of the gingival crevice caused by migration of the junctional epithelium along the root as the periodontal ligament is detached by a disease process.[1]

> **Intrabony/infrabony p.**—a periodontal pocket that extends into an intrabony peridontal defect.[1]

> **Pseudopocket**—a deepening of the gingival crevice resulting primarily from an increase in bulk of the gingiva without apical migration of the junctional epithelium or appreciable destruction of the underlying tissue.[1]

> **Suprabony p.**—a periodontal pocket that has a base coronal to the alveolar bone.[1]

Peridontal space—the space between the tooth root and alveolar bone containing the periodontal ligament.[1]

Periodontalgia—pain arising in the periodontal structures.[1]

Periodontics—that specialty of dentistry which encompasses the prevention, diagnosis, and treatment of diseases of the supporting and surrounding tissues of the teeth or their substitutes; the maintenance of the health, function, and esthetics of these structures and tissues; and the replacement of lost teeth and supporting structures by grafting or implantation of natural and synthetic devices and materials.[1]

Periodontitis—inflammation of the supporting tissues of the teeth. Usually a progressively destructive change leading to loss of bone and periodontal ligament. An extension of inflammation from gingiva into the adjacent bone and ligament.[1]

> **Necrotizing ulcerative p.**—severe and rapidly progressive disease that has a distinctive erythema of the free gingiva, attached gingiva, and alveolar mucosa; extensive soft tissue necrosis; severe loss of periodontal attachment; deep pocket formation is not evident.[1]

> **Refractory p.**—includes patients who are unresponsive to any treatment provided—whatever the thoroughness or frequency—as well as patients with recurrent disease at single or multiple sites.[1]

Periodontium—The collection of structures surrounding the tooth including the gingiva, the cementum, the periodontal ligaments, and the alveolar bone which forms the jaw and tooth sockets.

Periodontology—the scientific study of the periodontium in health and disease.[1]

Periodontometry—the measurement of tooth mobility.[1]

Periradicular—around or surrounding a tooth root.[1]

Petechiae—hemorrhagic spots of pinpoint to pinhead size in the skin or mucous membrane.[1]

Phenytoin (diphenylhidantoin)—an anticonvulsant drug used in the control of epilepsy and other disorders. Often associated with gingival overgrowth.[1]

PID—position-indicating device, cone.

Plaque—an organized mass, consisting mainly of microorganisms, that adheres to teeth, prostheses, and oral surfaces and is found in the gingival crevice and periodontal pockets. In addition to microorganisms, plaque consists of an organic, polysaccharide-protein matrix consisting of bacterial by-products such as enzymes, food debris, desquamated cells, and inorganic components such as calcium and phosphate.[1]

Plasma cell—an antibody-producing B-lymphocyte that has reached the end of its differentiation pathway.[1]

Polyp—a pedunculated tumor arising in a mucous membrane.[1]

Porcelain—in dentistry, a ceramic material made of kaolin, feldspar, silica, and various pigments.[2]

Porphyromonas gingivalis—formerly called *Bacteroides gingivalis*. Gram-negative, nonmotile, anaerobic, non–spore-forming bacillus that occurs primarily in the oral cavity and is associated with some forms of severe periodontal disease. It is a non-fermentative, pigmented *Porphyromonas* isolated principally from the gingival sulcus.[1]

Premaxilla—that part of the maxilla in which the incisor teeth develop and erupt.[2]

Premolars—the cheek teeth situated in the jaws between the canine and molars.

Primary dentin—a form of dentin formed prior to eruption of the tooth and comprising the bulk of the tooth.

Probe—a slender instrument with a blunt end suitable for use in exploring a channel, wound, sinus, pocket, etc.[1]

> **Clinical attachment level p.**—the distance from the cementoenamel junction to the tip of the periodontal probe (i.e. most apical insertion site) during usual periodontal diagnostic probing. The health of the attachment apparatus can affect the measurement.[1]

> **Periodontal p.**—a calibrated probe used to measure the depth and determine the configuration of a periodontal pocket.[1]

Probing depth—the distance from the soft tissue (gingiva or alveolar mucosa) margin to the tip of the periodontal probe (i.e., most apical insertion site) during usual periodontal diagnostic probing. The health of the attachment apparatus can affect the measurement.[1]

Prognathic—a forward relationship of the jaws, usually used with reference to the mandible.[1]

Prophylaxis, oral—the removal of plaque, calculus, and stains from the exposed and unexposed surfaces of the teeth by scaling, root planing and polishing as a preventative measure for the control of local irritational factors.

Protrusion—indicating teeth or other maxillary and mandibular structures that are positioned anterior to the normal or to the generally accepted standard.[1]

Proximal—nearest to the center. In dentistry, the surface of a tooth adjacent to another tooth.[1]

Ptyalism—condition in which there is an excess of saliva in the mouth, due to excessive secretion or to inability to swallow.[2]

Pulp—soft tissue lying within the dentine of a tooth and containing fibers, cells, and structures such as blood vessels, sensory nerves, and lymphatics.[2]

Pulp chamber—the area within the tooth structure that contains the pulp tissue.

Pulp obliteration—complete removal of the pulp by disease, degeneration or inflammation. Also secondary to trauma or the physiologic aging process.

Pulpectomy—the complete or partial removal of the dental pulp.

Pulpitis—inflammation of the dental pulp.[1]

Pulpotomy—surgical amputation of the coronal portion of the dental pulp.[1]

Pus—a product of inflammation consisting of leukocytes, degenerated tissue elements, tissue fluids, and microorganisms.[1]

Q

Quadrant—one of the four sections of the dental arches.[1]

R

Radicular—pertaining to the root of a tooth and its adjacent structures.[1]

Radicular pulp—the part of the dental pulp contained in the root canal of a tooth.

Radiolucent—permitting the passage of x-rays so that the image generated on film is relatively darker than adjacent structures.

Radiopaque—permitting the passage of x-rays but with attenuation, so that the image generated on film is relatively lighter than adjacent structures.

Radiosurgery—a method of cutting and coagulating soft tissues by means of passing high frequency radiowaves through the tissue (3.5 to 4.0 MHz).

Ranula—retention cyst, usually under the tongue, occurring when a sublingual salivary gland duct or mucous gland is blocked.[2]

Reattachment—to attach again. The reunion of epithelial and connective tissues with root surfaces and bone such as occurs after an incision or injury. Not to be confused with new attachment.[1]

Recession—location of marginal periodontal tissues apical to the cementoenamel junction.[1]

> **Gingival r.**—location of the gingival margin apical to the cementoenamel junction.[1]

Recipient site—the site into which a graft or transplant material is placed.[1]

Regeneration—reproduction or reconstitution of a lost or injured part.[1]

> **Guided tissue r.**—procedures attempting to regenerate lost periodontal structures through differential tissue responses. Barrier techniques, using materials such as expanded polytetrafluoroethylene, polyglactin, polylactic acid, bone allografts, and collagen, are employed in the hope of excluding epithelium and the gingival corium from the root surface in the belief that they interfere with regeneration.[1]

Registration (bite)—a record of jaw relationships used in the mounting of casts on an articulator.[1]

Resorption—the loss of substance from tissues that normally are calcified, such as the dentin or cementum of teeth, or of the alveolar process. The condition may be physiologic or pathologic.[1]

> **Bone r.**—bone loss due to osteoclastic activity.[1]

> **External r.**—resorption of tooth structure beginning on the external surface.[1]

> **Internal r.**—tooth resorption beginning from within the pulp.[1]

Retention—1. Maintenance of orthodontically-moved teeth until stability of the attachment apparatus in established. 2. Fixation and stabilization of a dental prothesis.[1]

Reticulation—"grainy-like" texture to an x-ray.

Retrofilling—a method of sealing the root canal of a tooth by an apical approach.[1]

Retrognathism—a condition of facial disharmony in which one or both jaws are posterior to normal in their craniofacial relationships; usually used in reference to the mandible.

Retrograde—directed backward.[2]

> **R. (or reverse) root filling**—filling inserted into the apical end of a tooth immediately following an apicoectomy.[2]

Reversible pulpitis—the returning of the pulp to a normal state after inflammation caused by trauma, pressure, or other abnormal physical forces to the pulpal tissues. This condition can proceed to the irreversible state.

Root—1. The anatomic portion of the tooth usually covered with cementum. 2. The anatomic part of a tooth normally within the alveolar bone and attached to it by the periodontal ligament.[1]

> **R. amputation**—the removal of a root from a multirooted tooth.[1]

> **R. canal**—the space within the root of a tooth containing connective tissue, nerves, and blood vessels, and connecting the pulp chamber with the apex of the root.[1]

> **R. canal therapy (endodontic therapy)**—treatment of a tooth, usually performed by completely removing the pulp, sterilizing the pulp chamber and root canal, and filling these spaces with inert sealing material. Usually done in a tooth with an irreversibly damaged pulp.[1]

> **R. denudation**—exposure of a portion of a root as the result of recession.[1]

> **R. fragment**—a portion of the root, usually the root tip, retained in the jaw following the incomplete extraction or failure of resorption of a primary tooth.[1]

> **R. fusion**—a union of merging roots of multirooted teeth. If roots from adjacent teeth are fused the condition is called concrescence.[1]

R. planing—a treatment procedure designed to remove cementum or surface dentin that is rough, impregnated with calculus, or contaminated with toxins or microorganisms. *See* Scaling.[1]

R. remnant—a piece of the tooth root structure left in the alveolar bone as a result of root resorption.

R. resection—surgical removal of all or a portion of a tooth root.[1]

R. resorption—loss or blunting of some portion of a root, sometimes idiopathic, but also associated with orthodontic tooth movement, inflammation, trauma, and neoplasia.[1]

Rostral (anterior) cross bite—mandibular incisor(s) deviated in buccal (anterior) version to the maxillary incisor(s) or one or more of the maxillary incisors are displaced lingual to the lower incisors when teeth are in occlusion.

Rotation—turning a tooth orthodontically either around a vertical axis from the cusp to the apex or around a horizontal axis midway between the cementoenamel junction and the tooth apex.

Rugae—the irregular ridges in the masticatory mucosa covering the anterior part of the hard palate.[1]

S

Sarcoma—a malignant neoplasm composed of cells derived from connective tissue such as bone and cartilage, muscle, blood vessel, or lymphoid tissue.

Scaler—an instrument for removing calculus or other deposits from the surfaces of teeth.

> **Sonic s.**—an instrument vibrating in the sonic range (approximately 6,000 CPS to 8,000 CPS) which, accompanied by a stream of water, can be used to remove adherent deposits from teeth.[1]

> **Ultrasonic s.**—an instrument vibrating in the ultrasonic range (approximately 30,000 CPS to 40,000 CPS) which, accompanied by a stream of water, can be used to remove adherent deposits from teeth.[1]

Scaling—instrumentation of the crown and root surfaces of the teeth to remove plaque, calculus, and stains from these surfaces. *See* Root planing.[1]

Scissors bite—normal occlusion of the lower incisor's cusps striking the cingulum of the upper incisors, normal interdigitation of the lower cuspids into their diastema between the upper lateral incisors and the upper cuspids, and normal alignment of the premolar teeth in nonoccluding saw blade interdigital fashion.

Sclerosing osteomyelitis—inflammation of the bone characterized by a diffuse inflammatory reaction, increased density, and sclerotic thickening of the cortex. Can be focal or diffuse.

Secondary dentin—1. Physiologic: a regular layer of uniform dentin that is manufactured routinely throughout the life of the tooth. 2. Reparative or tertiary dentin: a form of dentin that is produced in response to attrition, erosion, or other irritants.

Sequestration—the separation of necrotic bone from the surrounding healthy bone, forming a sequestrum.[1]

Sequestrum—a mass of nonvital bone that has become separated from healthy bone.[1]

Sharpey's fibers—those portions of the principal fibers of the periodontal ligament that are embedded in root cementum and alveolar bone proper and which contribute to the anchorage of the tooth.[2]

Sialadenitis—inflammation of a salivary gland.[1]

Sialolith—a salivary stone (calculus).[1]

SLOB Rule—also referred to as Clark's Rule; a system to allow identification of tooth roots on x-ray when two roots are superimposed on each other. The rule states that when a horizontal tube shift technique is utilized the most lingual or palatal root will shift in the same direction toward the tube head; i.e. SAME-lingual; OPPOSITE-buccal. In the cranial oblique tube shift the palatal or lingual root shifts cranial toward the tube head; in the caudal oblique the palatal or lingual root shifts caudally toward the tube head. This technique is very important in visualizing the roots of the upper fourth premolar in the canine and feline.

Splint—any apparatus, appliance, or device employed to prevent motion or displacement of fractured or movable parts.[1]

> **Dental s.**—an appliance designed to immobilize and stabilize loose teeth.[1]

Squamous cell carcinoma—a malignant tumor arising from squamous (flat, scalelike) epithelium.

Stent—1. A device used in conjunction with a surgical procedure to immobilize hard or soft tissue and to protect a healing wound. 2. An acrylic appliance used as a positioning guide or support.[1]

Stomatitis—inflammation of the soft tissues of the oral cavity.[1]

Subgingival curettage—removal of the junctional epithelium and the epithelial lining of a periodontal pocket, often accompanied by scaling and root planing.[2]

Subluxation—partial dislocation of a tooth within the alveolus.

Subtraction radiography—a photographic or digital method of eliminating background anatomical structures from the final image thus bringing out the differences between the pre- and postprocedure radiographic images.[1]

> **Digital s. r.**—a radiographic image subtraction method in which the pre- and postprocedure radiographic images are subtracted from each other within the computer memory and the resulting subtracted image is displayed on the monitor.[1]

Summation—when the images of two structures appear either relatively more radiolucent or more radiopaque because of overlap or superimposition of their images on the radiograph.

Supereruption—excess eruption of a tooth or extrusion, generally related to either cementosis, increased osteoblast activity in the apical periradicular alveolar bone or periapical inflammation.

Superimposition—when two subjects overlap one another in the path of the x-ray beam.

Supernumerary—in excess of the regular or normal number.[1]

Supportive periodontal treatment (periodontal maintenance, preventive maintenance, recall maintenance)—an extension of periodontal therapy. Procedures performed at selected intervals to assist the periodontal patient in maintaining oral health. These usually consist of examination, evaluation of oral hygiene and nutrition, and scaling, root curettage, and polishing the teeth.[1]

Supraeruption—the eruption of teeth beyond the normal occlusal plane.[1]

Symphysis—a type of cartilaginous joint in which the opposed bony surfaces are firmly united by a plate of fibrocartilage, also called a fibrocartilaginous joint. The mandibular symphysis.

T

Taurodontia—teeth with a large crown and pulp chamber, but with short roots. Most commonly seen as a hereditary problem in humans and occasionally seen in animals.

Taurodontism—a variation in tooth form affecting some or all of the primary and secondary molars, marked by elongation of the body of the tooth so that the pulp chambers are large apicoocclusally and the roots are reduced in size.[1]

Temporomandibular joint (TMJ)—the connecting sliding hinge mechanism between the mandible and the temporal bone.[1]

Tetracyclines—a group of similar bacteriostatic, broad-spectrum antibiotics differing in lipid solubility, hepatic extraction ratios, and half-lives. They deposit in all mineralizing tissues.[1]

Tic—a spasm; involuntary contraction or twitching usually of the facial and shoulder muscles.[1]

Titanium—a uniquely biocompatible metal commonly used for dental implants and full jacket crowns either in the commercially pure form or as an alloy.[1]

Titanium alloy—the most common titanium alloy (Ti-6Al-4V) used for dental implants and full jacket crowns; contains 6 percent aluminum to increase strength and decrease weight and 4 percent vanadium to prevent corrosion.[1]

Tonsillar lymphosarcoma—lymphoma affecting the tonsils.

Tooth extrusion—overeruption, supraeruption.[1]

Transillumination—the passage of light through body tissues for the purpose of examination.[1]

Transplant—to transfer the tissue from one part to another, from an autogenous, a heterogeneous, or homogenous donor site.[1]

Trigeminal—relating to the fifth cranial (trigeminal) nerve.[1]

> **Mandibular t.**—supplies the muscles of mastication, the lower part of face, the mandibular teeth and gingiva, the anterior two-thirds of tongue, the mylohyoid muscle, the cheek, the skin of temporal region, the temporomandibular joint, and the external ear.[2]

> **Maxillary t.**—supplies the middle part of the face, the upper lip, and the lower eyelid; the maxillary teeth and gingiva; and the soft palate and roof of the mouth, the maxillary sinus, and the mucous membrane of the nasopharynx.[2]

> **Ophthalmic t.**—supplies the eyeball, conjunctiva, and lachrymal gland; the skin of the forehead; the eyelids and nose; the mucous membranes of the nose and paranasal sinuses; and the dura mater.

Trismus—inability to open the mouth due to spasm of the muscles of mastication.[1]

U

Useful beam (or radiation)—that part of the primary beam which is limited by a filter or collimator and which is effective in producing a radiographic image.[2]

V

Ventrodorsal view—referring to the passage of the x-ray beam from the ventral aspect to the dorsal aspect of the animal.

Vertical bone loss (VBL)—a bone loss seen in advanced periodontal disease which has its base apical to the alveolar crest and is commonly associated with infrabony/intrabony pocket formation. With vertical bone loss, infrabony pockets are classified in reference to specific configurations of pocket morphology. (See infrabony/intrabony pockets and periodontal bony defects in this Glossary.)

W

Wry bite—malocclusion manifested by significant bilateral asymmetry in the relative size of the maxilla, or the cranium resulting in varying combinations of deviations including, but not limited to, cross bite, base narrow canines, rotations, micrognathia, prognathia, and temporomandibular joint symmetry.

X

Xenograft—a bone grafting material from one species to another species.

Xerostomia—dryness of the mouth due to inadequate salivary secretion.[1]

Z

Zinc oxide–eugenol cement—cement formed by mixing zinc oxide and eugenol (the principal constituent of oil of cloves). Modifiers may be added to speed up the setting reaction. Used as an obtundent, antiseptic temporary dressing in a cavity, or as a means of temporarily cementing crowns, bridges, and splints into place. May also be used as a root canal filling material.[2]

Zygomatic arch—the arch formed by the articulation of the broad temporal process of the zygomatic bone and the slender zygomatic process of the temporal bone. Also called the malar arch.

Sources

1. American Academy of Periodontology. Rita Shafer, Director of Publications. *The Glossary of Periodontal Terms*, 1992, 3rd Edition.

2. Butterworth-Heinemann Publishers. Mary Seager—Commissioning Editor—Medical Books Division. *Concise Illustrated Dental Dictionary*, 2nd Edition, by F. J. Harty.

INDEX

tooth buds, 136
410, canine
    endodontic disease, 38
    normal anatomy, 11
    tooth buds, pre-eruption
        identification, 18
411, canine
    normal anatomy, 11
    tooth buds, pre-eruption
        identification, 18

Abscess
    apical, 150
    camel, 245
    canine, 100
    crab seal, 239
    Dall sheep, 244
    deer, 233
    kangaroo, red, 242
    nyala, 243
    rabbit mandible, 254–255
    rhinoceros, 236
    wallaby, 242–243
Acanthomatous epulis, 89, 91–93
Adumbration, 203
Aging, feline
    radiographic features of, 119
    x-ray plates, 125–131
Alveolar bone, 59. *See also* Bone loss
Alveolar crest, 59
Alveolus, 4, 118, 249
Amalgam restoration, 54, 55, 71, 72, 73
Ameloblastic fibroma, 159
Ameloblastoma, 88, 89, 99
Ameloblasts, 3
Anisognathism, 251
Ankylosis
    canine, 66, 83
    feline, 157, 178–180, 188, 191–192, 196,
        198
Apex
    apexification, 4, 30, 53, 157
    apicoectomy, 56, 57, 237, 338
    blunderbuss, 142
    open, 19, 29, 79, 141, 153, 229
    resorption, 178
Apexification, 4, 30, 53, 157
Apexogenesis (apical closure), 29
Apical delta, 119
Apical formation, 36, 47–48
Apical granuloma, 60
Apical lysis, 35, 38–41, 44
Apical puff, 155, 229
Apicoectomy, 56, 57, 237, 238, 338
Aradicular hypsodont teeth, 247, 248

Artifacts, 210–214
    adumbration, 203
    black marks, 206
    cervical burnout, 118, 120, 127, 203, 222
    cone cut, 203
    curvature of film, 204
    developer, 209
    double image, 206
    elongation of tooth, 201
    endotracheal tube, 213–214
    fingerprint, 195
    fixer, 208, 209, 210
    fogging, 206
    foreshortening of tooth, 202
    graying film, 211
    human finger exposure, 213
    light leak, 207
    manufacturer's dimple, 204
    overlapping contacts, 211
    positional errors, 195, 201–203, 211
    reticulation, 211
    reversed film, 205
    scratched emulsion, 145, 147, 207
    static electricity, 208
    superimposition, 211–212
    tooth elongation, 85
Avulsion, 65, 107, 113, 176

Bengal tiger, 241
Biopsy, 87
Bisecting angle technique, xxi, xxii, xxv, 85
Black buck, 235
Blade implant, 224
Blunderbuss apex, 142
Bone loss
    abscess and, 100–101
    apical lysis, 35, 38–41, 44
    bone replacement, 60
    camel periodontitis, 245
    canine
        horizontal, 59, 60, 64, 66, 69, 101
        neoplasia, 87, 88, 91–97
        periodontitis, 102–103
        stomatitis, 102
        vertical, 84, 101
    digital image analysis, 68–70
    feline
        differential diagnosis, 185
        horizontal, 182–184, 186–189
        periodontitis, 178–198
    furcation exposures, 60, 63, 65, 66
    horizontal
        canine, 59, 60, 64, 66, 69, 101
        feline, 182–184, 186–189
        orangutan, 222
    imaging modalities and, 261

neoplasia, oral, 159, 161, 163–165, 167, 169,
    183
periapical lysis, 35, 40, 43–44
periodontitis, 101
pocket formation, 59–60
vertical, 59, 61–63, 65, 222
Brachycephalic breeds, xxii, xxiii
Brachygnathia, 77
Brachyodont teeth, 248
Bridge, 224
Buccal object rule, xxii

Cage biter syndrome, 228
Calcification
    canine oral neoplasia, 87, 88
    epithelial odontogenic tumors, 161
    pulp, 151, 157, 222
Calculus, 180, 184, 188
Camel, 245
Canadian lynx *(Felis lynx canadensis),* 228
Canals
    lateral (accessory), 29, 158
    mandibular, 10, 118, 120
    occluded, 36, 48
    pulp, 9–10, 37, 49–51
Canine
    endodontics, 35–58
    Modified Triadan Numbering System, 266
    neoplasia, 87–104
    normal anatomy, 3–13
        discussion, 3–5
        pedodontics, 16–20
            deciduous root resorption, 18
            intraradicular groove, 20
            mixed dentition, 19
            permanent immature teeth, 19
            tooth buds, pre-eruption identifica-
              tion of, 16–18
        periodontal tissue, 59
        radiographs, 6–13
    orthodontics, 77–85
    pedodontics, 15–33
    periodontics, 59–70
    restorative dentistry, 71–75
    trauma, oral, 105–113
Carcinoma, 87, 88
Caries, 221
Cementoenamel junction, 3, 4, 188
    alveolar crest height and bone loss, 59
    normal anatomy, 118, 120
Cementum
    hypercementosis, 155, 179, 181, 184
    normal anatomy, 118
    odontoma, 104
    overview, 3, 4
Cerclage wire, 108–109, 111–112